Review of
Medical Laboratory Techniques

Review of
Medical Laboratory Techniques

MCQs Based on Theoretical Knowledge and Clinical Practice

Reetika Menia DNB (Pathology)
Assistant Professor
Department of Pathology
All India Institute of Medical Sciences
Vijaypur, Jammu (J&K), India

Shivani Gandhi MD (Pathology)
Assistant Professor
Department of Pathology
All India Institute of Medical Sciences
Vijaypur, Jammu (J&K), India

Ishani Gupta MD (Pathology)
Assistant Professor
Department of Pathology
All India Institute of Medical Sciences
Vijaypur, Jammu (J&K), India

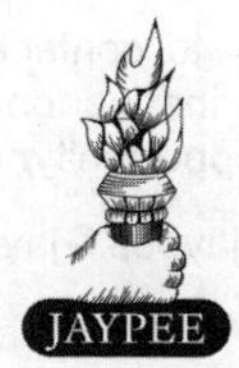

JAYPEE BROTHERS MEDICAL PUBLISHERS
The Health Sciences Publisher
New Delhi | London

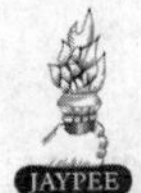 **Jaypee Brothers Medical Publishers (P) Ltd**

Headquarters

Jaypee Brothers Medical Publishers (P) Ltd
EMCA House, 23/23-B
Ansari Road, Daryaganj
New Delhi 110 002, India
Landline: +91-11-23272143, +91-11-23272703
+91-11-23282021, +91-11-23245672
Email: jaypee@jaypeebrothers.com

Corporate Office

Jaypee Brothers Medical Publishers (P) Ltd
4838/24, Ansari Road, Daryaganj
New Delhi 110 002, India
Phone: +91-11-43574357
Fax: +91-11-43574314
Email: jaypee@jaypeebrothers.com

Overseas Office

J.P. Medical Ltd
83 Victoria Street, London
SW1H 0HW (UK)
Phone: +44 20 3170 8910
Fax: +44 (0)20 3008 6180
Email: info@jpmedpub.com

Website: www.jaypeebrothers.com
Website: www.jaypeedigital.com

Inquiries for bulk sales may be solicited at: jaypee@jaypeebrothers.com

Review of Medical Laboratory Techniques

First Edition: **2024**

ISBN: 978-93-5696-530-0

Printed at: Sterling Graphics Pvt. Ltd.

Contributors

Harsimran Jit Singh
Assistant Professor
Department of Anatomy
All India Institute of Medical Sciences
Vijaypur, Jammu (J&K), India

Ishani Gupta
Assistant Professor
Department of Pathology
All India Institute of Medical Sciences
Vijaypur, Jammu (J&K), India

Juhi Taneja
Assistant Professor
Shri Atal Bihari Vajpayee Government
Medical College
Faridabad, Haryana, India

Mehak Mahajan
Assistant Professor
Department of Physiology
Government Medical College
Udhampur, Jammu (J&K), India

Navneet Kour
Assistant Professor
Department of Physiology
ASCOMS Medical College
Jammu (J&K), India

Rajani
Assistant Professor
Department of Biochemistry
All India Institute of Medical Sciences
Bathinda, Punjab, India

Reetika Menia
Assistant Professor
Department of Pathology
All India Institute of Medical Sciences
Vijaypur, Jammu (J&K), India

Shivani Gandhi
Assistant Professor
Department of Pathology
All India Institute of Medical Sciences
Vijaypur, Jammu (J&K), India

Preface

Welcome to *Review of Medical Laboratory Techniques*, a comprehensive and invaluable resource designed to enhance the understanding and mastery of essential concepts in the field of medical laboratory science. This book has been meticulously crafted to serve as a reliable companion for students, practitioners, laboratory technicians, and anyone seeking to deepen their knowledge of the diverse techniques employed in medical laboratories.

As medical laboratory professionals play a crucial role in diagnosing, monitoring, and managing various medical conditions in the healthcare field, their contributions' importance cannot be overstated, as accurate and timely laboratory results are fundamental to clinical decision-making. Recognizing the significance of a solid understanding of laboratory techniques, this book focuses on providing a wide array of multiple-choice questions (MCQs) to test and reinforce your knowledge.

Our aim is to cover a broad spectrum of medical laboratory techniques, encompassing areas such as Human Anatomy, Physiology, Biochemistry, Hematology, Histopathology, Cytology, Microbiology, Immunology, and Molecular Diagnostics. Each section is meticulously organized to align with the curriculum and requirements of medical laboratory science programs.

The MCQs in this book are thoughtfully curated to encompass a variety of question types, ranging from basic knowledge recall to critical thinking and problem-solving scenarios. This diversity challenges readers and fosters a deeper understanding of the subject matter. By presenting questions in a practical context, readers can better appreciate the application of theoretical knowledge to clinical practice.

This book serves as a practical self-assessment tool not only for the students preparing for the examination but also for a seasoned professional seeking to refresh their knowledge and an educator looking for supplementary materials to reinforce their understanding and boost their confidence in tackling challenging scenarios.

As you embark on this educational journey through *Review of Medical Laboratory Techniques*, we encourage you to approach each question with curiosity and an eagerness to learn. May this book serve as a valuable resource in your pursuit of excellence in the fascinating and vital field of medical laboratory science.

Best wishes for a rewarding and enriching learning experience!

Reetika Menia
Shivani Gandhi
Ishani Gupta

Acknowledgments

The creation of *Review of Medical Laboratory Techniques* has been a collaborative effort that would not have been possible without numerous individuals' support, guidance, and contributions. As we take a moment to reflect on the completion of this project, we extend our heartfelt gratitude to those who have played a pivotal role in its development.

First and foremost, we express our deepest appreciation to the Executive Director and CEO, Professor (Dr) Shakti Kumar Gupta, of our prestigious institute, All India Institute of Medical Sciences (AIIMS), Vijaypur, Jammu (J&K), India, an institution renowned for its dedication to excellence in healthcare and medical education. His continuous expertise and dedication have inspired this endeavor. Also, his commitment to advancing knowledge and fostering a passion for learning has been a guiding light throughout the writing process.

We extend our acknowledgment to the Medical Superintendent and Dean of Research, Lt Gen (Dr) Sunil Kant, SM, VSM (Retd) for providing valuable insights and feedback throughout this project; your enthusiasm and constructive input have greatly contributed to the refinement of this resource. Your commitment to excellence in your studies is truly commendable.

We would like to express our gratitude to our family and loved ones for their continuous support, understanding, patience, and encouragement that have sustained us throughout this project. Your recognition of the importance of accessible and comprehensive learning resources for medical laboratory science is deeply appreciated.

Special thanks are extended to our seniors, colleagues, and fellow researchers for their tireless efforts that have transformed this project from concept to reality. Your attention to detail, organizational skills, and commitment to quality have been instrumental in shaping the final product.

We also extend our acknowledgment to the contributors of this book, who have played a vital role in the final shaping of this project.

Last but certainly not least, we acknowledge the unwavering support of M/s Jaypee Brothers Medical Publishers (P) Ltd, New Delhi, India, especially Shri Jitendar P Vij (Group Chairman), Mr Ankit Vij (Managing Director), Mr MS Mani (Group President), Dr Madhu Choudhary (Director–Educational Publishing), Ms Pooja Bhandari [Director–Production (Books and Journals)], Ms Sunita Katla (Executive Assistant to Group Chairman and Publishing Manager), Mr Ajay Kumar Sharma [Deputy General Manager (Books and Journals)], Dr Sangeeta Yadav (Development Editor), Mr Rajesh Sharma (Production Coordinator), Ms Seema Dogra (Cover Visualizer), Mr Laxmidhar Padhiary (Quality Controller), Mr Mahesh Joshi (Typesetter), Mr Satender Singh (Graphic Designer) and their team, whose patience and encouragement have sustained us throughout the demanding process of creating this book. Your belief in our commitment to education and professional development has been a source of strength.

We sincerely thank everyone who has contributed, directly or indirectly, to the realization of *Review of Medical Laboratory Techniques*.

We hope this book proves to be a valuable asset in the educational journey of students and practitioners alike, fostering a deeper understanding and appreciation for the critical role of medical laboratory science in healthcare.

Reetika Menia
Shivani Gandhi
Ishani Gupta

Contents

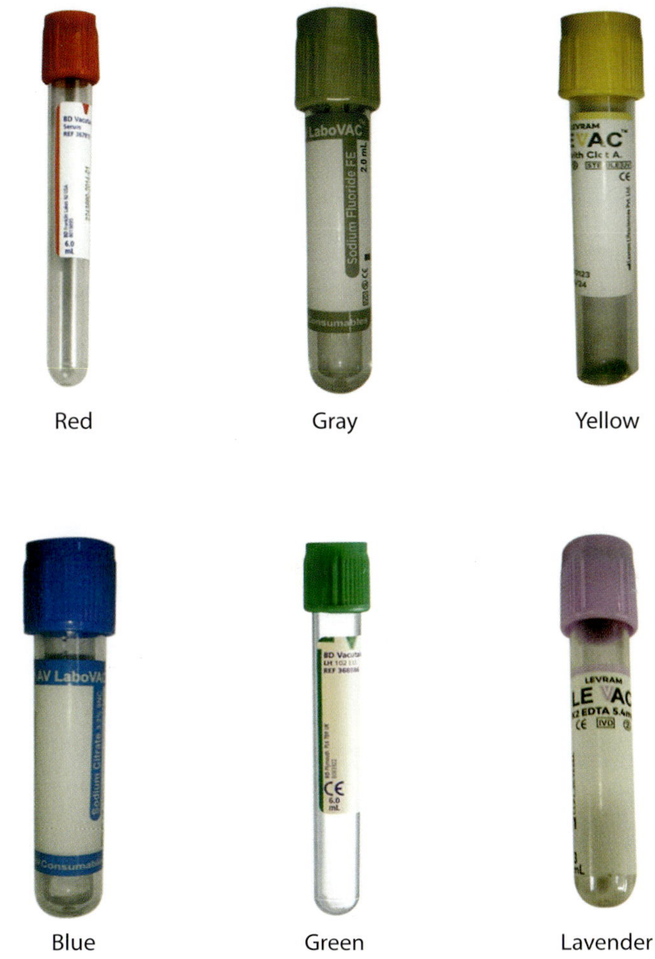

Table 4.2: Different vacutainers used in hematology (Page 234–236).

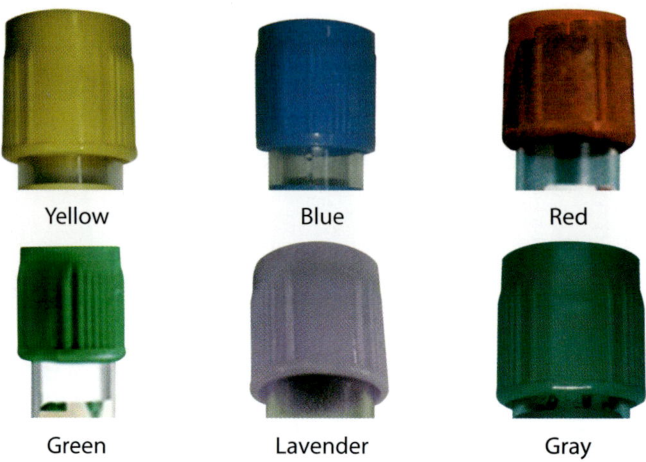

Sequence of filling the tubes (Page 237).

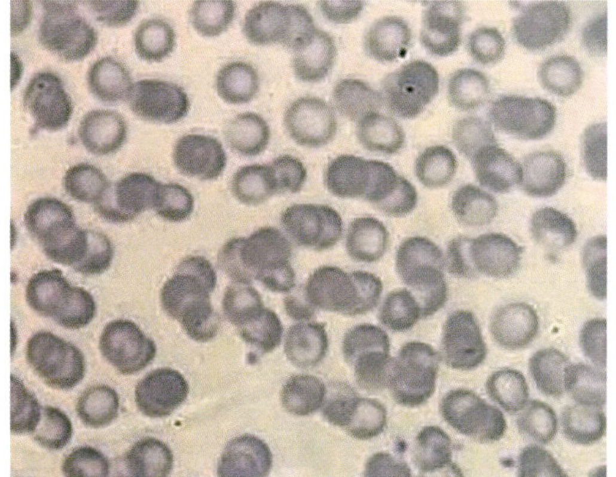

Fig. 4.2: Red blood cells (RBCs) in the blood smear.

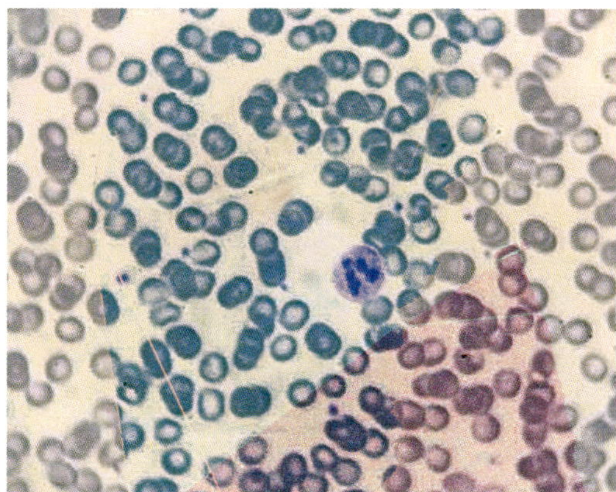

Fig. 4.3: A bilobed neutrophil in the center of the blood smear.

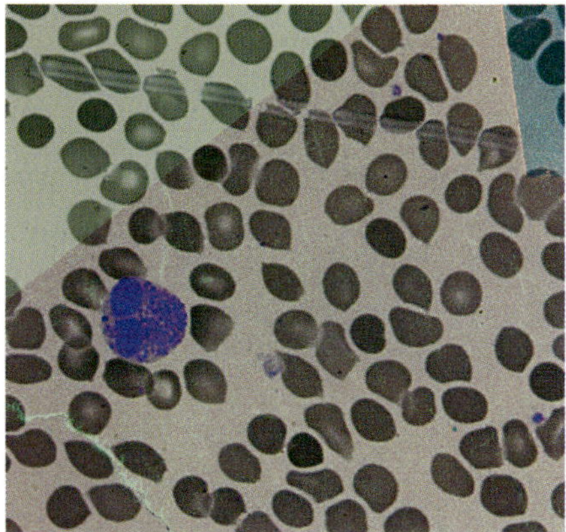

Fig. 4.4: Bilobed eosinophil in the center of the blood smear.

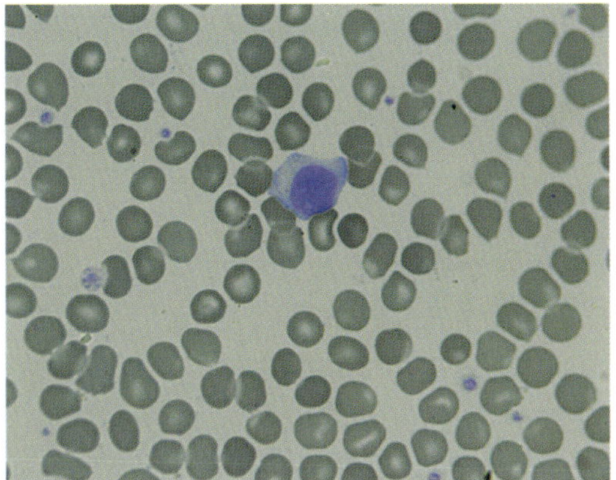

Fig. 4.5: Monocyte in the center of the blood smear.

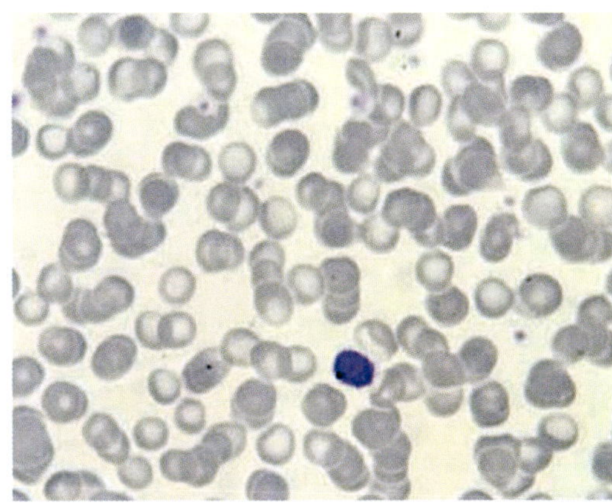

Fig. 4.6: Large lymphocyte in the center of the blood smear.

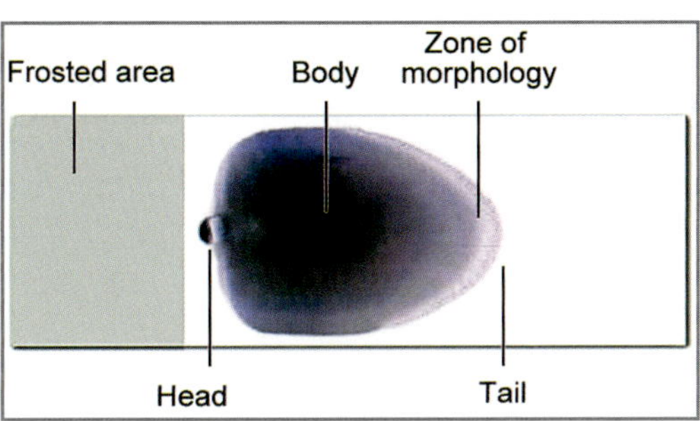

Fig. 4.7: A well prepared blood smear.

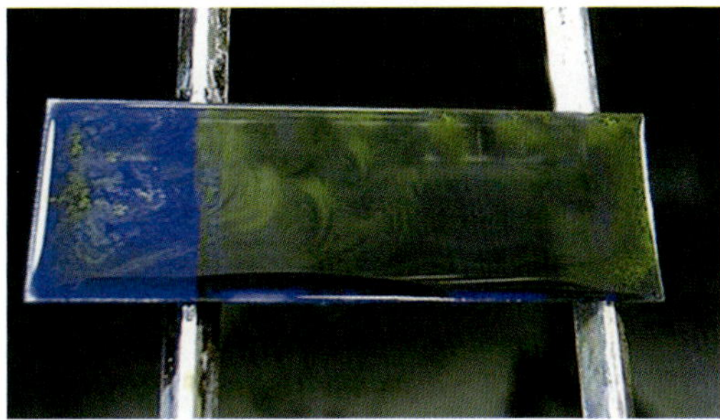

Fig. 4.8: A metallic sheen on the slide.

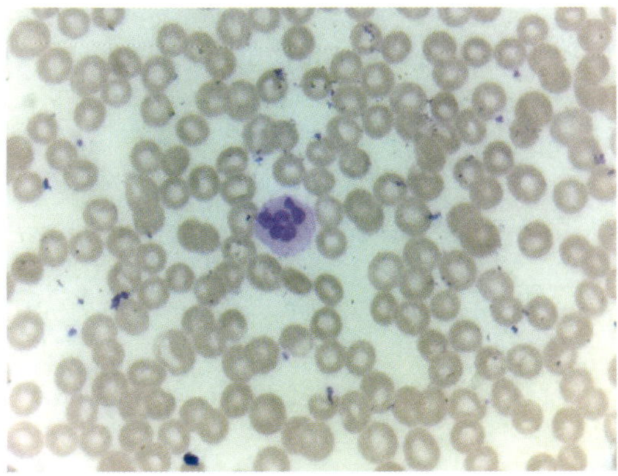

Fig. 4.9: Hypersegmented neutrophil having 6 lobes present in the center of the blood smear.

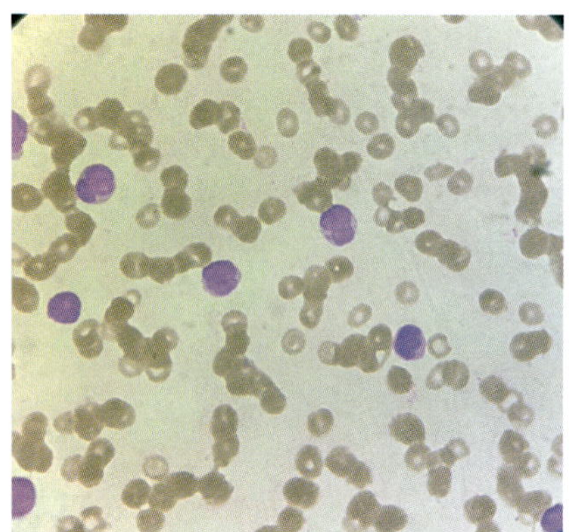

Fig. 4.10: Showing the multiple blasts that are larger in size with high N:C ratio with prominent nucleolus in some of them.

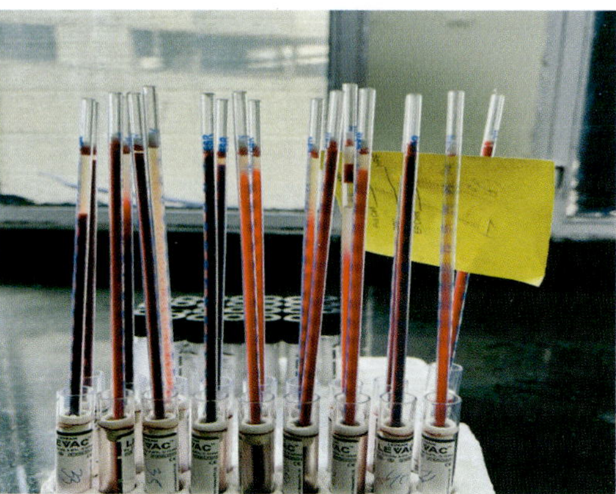

Fig. 4.14: Showing Westergren's pipette for ESR estimation.

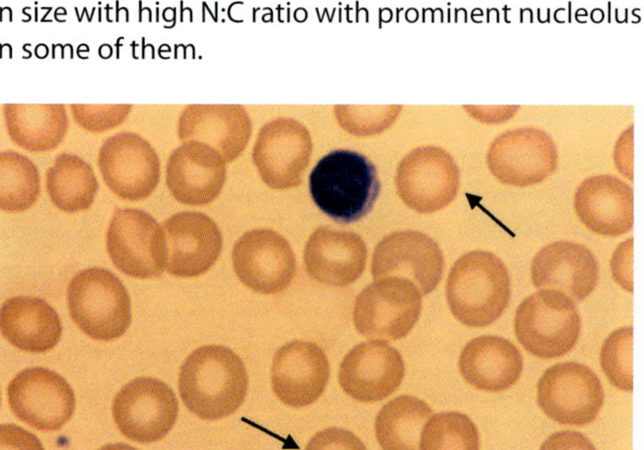

Fig. 4.16: Peripheral blood smear showing normal RBCs.

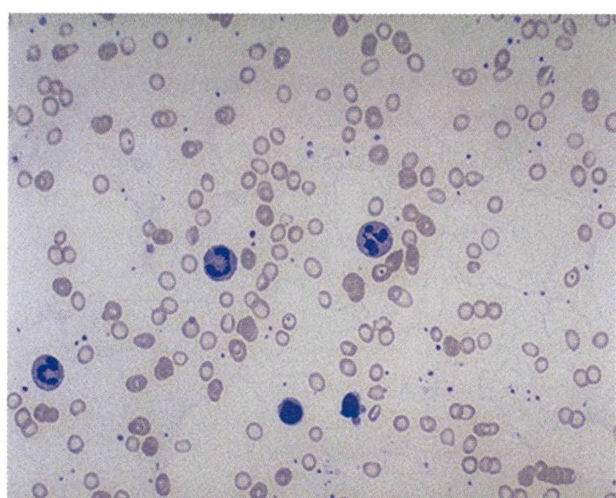

Fig. 4.17: Peripheral blood smear showing microcytes, hypochromic RBCs, and pencil cells.

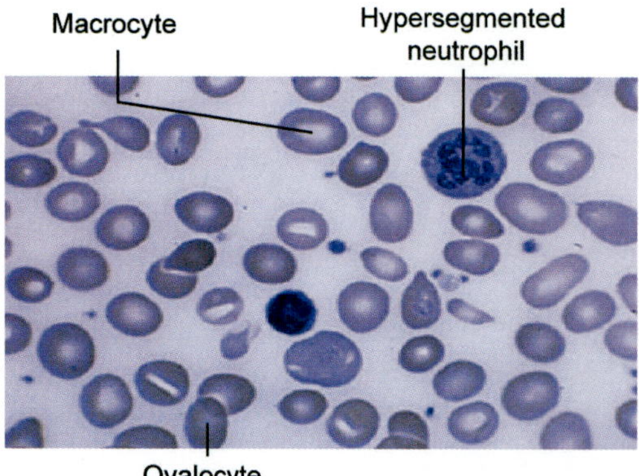

Fig. 4.18: PBS of macrocytic anemia showing macrocytes and a hypersegmented neutrophil.

Morphology	Classification	Nucleus	Nucleolus	Chromatin	Cytoplasm
	L1 acute lymphoblastic (principally pediatric)	Uniformly round, small	Single, indistinct	Slightly reticulated with pennucleolar clumping	Scant, blue
	L2 lymphoblastic (principally adult)	Irregular	Single to several indistinct	Fine	Moderate, pale
	L3 burkitt-type	Round to oval	Two to five	Course with clear parachromatin	Moderate blue, prominently vacuolated

Fig. 4.19: Morphological, immunophenotypic and cytogenetic features of lymphoblasts.

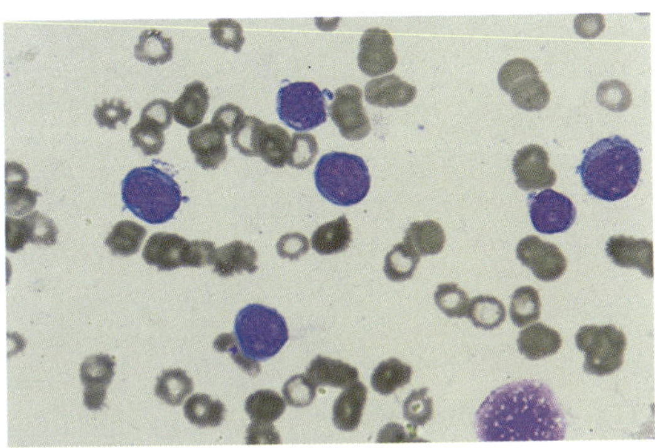

Fig. 4.20: Peripheral blood smear showing blasts.

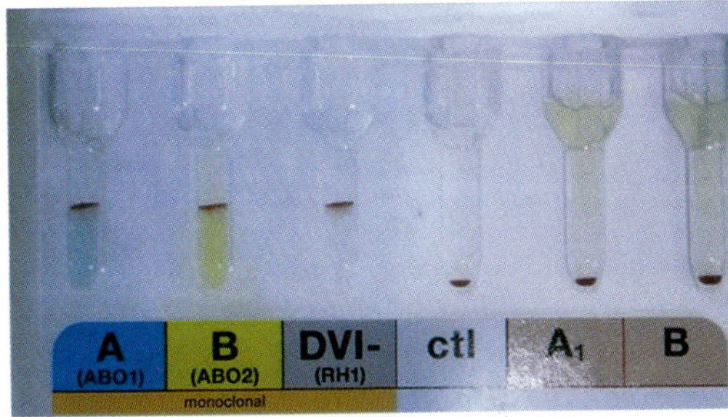

Fig. 4.29: Blood group AB +ve by forward cell typing method.

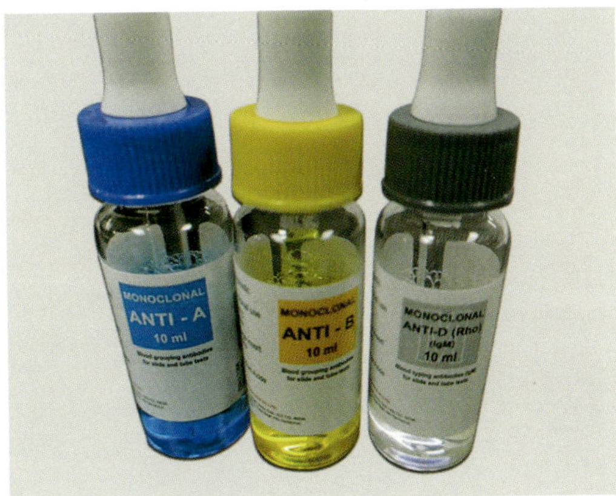

Fig. 4.30: Antisera A, B and D.

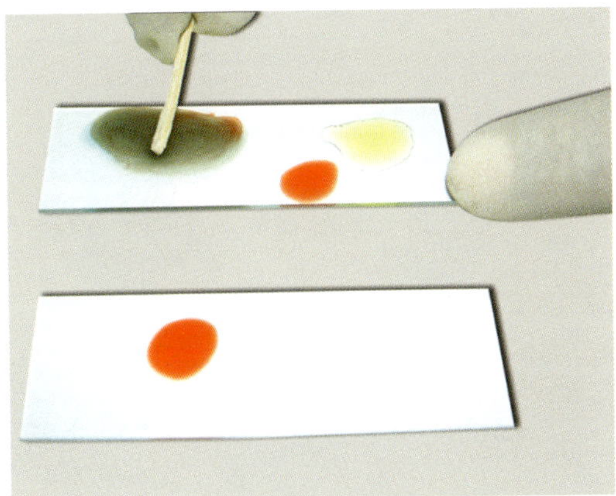

Fig. 4.31: Method of mixing of antisera and blood sample.

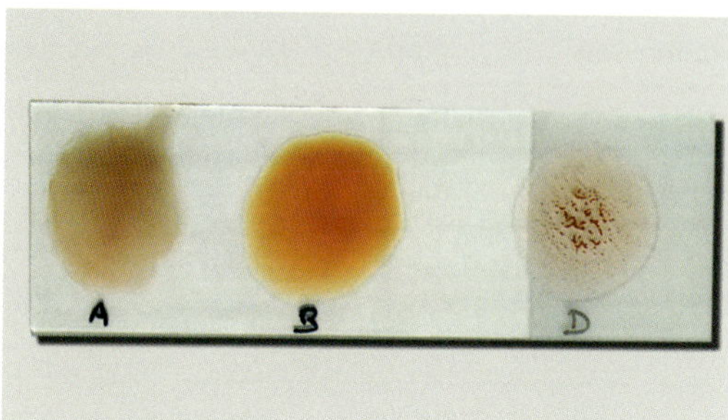

Fig. 4.32: Depicting O +ve blood group.

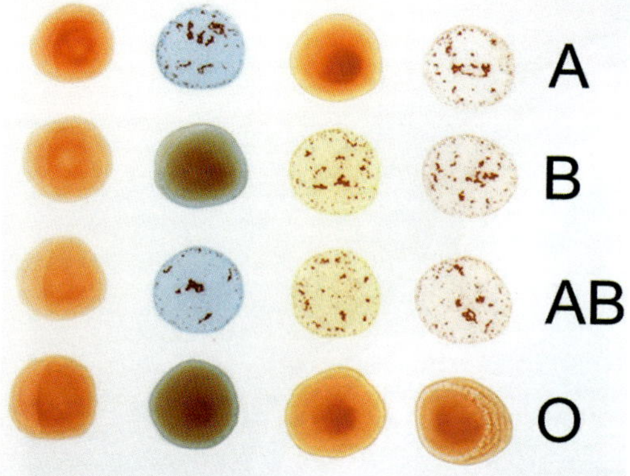

Fig. 4.33: Blood grouping based on agglutination.

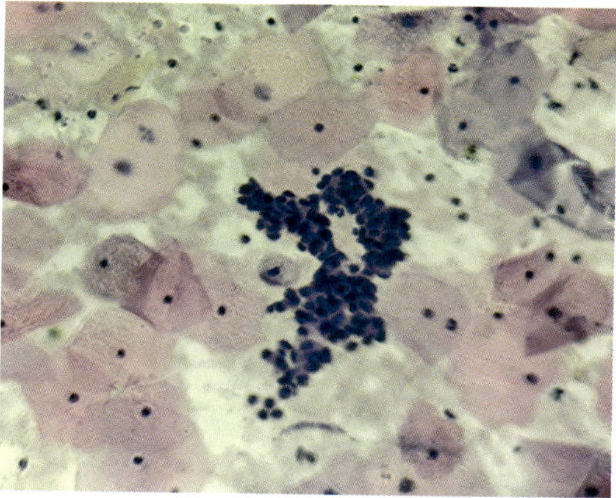

Fig. 6.3: Pap smear with squamous cells in the background and endocervical cells (in honeycomb pattern) in the center.

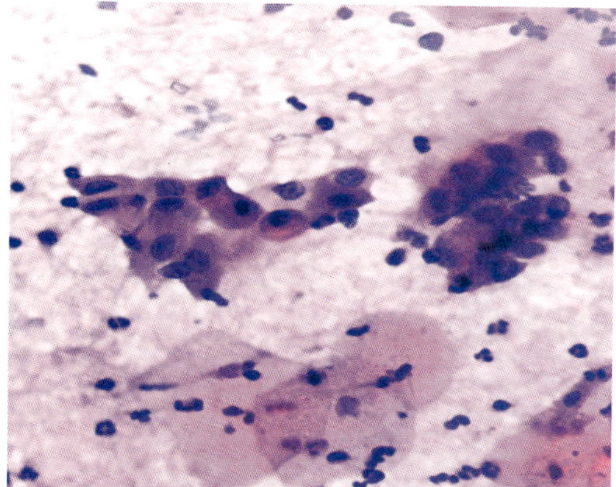

Fig. 6.4: Low-grade squamous intraepithelial lesion (LSIL).

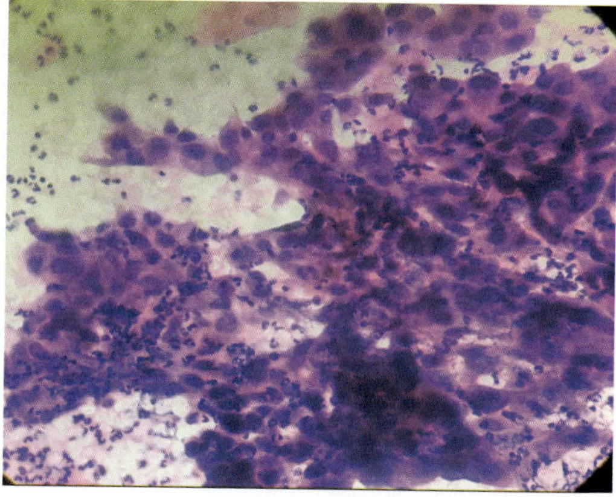

Fig. 6.5: High-grade squamous intraepithelial lesion (HSIL).

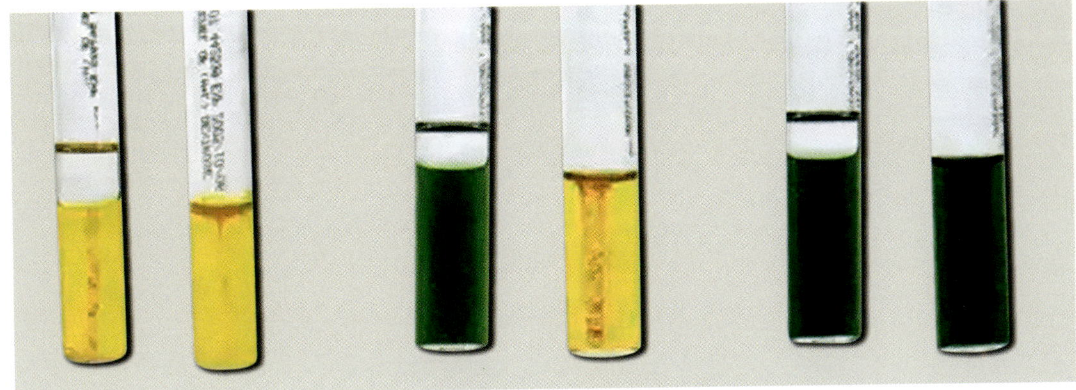

Fig. 7.8: Oxidative fermentation test.

SECTION 1

Anatomy and Physiology

1

Human Anatomy

CHAPTER

INTRODUCTION AND OVERVIEW

Human anatomy is the branch of medical science that deals with the human body's structure from macroscopic to microscopic levels. The term, 'anatomy', is derived from a Greek word, "anatome", meaning cutting up. The human body consists of cells that are composed of cytoplasm (which contains the cytosol and different organelles), nucleus and the surrounding plasma membrane.

The plasma membrane is a double layer of phospholipid molecules with a hydrophilic and a hydrophobic end. It contains proteins, including the ATPase (the sodium-potassium pump), which moves sodium ions out of the cell while moving potassium ions into the cell.

Tissue

Cells join to form the tissue in the body. Four major types of tissue are identified in the body—epithelial, connective, muscle and neural tissues.

Further epithelial tissue may be subdivided into squamous, cuboidal, columnar or glandular, depending on their role in the body. Muscle may be skeletal, smooth or cardiac. Connective tissue is quite varied and may be categorized under blood, bone, dermis, cartilage and tendon.

Bone

An adult skeleton contains 206 individual bones. They are classified as part of the axial or appendicular skeleton. Bone may be termed compact (dense) or spongy (cancellous).

- *Compact bone* is found in the shaft (the diaphysis) of long bones and is composed of microscopic cylindrical structures called osteons. These are lamellar structures with osteocytes within lacunae surrounding a central canal containing blood vessels. The central canal can exchange material with the lacunae via small channels called canaliculi.
- *Spongy bone* is found in the ends (the epiphyses) of long bones and is composed of bony trabeculae. Marrow is found in the shaft of long bones and between the trabeculae of spongy bones. Active marrow produces red and white blood cells by hemopoiesis. Yellow marrow is inactive.

Bone is a storage place for calcium and is continually being remodelled by osteoclasts (which remove bone) and osteoblasts (which deposit bone). In the process, calcium is released or stored.

The surface of bones is marked by the presence of projections or roughening or indented below the surface. The features mark attachment points for tendons and ligaments, places where a bone articulates with another, grooves where tendons may lie, or an opening for nerves and blood vessels to pass through. These features are given names such as tuberosity, condyle, foramen, tubercle, etc.

Joint

A bone is connected to an adjacent bone at an articulation (a joint), and they are bound to each other by ligaments. All the joints in the appendicular skeleton are freely moveable (synovial) joints and stabilized by tendons and intracapsular menisci.

Their free movement is produced when the muscles attached to them contract and is ensured by the smooth hyaline cartilage that covers the articulating bone surfaces and the lubricating synovial fluid within the joint capsule.

Muscle

Skeletal muscle is voluntarily controlled and contains multinucleated and striated cells with long fibers, plasma membrane (sarcolemma), cytoplasm (sarcoplasm), endoplasmic reticulum (sarcoplasmic reticulum) and sarcomeres (contractile myofibrils). Within a sarcomere are bundles of thick and thin myofilaments. Sarcomeres are joined end to end to form a long strand called a myofibril. The thick myofilaments are composed of the protein myosin. The thin myofilaments are composed of the protein actin, while the proteins troponin and tropomyosin, along with calcium ions and ATP, participate in the physiology of contraction of a sarcomere.

Each cell/fiber is surrounded by a membrane called the endomysium which overlies the sarcolemma.

The endomysium contains nerve axons and capillaries. A bundle of muscle fibers is called a fascicle and is surrounded by a connective tissue membrane called the perimysium.

A muscle is a bundle of fascicles, and the membrane surrounding a muscle is called the epimysium.

Respiratory System

Respiration is a term that is variously applied to:

○ The acts of inhalation and exhalation.
○ Movement of gas molecules in the lungs between alveolar air and blood in the alveolar capillaries.
○ Exchange of dissolved gases in the tissue between the systemic capillaries and the surrounding interstitial fluid.
○ The process conducted within the mitochondria of cells that results in the production of ATP (and CO_2) from small organic molecules by using O_2.

The respiratory system is a set of tubes that increase in number and decrease in size within an elastic structure that is moved by muscles.

The lungs and chest wall together act like bellows to move air into and out of the alveoli. The walls of the alveoli are part of the respiratory membrane that separates the air in the alveoli from the blood in the alveolar capillaries. The capillary walls are also part of the respiratory membrane. Air passes through the respiratory passage, which includes nostrils, the meatus of the nasal cavity, the pharynx, the larynx, the glottis, the trachea, the bronchi, and then into the secondary and tertiary (and smaller) bronchi, eventually into the bronchioles, then into smaller airways to reach the alveoli finally. Here, oxygen diffuses through the membrane from the alveoli to the blood, and carbon dioxide diffuses from the blood to the alveoli.

Bronchi are held open by the cartilage in their walls, while bronchioles are without cartilage but may dilate and constrict as the smooth muscle in their wall relaxes or contracts.

Nervous System

The brain and spinal cord are enclosed by membranes called meninges: the dura mater, the arachnoid mater and the pia mater. Together brain and spinal cord are the "Central Nervous System" (CNS). The peripheral nervous system includes motor nerves that leave the CNS from the brain or the spinal cord and sensory nerves that bring information to the CNS. Sensory nerves are "afferent", i.e., carry information from sensory organs to the brain—often via the spinal cord. Motor nerves are "efferent", i.e., they carry commands from the brain (usually) to the muscles (usually). Motor and sensory nerve fibers attached to the brain are called cranial nerves, and those attached to the spinal cord are called spinal nerves.

The brain consists of the cerebrum, diencephalon, brainstem and cerebellum, while cerebrospinal fluid (CSF) rather than blood circulates through the four ventricles within the brain, through the central canal of the spinal cord and between the arachnoid and pia maters. CSF is formed from blood at the choroid plexuses and returns to the blood in the superior sagittal sinus. The surface of the cerebrum is folded into gyri (ridges) and sulci (valleys) and divided into "lobes": frontal, two parietal, occipital, two temporal and two insula.

The central sulcus separates the frontal lobe from the parietal lobes while the precentral gyrus (of the frontal lobe) is noteworthy for being the primary motor area, and the post-central gyrus (of the parietal lobe) for being the primary somatosensory area.

In cross-section, the spinal cord displays its characteristic butterfly-shaped central gray matter region surrounded by the white matter of myelinated nerves. This white matter is either ascending tracts (carrying sensory information to the brain) or descending tracts (carrying motor instructions to muscles and glands).

The axons of sensory neurons within a spinal nerve enter the spinal cord from the dorsal side, while the axons of motor neurons within a spinal nerve exit the spinal cord from the ventral side. This "dorsal root" and the "ventral root" meet and join to form the spinal nerve that then passes through the vertebral foramina.

MUSCULOSKELETAL SYSTEM

Introduction

The musculoskeletal system is a complex network of bones, muscles, joints, and connective tissues that work together to support the body, provide movement, and protect vital organs. It is crucial to understand the structure and function of this system, as it plays a significant role in assessing and treating various medical conditions. In this chapter, we will explore the anatomy of the musculoskeletal system and gain insights into its remarkable capabilities.

Bones

Structure of Bones

Bones are the body's structural framework, providing support, protection, and a site for muscle attachment. They are classified into long, short, flat, and irregular bones based on their shape. The structure of a typical long bone consists of a shaft (diaphysis), two ends (epiphyses), compact bone, spongy bone, periosteum, and marrow cavity.

Bone Growth and Development

Bones undergo continuous growth and remodelling throughout life. During early development, bone formation occurs through two processes: intramembranous ossification and endochondral ossification. Factors such as nutrition, hormones, and physical activity influence bone growth. Knowing bone development helps in understanding conditions like fractures, osteoporosis, and skeletal abnormalities.

Classifications of Bones

Bones are classified, according to shape, into long, short, flat, irregular, and sesamoid bones and, according to their development, into endochondral and membranous bones, discussed as under.

Long Bones

Long bones include the humerus, radius, ulna, femur, tibia, fibula, metacarpals, and phalanges. They develop by replacement of hyaline cartilage plate (endochondral ossification). Long bones have a shaft (diaphysis) and two ends (epiphyses). The metaphysis is a part of the diaphysis adjacent to the epiphyses.

- **Diaphysis:** Forms the shaft (central region) and is composed of a thick tube of compact bone that encloses the marrow cavity.
- **Metaphysis:** Part of the diaphysis, the growth zone between the diaphysis and epiphysis during bone development.
- **Epiphyses:** Expanded articular ends, separated from the shaft by the epiphyseal plate during bone growth and composed of a spongy bone surrounded by a thin layer of compact bone.

Short Bones

Short bones include the carpal and tarsal bones and are approximately cuboid-shaped. They are composed of spongy bone and marrow surrounded by a thin outer layer of compact bone.

Flat Bones

Flat bones include the ribs, sternum, scapulae, and bones in the vault of the skull. It consists of two layers of compact bone enclosing spongy bone and marrow space (diploë). They have articular surfaces that are covered with fibrocartilage and grow by the replacement of connective tissue.

Irregular Bones

These include bones of mixed shapes such as bones of the skull, vertebrae, and coxa. It contains mostly spongy bone enveloped by a thin outer layer of compact bone.

Sesamoid Bones

These develop in certain tendons and reduce friction on the tendon, thus protecting it from excessive wear. Sesamoid bones are commonly found where tendons cross the ends of long bones in the limbs, as in the wrist and the knee (i.e. patella).

Joints

Classification of Joints

Joints are formed between union of two or more bones. They are classified on the basis of their structural features into fibrous, cartilaginous, and synovial types, discussed as under.

- **Fibrous joints (synarthroses):** Joined by fibrous tissue, have no joint cavities and permit little movement. Fibrous joints are further subdivided into:

  Sutures: Connected by fibrous connective tissue and found between the flat bones of the skull.

  Syndesmoses: Connected by fibrous connective tissue. Occur as the inferior tibiofibular and tympanostapedial syndesmoses.

- **Cartilaginous joints:** Cartilaginous joints are united by cartilage and have no joint cavity. They may be divided as follows:

  Primary cartilaginous joints (synchondroses): United by hyaline cartilage and permits no movement but growth in length. It includes epiphyseal cartilage plates (the union between the epiphysis and the diaphysis of a growing bone) and sphenoid-occipital and manubriosternal synchondroses.

  Secondary cartilaginous joints (symphyses): Joined by fibrocartilage and are slightly movable joints. It includes the pubic symphysis and the intervertebral discs.

- **Synovial (diarthrodial) joints:** They permit a great degree of free movement and are classified according to the shape of the articulation and/or the type of movement. They are characterized by four features—joint cavity, articular (hyaline) cartilage, synovial membrane (which produces synovial fluid), and articular capsule.

Different types of synovial joints are summarized below as:

i. **Plane (gliding) joints:** United by two flat articular surfaces, allowing simple gliding or sliding of one bone over the other. Occur in the proximal tibiofibular, intertarsal, intercarpal, intermetacarpal, carpometacarpal, sternoclavicular, and acromioclavicular joints.

ii. **Hinge (ginglymus) joints:** Resemble door hinges and allow only flexion and extension. Occur in the elbow, ankle, and interphalangeal joints.

iii. **Pivot (trochoid) joints:** Formed by a central bony pivot turning within a bony ring and allow only rotation (movement around a single longitudinal axis). It occurs in the superior and inferior radioulnar joints and in the atlantoaxial joint.

iv. **Condylar (ellipsoidal) joints:** Have two convex condyles articulating with two concave condyles (the shape of the articulation is ellipsoidal). It allows flexion and extension and occurs in the wrist (radiocarpal), metacarpophalangeal, knee (tibiofemoral), and atlantooccipital joints.

v. **Saddle (sellar) joints:** Resemble a saddle on a horse's back and allow flexion and extension, abduction and adduction, and circumduction but no axial rotation. It occurs in the carpometacarpal joint of the thumb and between the femur and patella.

vi. **Ball-and-socket (spheroidal or cotyloid) joints:** Formed by the reception of a globular (ball-like) head into a cup-shaped cavity and allow movement in many directions. It allows flexion and extension, abduction and adduction, medial and lateral rotations, and circumduction and occurs in the shoulder and hip joints.

Muscles

Types of Muscles

Muscles are responsible for movement and maintaining body posture. There are three types of muscles—skeletal, smooth, and cardiac. Skeletal muscles are attached to bones and produce voluntary movements, while smooth muscles control involuntary actions of internal organs, and cardiac muscles form the heart and pump blood.

Structure and Function of Skeletal Muscles

Skeletal muscles are composed of bundles of muscle fibers and are surrounded by connective tissues. They are attached to bones via tendons and work in pairs or groups to create movement. The contraction and relaxation of muscles are controlled by nerve impulses, allowing precise control over body movements.

Classification of Muscle

A muscle consists predominantly of contractile cells and produces the movements of various parts of the body by contraction. It is divided into three types:

1. **Skeletal muscle:** It is voluntary and striated; makes up approximately 40% of the total body mass and functions to produce movement of the body, generate body heat, and maintain body posture. It has two attachments—an origin (usually the more fixed and proximal attachment) and an insertion (the more movable and distal attachment). Muscles are enclosed by epimysium, a thin layer of connective tissue. Smaller bundles of muscle fibers are surrounded by perimysium. Each muscle fibre is enclosed by an endomysium.

2. **Cardiac muscle:** It is involuntary and striated and forms the myocardium, the

middle layer of the heart. Cardiac muscles are innervated by the autonomic nervous system but contract spontaneously without any nerve supply. It includes specialized myocardial fibers that form the cardiac conducting system.

3. **Smooth muscle:** It is involuntary and nonstriated and generally arranged in circular and longitudinal layers in the walls of many visceral organs. They are innervated by the autonomic nervous system, regulating the size of the lumen of a tubular structure. They undergo rhythmic contractions called peristaltic waves in the walls of the gastrointestinal (GI) tract, uterine tubes, ureters, and other organs.

NERVOUS SYSTEM

Introduction

The nervous system is a complex network of cells and tissues that coordinates and regulates the activities of the body. It is divided into two main parts—the central nervous system (CNS), consisting of the brain and spinal cord, and the peripheral nervous system (PNS), including nerves and ganglia throughout the body. The anatomy of the nervous system is crucial for recognizing neurological conditions, assessing injuries, and providing appropriate care. In this chapter, we will explore the general anatomy of the nervous system.

Central Nervous System

The central nervous system (CNS) is a complex network comprising the brain or encephalon, housed within the cranial cavity and serving as the hub for higher governing centres. Additionally, the spinal cord, known as the spinal medulla, occupies the upper two-thirds of the vertebral canal, featuring numerous reflex centers.

The Brain

The brain is the command center of the nervous system enclosed within the cranium or braincase and controls almost all body functions. It consists of several interconnected regions, each with specialized functions. The cortex is the outer part of the cerebral hemispheres composed of gray matter (consisting largely of the nerve cell bodies, dendrites, and neuroglia) and an interior part is composed of white matter (consisting largely of axons forming tracts or pathways, and ventricles, which are filled with cerebrospinal fluid).

Spinal Cord

It is a cylindrical structure that occupies approximately the upper two-thirds of the vertebral canal and is enveloped by the meninges. Conical end of the spinal cord is known as the conus medullaris and ends at the level of L2 (or between L1 and L2) in the adult and at the level of L3 in the newborn.

Neurons

Neurons are the structural and functional units of the nervous system (neuron doctrine). They are specialized for the reception, integration, transformation, and transmission of information. The components of neurons are as under:

○ Cell bodies are located in the gray matter of the CNS, and their collections are called ganglia in the PNS and nuclei in the CNS.
○ Dendrites (dendron means "tree") are usually short and highly branched and carry impulses toward the cell body.
○ Axons are usually single and long, have fewer branches (collaterals), and carry impulses away from the cell body.

Classification of Neurons

1. **Unipolar (pseudounipolar) neurons:** They have one process, which divides into a central branch that functions as an axon and a peripheral branch that serves as a dendrite.

2. **Bipolar neurons:** They have two processes (one dendrite and one axon), are sensory and are found in the olfactory epithelium, the retina, and the inner ear.
3. **Multipolar neurons:** They have several dendrites and one axon and are most common in the CNS (e.g., motor cells in anterior and lateral horns of the spinal cord, autonomic ganglion cells).

Other Components of the Nervous System

○ **Cells that support neurons:** Include Schwann cells and satellite cells in the PNS.
○ **Myelin:** Fat-like substance forming a sheath around certain nerve fibers. It is formed by Schwann cells in the PNS and oligodendrocytes in the CNS.
○ **Synapses:** Sites of functional contact of a neuron with another neuron, an effector (muscle, gland) cell, or a sensory receptor cell.

Peripheral Nervous System (PNS)

Components of PNS

Peripheral nervous system includes all the neural structures present outside the CNS discussed as under.

○ **Peripheral nerves**
  Cranial nerves: Consist of 12 pairs and are connected to the brain rather than to the spinal cord. PNS have motor fibers with cell bodies located within the CNS and sensory fibers with cell bodies that form sensory ganglia located outside the CNS. It emerges from the ventral aspect of the brain (except for the trochlear nerve, cranial nerve IV).
  Spinal nerves: They are a series of nerves that emerge from the spinal cord and branch out to various regions of the body. Based on their origin, they are classified into cervical, thoracic, lumbar, sacral, and coccygeal nerves.
○ **Ganglia (autonomic and sensory):** A ganglion is a collection of neuron cell bodies outside the CNS, and a nucleus is a collection of neuron cell bodies within the CNS.
○ **Autonomic nervous system (sympathetic and para-sympathetic nervous systems).**

Classification of PNS

The peripheral nervous system (PNS) consists of two major components:

Cerebrospinal Nervous System

○ Representing the somatic division of the PNS, it comprises 12 pairs of cranial nerves and 31 pairs of spinal nerves.
○ Functionally, it innervates somatic structures in the head, neck, limbs, and body wall, facilitating sensory and motor functions.

Peripheral Autonomic Nervous System

○ Serving as the visceral component of the PNS, it involves visceral or splanchnic nerves connected to the CNS via somatic nerves.
○ Its primary role is to innervate viscera, glands, blood vessels, and nonstriated muscles, mediating various visceral functions.

The cerebrospinal and autonomic nervous systems exhibit distinctions in their efferent pathways, as summarized here.

Comparison of cerebrospinal and peripheral autonomic nervous systems

Aspect	Cerebrospinal nervous system	Peripheral autonomic nervous system
Efferent pathway	Comprised of one neuron passing directly to the effector organ (skeletal muscles)	Characterized by two neurons (preganglionic and postganglionic) with an intervening ganglion for relay
Effector organ (viscera)	–	Effectively supplied by the postganglionic fiber

CARDIOVASCULAR SYSTEM

Introduction

The cardiovascular system, also known as the circulatory system, is responsible for the transportation of oxygen, nutrients, hormones, and waste products throughout the body. It comprises the heart, blood vessels, and blood. The blood serves as a medium for the transportation of various agents like nutrients, CO_2, O_2, etc., from the tissue to the heart and vice versa.

Essential Components of CVS

- **Heart:** It is a vital, four-chambered muscular organ responsible for pumping blood throughout the body. Each half comprises an atrium (receiving chamber) and a ventricle (pumping chamber).
- **Arteries:** The word is derived from the Greek word "Angeion," meaning vessel, leading to terms like angiology, angiography, hemangioma, and thromboangitis obliterans. These are the distributing channels with important features listed under:
  - Serve as conduits carrying blood away from the heart.
  - Branch extensively, resembling trees, as they transport blood to various body parts.
  - Large arteries feature elastic tissue, with an increasing presence of smooth muscle in smaller branches (arterioles).
- **Veins:** They are the draining channels that:
  - Functions as channels returning blood from different body regions to the heart.
  - Analogs to rivers, veins are formed by merging tributaries.
  - Small veins (venules) combine to create larger veins, ultimately forming major veins known as venae cavae.
- **Capillaries:** These are the networks of microscopic vessels that serve as intricate networks connecting arterioles with venules. Positioned closely to tissues, they facilitate the exchange of nutrients and metabolites between blood and tissue fluid. This exchange involves capillaries draining metabolites, with lymphatics also playing a role. In certain organs like the liver and spleen, capillaries are replaced by sinusoids, reflecting their functional adaptability.

Blood Vessels

These closed tubular structures carry blood from the heart to tissues and back to the heart from the tissues.

Functional Classification of Blood Vessels

Blood vessels can be functionally categorized into five groups:

1. **Distributing vessels (arteries):** These vessels, notably arteries, distribute oxygenated blood away from the heart to various body parts.
2. **Resistance vessels:** Arterioles and precapillary sphincters fall into this category, regulating blood flow and exerting control over peripheral resistance.
3. **Exchange vessels:** Including capillaries, sinusoids, and postcapillary venules, these vessels enable the exchange of nutrients, gases, and metabolites between blood and tissues.
4. **Reservoir (capacitance) vessels:** Larger venules and veins serve as reservoirs, accommodating varying blood volumes.
5. **Shunts:** Various types of anastomoses, including arterial, venous, or arteriovenous connections, contribute to shunting blood in specific circumstances.

Blood Circulation

- **Systemic (greater) circulation:** Blood flows from the left ventricle through the body to the right atrium, encompassing the entire systemic pathway.

○ **Pulmonary (lesser) circulation:** Blood travels from the right ventricle through the lungs to the left atrium, completing the pulmonary circuit.

○ **Portal circulation:** A subset of systemic circulation involves blood passing through two sets of capillaries before draining into a systemic vein. Examples include hepatic, hypothalamo-hypophyseal, and renal portal circulation.

Arteries

Characteristic Features and Types

Arteries exhibit distinct characteristics, such as thick walls, absence of valves, and association with veins and nerves in neurovascular bundles. They can be broadly classified into large elastic arteries, medium and small muscular arteries, and smallest muscular arteries, known as arterioles. Arterioles further branch into terminal arterioles and metarterioles, with precapillary sphincters regulating blood flow into capillary beds.

Microscopic Structure of Arteries

Microscopically, all arteries consist of three coats: tunica intima, tunica media, and tunica adventitia. The relative thickness and composition of these coats vary among different artery types. Large arteries are supplied with blood vessels called vasa vasorum, which form a dense capillary network in the tunica adventitia.

Palpable Arteries and Nerve Supply

Certain arteries, like the common carotid, brachial, and femoral, are palpable through the skin. Arteries receive nerve supply from nervi vascularis, mainly non-myelinated sympathetic fibers with vasoconstrictor functions, along with some myelinated sensory fibers.

Veins

Characteristic Features and Structure

Veins, distinguished by thin walls, larger lumens, and the presence of valves, play a crucial role in maintaining unidirectional blood flow. The structure of veins includes three coats, but they are less defined compared to arteries. Larger veins have dead spaces for dilation during increased venous return.

Blood and Nerve Supply of Veins

Similar to arteries, larger veins are supplied with vasa vasorum, and nerves (nervi vascularis) are distributed to veins. Venous return is aided by factors like overflow from capillaries, negative intrathoracic pressure, and muscular contractions.

Capillaries (Networks for Nutrient Exchange)

Capillaries are microscopically small endothelial tubes that connect arterioles and venules, facilitating the exchange of nutrients and metabolites between blood and tissue fluid. Continuous and fenestrated capillaries exhibit different types of junctions between endothelial cells, enabling the passage of molecules of varying sizes.

Sinusoids (Specialized Vascular Spaces)

Sinusoids replace capillaries in specific organs, featuring larger, irregular vascular spaces surrounded closely by organ parenchyma. Sinusoids differ from capillaries in lumen width, wall thickness, and the absence of adventitial support.

Anastomoses (Navigating Alternate Pathways in the Cardiovascular Network)

Definition

Within the cardiovascular context, anastomoses denote the intricate network of interconnected vessels that provide alternative routes for blood flow. These vital communications, occurring either before or after the capillary bed, play a pivotal role in maintaining circulation, especially in the face of potential vascular compromise.

Types of Anastomoses

Arterial anastomoses: Arterial anastomoses involve connections between arteries or their branches, offering diverse strategies for blood rerouting.

These can be categorized into two main types:

1. **Actual arterial anastomoses:** This type involves direct connections where arteries meet end to end. Notable examples include the palmar arches, plantar arch, circle of Willis, intestinal arcades, and labial branches of facial arteries.
2. **Potential arterial anastomoses:** Communication occurs between terminal arterioles in potential arterial anastomoses. While providing a gradual dilation for collateral circulation, these anastomoses may fail to compensate for sudden arterial occlusion, as observed in the coronary arteries and cortical branches of cerebral arteries.

Venous anastomoses: Venous anastomoses refer to communications between veins or their tributaries. A well-known example includes the dorsal venous arches found in the hand and foot, showcasing the adaptability of venous networks.

Arteriovenous anastomoses (shunts): Arteriovenous anastomoses, commonly known as shunts, signify the communication between an artery and a vein. These shunts play a crucial role in regulating the phasic activity of organs. During activity, these shunts are closed, directing blood through capillaries, while at rest, blood is shunted back through these connections, bypassing the capillary bed. The shunt vessel typically possesses a thick muscular coat and is under the influence of the sympathetic system.

○ **Specialized arteriovenous anastomoses:** These unique connections, found in regions like digital pads and nail beds, form smaller units known as glomera, contributing to the complexity of the circulatory network.
○ **Thoroughfare channels:** Another type of shunt, known as "thoroughfare channels," courses through the capillary network. Many true capillaries arise as side branches from these channels, further enhancing the adaptability of the cardiovascular system.

End Arteries

In contrast to anastomoses, end arteries represent vessels that do not anastomose with neighboring counterparts. Examples include the central artery of the retina and labyrinthine artery of the internal ear, highlighting their critical role in specific regions where alternate pathways are limited.

Applied Anatomy of the Cardiovascular System

○ **Blood pressure:** Systolic and diastolic pressures and pulse pressure are key indicators of cardiovascular health.
○ **Hemorrhage:** Bleeding can result from venous or arterial sources, leading to different patterns like oozing or spurting.
○ **Vascular catastrophes:** Thrombosis, embolism, and hemorrhage pose risks to blood vessel integrity, emphasizing the importance of collateral circulation.
○ **Arteriosclerosis:** The stiffening of arteries in old age impacts blood supply and contributes to increased systolic pressure.
○ **Arteritis, phlebitis, and atheroma:** Inflammation of arteries or veins and atheroma formation affects vascular health.

○ ***Coronary artery blockage:*** Clinical interventions like stents or grafts may be employed to address coronary artery blockages.

○ ***Aneurysms:*** Swelling or dilation of blood vessels poses a serious risk due to weakened walls.

○ ***Other conditions:*** Diseases like Buerger's disease, Raynaud's phenomenon, acute phlebothrombosis, and varicose veins highlight diverse vascular pathologies.

LYMPHATIC SYSTEM

Introduction

The lymphatic system comprises an extensive network of lymph vessels and lymph nodes through which lymph circulates. The fluid coursing through the lymphatic vessels is referred to as lymph. As it traverses the lymphatics, it undergoes filtration in structures known as lymph nodes, ultimately converging into the venous blood. It constitutes the body's defence mechanism against pathogens and also forms the drainage system for lymph.

Certain segments of the lymphatic system, termed lymphoreticular organs, are primarily dedicated to functions such as phagocytosis, orchestrating immune responses, and contributing to the cellular composition of both blood and lymph.

Components of the Lymphatic System

The components constituting the lymphatic system encompass:

○ Lymph vessels
○ Central lymphoid tissues
○ Peripheral lymphoid organs
○ Circulating lymphocytes.

Lymph Vessels

Lymph capillaries initiate as blind-ended structures within tissue spaces, forming intricate networks and unite to form lymph vessels. Their caliber surpasses that of blood capillaries, and their endothelial walls exhibit permeability to substances of significantly larger molecular size. Notably, lymph capillaries are absent from cellular structures such as the brain, spinal cord, splenic pulp, and bone marrow. The larger lymph vessels, called lymph ducts, are formed by the union of the smaller lymph vessels. A comparative analysis between lymph and blood capillaries highlights their distinctions **(Table 1.1)**.

Types of Lymph Ducts

Principal lymph ducts are of two types:

1. ***Thoracic duct:*** The largest lymphatic duct in the body that begins from the L1–L2

Table 1.1: Comparison of lymph and blood capillaries.		
Criteria	*Lymph capillaries*	*Blood capillaries*
Appearance	Colourless, difficult to observe	Reddish, easy to observe
Termination	Blind (closed at the tip)	Joined to arterioles at one end and to venules at another end
Diameter	Wider than blood capillaries	Narrower than lymph capillaries
Wall composition	Wall consists of thin endothelium and poorly developed basement membrane	Wall consists of normal endothelium and basement membrane
Fluid content	Contains colorless lymph	Contains red blood
Pressure	Relatively low pressure	Relatively high pressure
Function	Absorbs tissue fluid from intercellular spaces	Adds tissue fluid to intercellular spaces

vertebrae to the angle between the left jugular vein and the left subclavian vein. It drains the lymph from the left side of the head and neck, left thoracic region, left upper limb, lower extremities and abdomen.

2. **Right lymphatic duct:** It is a 1 cm long lymph vessel located in the root of the right side of the neck, formed by the fusion of the right jugular trunk, right subclavian trunk and right bronchomediastinal trunk. It drains the lymphatics from the right side of the head and neck, the right thoracic region and the right upper limb.

Lymphatic Drainage Patterns

○ **Superficial lymphatics:** Superficial lymphatics are often involved in assessing the spread of cancer. Lymphatic mapping helps identify the lymph nodes draining a particular area, aiding in cancer staging and treatment planning.

○ **Deep lymphatics:** Deep lymphatics are critical in understanding the spread of infections or tumors deep within tissues. In surgical procedures, preserving or removing specific deep lymph nodes is carefully considered to minimize complications.

Central Lymphoid Tissues

Central lymphoid tissues, encompassing the bone marrow and thymus, play pivotal roles in the overall functionality of the lymphatic system. The bone marrow serves as the primary site for the initial production of 'pluripotent' lymphoid stem cells, except during the early stages of fetal life when the liver takes on this crucial role.

Thymus and T-Lymphocyte Maturation

The thymus is a primary lymphoid organ located in the upper part of the chest, just behind the sternum. It is a crucial site for the maturation of T-lymphocytes, also known as T

cells. T-lymphocytes are white blood cells that play a central role in cell-mediated immunity, which involves the direct attack on infected or abnormal cells. The thymus is most active during childhood and adolescence, gradually decreasing in size and activity as a person ages. It consists of two lobes and is divided into lobules. Each lobule contains a cortex and a medulla, where different stages of T-cell maturation occur.

Stages of T-cell Maturation

○ **Thymic education:** T-cell precursors, originating from the bone marrow, enter the thymus and undergo a process of maturation and education. This involves T-cells' positive and negative selection based on their ability to recognize self-antigens. T-cells that are too reactive against self-antigens are eliminated (negative selection), ensuring that only T-cells capable of recognizing foreign antigens without attacking the body's own cells are allowed to mature.

○ **Positive selection:** T-cells that successfully navigate positive selection acquire the ability to recognize antigens presented by major histocompatibility complex (MHC) molecules on the surface of body cells. This is a crucial step in ensuring that T-cells are able to identify and respond to foreign invaders.

○ **Migration to peripheral organs:** Mature T-cells leave the thymus and migrate to peripheral lymphoid organs, such as lymph nodes, spleen, and other lymphoid tissues.

Functions of T-Lymphocytes

T-lymphocytes are versatile cells with various functions in the immune system:

○ **Cytotoxic T-cells (CD8+):** These T-cells directly kill infected or abnormal cells. They recognize foreign antigens presented on the surface of infected cells and induce their destruction.

○ **Helper T-cells (CD4+):** Helper T-cells play a central role in coordinating immune responses. They assist other immune cells, such as B-lymphocytes, in generating antibodies, and they stimulate the activity of cytotoxic T-cells and macrophages.

○ **Memory T-cells:** Some T-cells become memory T-cells, which "remember" specific antigens. If the body encounters the same antigen in the future, memory T-cells can mount a faster and more effective immune response.

○ **Regulatory T-cells (Tregs):** These cells help maintain immune system balance by suppressing excessive immune responses. They prevent autoimmune reactions and control the duration and intensity of immune responses.

Interconnection with Peripheral Lymphoid Organs

Mature T-lymphocytes leave the thymus and migrate to peripheral lymphoid organs. Here, they encounter antigens presented by antigen-presenting cells (APCs) and contribute to immune responses. This interconnection between the thymus and peripheral organs ensures a diverse and effective immune response against a wide range of pathogens.

Peripheral lymphoid organs: They include lymph nodes and spleen that are involved in the activation of lymphocytes and initiation of an immune response.

1. **Lymph nodes:** These are the oval bean-shaped structures present along the course of lymphatic vessels, with sizes varying from pinhead to large bean size. It has a fibrous capsule with an underlying subcapsular sinus. The small depression at the side is called the hilum. The outer darkly stained portion is the cortex that contains variable-sized lymphoid follicles with germinal centers. The central pale stained area is called the medulla and contains an anastomosing network of cords of cells.

○ **Palpation and examination:** Palpating lymph nodes is a routine part of clinical examinations. Enlarged, tender or fixed lymph nodes can indicate infection, inflammation, or malignancy.

○ **Sentinel lymph node biopsy:** In cancer treatment, identifying and biopsy of sentinel lymph nodes (the first nodes to receive drainage from a tumor) help assess cancer spread without the need for extensive lymph node dissection.

○ Clinical conditions associated with lymph nodes are:

➤ **Lymphadenopathy:** Abnormalities in lymph node size, consistency, and tenderness can be indicative of various medical conditions, including infections, autoimmune diseases, or cancers.

➤ **Lymphedema:** Lymphedema results from impaired lymphatic drainage, often secondary to surgery or radiation. It requires comprehensive management strategies, including physical therapy and compression garments.

➤ **Lymphadenitis:** It is the inflammation of lymph nodes that can occur in response to infections. Differentiating between bacterial and viral causes is crucial for appropriate treatment.

➤ **Lymphomas:** Lymphomas, lymphatic system cancers, have diverse clinical presentations. Diagnosis involves a combination of imaging, biopsy, and staging to determine the extent of the disease.

➤ **Lymphangiomas:** Lymphangiomas are benign tumors of lymphatic vessels. They may present as cystic masses, often in the neck or axilla, and their management may involve surgical intervention.

2. **Tonsils and peyer's patches:** They are components of mucosa-associated lymphoid tissue (MALT). Their inflammation or hypertrophy may contribute to recurrent infections, and their removal may be considered in certain clinical situations.
3. **Spleen:** The spleen is the largest lymphoid organ, located in the left hypochondrium between the fundus of the stomach and the diaphragm. It comprises of white pulp (lymphocytes and lymphatic vessels) and red pulp (consisting of a network of anastomosing splenic cords). Removal of the spleen (splenectomy) may be necessary in cases of trauma, certain hematological disorders, or splenic tumors. However, it poses risks of immunocompromised states, and alternative treatments are often considered.

RESPIRATORY SYSTEM

The respiratory system is dedicated to the vital process of breathing, encompassing the inhalation and exhalation of air during respiration. The respiratory tract serves as the gateway for oxygen to enter the blood and for carbon dioxide to exit the bloodstream into the atmosphere.

The respiratory cycle involves four interconnected processes:
1. **Ventilation:** Movement of air into and out of the lungs to facilitate the exchange of atmospheric air.
2. **Gaseous exchange:** The interchange of gases between the air in the lungs and the bloodstream.
3. **Transport of gases:** Conveyance of oxygen (O_2) and carbon dioxide (CO_2) in the blood.
4. **Cellular respiration:** Utilization of O_2 by cells for metabolic processes and CO_2 production as a metabolic byproduct.

Components of the Respiratory System

Anatomical Division
1. Upper respiratory tract (URT):
   - Nasal cavities
   - Pharynx and associated structures
2. Lower respiratory tract (LRT):
   - Larynx
   - Trachea
   - Bronchi
   - Lungs

Functional Division
1. Conducting portion
   - Nasal cavities
   - Pharynx
   - Larynx
   - Trachea
   - Bronchi
   - Bronchioles
   - Terminal bronchioles
2. Respiratory portion:
   - Respiratory bronchioles
   - Alveolar ducts
   - Alveolar sacs
   - Alveoli

The function of the conducting portions is an air conduit to provide a pathway for the movement of air to and from the lungs, and the function of the respiratory portion is the gaseous exchange to facilitate the exchange of oxygen and carbon dioxide between the air and the bloodstream.

- **Nasal cavity:** The nasal cavity is situated within the external nose and is divided into right and left nasal cavities by the nasal septum. It features external nostrils and internal choanae as openings. Three conchae, bony shelves, adorn the lateral wall, creating three meatuses. The vestibule, above the nostrils, is covered by skin with vibrissae. The olfactory region, for the sense of smell, is specialized. The respiratory region, the larger part, is lined with pseudostratified ciliated columnar epithelium, aiding in moistening and filtering air. The nose warms, moistens, and filters air, with cilia propelling particles to the nasopharynx.

○ *Pharynx:* A fibromuscular tube extending from the base of the skull to the 6th cervical vertebra, the pharynx facilitates both digestive and respiratory functions. It comprises three parts:

  ○ **Nasopharynx:** Exclusive to respiration, lined by respiratory epithelium, and houses the pharyngeal tonsils.

  ○ **Oropharynx:** Functions in both respiration and digestion, harboring palatine tonsils.

  ○ **Laryngopharynx:** Directs food to the esophagus and air to the larynx.

○ *Larynx ("voice box"):* It serves as the connecting passage between the laryngopharynx and the trachea. The laryngeal lumen's patency is maintained by rigid walls formed by hyaline and elastic cartilages interconnected by membranes. Comprising nine cartilages, three are unpaired—epiglottis, thyroid, and cricoid—while three are paired—arytenoid, corniculate, and cuneiform. In males, thyroid cartilage, the largest among them, prominently shapes the front of the neck, commonly known as the Adam's apple. The cricoid cartilage encircles the laryngeal lumen completely.

Internally, the larynx is lined with mucous membranes and externally covered by voluntary muscles. Two pairs of robust connective tissue bands traverse its lumen anteroposteriorly. The upper bands are termed false vocal cords, while the lower ones are the true vocal cords. The space between the false vocal cords is referred to as the rima vestibuli, and the space between the true vocal cords is known as the rima glottidis—the narrowest segment of the laryngeal cavity.

In the production of sounds, the true vocal cords play a vital role, while the false vocal cords provide support. The entire lining of the laryngeal cavity consists of pseudostratified squamous epithelium, except for the vocal cords, which are lined by stratified squamous epithelium.

○ *Trachea:* The trachea, or windpipe, is a flexible and fibroelastic cartilaginous tube measuring approximately 10 cm (4 inch) in length and 2.5 cm (1 inch) in diameter. Positioned in front of the esophagus, it extends partly within the neck and partly within the thoracic cavity. Roughly 5 cm (2 inch) below the jugular notch, the trachea divides into right and left bronchi. The trachea relies on 16–20 incomplete C-shaped rings composed of hyaline cartilage to maintain an open and patent structure. Bridging the gap between the posterior free ends of these C-shaped cartilages is a band of smooth muscle known as the trachealis, accompanied by a fibroelastic ligament. The trachea's inner lining is formed by pseudostratified ciliated columnar epithelium, housing numerous mucous-secreting goblet cells. The strategic arrangement of cartilages and elastic tissue within the trachea prevents kinking and airway obstruction during movements of the head and neck. Importantly, these cartilages prevent the collapse of the tube when internal pressure is lower than intrathoracic pressure, such as at the conclusion of forced expiration. This structural configuration ensures the unimpeded flow of air through the trachea, facilitating effective respiratory function.

○ *Bronchi, bronchioles, and terminal bronchioles:* Bronchi branch into bronchioles, eventually leading to terminal bronchioles, marking the end of the conducting portion.

○ *Respiratory bronchioles, alveolar ducts, alveolar sacs, and alveoli:* Gaseous exchange begins at respiratory bronchioles, progressing to alveolar ducts, sacs, and alveoli—functional units for gas exchange.

○ *Lungs:* The lungs, vital for oxygenating blood in adults, reside in the pleural cavity, flanking the mediastinum within the thorax. Each lung is divided into lobes, lobules, and bronchopulmonary segments supplied by bronchi. This intricate system functions to humidify, filter, and warm inspired air, enabling optimal respiratory processes. Composed mainly of spongy tissue, they possess an elastic texture akin to a rubber sponge. Within this elastic framework, bronchi, pulmonary arteries, and pulmonary veins form intricate branching networks.

Each lung is anatomically divided into lobes and further into smaller units called bronchopulmonary segments or lobules. This segmentation aids in the organization and functioning of the lungs:

- ○ **Right lung:** Separated by oblique and horizontal fissures, the right lung consists of three lobes—superior, middle, and inferior.
- ○ **Left lung:** A single oblique fissure divides the left lung into two lobes—superior and inferior.

Within each lobe are bronchopulmonary segments, totalling ten in each lung. Lobar bronchi supply the lobes, while tertiary bronchi cater to the bronchopulmonary segments.

The lungs are enveloped by a delicate, inseparable serous membrane known as visceral pleura. Another layer of serous membrane lines the thoracic cavity, diaphragm, and mediastinum, referred to as parietal pleura. These two layers maintain continuity at the root of the lungs, where structures enter and exit the lungs. The space between the visceral and parietal layers of the pleura is identified as the pleural cavity. This potential space is crucial for maintaining the integrity of the lungs, as it ensures a frictionless environment for respiratory movements. Consequently, each lung is encased by its own pleural cavity, contributing to the overall protection and functionality of the respiratory system.

Mechanics of Breathing

- ○ **Pulmonary ventilation:** Pulmonary ventilation refers to the process of breathing, which involves the movement of air in and out of the lungs.
- ○ **Gas exchange and transport:** Gas exchange occurs in the alveoli of the lungs, where oxygen from inhaled air enters the bloodstream and carbon dioxide is removed.

DIGESTIVE SYSTEM

Introduction

The digestive system comprises the digestive tract and associated organs, including teeth, tongue, salivary glands, liver, gallbladder, and pancreas. Collaborating with the circulatory system, it provides the body with water, electrolytes, vitamins, and nutrients. The digestive system functions as a coordinated system, ensuring the effective breakdown and absorption of nutrients for the body's sustenance.

The key functions of the digestive system encompass:

- ○ **Ingestion:** The intake of food through the mouth.
- ○ **Mastication:** Lower jaw movements to pulverize and mix food with saliva during chewing.
- ○ **Deglutition:** Swallowing food, allowing it to pass from the mouth to the stomach.
- ○ **Digestion:** Chemical breakdown of food material.

- ❍ **Absorption:** Absorption of nutrient molecules into the circulatory system through the small intestine's mucous membrane.
- ❍ **Peristalsis:** Rhythmic wave-like contractions in the intestines that move food through the digestive tract.
- ❍ **Defecation:** Elimination of solid/semisolid/liquid waste material (feces) through the anus.

The digestive tract extends from the mouth to the anus, measuring roughly 10 meters in length. Its parts include the mouth, pharynx, esophagus, stomach, small intestine, large intestine, rectum, and anal canal.

- ❍ *The mouth, or oral cavity,* serves as the initial segment of the digestive tract and is surrounded by lips, cheeks, palate, and a muscular floor.

Teeth: Embedded in the sockets of the mandible and maxilla, an adult has 32 teeth, divided into four types:

1. **Incisors (4 pairs):** Chisel-shaped for cutting and shearing.
2. **Canines (2 pairs):** Cone-shaped for holding and tearing.
3. Premolars/bicuspids (4 pairs)
4. **Molars/tricuspids (6 pairs):** Irregularly rounded surfaces for crushing and grinding.

- ❍ *Tongue:* A large muscular organ occupying most of the oral cavity proper, the tongue consists of intrinsic and extrinsic muscles. It plays a crucial role in taste sensation, with taste buds located on its dorsal surface. The tongue aids in manipulating food during mastication, swallowing, and holding food in place.
  - ❍ *Clinical correlation:* The sublingual route of drug administration involves placing certain lipid-soluble drugs under the tongue, allowing rapid absorption into the bloodstream. Nitroglycerin, a vasodilator used in angina pectoris, exemplifies this route.
- ❍ *Lips and cheeks:* Muscular folds and lateral walls, respectively, the lips and cheeks are internally lined by mucosa and externally by skin. The lips guard the oral orifice, and minor salivary glands in the mucus lining maintain moisture.
- ❍ *Salivary glands:* They are the major digestive (accessory) glands that produce saliva, containing enzymes, mucus, and lysozymes. The major salivary glands include the parotid, submandibular, and sublingual glands. In total, approximately 1–1.5 L of saliva is secreted daily.
- ❍ *Pharynx:* The pharynx serves as a funnel-shaped passageway, approximately 5 inches (12.5 cm) long, connecting the oral and nasal cavities to the esophagus and larynx. It receives a bolus of food from the oral cavity and transfers it to the esophagus, with the pharyngo-esophagal junction being the narrowest point of the digestive tract. It is divided into three parts: nasopharynx, oropharynx, and laryngopharynx, based on their locations behind the nasal cavity, oral cavity, and laryngeal cavity, respectively. While the nasopharynx is part of the respiratory system, the oropharynx and laryngopharynx are shared by both the respiratory and digestive systems.
- ❍ *Esophagus:* The esophagus, a collapsible muscular tube approximately 25 cm (10 inch) long, connects the pharynx to the stomach. It facilitates the transport of the bolus of food from the pharynx to the stomach through peristaltic movements. The upper half of the esophagus is composed of voluntary muscle, but it is not under voluntary control, while the lower half consists of involuntary muscle. The lower esophageal sphincter prevents the reflux regurgitation of food from the stomach into the esophagus. Upon the presence of food, the gastroesophageal sphincter relaxes, allowing food to enter the stomach.

The upper esophageal sphincter, formed by the pharynx's cricopharyngeus muscle, prevents air passage into the esophagus during inspiration. The esophageal lumen is lined with protective nonkeratinized stratified squamous epithelium.

○ **Stomach:** The stomach, positioned in the epigastric region below the diaphragm, is a highly distensible component of the gastrointestinal tract. It takes on a 'J-shaped' pouch form and links the esophagus with the duodenum. Gastric juice, secreted by the gastric mucosa, comprises water, mineral salts, mucus, hydrochloric acid, intrinsic factors, and pepsinogens. The stomach stores food, mechanically churning it with gastric secretions, initiating protein digestion, and propelling the partially digested material, known as chyme, into the small intestine.

○ **Small intestine:** Moving on to the small intestine is a hollow muscular tube approximately 6 meters (20 ft) long, connecting the stomach to the large intestine. The small intestine is divided into three segments: duodenum, jejunum, and ileum. The duodenum is a C-shaped tube receiving bile from the liver, gallbladder, and pancreatic secretions through the common bile duct and pancreatic duct. The jejunum and ileum are responsible for absorbing nutrients from digested food.

○ **Large intestine (colon):** The large intestine, measuring 1.5 meters (5 ft) in length, extends from the ileocecal junction to the anal orifice. It consists of the cecum, appendix, ascending colon, transverse colon, descending colon, sigmoid colon, rectum, and anal canal. While the large intestine has no digestive function, it absorbs water and electrolytes from chyme, forming feces. The mucous membrane lacks folds, with no villi present, but it features abundant goblet and absorptive cells. Peyer's patches, aggregations of lymphoid tissue, provide defence against microbes.

○ **Liver:** It is the largest internal organ, weighs about 1,500 g (1.5 kg) in adults and is reddish-brown. It is located in the upper right portion of the abdominal cavity, below the diaphragm. The liver is divided into left and right lobes, along with caudate and quadrate lobes. Hepatic cells arranged in plates form liver lobules, and bile secretion occurs through bile canaliculi, interlobular ducts, interlobar ducts, and hepatic ducts. The liver performs essential functions such as metabolism, detoxification, bile secretion, and heat production.

○ **Gallbladder:** It is a pear-shaped sac attached to the inferior surface of the right liver lobe, stores and concentrates bile received from the liver. The bile, containing bile salts and pigments, aids in fat digestion by emulsification.

○ **Pancreas:** It is a long and lobulated gland, acts as both an exocrine and endocrine organ. Pancreatic acini secrete pancreatic juice for digestion, while pancreatic islets of Langerhans produce insulin and glucagon for endocrine functions. The pancreatic duct joins the common bile duct to form the ampulla of Vater, releasing pancreatic juice into the duodenum.

URINARY SYSTEM

Introduction

The urinary system holds paramount importance as the primary excretory system in the body, playing a crucial role in maintaining water and electrolyte concentrations to uphold overall homeostasis.

Components of Urinary System

○ **Kidney:** The kidney is encapsulated by dense adipose tissue known as perinephric fat, offering mechanical protection. The renal fascia, a thin fascial sheath, surrounds the perinephric fat. The concave medial border of the kidney contains the hilum, through which the renal artery, nerves, renal vein, and ureter enter and exit.

○ **Ureter:** A tube that carries urine from the kidney to the urinary bladder.
○ **Urinary bladder:** Functions as a reservoir for urine storage.
○ **Urethra:** Serves as a common outlet for both urine and reproductive fluids in males.

Kidneys

The macroscopic structure of the kidney, as observed in a naked-eye examination of a coronal section, can be summarized as:

Pyramids and Cortex

○ The inner two-thirds of the kidney's cut surface is occupied by darkly stained pyramidal-shaped areas (8–15 in number).
○ The tips of these pyramids, known as papillae, project into the minor calyces.
○ The outer one-third of the cut surface, lying external to the bases of the pyramids, is termed the cortex. Renal columns, similar to cortical tissue, extend between the pyramids. The renal columns and pyramids together constitute the medulla.

Calyces and Renal Pelvis

○ Minor calyces surround the renal papillae, and these minor calyces from several pyramids join together to form two or three major calyces.
○ The major calyces converge to create a funnel-shaped channel called the renal pelvis.

Ureter

The renal pelvis narrows to form a narrow tube, the ureter, which leaves the kidney and connects it to the urinary bladder.

The microscopic structure of the kidney involves two main components:

1. **Excretory component:** Comprising about one million microscopic units called nephrons.
2. **Collecting component:** Comprising collecting tubules, minor, and major calyces. The collecting component includes collecting tubules, minor and major calyces, and the renal pelvis. The urinary system is a complex network of structures that ensures the filtration, collection, and elimination of waste products from the body.

Nephron

Nephrons are the structural and functional units of the kidney. Each nephron consists of two main parts:

1. **Glomerulus:** A spherical bunch of looped capillaries that invaginate the expanded blind end of the uriniferous tubule, known as the glomerular capsule or Bowman's capsule.
2. **Uriniferous tubule:** Consisting of the proximal convoluted tubule, Henle's loop, distal convoluted tubule, and finally, the junction.

Ureters

Each ureter is a slender, 25 cm (10 inch) long muscular tube connecting the renal pelvis to the urinary bladder. The renal pelvis, a funnel-shaped portion within the kidney, serves as the upper segment of the ureter. Urine is transported from the renal pelvis to the urinary bladder through peristaltic contractions of the smooth muscles in the ureter wall.

Observation through a cystoscope reveals jets of urine squirting into the bladder from ureteral orifices, driven by peristaltic waves initiated by the presence of urine in the renal pelvis. The ureter's lining is composed of transitional epithelium, which decreases in thickness as the urinary bladder expands, forming folds called rugae when empty.

The trigone of the urinary bladder develops from mesoderm, while the remainder of the bladder develops from endoderm. The trigone, a triangular area between two ureteric openings and a single urethral opening, maintains a smooth mucous membrane even when the bladder is empty.

In males, the internal urethral orifice may be obstructed by an enlarged uvula vesicae, a grape-like bulging produced by the median lobe of the prostate gland. This uvula vesicae can lead to obstruction if enlarged due to prostatic hypertrophy.

Urethra

The urethra is a tubular continuation of the urinary bladder's neck, responsible for conveying urine from the bladder to the external environment. It contains two muscular sphincters:

1. **Internal urethral sphincter:** Located at the bladder-urethra junction, formed by the detrusor muscle of the urinary bladder. It is involuntary and more developed in females.
2. **External urethral sphincter:** Formed by the sphincter urethrae muscle of the urogenital diaphragm. Composed of skeletal muscle fibers, it is voluntary in nature.

In females, the urethra is short (about 4 cm or 1.5 inch) and empties into the vestibule of the vagina, exclusively serving the urinary system. The male urethra will be discussed later in this chapter.

Clinical correlation: Cystitis, inflammation of the urinary bladder often caused by infections, is more common in females due to the shorter length of the female urethra, which opens in the vestibule of the vagina, making it more susceptible to bacterial entry from the outside.

ENDOCRINE SYSTEM

Introduction

The endocrine system forms the major control system of the body and plays an important role in maintaining homeostasis. It comprises various glands and organs that produce hormones, which regulate and coordinate numerous processes by acting as chemical messengers, influencing growth, metabolism, reproduction, and other essential functions. Diseases like diabetes mellitus, diabetes insipidus, thyroid disorders, etc., are associated with the dysfunction of the endocrine system.

Endocrine Glands

These are the ductless glands that directly pour their secretions into the bloodstream. Their secretion is called a hormone or chemical messenger that causes stimulation or inhibition of target tissues or organs. The secretions can be in the form of proteins, amino acid derivatives, steroids or peptides.

Some of the important endocrine glands of the body are:

- Pituitary gland (hypophysis cerebri)
- Thyroid gland
- Parathyroid glands
- Adrenal (suprarenal) glands
- Pineal gland
- Thymus gland

Pituitary Gland

The pituitary gland, often referred to as the "master gland," is a small pea-sized gland weighing 0.5 g located at the base of the brain at the pituitary fossa or hypophyseal fossa or sella turcica and is connected to the hypothalamus by a stalk of tissue called as infundibulum. It produces and releases various hormones that regulate other endocrine glands and influence growth, metabolism, and reproduction.

Pituitary gland is divided into two parts:

1. Anterior pituitary (adenohypophysis):
   - It is subdivided into pars anterior, pars intermedia and pars tuberalis.
   - The hormones secreted are growth hormone/GH (somatotrophs), adrenocorticotrophic hormone/

ACTH (corticotrophs), prolactin (mammotrophs), thyroid-stimulating hormone/TSH (thyrotrophs), follicle-stimulating hormone/FSH, luteinizing hormone/LH (gonadotrophs).
2. Posterior pituitary (neurohypophysis):
   ○ Oxytocin and antidiuretic hormones (ADH) or vasopressin are secreted by the posterior pituitary.
   ○ Oxytocin stimulates uterine contraction during pregnancy and childbirth and stimulates milk ejection by contractile action of myoepithelial cells of alveoli and mammary glands.
   ○ ADH promotes the reabsorption of water in tubules of the kidney to conserve the water in the body.

Thyroid Gland

The thyroid gland is the largest gland, weighing about 20 g and is located in the front of the neck and produces hormones that regulate metabolism, growth, and development. It has two lobes (right and left) that are connected by the isthmus. Blood supply is by the superior thyroid artery (a branch of the external carotid artery) and the inferior thyroid artery (a branch of the subclavian artery).

Some of the important features of the thyroid gland are:
○ The unit structure of the thyroid gland is called a follicle, comprising of the cuboidal epithelial cells with a cavity filled with colloid.
○ T3 (triiodothyronine or thyroxine) and T4 (tetraiodothyronine or thyroxine) are secreted by cuboidal cells of thyroid follicles.
○ Dietary iodine is essential for the synthesis of T3 and T4.
○ T3 and T4 are important for normal growth and maintaining the body's basal metabolic rate (BMR).
○ In between the follicles are the para-follicular cells that secrete calcitonin.

○ Calcitonin is important for maintaining the normal calcium homeostasis.

Parathyroid Glands

The parathyroid glands are small and oval, 4 in number, measuring roughly about $2 \times 3 \times 5$ mm, located on the back of the thyroid gland. It is supplied by the inferior thyroid artery. The hormone secreted by the parathyroid gland is parathyroid hormone (PTH), which functions to:
○ Regulate calcium and phosphorus levels in the body.
○ Inhibit osteoblastic activity and promote osteoclastic activity of the bone.
○ Convert vitamin D to 1,25-dihydroxychole-calciferol in the kidney (active form).
○ Increase the absorption of calcium in the kidney.

Adrenal Glands (Suprarenal Glands)

The adrenal glands are two in number (right and left), located retroperitoneal and situated on the upper pole of the kidneys. Structurally, it is divided into two main regions: the outer region, called the adrenal cortex (derived from mesoderm), and the inner region, the adrenal medulla (derived from neural crest). Some of the important features are as under:
○ The adrenal cortex forms the larger portion of the gland.
○ The adrenal cortex is subdivided into three zones—zona glomerulosa (outer zone), zona fasciculata (middle zone) and zona reticulata (inner zone).
○ The adrenal cortex produces hormones such as cortisol (zona fasciculata), aldosterone (from zona glomerulosa), and sex hormones (zona reticulata).
○ The adrenal medulla forms the inner soft part that contains chromaffin cells (so-called because the secretory granules present within the cytoplasm when treated with potassium dichromate solution turn brown).

○ Epinephrine and norepinephrine are secreted by the chromaffin cells of the adrenal medulla, which are released in fight or flight response.

Pineal Gland (Epiphysis Cerebri)

It is a photosensitive neuroendocrine gland about 10 mm in length, located below the splenium of the corpus callosum and is attached to the roof of the third ventricle by a stalk. It consists of epithelioid cells called pinealocytes, neuroglial cells and calcareous granules called brain sand. Melatonin and serotonin are secreted by the pineal gland. It is supplied by the posterior choroidal artery (a branch of a posterior cerebral artery).

Thymus Gland

It is a bilobed gland that weighs about 12–15 g at birth, 30–40 g at puberty and 10–15 g at 60 years, located in the superior mediastinum of thoracic cavity behind the sternum and extends upwards to the root of neck. Thymic epithelial cells, lymphocytes and macrophages constitute the cells of thymus. Epithelial cells are derived from the endoderm of the third pharyngeal pouch, and lymphocytes and macrophages are derived from the mesoderm. It is divided into an outer dark-staining zone called the cortex, and an inner light-stained zone called the medulla. The cortex contains lymphoblasts (immature lymphocytes) that undergo mitosis to produce small T lymphocyte clones in the deep portion of the cortex. The medulla contains thymic epithelial cells and a few lymphocytes along with Hassall's corpuscles. Hormone thymosin is produced by thymus that support the activity of T lymphocytes throughout the body.

Pancreas, Gonads, and Other Endocrine Organs

Pancreas

The pancreas is an organ with both exocrine and endocrine functions. The exocrine part is called pancreatic acini, which secrete digestive enzymes to help in digestion. The endocrine part of the pancreas, known as the islets of Langerhans, produces hormones such as insulin and glucagon, which regulate blood sugar levels. Islet cells are alpha (A) cells, beta (B) cells, delta cells, C cells. Alpha cells produce glucagon that increases the blood glucose level by promoting gluconeogenesis in the liver, and thus, it functions opposite to insulin. B cells produce insulin that decreases the blood glucose level to help in carbohydrate metabolism.

Gonads

The gonads, including the ovaries in females and testes in males, produce hormones such as estrogen, progesterone, and testosterone, which regulate sexual development and reproductive functions.

Testes are two small ovoid organs measuring approximately 5 × 2.5 cm situated within the scrotum. The exocrine function of the testes is to produce spermatozoa, and the endocrine function is to produce testosterone (steroid hormone).

Ovaries are small almond-shaped gonads located in the ovarian fossa of the lateral pelvic wall, one on each side attached to the broad ligament of the uterus by a peritoneal fold called mesovarium. The endocrine function of the ovary is to secrete steroid hormone (estrogen).

Diffuse Neuroendocrine Cells

The scattered neuroendocrine cells of the body are renin-producing juxtaglomerular cells of kidney and gut-associated endocrine (enteroendocrine) cells present in the epithelial layers of the stomach and small intestine. Enteroendocrine cells produce gastrin that act on the fundic glands of stomach to secrete hydrochloric acid and also act on the cells of duodenum to produce secretin (stimulate the secretion of pancreatic juices), cholecystokinin to stimulate the secretion of bile), pancreozymin (stimulate the secretion of pancreatic enzyme) and enterogastrone (reduce the acid secretion of stomach by inhibiting the peristaltic movement).

Other Endocrine Organs

Various other organs and tissues in the body, such as the pineal gland, thymus, and adipose tissue, also have endocrine functions and produce hormones that influence specific physiological processes.

REPRODUCTIVE SYSTEM

Introduction

The reproductive system is responsible for the production of gametes (sperm and ova), sexual differentiation, and the facilitation of reproduction. It consists of various organs and structures that work together to ensure the continuation of the species.

Male Reproductive System

The male reproductive system is comprised of the following organs:
- Testes
- Epididymis
- Ductus deferens
- Seminal vesicles (accessory glands)
- Ejaculatory ducts
- Prostate gland (accessory gland)
- Bulbourethral glands (accessory glands)

Penis, urethra and scrotum are the male external genitalia.

Testes

The testes are the primary male reproductive organs responsible for the production of sperm and testosterone. They are located one on each side within the scrotum. Each testis is ovoid, 4–5 × 2.5 cm in dimensions, comprising of 200–300 lobules and each lobule contains 1–4 seminiferous tubules. Seminiferous tubules contain germ cells and Sertoli cells. Germ cells produce spermatozoa, whereas Sertoli cells provide nourishment and mechanical support to the spermatozoa. Leydig's interstitial cells are present between the tubules that secrete testosterone at and after puberty. Seminiferous tubules open in the efferent ductules that open into the duct of epididymis.

Epididymis

The epididymis is a 6 cm long structure that is folded to form a comma-shaped body. It helps in the transportation and storage of sperm. The spermatozoa during the storage period become mature and motile.

Ductus Deferens

It is a 45 cm long fibromuscular tube that emerges from the tail of the epididymis. The muscular contractions of the wall of the duct help in the transportation of sperm from the epididymis to the ejaculatory duct.

Seminal Vesicles and Ejaculatory Duct

Seminal vesicles are 5 cm long, sac-shaped tubular structures originating from the last part of the ductus deferens. It joins with the ductus deferens to form the ejaculatory duct and form the common passage for urinary and genital systems.

Ejaculatory duct is 2.5 cm in length that opens into the urethra.

Prostate Gland and Bulbourethral Glands

The prostate is the largest accessory gland that weighs about 20 g in an adult male and is located below the neck of the urinary bladder and opens in the prostatic part of the urethra. It is partly glandular, partly muscular and partly fibrous. Mucosal, submucosal and prostatic glands are present in the glandular tissue. The secretions of the prostate contain citric acid, acid phosphatase, amylase, and prostatic-specific antigen (PSA).

Bulbourethral glands are two in number of pea size, located one on each side of membranous urethra. Their secretions are mucus-like that help in the lubrication of the penile urethra before ejaculation.

Penis

The word penis is derived from the Latin word that means a tail. It is involved in the transportation of the sperm to the female genital tract during copulation. The thick fibrous connective tissue that forms its lining is called tunica albuginea.

Urethra

The male urethra is about 20 cm long and provides the passage for urine and semen. It is divided into three parts: prostatic part (3 cm long), membranous part (2 cm long) and penile/spongy part (15 cm long).

Scrotum

It is divided into two internal compartments by a connective tissue septum and each compartment contains the testis and spermatic cord.

Female Reproductive System

The organs of the female reproductive system are:

- Ovaries
- Fallopian tubes/uterine tubes
- Uterus
- Vagina

The organs of the external genitalia include:

- Clitoris
- Labia majora
- Labia minora
- Greater vestibular (bartholin) glands
- Mons pubis
- Vaginal orifice

Ovaries

Ovaries are almond-shaped structures attached to the broad ligament's posterior surface with the help of a peritoneal fold called mesovarium. They are the primary female reproductive organs responsible for the production of ova (eggs) and female sex hormones, including estrogen and progesterone. Graafian follicles, also called ovarian follicles, are rounded structures that contain ova in the cortex. The inner zone of follicle is called theca interna and the outer zone is called theca externa. The cells of theca interna secrete estrogen to stimulate the proliferation of endometrium. Each ovary contains about 2 million immature ova at the time of birth and in the reproductive age group (15–45 years), one ovum is shed by the ovary each month into the peritoneal cavity.

Fallopian Tubes/Uterine Tubes/Oviduct

The fallopian tubes are about 10 cm long, two in number, one on each side of the uterus and uterus are structures involved in the transport of ova, fertilization, and the development of the fetus. They play important roles in reproduction and pregnancy.

It is divided into four parts: Intramural, isthmus, ampulla and infundibulum.

- **Intramural (interstitial) part:** Located within the myometrium of the uterus.
- **Isthmus:** Lateral continuation of the intramural part form the isthmus.
- **Ampulla:** It is the longest part of the tube with a thin wall and a wide lumen, where fertilization occurs.
- **Infundibulum:** Funnel-shaped distal end of the tube that contains finger-like projections called as fimbriae.

Uterus

It is a hollow, thick-walled muscular structure, present in the pelvic region between the urinary bladder and rectum. The rounder upper portion is called the fundus, and the inferior narrow portion is called the cervix. The body of the uterus is present between the fundus and cervix. The ovum after fertilization in the oviduct is transported to the uterine cavity for implantation and development into a fetus.

Vagina

It is a thin-walled, 7.5–10 cm long fibromuscular structure that forms the organ of copulation. The secretions and moist stratified squamous lining of the vagina provide protection and lubrication during copulation. The smooth muscle present in the lining of the vaginal wall help in stretching the vagina to allow the passage of baby during the childbirth.

External Genitalia

External genitalia, including the labia, clitoris, and Bartholin's glands, are structures involved in sexual intercourse, childbirth, and protection of the reproductive organs.

INTEGUMENTARY SYSTEM

Introduction

The integumentary system is the largest organ system in the body and serves as a protective barrier against external threats, regulates body temperature, and provides sensory information. It includes the skin, hair, nails, and associated glands discussed in brief as under.

Skin

Layers of the Skin

Skin is regarded as an important organ of the body and is composed of three main layers: the epidermis, dermis, and subcutaneous tissue (hypodermis). Each layer has distinct characteristics and functions.

○ **Epidermis:** The epidermis is derived from the ectoderm. It is a superficial and avascular layer of stratified squamous epithelium. It gives rise to skin appendages like nails, hair, sebaceous or sweat glands. It is comprised of a superficial cornified zone and a deep *germinative zone.* As the cells proliferate, they migrate from the deep layer to the superficial layer to replace the cells of the cornified layer that are lost due to wear and tear.

Layers of epidermis, from deep to superficial, are as under:

  ○ **Stratum basale/stratum germinatum:** Comprised of a single layer of cuboidal or columnar cells. It also contains melanocytes that synthesise and produce melanin.
  ○ **Stratum spinosum/prickle cell layer/ spiny layer:** It is the thickest of all the layers and is comprised of several layers of polygonal cells held together by cell junctions called desmosomes.
  ○ **Stratum granulosum/granular layer:** This is so-called because of the presence of keratohyalin granules in the cells. This layer is comprised of the flattened cells arranged in 3–4 layers.
  ○ **Stratum lucidum/clear layer:** It is a thin, clear, glossy, transparent layer found only in thick, glabrous skin such as the soles of feet and palms of hands.
  ○ **Stratum corneum:** It is the most superficial layer of the skin whose cells contain protein keratin.

○ The dermis, also known as corneum, derived from mesoderm, is the deep and vascular layer of the skin. It is divided into a superficial *papillary layer* and a deep *reticular layer*, both comprising of connective tissue admixed with lymphatics, blood vessels, nerves and elastic fibers.

Appendages of the Skin

The skin contains various appendages, including hair follicles, sebaceous glands, sweat glands, and nails. These appendages play important roles in protection, temperature regulation, and sensory perception.

Hair and Nails

Hair Structure and Growth

Hair is a thin, elongated keratinized structure of cells that is present all over the body surface except on palms, soles, lips, glans penis, clitoris and labia minora. It grows from hair follicles in the skin.

Hair is divided into three parts:
1. **Shaft:** The dead portion of the hair projects over the skin surface.
2. **Root:** Embedded within the skin surrounded by the hair follicle.
3. **Bulb:** Enlarged base of the root within the hair follicle. It is invaginated by highly vascular connective tissue that provides nutrition to the developing hair.

Nail Structure and Growth

Nails, also known as onych or onycho or ungues, are composed of keratinized cells and grow from the nail matrix located at the base of the nail. It is comprised of the following parts:
- **Root:** The proximal part that is hidden and buried into the mail groove.
- **Body:** It is the exposed part adherent to the underlying skin. The white opaque crescent present on the proximal part of the body is called the lunula.
- **Free border:** The distal part that is free from the skin.
- Hidden border.

The growth of the nails is by the proliferation of the germinal matrix and the transformation of the superficial cells of the matrix into the nail cells. The rate of growth of fingernails is about 1 mm per week.

Glands of the Skin

Sebaceous Glands

Sebaceous glands develop from the follicular epithelium of the hair. They produce sebum, an oily substance that helps moisturize, protect, lubricate and waterproof the skin's surface and prevents the hair from being brittle. They are distributed all over the body except palm and soles.

Sweat Glands

Also called sudoriferous glands. Each sweat gland has a secretory portion, present in the form of a twisted coil in the deep dermis and an excretory duct, a long portion that extends from the secretory position to the skin surface. Sweat glands produce sweat, which helps regulate body temperature and excrete waste products. There are two types of sweat glands: eccrine glands and apocrine glands.

The eccrine glands, by causing evaporation of sweat and excretion of body salts, help to regulate body temperature. They are stimulated by cholinergic fibers of sympathetic nerves. Eccrine glands are distributed throughout the body except for lip margins, eardrums, nail beds, an inner surface of the prepuce and glans penis.

The apocrine sweat glands are much larger and are stimulated by adrenergic fibers of sympathetic nerves. They are found in the axilla, pubic regions, areolae of breasts, labia minora and perianal region.

Functions of the Integumentary System

Protection and Sensation

The integumentary system serves as a protective barrier against physical, chemical, and microbial threats. It also contains sensory receptors that provide information about touch, temperature, and pain.

Temperature Regulation

The integumentary system helps regulate body temperature through sweat production and blood vessel dilation or constriction. The optimal body temperature is maintained by combined effect of sweating and shivering.

Synthesis

It also plays a role in vitamin D synthesis when exposed to sunlight. In addition to vitamin D, keratin and melanin are also synthesized in the skin.

Maintenance of Homeostasis

In addition to protecting the body from pathogens and external injury, it also plays a major role in maintaining body homeostasis.

Excretion

It plays an important role in removing excess water, salts and waste products such as ammonia and urea through excretion in the form of sweating.

MULTIPLE CHOICE QUESTIONS

1. **Which of the following is NOT a axial skeleton bone?**
   a. Ulna
   b. Ethmoid
   c. Sphenoid
   d. Sacrum

2. **Identify the bone structure in which osteocytes are present structures?**
   a. Osteons
   b. Canaliculi
   c. Lacunae
   d. Lamellae

3. **The process of the formation of blood cells by the bone is known as?**
   a. Hemolysis
   b. Hemostasis
   c. Hematuria
   d. Hemopoiesis

4. **Which of the following is NOT an example of "long" bone?**
   a. Humerus
   b. Tibia
   c. Carpal
   d. Metacarpal

5. **Bone which develops in the muscle's tendon is known as?**
   a. Sphenoid
   b. Hyoid
   c. Ethmoid
   d. Sesamoid

6. **Which of the following term refers to a depression in a bone?**
   a. Tuberosity
   b. Fossa
   c. Tubercle
   d. Condyle

7. **Synovial joint in the body is also known as?**
   a. Synarthrosis
   b. Immovable joint
   c. Slightly moveable joint
   d. Freely moveable joint

8. **The epiphyseal plate of a long bone is located at?**
   a. In the diaphysis
   b. Between the diaphysis and the epiphysis
   c. In the epiphysis
   d. In the medullary canal

9. **Which of the listed bones is superior to the rest of the bones?**
   a. Manubrium
   b. Xiphoid process
   c. Coccyx
   d. Femur

10. **Which of the following bone markings is NOT a projection?**
    a. Fossa
    b. Tuberosity
    c. Tubercle
    d. Trochanter

11. **Which of the following bones is part of the cranium?**
    a. Occipital
    b. Mandible
    c. Hyoid
    d. Cervical vertebrae

12. **Which of the following is not part of the appendicular skeleton?**
    a. The pectoral girdle
    b. The thoracic cage
    c. The phalanges
    d. The lower limbs

13. **Cells found in the lacunae of compact bone known as?**
    a. Osteocytes
    b. Osteons
    c. Osteoblasts
    d. Osteoclasts

Answers:

1. a	2. c	3. d	4. c
5. d	6. b	7. d	8. b
9. a	10. a	11. a	12. b
13. a			

14. What does the term "haversian canal" refer?
- a. The larger examples of foramina or canal
- b. A groove that receives a muscle's tendon
- c. The center of an osteon that contains blood capillaries
- d. The space within a long bone that contains marrow

15. Which structure attaches one bone to another bone?
- a. Ligament
- b. Cartilage
- c. Tendon
- d. Diaphysis

16. What is the role of hyaline cartilage in the body?
- a. It attaches muscle to bone
- b. It helps joints by tying one bone to another
- c. It covers articulating bone surfaces
- d. It produces synovial fluid

17. Bone forming cells are known as?
- a. Osteons
- b. Osteocytes
- c. Osteoclasts
- d. Osteoblasts

18. Which of the following parts of a long bone, are involved in an articulation?
- a. Epiphysis
- b. Metaphysic
- c. Diaphysis
- d. Symphysis

19. What is the metaphysis?
- a. The shaft of a long bone
- b. The region that separates the narrow shaft of a long bone from its end
- c. The end of a long bone
- d. The canal inside a long bone that contains marrow

20. Term is applied to moving the thigh laterally away from the midline of the body?
- a. Extension
- b. Adduction
- c. Abduction
- d. Flexion

21. The plasma membrane of a muscle cell is known as?
- a. Sarcoplasm
- b. Sarcomere
- c. Sarcoplasmic reticulum
- d. Sarcolemma

22. Which of the following character of the smooth muscle is different from cardiac muscle?
- a. Is found in the walls of arteries
- b. Cannot be voluntarily contracted
- c. Has many nuclei in a cell
- d. Has intercalated discs between cells

23. Which of the following muscles is named according to its origin and insertion?
- a. Pectoralis major
- b. Semimembranosus
- c. Sternocleidomastoid
- d. Deltoid

24. Which of the following is the smallest structure within a muscle fiber?
- a. Myosin
- b. Myofilament
- c. Myofibril
- d. Sarcomere

25. A single unit of a myofibril that contracts is known as?
- a. Sarcoplasm
- b. Sarcomere
- c. Sarcolemma
- d. Sarcoplasmic reticulum

Answers:

14. c	**15.** a	**16.** c	**17.** d
18. a	**19.** b	**20.** c	**21.** d
22. d	**23.** c	**24.** b	**25.** b

26. **What characteristic of a smooth muscle cell distinguishes it from cardiac and from skeletal muscle?**
    a. Being branched
    b. Being under involuntary control
    c. Lack of striations
    d. Being uninucleate

27. **Which of the following muscles is a common site for intramuscular injection?**
    a. Deltoid
    b. Gluteus maximus
    c. Vastus medialis
    d. Latissimus dorsi

28. **Which one of the following is NOT a characteristic of skeletal muscle?**
    a. Excitability
    b. Autonomic innervations
    c. Contractility
    d. Extensibility

29. **Which of the following feature is shared by cardiac muscle and skeletal muscles cells?**
    a. Striations
    b. Intercalated discs
    c. Branching
    d. Involuntary nature

30. **Cytoplasm of a skeletal muscle cell called as?**
    a. Sarcolemma
    b. Sarcomere
    c. Sarcoplasm
    d. Fasciculus

31. **The space between the ribs is filled with which muscles:**
    a. Intercostal muscle
    b. Costal cartilage muscles
    c. Intercostal space
    d. Pleura

32. **Units joined end to end within a myofibril called as?**
    a. Myofilament
    b. Motor unit
    c. Myosin
    d. Sarcomere

33. **The part of a skeletal muscle cell that is able to contract is known as:**
    a. Sarcoplasm
    b. Sarcolemma
    c. Sarcomere
    d. Sarcoplasmic reticulum

34. **Term used to describe the muscle wasting in a part of the body?**
    a. Disuse atrophy
    b. Denervation atrophy
    c. Muscle dystrophy
    d. Muscle hypertrophy

35. **Which type of cell produces hydrochloric acid in the stomach?**
    a. Zymogenic cells
    b. Parietal cells
    c. Chief cells
    d. Enteroendocrine cells

36. **Which of the following glands are accessory organs of the digestive system?**
    a. Adrenal glands
    b. Pancreatic islets
    c. Gastric glands
    D. Salivary glands

37. **What is the role of gastrin in the digestive system?**
    a. To stimulate release of bile and pancreatic juice
    b. To stimulate gastric secretion
    c. To activate pepsinogen
    d. To hydrolyse proteins to polypeptides

Answers: 26. b   27. a   28. b   29. a
          30. c   31. a   32. d   33. a
          34. a   35. b   36. d   37. b

38. Bile is produced by the cells of the liver?
a. Kupffer cells
b. Sinusoids
c. Hepatocytes
d. The acini

39. What are the end products of carbohydrate metabolism?
a. Chylomicrons
b. Amino acids
c. Free fatty acids
d. Monosaccharides

40. What feature of the small intestine enhances its ability to absorb digested food?
a. Its large surface area
b. The gaps between adjacent epithelial cells
c. Secretion of the hormone absorptin
d. Its longer length compared to the large intestine

41. Which statement about the layers of the alimentary canal is correct?
a. The serosa absorbs the products of digestion
b. The mucosa protects against self-digestion
c. The submucosa is involved in segmentation and peristalsis
d. The muscularis externa is dense connective tissue

42. Which of the following pairs of substances are NOT secreted by the stomach as part of "gastric juice"?
a. Hydrochloric acid and pepsinogen
b. Hormones and intrinsic factor
c. Nuclease and amylase
d. Mucus and gastrin

43. What are some products of lipid metabolism?
a. Free bases and pentose sugars
b. Fructose and glucose
c. Amino acids and small peptides
d. Free fatty acids and monoglycerols

44. Absorption of the digested food occurs in?
a. Duodenum   b. Stomach
c. Ileum   d. Ascending colon

45. Which of the following is an active enzyme?
a. Procarboxypeptidase
b. Pepsin
c. Telophase
d. Trypsinogen

46. Which of the following is a function of the liver?
a. Recycling of non-viable red blood cells
b. Conversion of pyruvic acid to lactic acid
c. Synthesis of plasma proteins
d. Production of rennin

47. What is the term applied to glucose production from non-carbohydrate molecules?
a. Deamination
b. Transamination
c. Glycogenolysis
d. Gluconeogenesis

48. Which of the following terms is used to describe the changing of large food molecules into smaller molecules?
a. Mechanical digestion
b. Deglutition
c. Segmentation
d. Hydrolysis

Answers: 38. c   39. d   40. a   41. b
                       42. c   43. d   44. c   45. b
                       46. c   47. d   48. d

49. **Role of "intrinsic factor" in gastric juice?**
    a. To activate pepsinogen
    b. To assist with the absorption of vitamin B12
    c. To protect the stomach lining against hydrochloric acid
    d. It stimulates the release of gastrin

50. **Which of the following feature does NOT contribute to increasing the surface area of the small intestine?**
    a. The brush border
    b. Plicae circulars
    c. Intestinal crypts
    d. Villi

51. **Which of the following is TRUE for bile juice?**
    a. It converts inactive pancreatic enzymes to active form
    b. Needed in the small intestine for the digestion of fats
    c. Synthesized by the gallbladder
    d. Needed in the small intestine for the emulsification of fats

52. **Which layer of the gastrointestinal tract is in contact with the contents of the gut?**
    a. Muscularis externa
    b. Mucosa
    c. Serosa
    d. Submucosa

53. **What is the name for moving the gut contents along the tract in the right direction?**
    a. Peristalsis
    b. Emesis
    c. Segmentation
    d. Deglutition

54. **Which hormone stimulates the release of bile and pancreatic juice?**
    a. Cholecystokinin
    b. Secretin
    c. Intestinal gastrin
    d. Pepsin

55. **What molecules are the products of protein hydrolysis?**
    a. Monoglycerols and free fatty acids
    b. Monosaccharides and disaccharides
    c. Amino acids
    d. Amino acids and small peptides

56. **One of these processes is NOT part of carbohydrate metabolism in the liver?**
    a. Production of ATP from glucose
    b. Production of glucose from glycogen
    c. Production of glucose from amino acids
    d. Production of glycogen from glucose

57. **The liver contains "leaky capillaries" known as sinusoids. This enables what liver product to enter the blood stream?**
    a. Angiotensinogen
    b. Kupffer cells
    c. Plasma proteins
    d. Cholesterol

58. **What is the function of bile salts?**
    a. To assist the absorption of digested lipids
    b. To emulsify lipids
    c. To hydrolyze lipids
    d. To digest lipids

Answers: 49. b 50. c 51. d 52. b
53. a 54. a 55. d 56. a
57. c 58. b

59. Which enzyme below digests proteins?
a. Nuclease
b. Maltase
c. Carboxypeptidase
d. Transaminase

60. Term "gluconeogenesis" refer to?
a. The conversion of non-carbohydrate molecules to glucose
b. The formation of non-essential amino acids from a keto-acid
c. The removal of an amine group from a molecule
d. The release of glucose from stored glycogen

61. What is the purpose of "intrinsic factor" in gastric juice?
a. To activate pepsinogen
b. To assist with the absorption of vitamin B12
c. To protect the stomach lining against hydrochloric acid
d. It stimulates the release of gastrin

62. What is the function of the esophagus in digestion?
a. It is a site of mechanical digestion
b. It transfers food from the mouth to the stomach
c. The esophagus secretes amylase to begin carbohydrate digestion
d. The esophagus secretes hydrochloric acid

63. What is the function of bile juice in the body?
a. Bile hydrolyzes polypeptides
b. Bile emulsifies fats and oils
c. Bile activates procarboxypeptidase
d. Bile stimulates the pancreas to secrete pancreatic juice

64. If blood glucose is high, what does the liver do about it?
a. The liver converts glucose to glycogen or triglycerides
b. The liver performs glycogenolysis
c. The liver performs gluconeogenesis
d. The liver transaminates glucose to produce amino acids

65. Which is an enzyme secreted by the gastric glands?
a. Pepsin
b. Gastrin
c. Cholecystokinin
d. Intrinsic factor

66. Which three sections does the small intestine consists of?
a. Ileum, duodenum, cecum
b. Antrum, jejunum, duodenum
c. Rectum, ileum, duodenum
d. Ileum, duodenum, jejunum

67. What name is given to the movement of food material through the gastrointestinal tract?
a. Peristalsis
b. Segmentation
c. Deglutition
d. Bowel movement

68. Emulsification is the name of the process carried out by:
a. Lipase
b. Bile
c. Micelles
d. Lacteals

69. Protein is digested to polypeptides by which of the following?
a. Pepsinogen
b. Intrinsic factor
c. Hydrochloric acid
d. Pepsin

Answers:

59. c	60. a	61. b	62. b
63. b	64. a	65. a	66. d
67. a	68. b	69. d	

70. **One of the following is NOT a function of the liver?**
    a. Recycling of red blood cells
    b. Storage of fat-soluble vitamins
    c. Removal and recycling of lactic acid
    d. Activation of vitamin D

71. **Which of the following is NOT a part of the gastrointestinal tract?**
    a. Ileum
    b. Pancreas
    c. Rectum
    d. Cecum

72. **What is the function of gastrin?**
    a. To facilitate the absorption of vitamin B12 from the gut
    b. To inhibit gastric secretion
    c. To stimulate gastric secretion
    d. To stimulate pancreatic secretion

73. **What are the cells in the pancreas that secrete "pancreatic juice" or enzymes?**
    a. Hepatocytes
    b. Peyer's patches
    c. The acini
    d. Islets of Langerhans

74. **The lowest pH is found in which of the listed body sites?**
    a. Pancreas
    b. Stomach
    c. Duodenum
    d. Blood

75. **The surface area available for absorption in the small intestine is increased by all of the following structures, *except*:**
    a. Villi
    b. Haustra
    c. Plicae circularis
    d. Microvilli

76. **Kupffer cells are macrophages. Where are they found?**
    a. In the lymphatics of the submucosa and devour bacteria that escape the gut
    b. In the lumen of the large intestine and feed on our normal flora to produce vitamin K
    c. They are in the stomach wall as part of the mucosal barrier
    d. They occur in liver sinusoids and engulf bacteria in blood coming from the gut

77. **One of the following is NOT a function of the large intestine?**
    a. Absorption of electrolytes
    b. Synthesis of some vitamins
    c. Absorption of water
    d. Digestion of fats

78. **Which of the following structures produce bile?**
    a. The gallbladder
    b. The liver
    c. The pancreas
    d. The duodenum

79. **What role do the Kupffer cells of the liver perform?**
    a. They are sinusoids
    b. They are hepatocytes
    c. They are macrophages
    d. They deaminate amino acids

80. **Fatty acids are transported around the body by the blood in structures known as:**
    a. Micelles
    b. Chylomicrons
    c. Triglycerols
    d. Low density lipoproteins

Answers: 70. **a** 71. **b** 72. **c** 73. **c**
74. **b** 75. **b** 76. **d** 77. **d**
78. **b** 79. **c** 80. **b**

81. **Which digestive enzyme in saliva breaks down starch?**
   a. Trypsin
   b. Lipase
   c. Pepsin
   d. Amylase

82. **Which of the following is a function of the normal flora of the large intestine?**
   a. To hydrolyse cellulose
   b. To synthesise blood clotting proteins
   c. To synthesise B vitamins and vitamin K
   d. To secrete intrinsic factor

83. **Why is insulin not given as an oral drug?**
   a. It is too irritating to the gastrointestinal mucosa
   b. It is altered by passing through the liver
   c. It is too big a molecule to be absorbed through the plasma membrane
   d. It would be digested by enzymes in the stomach

84. **Which of the following terms describes the body's ability to maintain its normal state?**
   a. Anabolism
   b. Catabolism
   c. Tolerance
   d. Homeostasis

85. **Which of the following best describes the human body's defense mechanism against environmental bacteria?**
   a. Hair in the nose
   b. Mucous membranes
   c. Osteoblasts
   d. Saliva

86. **Which cells in the blood cells do not have a nucleus?**
   a. Lymphocyte
   b. Monocyte
   c. Erythrocyte
   d. Basophil

87. **Which of the following is flexible connective tissue that is attached to bones at the joints?**
   a. Adipose
   b. Cartilage
   c. Epithelial
   d. Muscle

88. **Which of the following closes and seals off the lower airway during swallowing?**
   a. Alveoli
   b. Epiglottis
   c. Larynx
   d. Uvula

89. **Which of the following is located beneath the diaphragm in the left upper quadrant of the abdominal cavity?**
   a. Appendix
   b. Duodenum
   c. Gallbladder
   d. Spleen

90. **Which of the following cavities are separated by the diaphragm?**
   a. Abdominal and pelvic
   b. Cranial and spinal
   c. Dorsal and ventral
   d. Thoracic and abdominal

91. **Which of the following is a structural, fibrous protein found in the dermis?**
   a. Collagen
   b. Heparin
   c. Lipocyte
   d. Melanin

92. **Which of the following is the large bone found superior to the patella and inferior to the ischium?**
   a. Calcaneus
   b. Femur
   c. Symphysis pubis
   d. Tibia

Answers:
81. d   82. c   83. d   84. d
85. b   86. c   87. b   88. b
89. d   90. d   91. a   92. b

93. **Which of the following controls body temperature, sleep, and appetite?**
    a. Adrenal glands
    b. Hypothalamus
    c. Pancreas
    d. Thalamus

94. **Which of the following cranial nerves is related to the sense of smell?**
    a. Abducens
    b. Hypoglossal
    c. Olfactory
    d. Trochlear

95. **Which of the following is a substance that aids the transmission of nerve impulses to the muscles?**
    a. Acetylcholine
    b. Cholecystokinin
    c. Deoxyribose
    d. Oxytocin

96. **Blood flows from the right ventricle of the heart into which of the following structures?**
    a. Inferior vena cava
    b. Left ventricle
    c. Pulmonary arteries
    d. Pulmonary veins

97. **Blood flows from the right ventricle of the heart into which of the following structures?**
    a. Inferior vena cava
    b. Left ventricle
    c. Pulmonary arteries
    d. Pulmonary veins

98. **At which of the following locations does bile enter the digestive tract?**
    a. Gastroesophageal sphincter
    b. Duodenum
    c. Ileocecum
    d. Jejunum

99. **Which of the following is an accessory organ of the gastrointestinal system that is responsible for secreting insulin?**
    a. Adrenal gland
    b. Gallbladder
    c. Liver
    d. Pancreas

100. **Which of the following is the lymphoid organ that is a reservoir for red blood cells and filters organisms from the blood?**
    a. Appendix
    b. Gallbladder
    c. Pancreas
    d. Spleen

101. **Saliva contains an enzyme that acts upon which of the following nutrients?**
    a. Starches
    b. Proteins
    c. Fats
    d. Minerals

102. **Which of the following describes the cluster of blood capillaries found in each nephron in the kidney?**
    a. Afferent arteriole
    b. Glomerulus
    c. Loop of Henle
    d. Renal pelvis

103. **Fertilization of an ovum by a spermatozoon occurs in which of the following structures?**
    a. Cervix
    b. Fallopian tube
    c. Ovary
    d. Uterus

104. **The innermost layer of epidermis is called as:**
    a. Cornium
    b. Lucidum
    c. Granulosum
    d. Germinative

105. **The pigment which is responsible for color of the skin is:**
    a. Melanin
    b. Carotene
    c. Red pigment
    d. All of the above

Answers:	93. b	94. c	95. a	96. c
	97. d	98. b	99. d	100. d
	101. a	102. b	103. b	104. d
	105. a			

106. Most part of heat loss from the body occurs through the:
   a. Lungs
   b. Kidney
   c. Skin
   d. Brain

107. Epidermis is thickest on the:
   a. Elbow
   b. Palms oh the hands
   c. fingers
   d. Head

108. The most abundant tissue in human body:
   a. Epithelial
   b. Connective
   c. Muscle
   d. Nervous

109. In following which substance is not transported across the cell membrane by simple diffusion?
   a. Fatty acids
   b. Oxygen
   c. Glucose
   d. Steroids

110. The epithelial tissue which is found in the uterine tubes is:
   a. Squamous
   b. Ciliated
   c. Columnar
   d. Simple

111. What is the function of the smooth endoplasmic reticulum in the cell?
   a. They form protein
   b. They synthesize lipids
   c. They synthesize ATP
   d. All of the above

112. In which body structure keratinized stratified squamous epithelium is found?
   a. Conjunctiva of the eyes
   b. Hair
   c. Airway
   d. Stomach

113. Extrusion of waste material through the plasma membrane of a cell is known as:
   a. Pinocytosis
   b. Phagocytosis
   c. Exocytosis
   d. Leukocytosis

114. Which statement below about hormones is true?
   a. Hormones are enzymes that catalyze reactions
   b. Hormones are released into the blood circulation
   c. Hormones affect all cells of the body
   d. Hormones are released by neurons at synapses

115. Which statement about the hypothalamus is correct?
   a. The hypothalamus is connected to the brain by the infundibulum
   b. The hypothalamus is composed of glandular epithelial tissue
   c. The hypothalamus secretes "releasing hormones"
   d. The hypothalamus secretes epinephrine and norepinephrine

116. What hormone does the thyroid produce?
   a. Thyroid stimulating hormone
   b. Calcitriol
   c. Thyroxine
   d. Parathyroid hormone

117. What hormone(s) does the adrenal medulla produce?
   a. Aldosterone
   b. Epinephrine and norepinephrine
   c. Corticosteroids
   d. Glucocorticoids

Answers:

106. c	107. b	108. b	109. c
110. b	111. a	112. b	113. c
114. b	115. c	116. c	117. b

118. What is produced by the beta cells of the pancreas?
a. Angiotensin converting enzyme
b. Glucocorticoids
c. Glucagon
d. Insulin

119. Which gland or organ releases erythropoietin?
a. The kidneys
b. The adrenal glands
c. The anterior pituitary
d. The pancreas

120. What effect does parathyroid hormone have?
a. It increases plasma Ca^{2+} concentration
b. It decreases plasma Ca^{2+} concentration
c. It increases the rate of ATP formation
d. It stimulates the thyroid gland to produce thyroxine

121. Which one of the following is NOT part of the endocrine system?
a. The islets of Langerhans (pancreatic islets)
b. The thyroid gland
c. The acini cells of the pancreas
d. The parathyroid glands

122. From where are antidiuretic hormone and oxytocin released?
a. The anterior pituitary
b. The posterior pituitary
c. The adrenal cortex
d. The adrenal medulla

123. Which hormone has the element iodine as part of its molecule?
a. Calcitonin
b. Hemoglobin
c. Thyroxine
d. Parathyroid hormone

124. Which of the following is a part of the endocrine system?
a. The thalamus
b. The pancreatic islets (islets of Langerhans)
c. The renal glands
d. The salivary glands

125. Which of the following is an amino acid derivative hormone?
a. Epinephrine
b. Tyrosine
c. Testosterone
d. Prostaglandin

126. Which structure controls the endocrine system and integrates the activities of the nervous and endocrine systems?
a. The infundibulum
b. The pituitary gland
c. The thalamus
d. The hypothalamus

127. What effect does aldosterone have? It causes:
a. Angiotensin to be formed from angiotensinogen
b. Na^+ to be absorbed from the filtrate
c. Na^+ and Ca^{++} to be absorbed from the filtrate and K^+ to be secreted into the filtrate
d. Na^+ to be absorbed from the filtrate and K^+ to be secreted into the filtrate

---

Answers: 118. d   119. a   120. a   121. c
122. b   123. c   124. b   125. a
126. d   127. d

128. **Peptide hormones are produced (and/or released) by which structure?**
a. The adrenal cortex
b. The gonads
c. The hypothalamus
d. The kidneys

129. **Which endocrine organ produces "releasing hormones" and "inhibitory hormones"?**
a. Thyroid
b. Anterior pituitary
c. Hypothalamus
d. Thalamus

130. **What hormone is produced by the parafollicular cells of the thyroid gland?**
a. Parathyroid hormone
b. Calcitonin
c. Thyroid hormone
d. Thyroxine

131. **What hormones are produced by the adrenal medulla?**
a. Epinephrine and norepinephrine
b. Insulin and glucagon
c. Aldosterone and erythropoietin
d. Testosterone and estrogen

132. **Which structure integrates the activities of the endocrine system and the nervous system?**
a. The hypothalamus
b. The thalamus
c. The posterior pituitary
d. The anterior pituitary

133. **To which group of hormones does aldosterone belong?**
a. Catecholamines
b. Glucocorticoids
c. Mineralocorticoids
d. Gonadocorticoids

134. **The hypothalamus produces "releasing hormones". What do these releasing hormones do?**
a. They direct the posterior pituitary to release hormones
b. They direct the anterior pituitary to release hormones
c. They direct the gonads to release hormones
d. They act as "second messengers" when hormones bind to their receptor site

135. **What effect does insulin have?**
a. It increases metabolic rate
b. It causes the breakdown of glycogen to glucose
c. It lowers blood sugar level
d. It stimulates gluconeogenesis

136. **Which cells produce insulin?**
a. The acini cells of the pancreas
b. Parafollicular cells of the thymus
c. Alpha cells of the islets of Langerhans
d. Beta cells of the islets of Langerhans

137. **One of the following groups of hormones has their receptor inside the cell. Which one?**
a. Steroid hormones
b. Catecholamines
c. Adrenaline and noradrenaline
d. Peptide hormones

Answers: 128. c   129. c   130. b   131. a
132. a   133. c   134. b   135. c
136. d   137. a

138. What is the difference between endocrine glands and exocrine glands?
a. Endocrine glands produce hormones whereas exocrine glands do not
b. Exocrine glands secrete into the bloodstream whereas endocrine glands do not
c. Endocrine glands are controlled by the autonomic nervous system whereas exocrine glands are not
d. Exocrine glands secrete steroid hormones whereas endocrine glands secrete amino acid-based hormones

139. Which of the following secretes growth hormone?
a. The adrenal glands
b. The thyroid gland
c. The posterior lobe of the pituitary gland
d. The anterior lobe of the pituitary gland

140. What is the name for the entry point to the kidney for nerves, blood vessels, ureters and lymphatics?
a. Calyx
b. Hilum
c. Pelvis
d. Pyramid

141. Where are all of the glomeruli of the kidney located?
a. In the medulla
b. In the columns
c. In the pyramids
d. In the cortex

142. Which part of the nephron is impermeable to water?
a. Proximal convoluted tubule
b. Distal convoluted tubule in the presence of ADH
c. Ascending limb of the loop of Henle
d. Descending limb of the loop of Henle

143. Which material is actively reabsorbed from the filtrate in the kidney tubule?
a. Na^+
b. HCO
c. 3 – C. Cl^-
d. H_2O

144. Which material is secreted into the filtrate in the kidney tubule?
a. H_2O
b. Urea
c. Na^+
d. Albumin

145. In the glomerulus, what is the method by which solutes are transferred from the blood to the Bowman's capsule?
a. Diffusion
b. Active transport
c. Secretion
d. Filtration

146. Which one of the following is NOT produced by the kidneys?
a. Aldosterone
b. Renin
c. Erythropoietin
d. Calcitriol

147. What is the name of the tube that connects the bladder to the kidney?
a. Renal tubule
b. Ureter
c. Urethra
d. Collecting duct

Answers: 138. a 139. d 140. b 141. d
142. c 143. a 144. b 145. d
146. a 147. b

148. In which part of the nephron does most of the reabsorption of water and solutes occur?
a. The collecting duct
b. The nephron loop (loop of Henle)
c. The vasa recta
d. The proximal convoluted tubule

149. Which of the following statement about kidney anatomy is correct?
a. The cortex is superficial to the medulla and contains all of the glomeruli
b. The cortex is deep to the medulla and contains the collecting tubules
c. The pyramids are in the cortex and contain the collecting tubules
d. The pyramids are in the medulla and contain all of the glomeruli

150. Which hormone causes increased sodium reabsorption in the kidney?
a. Angiotensin I
b. Antidiuretic hormone
c. Vasopressin
d. Aldosterone

151. The filtrate that is formed in the kidney contains all of the following except one. Which one?
a. Metabolic wastes
b. Electrolytes
c. Plasma proteins
d. Nutrients

152. What is the term applied to the first process in urine formation, where some components of blood pass into the Bowman's capsule?
a. Filtration
b. Active transport
c. Dialysis
d. Osmosis

153. What is the term used to describe the production of an insufficient volume of urine?
a. Polyuria
b. Uremia
c. Anuria
d. Oliguria

154. The functional unit of the kidney that filters blood and produces urine is called the:
a. Medulla
b. Glomerulus
c. Neuron
d. Nephron

155. Which of the following are organic wastes produced by the body?
a. Uric acid and ammonium ions
b. Amino acids and potassium ions
c. Albumin and globulin
d. Urea and sodium ions

156. What feature does cardiac muscle possess that is missing in skeletal muscle?
a. Striations
b. Multiple nuclei
c. Voluntary control
d. Intercalated discs

157. What is the name of the valve between the left atrium and the left ventricle?
a. Mitral valve
b. Tricuspid valve
c. Semi-lunar valve
d. Aortic valve

158. What is the main function of mitral valve?
a. To increase the pressure inside the left atrium during systole
b. To prevent a drop in pressure in the aorta during diastole
c. To prevent backflow from left ventricle to left atrium during systole
d. To add additional blood from left atrium to left ventricle during atrial systole

Answers: 148. d   149. a   150. d   151. c
           152. a   153. d   154. d   155. a
           156. d   157. a   158. c

159. **How are cardiac cells mechanically attached to each other? By their:**
    a. Mitochondria
    b. Intercalated discs
    c. Gap junctions
    d. Sarcolemma

160. **Which period of the heart cycle is completely occupied by the ventricles relaxing?**
    a. Atrial systole
    b. Atrial diastole
    c. Ventricular systole
    d. Ventricular diastole

161. **Through which valve does blood flow when it moves from the right atrium into the right ventricle?**
    a. The tricuspid valve
    b. The mitral valve
    c. The pulmonary valve
    d. The bicuspid valve

162. **How is the fibrous pericardium attached to the surrounding structures?**
    a. Laterally to the pleural surfaces of the lungs
    b. Posteriorly to the sternum
    c. Anteriorly to trachea, main-stem bronchi and esophagus
    d. Inferiorly to the diaphragm

163. **Through which valve does blood flow when it moves from the left atrium into the left ventricle?**
    a. The semilunar valve
    b. The mitral valve
    c. The tricuspid valve
    d. The bicuspid valve

164. **Which period of the heart cycle is completely occupied by the ventricles contracting?**
    a. Atrial systole
    b. Atrial diastole
    c. Ventricular systole
    d. Ventricular diastole

165. **Which structure has the thickest wall?**
    a. The aorta
    b. The inter-atrial septum
    c. The left ventricle
    d. The right ventricle

166. **Which tissue is supplied with blood via the coronary arteries?**
    a. The lungs
    b. The myocardium
    c. The corona
    d. The aorta

167. **What is the innermost layer of the heart wall known as?**
    a. Epicardium
    b. Pericardium
    c. Visceral pericardium
    d. Endocardium

168. **Choose the structure known as the pacemaker of the heart from the following:**
    a. Atrioventricular node
    b. Sinoatrial node
    c. Atrioventricular bundle
    d. The bundle of His

169. **By what name is the heart muscle known?**
    a. Epicardium
    b. Myocardium
    c. Pericardium
    d. Endocardium

Answers:

159. b	160. d	161. a	162. d
163. b	164. c	165. c	166. b
167. d	168. b	169. b	

170. The heart receives its own oxygenated blood supply via the:
a. Coronary arteries
b. The pulmonary veins
c. The coronary sinus
d. The foramen ovale

171. Where does the pulmonary trunk deliver its blood to?
a. The left atrium
b. The right ventricle
c. The lungs
d. The left ventricle

172. What is the outermost layer of the heart wall known as?
a. Epicardium
b. Pericardium
c. Parietal membrane
d. Endocardium

173. What is the name given to the remnant of the opening in the fetal heart that allowed the fetal lungs to be bypassed?
a. Coronary sinus
b. Foramen ovale
c. Interatrial septum
d. Fossa ovalis

174. Which chamber of the heart has the thickest myocardium?
a. Left ventricle
b. Right ventricle
c. Left atrium
d. Right atrium

175. What supplies blood to the myocardium?
a. The coronary circulation
b. The vena cavae
c. The vasa recta
d. The pulmonary circulation

176. What structure in the heart prevents backflow of blood into the right atrium?
a. The tricuspid valve
b. The bicuspid valve
c. The mitral valve
d. The foramen ovale

177. What causes venous blood to return to the heart?
a. The pumping action of the heart
b. The squashing action of muscles, and valves in the veins
c. Rhythmic vasoconstriction and valves in the veins
d. Gravity, valves and the negative pressure generated by the atria emptying

178. In which organs would be found continuous, fenestrated, and sinusoid capillaries, respectively?
a. Brain, small intestine, liver
b. Bone marrow, brain, spleen
c. Liver, bone marrow, brain
d. Small intestine, liver, brain

179. Which capillaries allow cells and plasma proteins to enter or leave their lumen?
a. Continuous
b. Fenestrated
c. Sinusoidal
d. Anastomotic

180. Which of the following materials is found in the walls of capillaries?
a. Endothelium
b. Elastic fibers
c. Collagen fibers
d. Smooth muscle

Answers: 170. a   171. c   172. a   173. d
174. a   175. a   176. a   177. b
178. a   179. c   180. a

181. Which type of capillary is required to allow the liver to perform its function of producing plasma proteins?
a. Continuous
b. Fenestrated
c. Sinusoidal
d. Anastomotic

182. Which of the following is found in the walls of capillaries?
a. Endothelial cells and basement membrane
b. Tunica externa
c. Tunica media
d. Smooth muscle

183. Why do arteries have more elastic and muscular tissue than veins?
a. Arteries need to expand and contract as blood flows through them
b. Arteries need carry a greater volume of blood than do veins
c. To ensure that blood flows only in the direction away from the heart
d. In order to support the larger diameter of arteries compared to veins

184. Which factor below does NOT assist venous return of blood?
a. Breathing
b. Gravity
c. Smooth muscle contraction
d. Skeletal muscle contraction

185. Vasoconstriction and vasodilation of blood vessels is facilitated by the:
a. Elastic fibers in vessel walls
b. Parasympathetic division of the nervous system
c. Smooth muscle in vessel walls
d. Tunica intima of the blood vessel

186. Exchange between the blood and the interstitial fluid occurs most readily through which type of capillary?
a. Venules
b. Fenestrated capillaries
c. Sinusoids
d. Arterioles

187. What is meant by the "pulmonary circulation"? The flow of blood:
a. Out the aorta and back through the vena cavae
b. From the heart through the lungs and back to the heart
c. Into the coronary arteries and back through the coronary sinus
d. Into the vena cavae and out to the pulmonary trunk via the right ventricle

188. The wall of a capillary consists of one layer (or coat). What is it called?
a. Tunica intima   b. Tunica externa
c. Lamina propria   d. Tunica media

189. In which two anatomical structures does the larynx lie?
a. The nares and the choanae
b. The epiglottis and the trachea
c. The choanae and the glottis
d. The glottis and the epiglottis

190. What is the function of the ciliated cells of the respiratory epithelium?
a. To trap inhaled particles not removed by the nasal cavity
b. To secrete a mucus layer onto the epithelium
c. To move mucus and trapped particles up the bronchial tree
d. To secrete surfactant that decreases water surface tension

Answers: 181. c   182. a   183. a   184. c
185. c   186. c   187. b   188. a
189. b   190. c

191. The walls of the following structures are all supported by cartilage except for one of them. Which one?

a. Bronchioles   b. Trachea

c. Bronchi   d. Larynx

192. What distinguishes bronchioles from the larger bronchi?

a. Bronchioles have no cartilage in their walls

b. Bronchioles have smooth muscle in their walls

c. Bronchioles collapse between exhalation and inhalation

d. The alveoli open onto these air passages

193. Which structures constitute the "upper respiratory tract"?

a. Nose, pharynx and larynx

b. Larynx, epiglottis and bronchi

c. Trachea, bronchi and bronchioles

d. Terminal bronchioles, alveoli and pleurae

194. What is a cavity in a skull bone that is lined with mucus membrane?

a. Sinus   b. Bronchiole

c. Glottis   d. Larynx

195. Which structures comprise the lower respiratory tract?

a. Pharynx, larynx, trachea

b. Larynx, trachea, bronchi

c. Nose, pharynx, larynx

d. Trachea, bronchi, lungs

196. What are the cells that produce surfactant called?

a. Mucus cells

b. Ciliated cells

c. Alveolar macrophages

d. Type II pneumocytes

197. What happens when carbon dioxide levels in the blood increase?

a. pH of the blood increases

b. The blood becomes more alkaline

c. The number of hydrogen ions in the blood decreases

d. The blood becomes more acidic

198. Where does the actual gas exchange between inspired air and the blood in the capillaries occur? In the:

a. Bronchi

b. Bronchioles

c. Alveolar ducts and alveoli

d. Respiratory bronchioles

199. The walls of the trachea are held open by which of the following?

a. Nerve impulses

b. Rings of cartilage

c. Fine bones

d. Smooth muscle contractions

200. Normal expiration in a person at rest is due to:

a. Elastic tissue in the lung

b. Contraction of abdominal muscles

c. Contraction of the expiratory muscles

d. Diffusion

201. What is the number of breaths per minute called? The:

a. Respiratory rate

b. Respiratory speed

c. Pulmonary index

d. Respiratory volume

202. What are the membranes that surround each lung called? The:

a. Parietal and visceral membranes

b. Parietal and visceral meninges

c. Pleura

d. Peritoneum

Answers: 191. a   **192. a**   **193. a**   **194. a**

195. d   **196. d**   **197. d**   **198. c**

199. b   **200. a**   **201. a**   **202. c**

203. What are the main muscles involved in normal inspiration?
a. Muscles of the neck
b. Abdominal muscle
c. SC intercostal muscles
d. Intercostals and the diaphragm

204. Which is the major type of nerve cell in the CNS?
a. Anaxonic
b. Unipolar
c. Bipolar
d. Multipolar

205. What is the purpose of the myelin sheath around an axon?
a. To control the chemical environment around the nerve cell
b. To phagocytose microbes
c. To prevent movement of ions through the nerve cell membrane
d. To form the blood-brain barrier

206. Which nerve cells carry impulses from the brain to the muscles?
a. Sensory b. Motor
c. Afferent d. Association

207. What is the type of neuroglia that forms the myelin sheath on neurons outside of the CNS?
a. Oligodendrocytes
b. Satellite cells
c. Schwann cells
d. Microglia

208. Which of the following is NOT composed of "gray matter"?
a. Spinothalamic tract
b. Cerebral cortex
c. Basal nuclei
d. Post-central gyrus

209. Where in the brain is the "primary motor area"?
a. Midbrain
b. Thalamus
c. Basal nuclei
d. Pre-central gyrus

210. The hypothalamus does ALL of the following except one. Which one?
a. It is the autonomic control center
b. It directs lower CNS centers to perform actions
c. It produces the rigidly programmed, automatic behaviors necessary for survival
d. It performs many homeostatic roles

211. Which of the following structures together make up the brainstem?
a. Medulla oblongata, pons, midbrain, cerebellum
b. Medulla oblongata, pons, midbrain
c. Medulla oblongata, pons, midbrain, thalamus
d. Medulla oblongata, pons, midbrain, pineal gland

212. In which of the following places would you NOT find cerebrospinal fluid?
a. The subarachnoid space
b. The third ventricle of the brain
c. The epidural space
d. The central canal of the spinal cord

213. What is the name of the lobe of the brain that is immediately superior to the cerebellum?
a. Dorsal
b. Occipital
c. Posterior
d. Parietal

Answers: 203. d 204. d 205. c 206. b
207. a 208. a 209. d 210. c
211. b 212. c 213. b

214. **Which of the following statements about the blood-brain barrier (BBB) is correct?**
   a. The BBB prevents fluctuations of hormone and ion concentrations in blood from affecting the brain
   b. It is formed by Schwann cells wrapping around capillaries
   c. The brain is supported by (it floats in) the BBB
   d. The BBB is formed by the choroid plexus

215. **In which part of the brain is the thalamus found?**
   a. Diencephalon   b. Cerebrum
   c. Cerebellum   d. Brainstem

216. **Where is the autonomic control center for most of body homeostasis located?**
   a. In the limbic system
   b. In the brainstem
   c. In the hypothalamus
   d. In the cerebellum

217. **Which part of the brain allows us to control skilled voluntary muscle movements?**
   a. Basal nuclei
   b. Cerebellum
   c. Pre-central gyrus
   d. Thalamus

218. **Corticospinal pathways cross-over from one side of the brain to the other side. Where does this cross-over occur?**
   a. In the medulla oblongata
   b. In the cerebellum
   c. In the hypothalamus
   d. In the reticular formation

219. **Which layer of membrane around the brain is the most superficial?**
   a. Dura mater
   b. Meningeal mater
   c. Arachnoid mater
   d. Pia mater

220. **What part of the brain contains the motor areas and the sensory areas?**
   a. Cerebrum
   b. Diencephalon
   c. Brainstem
   d. Cerebellum

221. **What part of the brain subconsciously provides precise timing for the movements of learned skeletal muscle contraction?**
   a. Cerebrum
   b. Diencephalon
   c. Brainstem
   d. Cerebellum

222. **Where does the spinal cord start and finish?**
   a. It extends from the foramen magnum to L1–L2
   b. It extends from the foramen magnum to the sacrum
   c. It starts at the superior part of the medulla oblongata and extends to the inferior part of the cauda equina
   d. It extends from C7 to L5

223. **What part of the brain receives sensory input before passing it on to another part of the brain for interpretation or action?**
   a. Pons
   b. Hypothalamus
   c. Post-central gyrus
   d. Thalamus

Answers:
214. a   215. a   216. c   217. c
218. a   219. a   220. a   221. d
222. a   223. d

224. What is the primary function of the cerebellum?
a. It regulates such things as body temperature, water balance and emotional responses
b. It refines/adjusts learned motor movements so that they are performed smoothly
c. It controls our automatic functions such as breathing, digestion and cardiovascular functions
d. It is the origin of our conscious thoughts and intellectual functions

225. What part of the brain subconsciously provides the appropriate pattern of smooth coordinated skeletal muscle contraction for movements that we have learned?
a. The cerebellum
b. The brainstem
c. The cerebrum
d. The diencephalon

226. Which part of the brain controls breathing, heart function, vasoconstriction and swallowing?
a. Mesencephalon
b. Cerebellum
c. Diencephalon
d. Brainstem

227. What is found between the arachnoid and pia mater?
a. Adipose tissue
b. Venous sinuses
c. Choroid plexus
d. Cerebrospinal fluid

228. Which one of the following is NOT a function of the cerebral spinal fluid?
a. To produce hormones
b. To transport nutrients around the brain
c. To protect the spinal cord
d. To cushion the brain

229. Which best describes the function of the association area of the temporal lobe?
a. It perceives of movement
b. It interprets the meaning of sound patterns
c. It recognizes of geometric shapes and faces
d. It perceives meaningful information from different senses

230. What innervates the diaphragm?
a. The spinal nerves from T6 to T12
b. The vagus nerve
c. The phrenic nerve
d. The sciatic nerve

231. Which neurotransmitter do all motor neurons release at their synapses with skeletal muscle cells?
a. ACh
b. ATP
c. GABA
d. Norepinephrine

Answers: 224. **b**   225. **a**   226. **d**   227. **d**
228. **a**   229. **b**   230. **c**   231. **a**

232. **What is the parasympathetic division of the autonomic nervous system responsible for?**
   a. Rapid predictable motor responses without processing by the brain
   b. Conserving energy and maintaining body activities without conscious brain control
   c. Preparing the body for energetic activity without conscious brain control
   d. Gathering sensory information from the viscera that is not interpreted by the brain

233. **What is a spinal reflex?**
   a. It involves rapid processing by the brain and a predictable response
   b. It involves stimulation of a motor neuron by a sensory neuron without a synapse
   c. It is a rapid, predictable, learned and involuntary motor response
   d. It is a predictable, unlearned and involuntary motor response

234. **Which part of the nervous system prepares you for vigorous activity ("to fight or flee")?**
   a. Sympathetic
   b. Parasympathetic
   c. Somatic
   d. Autonomic

235. **What is that part of the nervous system that carries commands to the skeletal muscles called?**
   a. Somatic nervous system
   b. Autonomic nervous system
   c. Central nervous system
   d. Sympathetic division

236. **Which neurotransmitter do all motor neurons release at their synapses?**
   a. Acetylcholine
   b. Norepinephrine
   c. Dopamine
   d. Adenosine triphosphate

237. **What is the nerve that that carries most of the parasympathetic signals?**
   a. Phrenic   b. Vagus
   c. Sciatic   d. Trigeminal

238. **Which part of the retina has the greatest sensitivity to light?**
   a. The optic disc
   b. Macula lutea
   c. The choroid
   d. Fovea centralis

239. **The deterioration of sight with age is known by which term?**
   a. Protanopia   b. Presbyopia
   c. Hyperopia   d. Scotopia

240. **What is the place where the blood vessels and nerve fibers come together and leave the posterior chamber of the eye called?**
   a. Macula lutea   b. Optic disc
   c. Fovea centralis   d. Choroid

241. **Accommodation refers to the eye's ability to focus light from objects whatever their distance from the eye. How is this achieved?**
   a. By altering the distance between the cornea and the eye's lens
   b. By altering the distance between the lens and the retina
   c. By altering the shape of the eye's lens
   d. By altering the shape of the cornea

Answers: 232. b   233. d   234. a   235. a
          236. a   237. b   238. d   239. b
          240. b   241. c

242. Which cells of the retina are responsible for detecting light in scotopic (i.e., low light) conditions?
a. Bipolar cells
b. Rod cells
c. Ganglion cells
d. Cone cells

243. What is the purpose of the optic chiasma?
a. To allow images from each eye to cross over to the other side of the brain prior to crossing back at the decussation of pyramids
b. To allow fibers from the medial aspect of one eye to join fibers from the lateral aspect of the other eye to form an optic tract
c. To allow the fibers from the lateral aspect of each eye to come together as an optic tract
d. To allow light entering the left eye to be interpreted by the right hand side of the occipital lobe (and vice versa)

244. What is presbyopia (old-age vision) due to?
a. The loss of elasticity of the lens of the eye
b. The change in the curvature of the cornea
c. The gradual loss of cone cells from the retina
d. The deviation from a spherical eye-ball shape with aging

245. In which region of the eye does the most detailed vision occur? The:
a. Fovea centralis
b. Optic disc
c. Macula lutea
d. Ciliary body

246. What is the light sensitive cell in the retina that responds to color called?
a. Macula
b. Macula lutea
c. Cone
d. Rod

247. Glaucoma is an eye disease which affects vision. It is caused by:
a. Blockage of the flow of aqueous humor through the canal of Schlemm and loss of intraocular pressure in the vitreous humor
b. Detachment of the retina and subsequent loss of vision in this part of the eye
c. Cataracts that form in the eye's lens which prevent light from reaching the retina
d. Increased intraocular pressure which collapses the blood capillaries that perfuse the retina so part of it dies

248. Myopia may be corrected with a lens that is:
a. Bifocal
b. Concave
c. Cylindrical
d. Convex

249. The change in vision that occurs with ageing is called:
a. Protanopia
b. Hyperopia
c. Deuteranopia
d. Presbyopia

250. Which part of the ear contains the apparatus that we use to distinguish between different frequencies of sound?
a. The cochlea
b. The Eustachian (or auditory) tube
c. The tensor tympani
d. The auditory meatus

Answers: 242. b 243. b 244. a 245. a
246. c 247. d 248. b 249. d
250. a

251. **Sound produces vibrations in the cochlear fluid of the inner ear. The movement of the fluid then produces motion in which of the following?**
   a. Tectorial membrane
   b. Basilar membrane
   c. Otolithic membrane
   d. Crista ampullaris

252. **Lungs are enclosed within:**
   a. Perichondrium
   b. Periosteum
   c. Pleural membrane
   d. Pericardium

253. **Which of the following organs contains the 'bundle of His'?**
   a. Pancreas   b. Brain
   c. Kidney   d. Heart

254. **The following artery is a content of the upper triangular space:**
   a. Circumflex scapular artery
   b. Axillary artery
   c. Brachial artery
   d. Musculocutaneous nerve

255. **Superficial palmar arch is formed mainly by the continuation of:**
   a. Radial artery
   b. Posterior interosseous artery
   c. Ulnar artery
   d. Common interosseous branch of ulnar artery

256. **Biceps brachii is inserted into the:**
   a. Ulnar tuberosity
   b. Bicipital groove
   c. Radial tuberosity
   d. Deltoid tuberosity

257. **The commonest site of shoulder joint dislocation is:**
   a. Superior   b. Inferior
   c. Anterior   d. Posterior

258. **The outer covering of the peripheral nerve is called:**
   a. Epineurium   b. Perineurium
   c. Endoneurium   d. Neurilemma

259. **Nerve supply of adductor magnus is through:**
   a. Tibial part of sciatic nerve
   b. Common peroneal part of sciatic nerve
   c. Obturator nerve
   d. Both a and c

260. **Which joint is immovable?**
   a. Synovial joint
   b. Ball and socket joint
   c. Fibrous joint
   d. Cartilaginous joints

261. **Foot drop result as a result of injury of:**
   a. Deep peroneal nerve
   b. Superficial peroneal nerve
   c. Tibial nerve
   d. Obturator nerve

262. **The strongest ligament in the body is:**
   a. Inguinal ligament
   b. Lacunar ligament
   c. Ligamentum flavum
   d. Iliofemoral ligament

263. **Muscle causing abduction of vocal cords is:**
   a. Aryepiglotticus
   b. Transverse arytenoids
   c. Lateral cricoarytenoid
   d. Posterior cricoarytenoid

264. **All structures pass through jugular foramen, *except*:**
   a. Jugular vein
   b. Glossopharyngeal nerve
   c. Hypoglossal nerve
   d. Accessory nerve

Answers: 251. b   252. c   253. d   254. a
255. c   256. c   257. b   258. a
259. d   260. c   261. a   262. d
263. d   264. d

265. The muscle which divides the neck into anterior and posterior triangles:
a. Sternocleidomastoid muscle
b. Platysma
c. Digastric
d. Trapezius

266. The root value of phrenic nerve:
a. C1, C2, C3
b. C2, C3, C4
c. C3, C4, C5
d. C3, C4, C5, T1

267. Largest cartilage of larynx is:
a. Thyroid
b. Epiglottis
c. Cricoids
d. Arytenoid

268. Parotid duct opens at:
a. Upper 1st molar teeth
b. Upper 2nd molar teeth
c. Upper 3rd molar teeth
d. Upper 1st premolar teeth

269. Which of the following is forming the roof of the posterior triangle:
a. Investing layer
b. Pretracheal layer
c. Prevertebral layer
d. Buccopharyngeal fascia

270. Dangerous area of face is:
a. Upper lip
b. Lower part of nose
c. Lower lip
d. Upper lip and lower part of nose

271. Porter's tip or policeman's tip deformity occurs due to:
a. Klumpke's paralysis
b. Paralysis of median nerve
c. Paralysis of radial nerve
d. Erb's paralysis

272. Pericardium is situated in:
a. Superior mediastinum
b. Posterior mediastinum
c. Anterior mediastinum
d. Middle mediastinum

273. Apex of heart is formed by:
a. Left ventricle
b. Right ventricle
c. Left ventricle and left atrium
d. Left and right ventricle

274. Lateral boundary of cubital fossa is formed by:
a. Biceps brachii
b. Brachioradialis
c. Brachialis
d. Extensor carpi radialis longus

275. Eustachian valve is present at the opening of:
a. Superior vena cava
b. Inferior vena cava
c. Ascending aorta
d. Both a and b

276. The scapula is an example of:
a. Long bone
b. Flat bone
c. Irregular bone
d. Short bone

277. Structure that arches over hilum of right lung is:
a. Azygous vein
b. Thoracic duct
c. Superior vena cava
d. Arch of aorta

278. Anterior interventricular artery is a branch of:
a. Right marginal
b. Pulmonary trunk
c. Right coronary
d. Left coronary

279. All are forming stomach bed, *except:*
a. Left suprarenal gland
b. Right kidney
c. Pancreas
d. Left kidney

Answers:

265. a	266. c	267. a	268. b
269. a	270. d	271. d	272. d
273. a	274. b	275. b	276. b
277. a	278. d	279. b	

280. Free margin of lesser omentum contains:
a. Hepatic artery, bile duct and portal vein
b. Portal vein and bile duct
c. Portal vein, bile duct, hepatic vein
d. Only bile duct

281. Fixed part of small intestine is:
a. Jejunum
b. Ilium
c. Duodenum
d. Cecum

282. Accessory pancreatic duct opens into:
a. Minor duodenal papilla 2 cm distal to major duodenal papilla
b. Minor duodenal papilla 2 cm proximal to major duodenal papilla
c. At major duodenal papilla
d. None of the above

283. Broad ligament of uterus contains:
a. Uterine vessels
b. Uterine tube
c. Ovarian ligament
d. All of the above

284. Right adrenal vein drains into:
a. Right renal vein
b. Inferior vena cava
c. Lumbar veins
d. Left renal vein

285. Boundaries of Hesselbach's triangle are all, *except:*
a. Lateral border of rectus abdominis
b. Inguinal ligament
c. Inferior epigastric artery
d. Medial border of pyramidalis

286. Pouch of Douglas is situated between:
a. Bladder and uterus
b. Bladder and pubic symphysis
c. Bladder and rectum
d. Uterus and rectum

287. Pancreatic bed does not include:
a. Left kidney
b. Splenic artery
c. Left renal vein
d. Left crus of diaphragm

288. Falciform ligament contains:
a. Ligamentum teres
b. Ligamentum venosum
c. Bile duct and portal vein
d. Superior epigastric artery

289. Which of the following is the content of deep inguinal ring:
a. Suspensory ligament of ovary
b. Mesosalpinx
c. Spermatic cord
d. Round ligament of uterus

290. Rectus abdominis is inserted into:
a. Xiphoid process
b. Median plane
c. Linea alba
d. 1–4 ribs

291. Ejaculatory ducts opens into:
a. Membranous urethra
b. Prostatic urethra
c. Penile urethra
d. Seminal vesicles

292. Deep perineal pouch contains:
a. Bulb of penis
b. Crura of penis
c. Bulbospongiosus
d. Membranous urethra

293. Posterior relation of neck of pancreas:
a. Inferior vena cava
b. Origin of portal vein
c. Aorta
d. Common bile duct

Answers:

280. a	281. c	282. b	283. d
284. b	285. d	286. d	287. b
288. a	289. c	290. a	291. b
292. d	293. b		

294. Labyrinthine artery is a branch of:
a. Anterior inferior cerebellar artery
b. Vertebral artery
c. Posterior inferior cerebellar artery
d. Superior cerebellar artery

295. Entry channels of heart are all, *except:*
a. Superior vena cava
b. Inferior vena cava
c. 4 pulmonary veins
d. Pulmonary trunk

296. Which one is not a component of carotid sheath?
a. Internal carotid artery
b. Vagus nerve
c. Sympathetic trunk
d. Internal jugular vein

297. Investing layer of cervical fascia encloses all, *except:*
a. Two muscles
b. Two salivary glands
c. Axillary vessels
d. Two spaces

298. Which of the following is not a muscle of mastication?
a. Medial pterygoid
b. Masseter
c. Temporalis
d. Orbicularis oris

299. Ophthalmic artery is a branch of which of the following arteries?
a. Internal carotid
b. External carotid
c. Maxillary
d. Vertebral

300. Trapezoid body is concerned with:
a. Pain and temperature
b. Hearing
c. Touch and pressure
a. Proprioception

301. Which air sinus is most commonly infected?
a. Ethmoidal   b. Frontal
c. Maxillary   d. Sphenoidal

302. Haversian canal contains:
a. Blood vessels
b. Muscle
c. Some loose connective tissue
d. Few osteoblasts and osteoclasts

303. The intercalated disks are present in which muscle:
a. Smooth muscle   b. Skeletal
c. Cardiac   d. Voluntary

304. Nerve plexus in the submucosa of the gastrointestinal tract is called as:
a Meissner's plexus
b. Auerbach plexuses
c. There are no plexuses in submucosa
d. Meissner's and Auerbach plexuses both are present

305. Which of the following arteries is an end-artery?
a. Lacrimal artery
b. Zygomaticotemporal artery
c. Central artery of retina
d. Anterior ethmoidal artery

306. Left superior intercostal vein drains into:
a. Azygous vein
b. Hemiazygos vein
c. Left brachiocephalic vein
d. Internal thoracic vein

307. Which of the following will not drain into coronary sinus?
a. Great cardiac vein
b. Middle cardiac vein
c. Small cardiac vein
d. Anterior cardiac vein

Answers: 294. a   295. d   296. c   297. c
          298. d   299. a   300. b   301. c
          302. d   303. c   304. a   305. c
          306. c   307. d

308. Oblique sinus lies:
a. Behind the left atrium
b. Behind the ascending aorta
c. Behind the superior vena cava
d. Anterior to pulmonary trunk

309. Blood supply of lungs:
a. Pulmonary artery
b. Pulmonary vein
c. Bronchial artery
d. Intercostal artery

310. The esophagus:
a. Begins at the upper border of thyroid cartilage
b. Runs a straight course throughout
c. Is narrowed at its termination
d. Is narrowed at its beginning

311. Arch of aorta lies in which mediastinum:
a. Anterior   b. Posterior
c. Middle   d. Superior

312. A femoral hernia is more common in female due to:
a. Wider pelvis
b. Smaller size of femoral vessel
c. Femoral canal is wider
d. All of the above

313. Which of the following structure does not pass through superior aperture of thorax:
a. Right recurrent laryngeal nerve
b. Left common carotid artery
c. Subclavian vein
d. Thoracic duct

314. Fabella is:
a. A ligament
b. An accessory projection from fibula
c. A sesamoid bone
d. Other name for patella

315. Which muscle is known as Tailor's muscle:
a. Flexor carpi ulnaris
b. Quadrates femoris
c. Lateral head of gastrocnemius
d. Sartorius

316. Femoral artery is the continuation of which artery?
a. Popliteal   b. External iliac
c. Profunda femoris d. Obturator

317. Ischial tuberosity gives attachment to:
a. Obturator internus
b. Quadrates femoris
c. Gluteus maximus
d. Adductor magnus

318. The anterior division of obturator nerve innervates:
a. Hip joint   b. Knee joint
c. Sartorius   d. Pectineus

319. Where does the femoral artery becomes the popliteal artery:
a. At apex of femoral triangle
b. At the hiatus in adductor magnus
c. Within the adductor canal
d. None of the above

320. Peroneal artery is a branch of:
a. Anterior tibial artery
b. Posterior tibial artery
c. Popliteal artery
d. Arcuate artery

321. What is true about femoral canal:
a. Smaller in female
b. Contains femoral vein
c. Inferior epigastric artery lies medially
d. Medial most compartment of femoral sheath

Answers: 308. a   309. c   310. c   311. d
312. d   313. c   314. c   315. d
316. b   317. d   318. a   319. c
320. b   321. d

322. Short saphenous vein is the continuation of:
a. Medial marginal vein
b. Lateral marginal vein
c. Dorsal venous arch
d. Tibial vein

323. Which muscle is called peripheral heart?
a. Soleus
b. Gastrocnemius
c. Plantaris
d. Sartorius

324. Tibial nerve is a subdivision of which nerve?
a. Obturator
b. Sciatic
c. Femoral
d. Common peroneal

325. Which of the following is the thickest nerve of the body?
a. Sciatic
b. Pudendal
c. Superior gluteal
d. Nerve to quadratus femoris

326. Which is the main artery of anterior compartment of leg?
a. Anterior tibial
b. Dorsalis pedis
c. Peroneal
d. Popliteal

327. Which muscle is not undercover of gluteus maximus?
a. Piriformis
b. Quadratus femoris
c. Sartorius
d. Obturator internus with two gemelli

328. Out of following muscles which muscle acts as key of locked knee joint?
a. Popliteus
b. Flexor digitorum longus
c. Tibialis posterior
d. Flexor hallucis longus

329. Which muscle is one of the most powerful and bulkiest muscle in human?
a. Gluteus maximus
b. Obturator internus
c. Quadriceps femoris
d. Soleus

330. Which is not the content of popliteal fossa?
a. Popliteal artery and its branches
b. Popliteal vein and its tributaries
c. Tibial nerve
d. Long saphenous vein

331. Goblet cells are absent in which part of alimentary canal:
a. Duodenum
b. Stomach
c. Colon
d. Appendix

332. What type of muscle is arrector pilorum:
a. Skeletal
b. Smooth
c. Cardiac
d. None of these

333. An example of dense irregular connective tissue is:
a. Tendon
b. Myxomatous tissue
c. Areolar
d. Dermis

334. Which part of intestine contains Brunner's glands?
a. Ileum
b. Duodenum
c. Jejunum
d. Colon

Answers:

322. b	323. a	324. b	325. a
326. a	327. c	328. a	329. a
330. d	331. c	332. b	333. d
334. b			

335. Following are ventral branches of aorta, *except:*
a. Celiac axis
b. Superior mesenteric artery
c. Inferior mesenteric artery
d. Gonadal artery

336. At birth the lower end of spinal cord is at what level:
a. L1
b. L2
c. L3
d. L4

337. All of the following are features of veins, *except:*
a. Thin walls
b. Thin tunica adventitia
c. Thin tunica media
d. Wider lumen

338. All of the following are examples of end arteries, *except:*
a. Central branches of cerebral arteries
b. Central artery of retina
c. Facial artery
d. Splenic artery

339. Which of the following is not a characteristic feature of large intestine?
a. Sacculations
b. Villi
c. *Taenia coli*
d. Appendices epiploicae

340. Most common position of vermiform appendix is:
a. Pelvic
b. Retrocaecal
c. Preileal
d. Postileal

341. Superior rectal is a branch/continuation of:
a. Superior mesenteric
b. Inferior mesenteric
c. Internal iliac
d. External iliac

342. All of the following are the examples of synovial joint, *except:*
a. Pivot   b. Saddle
c. Syndesmosis   d. Ellipsoid

343. All of the following are examples of portal circulation, *except:*
a. Pulmonary circulation
b. Hepatic circulation
c. Renal circulation
d. Circulation in hypophysis cerebri

344. Which of the following is primary lymphoid tissue?
a. Lymph node
b. Spleen
c. Thymus
d. Palatine tonsil

345. A collection of nerve fibers outside the CNS is called:
a. Tract
b. Nerve
c. Ganglion
d. Nucleus

346. Hyaline cartilage is present in:
a. Intervertebral disc
b. Glenoidal labrum
c. Epiphyseal plate
d. Menisci

347. Buck's fascia is related to:
a. Ischiorectal fascia   b. Thigh
c. Neck   d. Penis

Answers: 335. d   336. c   337. b   338. c
339. b   340. a   341. b   342. c
343. a   344. a   345. c   346. b
347. d

348. Length of female urethra is:
a. 2 cm
b. 3 cm
c. 4 cm
d. 5 cm

349. Valve of Hasner is seen in:
a. Common bile duct
b. Common hepatic duct
c. Nasolacrimal duct
d. Pancreatic duct

350. All the muscles of eye are supplied by oculomotor nerve, *except*:
a. Lateral rectus
b. Superior oblique
c. Superior rectus
d. Lateral rectus and superior oblique

351. Which of the following is a part of the hindbrain?
a. Hypothalamus
b. Cerebellum
c. Spinal cord
d. Corpus callosum

352. Commonest site of fertilization:
a. Ampulla of uterine tube
b. Fundus of the uterus
c. Ovarian end of fallopian tubes
d. Lower part of the uterus

353. Which structure is not innervated by vagus nerve?
a. Small intestine
b. Heart
c. Stomach
d. Sternocleidomastoid

354. All of following are parts of basal ganglia, *except*:
a. Caudate nucleus
b. Thalamus
c. Putamen
d. Globus pallidus

355. Regarding spinal cord, the following are true, *except*:
a. It has cervical and lumbar enlargements
b. It ends in adults at lower border of 3rd lumbar vertebra
c. It is traversed by the central canal
d. It begins at level of foramen magnum as a continuation of medulla oblongata

356. Which is not a cranial nerve?
a. Vagus
b. Glossopharyngeal
c. Phrenic
d. Hypoglossal

357. Parkinsonism disease is due to lesion in:
a. Corpus luteum
b. Corpus striatum
c. Corpus callosum
d. Substantia nigra

358. Afferents to lateral geniculate body is:
a. Optic tract
b. Globus pallidus
c. Auditory fibers from inferior colliculus
d. Reticular formation of brainstem

359. Anterior spinal artery is a branch of which artery:
a. Vertebral
b. Internal carotid
c. Basilar
d. Labyrinthine

360. Which is not a part of limbic system?
a. Hypophysis cerebri
b. Amygdaloid nuclei
c. Olfactory nerve, bulbs, tracts and stria
d. Fornix

Answers:	348. c	349. c	350. b	351. b
	352. a	353. d	354. b	355. b
	356. c	357. d	358. c	359. a
	360. a			

361. **Myelin sheath in the central nervous system is formed by:**
  a. Schwann cell
  b. Microglia
  c. Oligodendrocytes
  d. Protoplasmic astrocytes

362. **Which type of epithelium is found in the Bowman's capsule of mammalian kidney?**
  a. Pseudostratified
  b. Stratified
  c. Squamous
  d. Cuboidal

363. **All structures pass through jugular foramen, *except:***
  a. Jugular vein
  b. Glossopharyngeal nerve
  c. Hypoglossal nerve
  d. Accessory nerve

364. **Which nucleus is not found in the floor of the fourth ventricle:**
  a. Abducens nucleus
  b. Dorsal vagal nuclei
  c. Facial nucleus
  d. Hypoglossal nucleus

365. **The root value of phrenic nerve:**
  a. C1, C2, C3
  b. C2, C3, C4
  c. C3, C4, C5
  d. C3, C4, C5, T1

366. **The excretory passages of the urinary system has a lining of epithelial:**
  a. Stratified squamous
  b. Glandular epithelium
  c. Squamous epithelium
  d. Transitional epithelium

367. **Stratified squamous epithelium is seen in:**
  a. Epidermis of skin, esophagus, anal canal
  b. Intestine, lungs, heart
  c. Blood and lymphatic vessels
  d. Ducts of salivary and mammary glands

368. **Exocrine glands containing glandular cells which shed themselves to secrete their products are known as:**
  a. ductless glands
  b. Apocrine glands
  c. Mesocrine glands
  d. Holocrine glands

369. **Parathyroid glands develop from............ branchial pouches.**
  a. 1st and 2nd
  b. 2nd and 3rd
  c. 3rd and 4th
  d. 5th and 6th

370. **Malleus and incus bones are derived from:**
  a. First arch
  b. Second arch
  c. Third arch
  d. Fourth arch

371. **The umbilical cord has:**
  a. Two arteries and one vein
  b. One arteries and two vein
  c. Two arteries and two veins
  d. One artery and one vein

372. **Polar bodies are formed during:**
  a. Spermatogenesis
  b. Organogenesis
  c. Oogenesis
  d. Morphogenesis

373. **Pharyngeal tonsil develop from which pharyngeal pouch:**
  a. First
  b. Second
  c. Third
  d. Fourth

Answers:
361. c	362. c	363. d	364. a
365. c	366. d	367. a	368. c
369. c	370. a	371. a	372. c
373. b			

374. Haversian system is seen in:
a. Cortical bone   b. lungs
c. Teeth   d. Nail

375. Which cranial nerve passes through stylomastoid foramen?
a. Facial nerve
b. Glossopharyngeal nerve
c. Vagus nerve
d. Hypoglossal nerve

376. Unpaired structure in the brain:
a. Basilar artery
b. Vertebral artery
c. Middle cerebral artery
d. Anterior cerebral artery

377. Pyramidal fibers are:
a. Projection fibers
b. Association fibers
c. Commissural fibers
d. Association and commissural fibers

378. Double Barr body is seen in............... syndrome:
a. Turners   b. Klinefelters
c. XXX   d. Downs

379. Space of Disse is seen in:
a. Spleen
b. Kidney
c. Liver
d. Small intestine

380. The epithelial tissue which form protective layer of the skin, buccal cavity and tongue is:
a. Squamous epithelium
b. Ciliated epithelium
c. Glandular epithelium
d. Stratified epithelium

381. The spinal nerves pairs are:
a. 28   b. 30
c. 31   d. 33

382. Brodmann's number given to auditosensory area is:
a. 41, 42   b. 44, 45
c. 3, 1, 2   d. 18, 19

383. Brunner's glands are located in the:
a. Duodenum
b. Jejunum
c. Ileum
d. Large intestine

384. Meckel's cartilage develops from:
a. Second pharyngeal arch cartilage
b. Third pharyngeal arch cartilage
c. Fourth pharyngeal arch cartilage
d. First pharyngeal arch cartilage

385. Inner lining of trachea is formed by:
a. Simple squamous epithelium
b. Pseudostratified epithelium
c. Stratified epithelium
d. Simple glandular epithelium

386. Melanoblasts are derived from:
a. Basal epidermal cells
b. Neural crest cells
c. Prickle cells of epidermis
d. Somatopleuric mesoderm

387. Area postrema functions as:
a. Chemoreceptor
b. Osmoreceptor
c. Nociceptor
d. None of the above

388. Broca's area is located in which lobe?
a. Parietal   b. Frontal
c. Temporal   d. Occipital

389. Ligamentous arteriosus is a remnant of:
a. Ductus arteriosus
b. Ductus caroticus
c. Ductus venosus
d. None

Answers: 374. a 375. a 376. a 377. a
378. b 379. a 380. d 381. c
382. a 383. a 384. d 385. b
386. b 387. a 388. a 389. a

390. Example for a holocrine gland is:
a. Salivary gland
b. Sweat gland
c. Sebaceous gland
d. Mammary gland

391. The ureter is lined by...........
epithelium:
a. Stratified squamous
b. Cuboidal
c. Ciliated columnar
d. Transitional

392. The epithelial lining of ovary and seminiferous tubules of the testes is:
a. Sensory
b. Cuboidal
c. Squamous
d. Glandular

393. Goblet cells are:
a. Unicellular mucous glands
b. Multicellular mucous glands
c. Cuboidal epithelial cells
d. Stratified cuboidal cells

394. Fasciculus gracilis and fasciculus cuneatus are parts of which of the following tracts in the spinal cord?
a. Dorsal column
b. Lateral spinothalamic tract
c. Spinocerebellar tract
d. Ventral spinothalamic tract

395. Which nerve does not arise from medulla:
a. Facial
b. Oculomotor
c. Vagus
d. Hypoglossal

396. Dentate nucleus is a part of:
a. Midbrain
b. Pons
c. Medulla
d. Cerebellum

397. Broca's area is:
a. 44 and 45
b. 40 and 42
c. 43 and 44
d. 41 and 42

398. Which area is devoid of blood- brain barrier:
a. Thalamus
b. Cerebral cortex
c. Fourth ventricle
d. Area postrema

399. Trapezoid body is concerned with:
a. Pain and temperature
b. Hearing
c. Touch and pressure
d. Proprioception

400. Fibers passing through crus cerebri are:
a. Corticonuclear and corticospinal fibers
b. Medial leminiscus
c. Spinothalamic
d. Both b and c

401. Haversian canal contains:
a. Blood vessels
b. Muscle
c. Some loose connective tissue
d. Few osteoblasts and osteoclasts

402. The intercalated disc are present in which muscle:
a. Smooth muscle
b. Skeletal
c. Cardiac
d. Voluntary

403. Nerve plexus in the submucosa of the gastrointestinal tract is called as:
a. Auerbach plexuses
b. There are no plexuses in submucosa
c. Meissner's and Auerbach plexuses both are present
d. Meissner's plexus

Answers:	390. c	391. d	392. b	393. a
	394. b	395. b	396. d	397. a
	398. d	399. b	400. a	401. d
	402. c	403. d		

404. Which of the following is not a feature of tetralogy of Fallot:
a. Overriding of aorta
b. Ventricular septal defect
c. Pulmonary stenosis
d. Left ventricular hypertrophy

405. Left superior intercostal vein drains into:
a. Azygous vein
b. Hemiazygos vein
c. Left brachiocephalic vein
d. Internal thoracic vein

406. The epithelial lining of ovary and seminiferous tubules of the testes is:
a. Sensory
b. Cuboidal
c. Squamous
d. Glandular

407. Oblique sinus lies:
a. Behind the left atrium
b. Behind the ascending aorta
c. Behind the superior vena cava
d. Anterior to pulmonary trunk

408. All are mesodermal in origin, *except*:
a. Iris stroma
b. Ciliary body
c. Dilator papillae
d. Vitreous

409. Corona radiata of ovum is formed from:
a. Cummulus ovaricus
b. Zona pellucida
c. Formative yolk
d. Follicular cells

410. The mammillothalamic tract terminates in which one of the following nuclei in the thalamus:
a. Anterior
b. Ventral lateral
c. Mediodorsal
d. Pulvinar

411. Corpora amylacea is found in:
a. Pineal
b. Prostate
c. Pituitary
d. Thyroid

412. The type of tissue that covers the surface of the body and lines vessels and body cavities is:
a. Connective tissue
b. Muscular tissue
c. Nerve tissue
d. Epithelial tissue

413. Proximal convoluted tubules develops from:
a. Mesonephric duct
b. Metanephric tubules
c. Mesonephric tubules
d. Ureteric buds

414. Which of the following is a holocrine gland?
a. Sweat gland
b. Breast
c. Pancreas
d. Sebaceous gland

415. Brunner's glands are seen:
a. Duodenum
b. Gastric
c. Gallbladder
d. Ileum

416. Through which part of internal capsule does auditory pathway pass:
a. Anterior limb
b. Posterior limb
c. Retrolentiform part
d. Sublentiform part

417. Stave cells are seen in:
a. Liver
b. Spleen
c. Pancreas
d. Gallbladder

Answers: 404. d | 405. c | 406. b | 407. a
408. c | 409. a | 410. c | 411. b
412. d | 413. b | 414. d | 415. a
416. d | 417. b

418. 4th ventricle develops from:
a. Telencephalon
b. Mesencephalon
c. Diencephalon
d. Rhombencephalon

419. In cuboidal epithelial cells, nuclei are situated:
a. Centrally
b. Apically
c. Basally
d. Eccentrically

420. Pseudociliated epithelium is a characteristic feature of mucous membrane of:
a. Liver
b. Heart
c. Trachea
d. Stomach

421. Appendix of epididymis is a remnant of:
a. Mesonephric duct
b. Paramesonephric duct
c. Mullerian duct
d. None

422. Pineal gland forms:
a. Floor of third ventricle
b. Anterior wall of third ventricle
c. Posterior wall of third ventricle
d. Roof of third ventricle

423. Diencephalon represents:
a. Lateral ventricle
b. Third ventricle
c. Fourth ventricle
d. Cerebral aqueduct

424. Nucleus ambiguus is related to all the cranial nerves, *except:*
a. 8th
b. 9th
c. 10th
d. 11th

425. In embryogenesis the blood vessels are derived from:
a. Endoderm
b. Ectoderm
c. Mesoderm
d. Mesothelium

426. Spermatogenesis takes place in the following tubules:
a. Straight tubules
b. Rete testis
c. Seminiferous tubules
d. Ductuli efferentes

427. The platysma is innervated by the which nerve:
a. Facial
b. Accessory
c. Trigeminal
d. Transverse cervical

428. Where are the parafollicular cells present:
a. Parathyroid
a. Suprarenal
b. Thyroid
c. Pancreas

429. Goblet cells are absent in which part of alimentary canal:
a. Duodenum
b. Stomach
c. Colon
d. Appendix

430. What type of muscle is arrector pilorum:
a. Skeletal
b. Smooth
c. Cardiac
d. None of these

431. An example of dense irregular connective tissue is:
a. Tendon
b. Myxomatous tissue
c. Areolar
d. Dermis

432. Nerve of 2nd pharyngeal arch is:
a. Facial
b. Glossopharyngeal
c. Vagus
d. Trigeminal

Answers:

418. d	419. a	420. c	421. a
422. c	423. b	424. a	425. c
426. c	427. a	428. c	429. a
430. b	431. d	432. d	

433. Pituitary gland develops from:
a. Telencephalon
b. Mesencephalon
c. Rathke's pouch
d. Metencephalon

434. At birth the lower end of spinal cord is at what level:
a. L1
b. L2
c. L3
d. L4

435. Derivative of midgut is:
a. Caecum
b. Stomach
c. Liver
d. Pancreas

436. Placenta previa is:
a. Abnormal attachment of chorionic villi to myometrium
b. Where umbilical cord is attached to the margin of placenta
c. Two or three incomplete lobes of placenta
d. Placenta has an abnormal implantation site

437. Down's syndrome is characterized by:
a. 19 trisomy
b. 21 trisomy
c. Only one X chromosome
d. Two X and one Y chromosome

438. The syndrome in which individual somatic cell contains three sex chromosomes XXX is called:
a. Down's syndrome
b. Super female
c. Turner's syndrome
d. Klinefelter's syndrome

439. Patau's syndrome occurs due to trisomy of:
a. 13th chromosome
b. 18th chromosome
c. 21st chromosome
d. 22nd chromosome

440. Which of the following nerves arises from the roots of the brachial plexus?
a. Dorsal scapular
b. Suprascapular nerve
c. Medial pectoral nerve
d. Nerve to subclavius

441. The nerve supply to latissimus dorsi is from the:
a. Thoracodorsal nerve
b. Axillary nerve
c. Long thoracic nerve
d. Dorsal scapular nerve

442. Which nerve endings are present in epithelium of skin:
a. Meissner's plexus
b. Paccinian
c. Krause's end bulb
d. Free nerve endings

443. The mandibular division of the trigeminal nerve exits the skull through:
a. Foramen ovale
b. Foramen lacerum
c. Foramen spinosum
d. Superior orbital fissure

444. The anterior end of neural tube forms:
a. Notochord
b. Gonads
c. Brain
d. Gut

445. Which structure does not pierce the clavipectoral fascia?
a. Cephalic vein
b. Lymphatics
c. Lateral thoracic artery
d. Lateral pectoral nerve

Answers: 433. c 434. a 435. a 436. a
437. b 438. c 439. a 440. a
441. a 442. d 443. a 444. a
445. c

446. **The median nerve lies in between two heads of which muscle?**
 a. Supinator
 b. Pronator teres
 c. Pronator quadratus
 d. Flexor digitorum superficialis

447. **What is the nerve that passes through foramen rotundum?**
 a. Olfactory
 b. Maxillary
 c. Mandibular
 d. Ophthalmic

448. **Which one of the following muscles abducts the vocal folds?**
 a. Cricothyroid
 b. Thyroarytenoid
 c. Lateral cricoarytenoid
 d. Posterior cricoarytenoid

449. **Coracoid process is a which kind of epiphysis:**
 a. Atavistic
 b. Pressure
 c. Traction
 d. Aberrant

450. **Carpal tunnel syndrome is due to compression of:**
 a. Ulnar nerve
 b. Median nerve
 c. Radial nerve
 d. Ulnar artery

451. **Which of the following structure is not supplied by left coronary artery?**
 a. SA node
 b. Posterior 1/3 of interventricular septum
 c. Left ventricle
 d. Apex of heart

452. **Which of the following structure does not form the boundary of triangle of auscultation?**
 a. Serratus anterior
 b. Scapula
 c. Trapezius
 d. Latissimus dorsi

453. **Hyaline cartilage of respiratory tree extends up to:**
 a. Tertiary bronchus
 b. Respiratory bronchiole
 c. Terminal bronchiole
 d. Bronchi

454. **Which of the following is not a tributary of azygos vein?**
 a. Right posterior intercostal vein
 b. Right superior intercostal vein
 c. Left superior intercostal vein
 d. Accessory hemiazygos vein

455. **The least dilatable part of the urethra:**
 a. Prostatic
 b. Membranous
 c. Spongy
 d. All are equally dilatable

456. **Which of the following is the example of saddle variety of synovial joint?**
 a. Knee joint
 b. Hip joint
 c. Elbow joint
 d. First carpometacarpal joint

457. **A surgeon was operating a case of cancer rectum, following areas need to be excised, *except:***
 a. Pelvic colon
 b. Anal skin
 c. Ischiorectal fossa
 d. Mesentery

458. **Following are the branches of profunda femoris artery, *except:***
 a. Lateral circumflex femoral
 b. Medial circumflex femoral
 c. Perforating
 d. Medial circumflex iliac

459. **Following cranial nerves are related to midbrain:**
 a. I, II
 b. III, IV
 c. IV, V
 d. V, VI

Answers:
446. b	447. b	448. d	449. a
450. b	451. b	452. a	453. d
454. c	455. b	456. d	457. d
458. d	459. b		

460. Which of the following possibilities is true if a woman carrying an autosomal recessive trait is married to a normal man?
a. All children affected
b. 25% children carrier
c. All children carrier
d. 50% normal and 50% carrier

461. A sudden onset of left third nerve palsy and right hemiplegia could be caused by:
a. Infarction in left internal capsule
b. Infarction in right intern capsule
c. Infarction in left half of midbrain
d. Infarction in right half of midbrain

462. The falciform process of the sacrotuberous ligament continues on the:
a. Ischial ramus
b. Lateral part of sacrum
c. Ischial spine
d. Tendon of biceps femoris

463. The fetal complement of 33 vertebrae become 24 in the adult because of:
a. Loss of vertebral bodies
b. Adhesion of upper vertebrae to skull
c. Fusion of some into composite bones
d. Shrinkage of intervertebral tissue

464. Following tendon grooves the inferior aspect of sustentaculum tali:
a. Peroneus longus
b. Flexor hallucis longus
c. Peroneus tertius
d. Flexor digitorum

465. In calcification of cartilage matrix hardens because of deposition of:
a. Calcium salts
b. Carbohydrates
c. Proteins
d. Chondroblasts

466. 'Crossing over' takes place during what stage of prophase?
a. Leptotene
b. Zygotene
c. Pachytene
d. Diplotene

467. Lesion of Brodmann's area 22 is associated with:
a. Auditory amnesia   b. Agnosia
c. Visual amnesia   d. Alexia

468. Under cover of flexor retinaculum, the tendon of flexor digitorum longus is:
a. Superior and medial to the tendon of flexor hallucis longus
b. Inferior and medial to the tendon of tibialis posterior
c. Inferior and lateral to the tendon of flexor hallucis longus
d. Superior and lateral to the tendon of tibialis posterior

469. Which of the following is not attached to lateral surface of medial condyle of femur?
a. Posterior cruciate ligament
b. Anterior cruciate ligament
c. Ligament of Humphrey
d. Ligament of Wrisberg

470. All the muscles of mastication develop from __________ branchial arch.
a. I   b. II
c. III   d. IV

Answers: 460. d   461. c   462. a   463. c
464. b   465. a   466. c   467. a
468. a   469. b   470. a

471. **Which artery gives rise to arteria radicularis magna (artery of Adamkiewicz)?**
   a. Vertebral
   b. 5th intercostal
   c. 11th intercostal
   d. 1st lumbar

472. **The vein formed near the medial malleolus and ascending up the medial side of leg is:**
   a. Posterior arch vein
   b. Medial arch vein
   c. Short saphenous vein
   d. Accessory saphenous vein

473. **Outer border of upper limb is called as:**
   a. Postaxial   b. Preaxial
   c. Medial border   d. None of above

474. **Cartilages of larynx develop from __________ pharyngeal arches.**
   a. 1st and 2nd   b. 2nd and 3rd
   c. 3rd and 4th   d. 4th and 6th

475. **Male trigger in a human embryo is first given by:**
   a. YPTER   b. XPTER
   c. SRY   d. MIF

476. **Muscle responsible for rectal continence:**
   a. Puborectalis
   b. Internal anal sphincter
   c. External anal sphincter
   d. Longitudinal muscle

477. **One of the following is not part of the neurohypophysis. Which is it?**
   a. Pars posterior
   b. Median eminence
   c. Infundibulum
   d. Pars glandularis

478. **Epigenetic influence on twins occurs:**
   a. During the neonatal period
   b. During childhood
   c. Throughout life
   d. During fourth and fifth decades of life

479. **Philtrum develops from __________**
   a. Mandibular process
   b. Medial nasal process
   c. Frontonasal process
   d. Lateral nasal process

480. **Which of the following is not attached to fibula?**
   a. Tibialis anterior
   b. Extensor hallucis longus
   c. Extensor digitorum longus
   d. Peroneus tertius

481. **The thoracic duct:**
   a. Continues as the right lymphatic duct
   b. Enters into the venous system
   c. Drains head and neck
   d. Is an arteriovenous shunt

482. **The ductus arteriosus develops from**
   a. Proximal segment of right sixth arch artery
   b. Proximal segment of left sixth arch artery
   c. Distal segment of right sixth arch artery
   d. Distal segment of left sixth arch artery

483. **Thoracic duct enters the thorax through __________ opening in the diaphragm.**
   a. Aortic
   b. Vena caval
   c. Esophageal
   d. Foramen of Morgagni

Answers: 471. c   472. a   473. b   474. d
475. c   476. a   477. d   478. c
479. c   480. a   481. b   482. d
483. a

484. All are branches from posterior cord of brachial plexus, *except:*
a. Ulnar nerve
b. Radial nerve
c. Axillary nerve
d. Thoracodorsal nerve

485. When the knee is flexed, plantar flexion is caused by:
a. Soleus alone
b. Gastrocnemius alone
c. Soleus and medial head of gastrocnemius
d. Soleus and both heads of gastrocnemius

486. Following are the uncrossed descending fibers, *except:*
a. Lateral corticospinal
b. Anterior corticospinal
c. Uncrossed lateral corticospinal
d. Vestibulospinal

487. The rectum begins in front of the following vertebra:
a. S2
b. S3
c. S4
d. S5

488. Couinaud's hepatic segment IV corresponds to:
a. Left lobe to the left of falciform ligament
b. Fossa for gallbladder
c. Caudate lobe
d. Quadrate lobe

489. Which of the following is not a fibrous joint?
a. Schindylesis
b. Symphysis
c. Gomphosis
d. Syndesmosis

490. What is false about axillary artery:
a. It is a continuation of subclavian artery
b. It is crossed by pectoralis minor
c. It is accompanied by axillary vein only in its distal third
d. It gives out the superior thoracic artery from its first part

491. The superficial lymphatic plexus of the lungs is otherwise called the:
a. Subvisceral plexus
b. Parenchymal plexus
c. Subliminal plexus
d. Subpleural plexus

492. The skin overlying the thenar eminence is supplied by:
a. Recurrent branch of median nerve
b. Palmar cutaneous branch of ulnar nerve
c. Palmar cutaneous branch of median nerve
d. Lateral proper digital branch of median nerve

493. The germinal epithelium of ovary:
a. Produces new germ cells
b. Produces ovarian stroma
c. Is continuous with peritoneum
d. Develops from endoderm

494. The vocal process is a part of:
a. Thyroid cartilage
b. Cricoid cartilage
c. Arytenoid cartilage
d. Epiglottis

Answers:

484. a	485. a	486. a	487. b
488. a	489. b	490. c	491. d
492. c	493. c	494. c	

495. **Which of the following statement is false?**
a. The trochlear articular surface on the talus is for articulation with tibia
b. The anterior tuberosity of the calcaneum is an extension of the lateral process of calcaneal tuberosity
c. The medial projecting aspect of the navicular bone is its tuberosity
d. Intermediate cuneiform is the smallest of the cuneiform group

496. **Why is the superior thoracic aperture called the thoracic outlet?**
a. Because air and food passages enter through this opening
b. Because it is often involved in thoracic outlet disease
c. Because important vessels and nerves emerge out of this aperture
d. It is the largest of the thoracic openings

497. **Juxtaglomerular cells are modified cells of following structure:**
a. Distal tubule
b. Afferent arteriole
c. Efferent arteriole
d. Proximal tubule

498. **Which of the following is not a derivative of the vitelline vein?**
a. Lower inferior vena cava
b. Inferior mesenteric vein
c. Superior mesenteric vein
d. Portal vein

499. **Which of the following veins pierces the fascial roof of posterior triangle?**
a. External jugular
b. Subclavian
c. Transverse cervical
d. Suprascapular

Answers: 495. **b** 496. **c** 497. **b** 498. **b**
499. **a**

2 Physiology

HOMEOSTASIS

Cell

The basic unit of living things is cell.

Some of the facts related to cells are as under:

- Humans are multicellular
- **Functions:** Several basic functions of all cells are to:
  - Obtain nutrients and O_2
  - Make energy, food $+ O_2 \rightarrow CO_2 + H_2O +$ energy
  - Eliminate wastes
  - Synthesize needed molecules
  - Respond to environmental changes
  - Control exchange of materials with the environment
  - Transport molecules
  - Reproduce
- In multicellular organisms, cells specialize to form tissue.

Tissues

It is a group of cells with similar structure and function.

Four major types are as follows:

Muscle

- Specialized in contraction and force generation
- **Skeletal:** Movement of body or body parts
- **Cardiac:** Pumps blood
- **Smooth:** Movement of organs

Epithelium

- Specialized for exchange between cell and the environment
- 2 general types—sheets and secretory glands
- Sheets are tightly joined cells covering or lining parts of the body
- Glands secrete products (exocrine glands have ducts leading to a body surface, e.g., sweat glands; endocrine glands release products to interstitial fluid and it goes into blood, e.g., adrenal glands)

Nervous Tissue

- Specialized for initiating and transmitting electrical impulses
- Brain, spinal cord, nerves

Connective Tissue

- Specialized for connecting and supporting
- Found all over body

Organs

It is a group of two or more tissues designed to perform specific functions.

Body System (Organ System)

It is a group of organs designed to perform particular functions.

Whole Organism

It is a group of organ systems.

Introduction and Overview

Homeostasis is a dynamic equilibrium where body conditions are maintained within narrow limits, necessary for each cell to survive. Each cell contributes, and all cells are in contact with an aqueous (watery) internal environment that connects all cells, and exchanges are made outside and inside the body.

Extracellular fluid: Comprised of:
- Plasma (fluid in the blood)
- Interstitial fluid (surrounding cells)

Major factors that maintain the homeostasis are:
- **The concentration of nutrient molecules:** Cells need energy and building blocks
- **Concentration of O_2 and CO_2**
  - O_2 is used to make usable energy (ATP)
  - CO_2 made must be removed
- **The concentration of waste products:** Become toxic at high levels
- **pH:** Acidity affects enzyme reactions and nerve cell impulses
- **Concentration of water, salt and other for electrolytes for:**
  - Maintaining cell volume
  - Various functions of electrolytes
- **Temperature:** Too cold or too much heat harmful to cells
- **Volume and pressure:** Blood must be at an appropriate volume and pressure to be transported around the body

Major Organ Systems

Control mechanisms: Body is controlled mainly by the nervous and endocrine systems. The parts of a control system (all interdependent) are:

Sensor
- Monitors variable (factor being regulated)
- Responds to changes (stimuli) by sending input to control system/integrator.

Integrator
- Determines the set point (an appropriate level of variable)
- Compares set point to input
- Sends the response to the effector

Effector
Responds to changes

Most of the control systems operate using negative feedback to:
- Decreases or shuts off the original stimulus
- Resists change

Positive feedback helps to:
- Enhances original stimulus
- Uterine contractions during childbirth
- Blood clotting

CELL PHYSIOLOGY

Cell Basics

A typical human cell is 10–20 µm in diameter. Cells have three major subdivisions:

Plasma Membrane (Cell Membrane)
Defines inside/outside of the cell and comprised of:
- **Intracellular fluid (ICF):** Inside cell
- **Extracellular fluid (ECF):** Outside cell
- **Selectively permeable:** Controls movement of molecules between ICF and ECF

Nucleus
- Usually near center of the cell.
- It is double layered membrane.
- Contains DNA, "genetic blueprint," directs protein synthesis, control center of cell.

Cytoplasm
- It is an area between nucleus and plasma membrane
- Contains organelles that
  - Help in chemical reactions
  - Are specialized for a particular function
- Cytosol is semiliquid, site of chemical reactions

Organelles

Endoplasmic Reticulum (ER)
- It is an interconnected fluid-filled membranous system.

○ It is of two types:
  ○ **Smooth:** Interconnected tubules
  ○ **Rough:** Interconnected flattened sacs

Rough ER

○ Synthesizes proteins and lipids, releases them to ER in the lumen.
○ Some will be secreted from the cell (hormones, enzymes), some will become new membranes for the cell or its organelles, or other protein parts of organelles.
○ Once in the lumen, the protein can be modified.

Smooth ER

○ In most cells, it packages and transports products of rough ER (sections pinch off and become transport vesicles; move to Golgi complex).
○ Some cells have extensive specialized smooth ER
○ The functions of smooth ER are:
  ○ Lipid synthesis (steroid hormone-secreting cells)
  ○ Detoxify harmful substances (liver cells)
  ○ Store calcium (muscle cells)

Golgi Complex

○ It is composed of layers of flattened membranous sacs (cisternae)
○ It helps to process ER products into the final form
○ It sorts and sends products to the appropriate place
○ It helps to transport vesicles (contain products) to locations in or outside the cell or various destinations, such as lysosomes, plasma membrane or secretion

Lysosomes

○ It is a membranous sac containing hydrolytic enzymes

○ It digests cellular debris and other substances (old organelles, bacteria). Material from outside the cell can be brought into digested by lysosome by a process of:
  ○ Endocytosis (membrane surrounds substance and vesicle pinches off)
  ○ Pinocytosis: Fluids, "cell drinking" or
  ○ Phagocytosis: Large particles, "cell eating" cells can use digested material.

Peroxisomes

○ It is a membranous sac containing oxidative enzymes to carry out oxidative reactions.
○ They also help in lipid production.
○ They also convert reactive oxygen species like hydrogen peroxide to safer molecules like oxygen and water with the help of catalases.

Mitochondria

○ It has a double membrane. The inner membrane has folds called cristae (folds increase surface area), and the inside matrix is gel-like.
○ It plays a role in apoptosis (programmed cell death)
○ It converts energy from food into usable energy for the cell—ATP (adenosine triphosphate)
  ○ Energy in chemical bonds of food molecules cannot be used directly
  ○ ATP → ADP + Pi + useful energy
○ Three major steps in forming ATP (called cellular respiration) are glycolysis, citric acid cycle and oxidative phosphorylation as discussed under:

Glycolysis

○ It occurs in cytosol
○ Glucose → 2 pyruvic acid (a series of steps)
○ Yields 2 ATP/glucose
○ Attach H to carrier molecules

Citric Acid Cycle (Also called Krebs Cycle or Tricarboxylic Acid Cycle)

- Pyruvic acid is transported to the mitochondrial matrix
- Pyruvic acid → acetyl CoA
- Acetyl CoA enters the citric acid cycle, which is a series of reactions
- CO_2 is produced
- Hydrogen atoms are attached to carrier molecules (NAD$^+$, nicotinamide adenine dinucleotide; FAD, flavine adenine dinucleotide; become NADH and FADH$_2$)
- 2 more ATP/original glucose

Electron Transport Chain/Oxidative Phosphorylation

- Occurs on the inner mitochondrial membrane, which contains electron carrier molecules (each H contains one electron; moving electrons means moving energy).
- NADH and FADH$_2$ from glycolysis and citric acid cycle enter the chain, and the electron is removed from each H and passed through the series of electron carriers in the membrane, finally ending up on O_2 (the final electron acceptor).
- The energy from the electrons is used to transport H$^+$ (across the inner membrane; this creates a concentration gradient—more H$^+$ on one side of the membrane than the other—so H$^+$ will flow back across the inner membrane.
- H$^+$ can only flow back across at certain points—it flows through channels that contain ATP synthase (the enzyme that makes ATP)
- Yields 28 ATP/original glucose
- Steps 3 and 4 are known as the chemiosmotic mechanism (chemical reaction coupled to the flow of a substance across a membrane)
- Because O_2 is used to make ATP, it is called oxidative phosphorylation

(Glycolysis can happen anaerobically—without O_2—but this alone is not very efficient)

Cytosol

- Constitutes 55% of cell volume
- Composition varies in different areas of the cell
- Involved in several kinds of cell activities such as:

Enzymatic regulation of intermediary metabolism

- Chemical reactions involving synthesizing and breaking down small organic molecules (e.g., sugars, amino acids, fatty acids).
- Provides raw material for structure and function.

Ribosome protein synthesis: Free ribosomes make enzymes for use in cytosol.

Storage of fat and glycogen (stored form of glucose)

- **Inclusions:** Masses of stored nutrients.
- Can be broken down when needed to make ATP.

Cytoskeleton

- Complex protein network running through cytosol that helps to:
  - Supports and organizes parts of a cell
  - Controls movements of cell and within a cell
- **It has three parts:** Microtubule, microfilaments and intermediate filaments

Microtubules

- It is the largest of cytoskeletal parts and is made mostly of the protein tubulin.
- It maintains the shape of a cell.
- It helps in the transport of vesicles.
- It contains special motor proteins (e.g., kinesin) attached to vesicles and microtubules, pulling vesicles along.
- It helps in the movement of cilia and flagella.

- ○ Cilia are shorter, hairlike, and many on a single cell; move substances across the surface of cell (respiratory tract, oviduct)
- ○ Flagella are long, one per human cell; move whole cell (sperm)
- ○ Both have the same basic structure of grouped microtubules; movement is produced when a motor protein (dynein) displaces tubules relative to one another
- ○ It is involved in the formation of the mitotic spindle, formed during mitosis (division of nucleus) and directs the movement of chromosomes (DNA).

Microfilaments

- ○ One of the smaller elements of the cytoskeleton
- ○ Many of these are made of the protein actin
- ○ It is involved in cellular contractile systems such as:
  - ○ Muscle cells
  - ○ **Contractile ring that divides a cell:** Pinches cell together and separates halves
  - ○ **Amoeboid movement:** Some cells can alternately form and break down actin filaments to move the whole cell (e.g., white blood cells)
  - ○ Provide mechanical support to the cell.
  - ○ **Support microvilli:** Extensions of cytoplasm important for increasing the surface area of cell

Intermediate Filaments

- ○ These are medium-sized and are made of different proteins depending on the cell.
- ○ They are very stable in comparison to other cytoskeletal elements.
- ○ They strengthen and stabilize cells.
- ○ They hold together contractile units in muscle cells.
- ○ Elements of the cytoskeleton are interconnected to support and provide rigidity and shape to the cell.

- ○ Organizes groups of enzymes to direct transport and movement

PLASMA MEMBRANE AND MEMBRANE POTENTIAL

Basics

The plasma membrane is selectively permeable, i.e., it controls what gets in and out of the cell.

Membrane Structure

The plasma membrane structure comprises phospholipids, cholesterol, protein, and carbohydrates.

Phospholipids

- ○ Basic membrane structure is a phospholipid bilayer having:
  - ○ Hydrophilic (water-loving) heads are polar, face outward toward water
  - ○ Hydrophobic (water-fearing) tails are nonpolar, face inward away from water
- ○ **Act as barrier to diffusion:** Stops water-soluble molecules from passing through
- ○ It is responsible for membrane fluidity

Cholesterol

- ○ It is located between phospholipids
- ○ Contributes to fluidity and stability

Proteins

- ○ Some span the membrane, acting as a selective channel to transport substances across the membrane (e.g., ions). Carrier proteins also transport specific molecules across the membrane
- ○ Some are on one side of the membrane, as discussed under
  - ○ **Receptors:** Bind with molecules on the outer surface and initiate changes in a cell.
  - ○ **Membrane-bound enzymes:** Chemical reactions at the inner or outer membrane surface

○ Filamentous meshwork on the inner side binds with the cytoskeleton to maintain cell shape and for movement

○ **Cell adhesion molecules (CAMs):** Stick out from the outer surface and secure cell to other cells (cadherins "zip" cells together in tissues/organs), also cell communication (growth, defense responses), integrins span the membrane and link cytoskeleton to the external environment and relay regulatory signals

○ Some allow cells to recognize "self" and interact with one another (often glycoproteins)

Carbohydrates

○ Are present on the outer surface, bound to membrane proteins and lipids (glycoproteins, glycolipids)

○ Important in the recognition of cells of the same type and tissue organization.

○ Involved in tissue growth

This structure is known as a fluid mosaic model.

Functions of Plasma Membrane

1. Cell-to-cell Adhesions

○ Carbohydrates on the membrane surface help arrange cells into groups, which are held together in various ways:

  ○ CAMs

  ○ Extracellular matrix (connective tissues) Cells may not be joined directly to other cells but embedded in a matrix of carbohydrates and protein fibers, such as:

Collagen: Resists tension (e.g., skin)

Elastin: Stretch and recoil (e.g., skin, lungs)

Fibronectin: Holds cells in position (all over body)

  ○ Specialised junctions like:

    ➤ **Desmosomes:** Cells join at particular spots, found all over the body, particularly where stretch occurs (e.g., skin, muscle).

➤ **Tight junctions:** Impermeable barrier, common in epithelial sheets where they prevent leakage.

➤ **Gap junctions:** Cells linked by protein tunnels, allow small molecule to pass between cells, important in some cells that transmit electrical activity (e.g., cardiac muscle).

2. Membrane Transport

Two important factors influencing transport are solubility of the substance in lipid and size of the substance

○ Small, uncharged or nonpolar molecules move through lipid bilayer (e.g., O_2, CO_2, fatty acids)

○ Ions and small polar molecules (like glucose) can move through channels or by carrier proteins if the right transporter exists.

○ Substances too big or without a special protein transporter need special mechanisms to get through the membrane.

Types of Transport

Transport (No ATP is used)

○ **Diffusion:** Molecules move down their concentration gradient (greater to lesser concentration), charged particles move down electrochemical gradients.

Types of diffusion

○ **Simple diffusion:** Substance moves through lipid bilayer or protein channels (e.g., O_2, CO_2, some ions)

○ **Osmosis:** Water moves down its concentration gradient

○ Facilitated diffusion uses a carrier protein that binds to the molecule to be transported and brings it to the other side of the membrane (e.g., glucose)

○ **Filtration:** Water and solutes forced through the membrane by pressure (e.g., in kidneys)

Active Transport (ATP is Used)

The carrier proteins transport substance against its concentrating gradient (needs ATP to change conformation)

- **Primary active transport:** Energy from ATP used directly to transport a substance (e.g., Na^+-K^+ pump, in all cells)
- **Secondary active transport:** Driven by gradients set up by primary active transport, e.g., in the digestive tract, glucose and amino acids are "dragged along" with Na^+ diffusing into cell (Na^+ gradient set up by Na^+-K^+ pump)
- **Vesicular transport (bulk transport):** Large molecules or multimolecular substances enclosed in pieces of membrane as in:
  - **Endocytosis (pino/phagocytosis):** Where lysosomes break down the substance and release the products into the cell. Vesicle travels to the opposite side of the cell and release the contents.
  - **Exocytosis:** Large polar molecules like hormones and enzymes are secreted.

3. Intercellular Communication and Signal Transduction

Cells must communicate so they can coordinate their activities (maintain homeostasis, control growth and development).

Types of Intercellular Communication

- **Gap junctions**
  - Small molecules and ions directly exchange between cells
  - Important in the spread of electrical signals (cardiac and smooth muscle, very rarely neurons)
- **Signal molecules on the cell surface allow direct interaction:** Phagocytes (body defense cells) recognize and kill invading cells
- **Chemical messengers**
  - A specific chemical is made by special cells that acts on target cells, which then respond appropriately
  - It is of four types:
    - **Paracrine:** Act locally (e.g., histamine in inflammatory response)
    - **Neurotransmitters:** Act locally; nerve cells release them to other nerve cells, muscles, or glands
    - **Hormones:** Acts over long distances, released into the blood by endocrine glands
    - **Neurohormones:** Act over long distances, released into the blood by special nerve cells (neurosecretory neurons)

Pathway of Chemical Messengers

It is explained in the following steps:

Binding

- Specialized protein receptors on the plasma membrane bind with a particular messenger to trigger a sequence of events that control a particular cell activity. The response is elicited in three ways:
  - Opening (most commonly) or closing chemically-gated receptor channels in the membrane (regulates the movement of ions in/out of the cell)
  - Activating receptor—enzymes
  - Transferring a signal to the second messenger (an intracellular chemical messenger), which initiates a series of events inside the cell

Channel Regulation

- Channel proteins can change shape and thus open/close (act like gates).
- Receptor binding site is part of the channel, and messenger binds $\rightarrow$ channel opens, e.g., neurotransmitters trigger movement of Na^+, K^+, or both across the membrane, which changes the electrical activity of cell (muscle and nerve cells).

Tyrosine Kinase Pathway

○ Messenger binds and activates a receptor enzyme (usually protein kinase that phosphorylates another protein)
○ Typically, a cascade is initiated, which ultimately activates a particular protein that brings about the response, e.g., insulin and growth factors

Second Messenger Systems (Most Common Pathway)

Second messenger pathway includes:
○ cAMP pathway
○ Ca²⁺ pathway

The general steps of second messenger pathway are as under:

Messenger binds to receptor (G-protein-coupled receptor)
↓
Enzyme on cytoplasmic side of membrane activated by G-protein
↓
Intracellular second messengers are activated, and diffuse through the cell to trigger appropriate response
↓
Typically a cascade is initiated and response accomplished by altering structure/function of particular proteins

cAMP Pathway (Cyclic Adenosine Monophosphate, Most Common)

Messenger binds to a receptor
↓
Activates G protein which activates adenylyl cyclase (on cytoplasmic side of membrane)
↓
ATP → cAMP, which diffuses through cell
↓
cAMP-dependent protein kinase activated, then phosphorylates a particular intracellular protein (this changes the protein's shape/function, bringing about the appropriate response)
↓
Can switch cellular processes on or off, e.g., heart rate changes, formation of sex hormones in typical female, breakdown of stored glucose in liver, water conservation in kidneys

Ca²⁺ Pathway

Messenger binds to a receptor
↓
Activates G protein which activates phospholipase C (on cytoplasmic side of membrane)
↓
$PIP_2 \rightarrow DAG + IP_3$
↓
IP_3 increases Ca^{2+} in cytosol (from stores in ER), Ca^{2+} diffuses. Through cell and binds to the protein calmodulin, which in turn activates another protein, bringing about the appropriate response

○ This pathway is important in cell movement, such as smooth muscle contraction.
○ **Very low concentrations of first messengers trigger large responses:** One messenger molecule can result in millions of product molecules.
○ Receptors can be regulated (number, affinity for messenger)

Apoptosis

Apoptosis is a programmed cell death that comes in function during:
○ Development
○ Tissue turnover
○ Immune system (infected cells and worn-out phagocytes)
○ Old, damaged or mutated cells

Membrane Potential

Membrane potential is maintained due to the separation of charges across a membrane as separated charges have the potential to do work—electrical and force of attraction can be harnessed.

It is measured in millivolts (mV). More the charges separated, greater the potential.

All plasma membranes have potential due to:
○ Unequal distribution of a few key ions involved, like:
○ Na^+
○ K^+
○ A^- (large anionic intracellular proteins)

○ Na⁺-K⁺ pump: It is responsible both directly and indirectly for establishing membrane potential.

Directly, it generates about 20% of potential (4 mv), explained as under

It actively transports 3 Na⁺ out for every 2 K⁺ in in order to:
- ○ Leave cell slightly negative inside
- ○ Establish concentration gradients (Na⁺ high outside, K⁺ high inside)
- ○ Passively, Na⁺ → in, K⁺ → out

Indirectly, it generates other 80% of membrane potential as under
- ○ Membrane is more permeable to K⁺ than to Na⁺ (more K⁺ channels open)
- ○ K⁺ will passively flow out, increasing membrane potential.
- ○ K⁺ flows out until the concentration gradient is balanced by the electrical gradient (negative charges inside attract K⁺)
- ○ Very little Na⁺ leaks back in (closed channels), leading to resting membrane potential of –70 mV in a typical nerve cell (sign means more negative inside)

○ **Other effects**
- ○ A⁻ cannot leave the cell (too large), which contributes to negative charges that balance the leakage of K⁺ out of cell.
- ○ Cl⁻ distribution influenced by membrane potential
- ○ High outside
- ○ Negative charge inside cell drives Cl⁻ out (cells permeable to Cl⁻, but most do not actively transport it)

Importance of Membrane Potential

○ Altering membrane potential results in nerve impulses and muscle contraction
○ May be involved in activity of secretory cells
○ Significance in other cells not understood

NEURONAL PHYSIOLOGY

Definitions

○ **Excitable tissues:** Capable of producing electrical signals (transient, rapid changes in membrane potential) in nerve and muscle.
○ **Resting membrane potential (RMP):** The membrane potential that exists when no net changes in potential are occurring.
○ **Graded potentials:** Local changes in membrane potential that vary in magnitude (flow of ions).
○ **Action potentials:** Brief, rapid reversals in membrane potential, which can spread throughout the membrane (flow of ions).
○ **Voltage-gated channels:** Membrane channels that open or close in response to changes in potential.
○ **Polarization:** A membrane that has the potential that is polarized.
○ **Depolarization:** A decrease in membrane potential (inside becomes more positive).
○ **Triggering event:** Event that initiates a depolarization (stimulus like light or touch, chemical messenger).
○ **Hyperpolarization:** An increase in membrane potential (inside becomes more negative).
○ **Repolarization:** Return to resting potential after a depolarization.

Graded Potentials

The magnitude of graded potential is related to:
○ The magnitude of the triggering event: Stronger trigger → greater magnitude of change in potential
○ Current flow (movement of charges)

When a graded potential occurs, a piece of the membrane (called the active area) has a different potential than the rest of the membrane. Inactive area of the membrane is called as the resting potential.

○ Current flows between the active area and adjacent inactive areas (opposite charges attract)

○ Previously inactive areas become active, and more current flow occurs

○ Spread of graded potential is decremental, i.e., it decreases as it moves along the membrane causing current to leak into ECF that function as signals over short distances

Action Potentials (AP) (Fig. 1.1)

It can be transmitted over long distances without losing strength.

The steps of action potential are discussed as under:

Depolarization

○ Triggering event causes depolarization to occur relatively slowly until threshold potential is reached (about –50 to –55 mV).

○ Once a threshold is reached, the membrane quickly depolarizes to +30 mV.

○ When the triggering event begins depolarization, some of the voltage-gated Na^+ channels open, and Na^+ flows into a cell (proteins that make up the channel have charged portions; shape change occurs as those charges interact with charges surrounding the membrane).

○ This further depolarizes the membrane, causing even more Na^+ channels to open.

○ At the threshold, all the Na^+ channels are open, and there is an explosive increase in Na^+ permeability (P Na^+).

○ At peak depolarization, the Na^+ channels close (the channel is constructed so that the same depolarization that opens them also closes them).

Repolarization Begins

○ As Na^+ channels close, K^+ channels open (K^+ increases) due to delayed voltage-gated response to the depolarization, K^+ flows out of the cell

○ This restores internal negativity as repolarization progresses Na channels resume original conformation (closed but capable of opening). Newly opened K channels close

○ Na^+ channels resume original conformation (closed but capable of opening)

○ Newly opened K^+ channels close

○ Hyperpolarization occurs before channels close (membrane even more negative than at resting potential)

○ Resting potential restored

Action potential lasts about 1 millisecond.

Neuron (Nerve Cell)

The three basic parts of neurons (**Fig. 1.2**) are:
1. Cell body
2. Dendrites
3. Axon

Cell Body

○ Houses nucleus and organelles

○ Receives signals from other cells (contains receptors for chemical messengers)

Dendrites

○ Projections from the cell body

○ Increase surface area for receiving signals

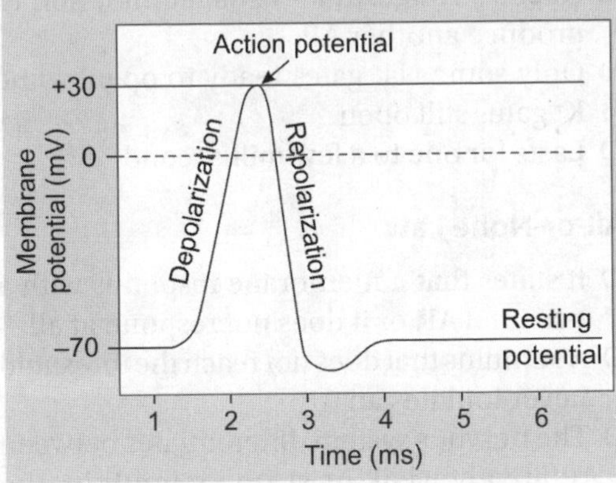

Fig. 1.1: Action potential graph.

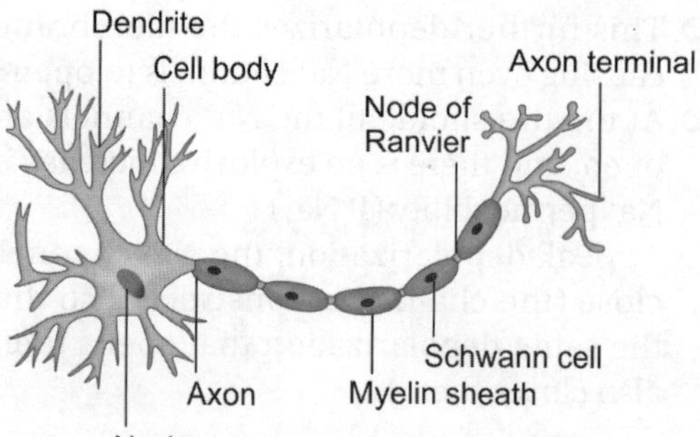

Fig. 1.2: Structure of a neuron.

Axon (Nerve Fiber)

- Single elongated projection
- Conducts APs away from cell body
- Often has collaterals (side branches)
- Axon hillock (part of cell body and first part of axon) is area where APs generated in most neurons.
- Ends in branches called axon terminals that release chemical messengers.
- May be less than a mm or more than a meter.

Propagation of an AP

It is the conduction by local current flow (contiguous conduction).

- AP propagates as a wave along the axon and is generated at the axon hillock.
- Local current flow between this active area and adjacent inactive area causes new AP.

Saltatory Conduction

- It is the propagation of AP that occurs in myelinated fibers from one node of Ranvier to the next node. There is rapid and efficient transmission of electrical signals along myelinated axons.
- Myelin sheath is formed by oligodendrocytes in central nervous system (CNS), by Schwann cells in peripheral nervous system (PNS).
- The myelin sheath acts as an electrical insulator, preventing the leakage of ions and electrical signals from the axon.

- **Nodes of Ranvier:** Between successive segments of myelin sheath are small gaps or exposed regions of the axon known as nodes of Ranvier. At these nodes, the axonal membrane is exposed and contains a high concentration of ion channels.
- Fiber diameter influences speed of propagation.
- Larger fiber diameter → faster conduction
- Large myelinated fibers found in areas where information must be transmitted quickly (e.g., fibers innervating skeletal muscle).
- Smaller unmyelinated fibers found in areas where speed not critical to function (e.g., fibers innervating digestive tract).

Refractory Period

- It ensures APs propagated in only one direction
- **It is of two types:** Absolute refractory period and relative refractory period

Absolute Refractory Period

- No amount of stimulation will induce another AP
- Time between when Na^+ gates first opened and when they are in their "ready to open" conformation

Relative Refractory Period

- Needs stronger than usual stimulation to produce another AP
- Only some Na^+ gates ready to open, some K^+ gates still open
- Lasts for one to a few millisecond

All-or-None Law

- It states that a membrane responds with a maximal AP, or it does not respond at all.
- A stimulus that does not reach the threshold never initiates an AP.
- The nervous system differentiates between relatively weak or strong stimuli by the frequency of APs.
- Stronger stimuli → more APs/sec.

Synapse

- It is junction between the axon terminal of one neuron and the dendrites or cell body of the next neuron.
- Most neurons have thousands of synaptic inputs.
- **Anatomy of a synapse:** Synapse is comprised of presynaptic neuron, post-synaptic neuron and synaptic cleft.

Presynaptic Neuron

- Conducts APs toward synapse.
- Ends in swelling called synaptic knob, which contains synaptic vesicles that store a specific neurotransmitter.

Postsynaptic Neuron

- Conducts APs away from synapse.
- Portion at synapse called subsynaptic membrane.

Synaptic Cleft

- Space between pre- and post-synaptic neurons.
- Generally operates in one direction (changes in membrane potential in presynaptic neuron bring changes in membrane potential of a postsynaptic neuron).

Synapse Function

The function of synapse is explained schematically in **Flowchart 2.1**.

Flowchart 2.1: Function of synapse.

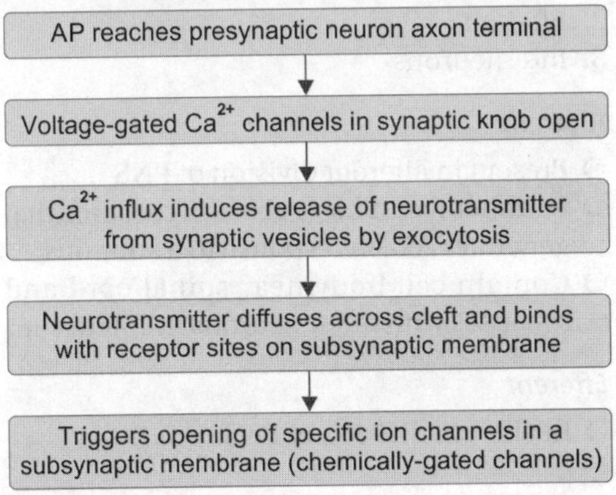

AP reaches presynaptic neuron axon terminal

↓

Voltage-gated Ca^{2+} channels in synaptic knob open

↓

Ca^{2+} influx induces release of neurotransmitter from synaptic vesicles by exocytosis

↓

Neurotransmitter diffuses across cleft and binds with receptor sites on subsynaptic membrane

↓

Triggers opening of specific ion channels in a subsynaptic membrane (chemically-gated channels)

Types of Synapses

- Excitatory synapse
  - Na^+ and K^+ channels open
  - Net movement of Na^+ inside
  - Results in small depolarization called an excitatory postsynaptic potential (EPSP), a kind of graded potential
  - Takes many EPSPs to bring the membrane to a threshold and generate an AP (each one brings the membrane closer to the threshold)
- Inhibitory synapse
  - Opens channels for K^+ or Cl^-
  - $K^+ \rightarrow$ out, or $Cl^- \rightarrow$ in
  - Results in small hyperpolarization called an inhibitory postsynaptic potential (IPSP)
  - Each IPSP moves the membrane further away from the threshold
- A given synapse is either always excitatory or always inhibitory
- The same neurotransmitter is generally released at a given synapse
- Some are always excitatory
- Some are always inhibitory
- Some produce an IPSP at one synapse and an EPSP at another synapse

Synaptic Delay

- Time taken for signal to cross synapse (0.5–1 msec)
- The more synapses a signal must cross, the longer the time needed for response to occur (total reaction time)

Removal of Neurotransmitter from the Synaptic Cleft

- As long as the neurotransmitter is bound to receptor, IPSP or EPSP continues
- It is removed from synapse by the following ways:
  - Diffuses away from synaptic cleft
  - Inactivated by enzymes in subsynaptic membrane
  - Actively transported back to presynaptic neuron

Neurotransmitters and Second Messenger Systems

- Most neurotransmitters change the conformation of chemically-gated channels
- Some use second messenger systems (cAMP), which work in short-term and long-term changes like memory

Grand Postsynaptic Potentials (GPSP)

- Composite of all EPSPs and IPSPs occurring on a cell at the same time
- Temporal summation is the summation of potentials occurring very close together in time from the same synaptic input
- Spatial summation is the summation of potentials from many different synaptic inputs at the same time

Classical Neurotransmitters and Neuropeptides

Classical Neurotransmitters

- Small, fast-acting
- Made in axon terminal
- Amino acids or related compounds

Neuropeptides

- Large (many amino acids)
- Made in cell body, stored in dense-core vesicles in the axon terminal
- One or more may be released along with a classical neurotransmitter
- Some act like classical neurotransmitter
- Most are neuromodulators
  - Do not cause EPSPs/IPSPs
  - Cause long-term changes in synapse
  - Often use second messenger systems

Convergence and Divergence

- In convergence, a single neuron is influenced by many other neurons synapsing on it
- In divergence a single neuron influences many other neurons

CENTRAL NERVOUS SYSTEM

Introduction

- CNS contain specific pathways for the transmission of signals between areas of the body
- In general, coordinates rapid, precise responses and interacts with the endocrine system ("wireless")

Organization of the Nervous System

- **Central nervous system (CNS):** Brain and spinal cord
- **Peripheral nervous system (PNS)**
  - Nerve fibers carry information between CNS and rest of the body
  - **Afferent (sensory) division:** Carries information toward CNS
  - **Efferent (motor) division:**
    - ➤ Carries information away from CNS to effector organs (muscles, glands)
    - ➤ Somatic nervous system: Motor neurons supplying muscles
    - ➤ Autonomic nervous system (innervates smooth and cardiac muscle, glands, sympathetic division, "fight or flight", parasympathetic division, "resting and digesting")

Classes of Neurons

Neurons are divided into three types as listed below:
1. Afferent
2. Efferent
3. Interneurons

Afferent

- Present in afferent division of PNS
- Peripheral end has a sensory receptor that generates APs in response to a stimulus
- Contain cell body near spinal cord and synapses with other neurons in spinal cord

Efferent

- In efferent division of PNS

○ Cell body in CNS
○ Terminates at a muscle or gland

Interneurons (Most Neurons)

○ In CNS, between afferent and efferent neurons
○ Interconnect with one another

Protection/Nourishment of the Brain

The protection or nourishment of the brain is done by:
○ Glial cells
○ Blood-brain barrier
○ CSF
○ Meninges
○ Bones

Glial Cells (Neuroglia)

○ Astrocytes:
  ○ Hold neurons together
  ○ Helps in repair of injury and scar formation
  ○ Induce changes in blood vessels (blood-brain barrier) and participate in transport across the barrier
  ○ Take up and break down some neurotransmitter (glutamate, GABA), take up excess K^+ in ECF
  ○ Enhance synapse formation and modify function, physical and chemical influences
  ○ Communicate with each other and neurons via gap junctions, neurotransmitters and other chemicals
○ Oligodendrocytes: Forms myelin sheath
○ Ependymal cells:
  ○ Line internal cavities of CNS (ventricles of brain, central canal of spinal cord)
  ○ Help to form cerebrospinal fluid (CSF)
  ○ Serve as stem cells in some areas of the brain
○ Microglia
  ○ Defense cells, role in phagocytosis
  ○ Secrete nerve cell growth factor

Blood-Brain Barrier

○ Capillaries in the brain have tight junctions joining cells to allow passage of lipid-soluble substances, e.g., O_2, CO_2, alcohol, steroid hormones and substances with specific carriers e.g., glucose, amino acids, ions).
○ Protects the brain from harmful substances.
○ Keeps out circulating hormones that act like neurotransmitters.

Cerebrospinal Fluid

○ Formed by choroid plexuses, surrounding brain and spinal cord.
○ Cushions CNS.
○ It is the interstitial fluid of the CNS and directly contacts CNS cells, and exchanges take place.
○ It is similar to plasma, but lower in K^+ and higher in Na^+.

Meninges: Connective Tissue Membranes

○ Dura mater is the outer layer that forms dural sinuses and venous sinuses (blood and CSF pool, return to circulation)
○ Arachnoid mater is the middle layer comprising of subarachnoid space that contains CSF and arachnoid villi to reabsorb CSF (return to blood in sinuses)
○ Pia mater is the inner layer, is well vascularized and important in forming CSF.
○ ***Bones offer physical protection***
  ○ **Cranium (skull):** Brain
  ○ **Vertebral column:** Spinal cord

Brain Structure

Cerebrum

○ Cortex is outer layer of gray matter (neuron cell bodies and dendrites, glial cells).
○ Underneath is white matter (tracts of myelinated fibers), which transmits signals between cortical areas, and to other CNS locations.

- Divided into functional areas (some degree of overlap) specialized for particular activities, but no area acts alone
- Contains two hemispheres, connected by corpus callosum
- Most functional areas occur in both hemispheres (except language areas)
- Some degree of specialization are as under
  - **Left:** Logical, analytical tasks like language, math; fine motor control
  - **Right:** Nonlanguage skills like spatial perception and art/music
- Generally involved in functions of opposite sides of body (contralateral)

Functional Area of the Brain

- Functional areas often contained within a lobe
- Three kinds of functional areas
  1. **Motor areas:** Control voluntary motor functions
  2. **Sensory areas:** Conscious awareness of sensation
  3. **Association areas:** Integrate diverse information

Selected Functional Areas

Primary Visual Cortex

- Receives visual information
- Surrounding higher-order visual cortex interprets

Primary Auditory Cortex

- Receives information on sound
- Surrounding higher-order auditory cortex interprets

Somatosensory Cortex

- Receives sensory input (somesthetic sensations from skin like touch, temperature and proprioception, etc.)
- Localizes source of input, perceives intensity of stimulus, capable of spatial discrimination

- **Sensory homunculus:** A particular region of the brain receives information from a certain part of the body

Posterior Parietal Cortex

- Integrates somatosensory and visual input
- Important in complex movement

Primary Motor Cortex

- Voluntary control of skeletal muscle
- **Motor homunculus:** Neurons controlling a particular body part tend to be grouped together

Supplementary Motor Area

Helps prepare "programs" for complex patterns of movement.

Premotor Cortex

- Plans movement based on body orientation, coordination of complex movements
- Interacts with posterior parietal cortex

Language Areas: Broca's Area, Wernicke's Area

- **Broca's area:** Important in ability to speak—interacts with motor areas for speech
- **Wernicke's area:** Important in language comprehension (written and spoken) and patterns of speech
- Broca's and Wernicke's usually in left hemisphere only, right side has affective language areas, which express and comprehend emotion in speech

Prefrontal Association Cortex

- Plans for voluntary activities
- Weighing consequences, making choices
- Personality
- Complex learning, intellect (cognition), conscience

Parietal-temporal-occipital Association Cortex

Integrates information from those lobes.

Limbic Association Cortex

Motivation, emotion, memory.

Subcortical Structures

Basal Nuclei (Basal Ganglia)

- Masses of gray matter within cerebral white matter
- Is functional aggregations of cell bodies that inhibit muscle tone, maintain purposeful motor activity and suppress unnecessary movement and monitor/coordinate muscle contractions in posture/support
- Complex aspects of motor control
- May be involved in cognitive functioning
- Receives input from all cortical areas
- Sends feedback via thalamus mainly to prefrontal and premotor areas (no direct connection to motor neurons)

Thalamus

- Preliminary processing of sensory input and screens out unimportant stimuli and passes on significant input to the somatosensory cortex and other brain regions
- Crude awareness of sensation
- Reinforces voluntary motor activity
- Some degree of consciousness
- "Gateway" to cerebral cortex—virtually all inputs to cortex pass-through
- Contains many nuclei, each with a functional specialty

Hypothalamus

- Many functionally grouped nuclei
- Integrating center for homeostasis, links ANS and endocrine system
- Regulates body temperature (monitors blood temperature)
- Regulates water balance (urine output) and thirst (contains osmoreceptors to test concentration of body fluids)
- Regulates food intake (monitors blood levels of nutrients and hormones)
- Controls endocrine functioning (produces hormones, regulates pituitary)
- Role in emotional and behavioral patterns
- Controls autonomic centers in brain and spinal cord (e.g., activity of smooth and cardiac muscle, exocrine glands)
- "Biological clock"

Limbic System

- Parts of cortex, basal nuclei, thalamus, hypothalamus
- Involved in all aspects of emotion (pleasure, fear, anger, etc.) and physical expressions of emotion (attacking when angered, laughing, crying, etc.)
- Contains "reward" and "punishment" centers
- Important in homeostatic drives—hunger, thirst, sex
- Secrete norepinephrine, dopamine and serotonin, important neurotransmitters (precise role unclear, more of these neurotransmitters associated with pleasure, less with depression)

Learning and Memory

- **Learning:** Acquisition of knowledge or skills as a consequence of experience, instruction, or both
- **Memory:** Storage of knowledge for later recall
- **Remembering:** A process of retrieving information from storage
- **Forgetting:** Inability to retrieve information
- **Memory trace:** Neural change responsible for the storage of information present throughout the brain. Particular areas appear to be important in certain kinds of memories, as under:
  a. **Hippocampus:** Short-term memories involving the integration of stimuli, consolidation (converting from short-term to long-term), declarative memories (facts and events).
  b. **Cerebellum:** Procedural memories (skill memories involving motor pathways, e.g., playing piano, typing, riding a bike).

Types of Memory

Short-term

❍ Immediately stored
❍ Limited capacity
❍ Retrieved rapidly
❍ Forgetting is permanent (unless consolidated)
❍ Transient changes in preexisting synapses (changes in amount of neurotransmitter released via modification of Ca^{2+} channels, may involve cAMP pathways)

Long-term

❍ Longer storage time, enhanced by practice
❍ Large storage capacity
❍ More slowly retrieved
❍ Quite stable, forgetting usually transient
❍ Permanent changes in neurons (formation of new synapses, synthesis of proteins in pre- or post-synaptic membranes, changes in amount of neurotransmitter released)

Cerebellum

❍ Different portions specialize in particular functions (mostly ipsilateral)
❍ Maintains balance and equilibrium, important in movement
❍ Enhances muscle tone
❍ Coordinates voluntary movements
  ➤ Input from cortical motor areas and peripheral receptors (indirect)
  ➤ Ensures smooth, precise movement
❍ Plans and initiates voluntary movement (output to cortical motor areas)
❍ Procedural memories

Brainstem

❍ All incoming and outgoing fibers pass through; most synapse here for processing
❍ Functions
  ○ Cranial nerve origin
  ○ Contains nuclei for control of autonomic activities
  ➤ Cardiovascular center (force and rate of heart contraction, blood pressure)
  ➤ Respiratory centers (rate and depth of breathing)
  ➤ Many others, such as vomiting, hiccupping, swallowing, coughing and sneezing.
❍ Modulates pain
❍ Regulates equilibrium and posture reflexes
❍ Contains reticular formation
  ○ Receives/integrates all synaptic input
  ○ Controls cortical alertness (reticular activating system—RAS)
  ○ Important in ability to direct attention
❍ Contains sleep centers

Sleep

It is an active process in which an individual is not consciously aware of surroundings but can be aroused by external stimuli.

Types of Sleep

Slow-wave Sleep

❍ From light sleep to deep sleep and back
❍ Characterized by frequent movement, small decrease in heart and respiratory rate, and blood pressure

Paradoxical (REM) Sleep

❍ Brain activity similar to an awake state
❍ Characterized by lack of movement (except eyes), irregular heart and respiratory rate and blood pressure, dreaming
❍ Probably controlled by three centers that interact to produce the stages of sleep (arousal system, slow-wave center, REM center)

Functions

❍ Time to restore chemical/physiological processes
❍ Accomplish changes for learning and memory

Spinal Cord

- Extends from brainstem
- It has paired spinal nerves that serves a particular body region
- Contain both afferent (sensory) and efferent (motor and ANS) fibers
- Spinal cord contains gray matter and white matter
- **Gray matter:** Present in:
  - Neuron cell bodies and dendrites, short interneurons, glial cells
  - Dorsal horns (cell bodies of interneurons, afferent neurons terminate)
  - Lateral horns (efferent ANS cell bodies)
  - Ventral horns (efferent motor neuron cell bodies)
- White matter in fiber tracts, ascending: cord → brain, descending: brain → cord

Reflexes

- Response that occurs without conscious effort
- It can be simple or acquired
- **Simple (basic):** Built-in, unlearned (e.g., pulling away from a painful stimulus)
- **Acquired (conditioned):** Learned through practice (e.g., typing, playing sports)

Reflex Arc

- The neural pathway involved
- Receptor responds to stimulus by generating an AP
- Afferent pathway relays information to integrating center (spinal cord or brainstem for simple reflexes, higher brain levels for acquired reflexes)
- Efferent pathway transmits information to effector (muscle or gland)

Spinal Reflexes

- Spinal cord is integrating center (no brain involvement needed)
- Afferent pathway terminates on three types of neurons:

1. Excitatory interneuron, which stimulates efferent motor neurons (muscle contracts)
2. Inhibitory interneuron, which inhibits efferent motor neurons leading to antagonistic muscle group (called reciprocal inhibition or innervation)
3. Interneurons carrying signal to brain (person becomes aware of stimulus)

- Brain can modify spinal reflex
- Consciously override by sending inhibitory signals to muscle group that would move, excitatory signals to antagonistic muscle.

PERIPHERAL NERVOUS SYSTEM; AFFERENT DIVISION

The peripheral nervous system (PNS) has two divisions:

1. Afferent division, also known as the sensory division
2. Efferent division.

Some basic details about the PNS afferent division are:

Function

It is responsible for carrying sensory information from the body's periphery (such as skin, muscles, organs, and sensory organs) to the central nervous system (CNS)—the brain and spinal cord.

Sensory Receptors

It consists of sensory receptors located throughout the body that detect various types of sensory stimuli, including touch, pressure, temperature, pain, proprioception (awareness of body position), and information from the special senses like vision, hearing, taste, and smell.

Types of Sensory Neurons

Sensory neurons within the PNS afferent division are categorized into different types based on the specific sensations they convey. For example, mechanoreceptors, thermoreceptors, nociceptors, and photoreceptors.

Types of Sensory Receptors

- **Mechanoreceptors:** These respond to mechanical forces like pressure, touch, and vibration.
- **Thermoreceptors:** These detect changes in temperature.
- **Nociceptors:** Also known as pain receptors, they respond to tissue damage or potentially harmful stimuli.
- **Photoreceptors:** Found in the eyes, these are responsible for detecting light and allowing us to see.
- **Chemoreceptors:** They sense changes in chemical concentrations, such as in taste and smell.
- **Proprioceptors:** These provide information about body position and movement, helping with balance and coordination.

Neuronal Pathways

Sensory information travels along specific neural pathways within the PNS afferent division. These pathways transmit signals from the peripheral sensory receptors to the CNS, where the brain processes and interprets the sensory input.

Unipolar Neurons

Most sensory neurons in the PNS have a unipolar structure that means they have a single long process (axon) that splits into two branches, with one branch receiving sensory input from the periphery and the other extending into the CNS.

Reflex Arcs

The PNS afferent division plays a crucial role in reflex arcs, which are rapid, automatic responses to sensory stimuli that help protect the body from harm. Sensory information

is processed in the spinal cord, and motor commands are sent back out to effectors (muscles or glands) without involving the brain in some reflexes.

Receptor Physiology

It is the study of understanding the role of sensory receptors in the body. Sensory receptors are specialized cells or structures that respond to specific stimuli from the external or internal environment, converting these stimuli into electrical signals that can be interpreted by the brain.

Some key aspects of receptor physiology:

Transduction

Sensory receptors transduce (convert) physical or chemical stimuli into electrical signals called action potentials. This process involves changes in the receptor's membrane potential, usually through the opening or closing of ion channels.

Receptor Specificity

Each type of sensory receptor is specialized to respond to a specific type of stimulus. For example, photoreceptors—sensitive to light, mechanoreceptors in the skin—pressure and touch.

Adaptation

Sensory receptors can adapt to sustained or repetitive stimuli. Some receptors become less responsive over time (phasic receptors), while others continue to generate signals as long as the stimulus is present (tonic receptors).

Receptive Fields

Sensory receptors have specific areas of the body or environment to which they are most sensitive, known as receptive fields. Receptive fields can vary in size and shape.

Sensory Pathways

Once sensory information is transduced into electrical signals, it is transmitted along specific neural pathways to the CNS. These pathways may involve relay stations like the spinal cord or the brainstem before reaching the cerebral cortex for perception and interpretation.

Modality and Coding

Sensory receptors convey information about the modality (type) and intensity of a stimulus. The brain interprets these signals based on the specific pathways and patterns of action potentials, allowing us to recognize different sensations.

Sensory Integration

The CNS integrates sensory information from multiple sources to create a coherent perception of our surroundings and internal states. This process involves comparing and combining signals from various sensory receptors.

Graded Receptor Potentials

Graded receptor potentials, also known as graded potentials, are electrical changes in the membrane potential of sensory receptor cells in response to a stimulus. These graded changes in membrane potential are subthreshold, vary in amplitude (size) depending on the strength of the stimulus.

Some of their key characteristics are:

Stimulus detection: Graded receptor potentials occur when specialized sensory receptors detect specific environmental stimuli.

Subthreshold: Graded potentials are subthreshold events, which means they do not result in the generation of an action potential on their own.

Amplitude reflects stimulus strength: The amplitude (size) of the graded receptor potential is directly proportional to the strength or intensity of the stimulus. A stronger stimulus will produce a larger graded potential, while a weaker stimulus generates a smaller one.

Local signaling: Graded potentials are typically localized responses that occur at the site of the sensory receptor. They do not travel along the entire length of a neuron. Instead, they influence nearby regions of the neuron.

Integration: In sensory systems, the graded receptor potentials may undergo further processing and integration before they can lead to the generation of action potentials and transmission of the sensory information to the central nervous system.

Threshold: If the amplitude of the graded receptor potential reaches a certain threshold, it may trigger the opening of voltage-gated ion channels and initiate an action potential. This action potential can then propagate along the sensory neuron for further signal transmission.

A receptor potential, or generator potential, is a type of graded potential that occurs in sensory receptor cells when they are stimulated by a specific sensory stimulus. Receptor potentials are a critical part of the sensory transduction process, where sensory information from the external or internal environment is converted into electrical signals that can be interpreted by the nervous system.

Stronger stimuli → greater frequency of APs (frequency code)

Somatosensory Pathways

These are neural pathways responsible for transmitting sensory information related to touch, pressure, vibration, temperature, pain, and proprioception (awareness of body position and movement) from the peripheral nervous system (PNS) to the central nervous system (CNS), specifically the brain. These pathways play a crucial role in allowing us to perceive and respond to sensory stimuli from our body and the external environment.

There are two main somatosensory pathways: The dorsal column-medial lemniscus pathway and the spinothalamic pathway.

Dorsal Column-Medial Lemniscus Pathway (DCML)

- **Primary sensory neurons:** Sensory information is initially detected by specialized sensory receptors (e.g., mechanoreceptors) located throughout the body.
- **First-order neurons:** These sensory signals are then transmitted through the PNS to the dorsal root ganglia and enter the spinal cord.
- **Ascend in the dorsal columns:** In the spinal cord, these signals ascend on the same side (ipsilateral) through the dorsal columns, which are specific regions of white matter.
- **Synapse in the medulla:** Upon reaching the medulla of the brainstem, the first-order neurons synapse with second-order neurons in a structure called the nucleus gracilis or nucleus cuneatus.
- **Crossing over:** The second-order neurons decussate (cross over) to the opposite side of the brainstem.
- **Medial lemniscus:** The crossed signals travel through a bundle of nerve fibers called the medial lemniscus.
- **Thalamus:** The medial lemniscus terminates in the ventral posterolateral nucleus of the thalamus.
- **Third-order neurons:** From the thalamus, third-order neurons project to the primary somatosensory cortex in the postcentral gyrus of the cerebral cortex, where conscious perception of the sensory stimulus occurs.

Spinothalamic Pathway

- **Primary sensory neurons:** Sensory information is detected by various receptors and transmitted to the spinal cord.
- **First-order neurons:** These neurons enter the spinal cord and synapse with second-order neurons almost immediately.
- **Decussation:** The second-order neurons decussate (cross over) to the opposite side of the spinal cord.
- **Anterolateral pathway:** The crossed signals travel up the spinal cord in the anterolateral pathway.
- **Thalamus:** Second-order neurons synapse in the thalamus (ventral posterolateral nucleus).
- **Third-order neurons:** Third-order neurons project to the primary somatosensory cortex for conscious perception.

Discriminative Ability

- **Tactile discrimination:** Discriminative ability is primarily associated with the sense of touch, and it involves recognizing differences in texture, shape, size, temperature, and pressure of objects by touch alone.
- **Highly innervated areas:** Areas of the body with a high concentration of sensory receptors, such as Meissner's corpuscles and Merkel cells, contribute to high tactile discriminative ability. The fingertips are especially rich in these receptors, making them highly sensitive.
- **Importance for fine motor skills:** Discriminative ability acuity is essential for tasks that require fine motor skills and precision, such as typing, playing musical instruments, and performing surgical procedures.
- **Training and development:** Discriminative acuity can be improved with training and practice. Individuals who regularly engage in tasks that demand tactile discrimination often develop higher levels of acuity.
- **Clinical significance:** Reduced tactile discriminative ability can be a symptom of neurological disorders or peripheral nerve damage. It is evaluated by clinicians in neurological assessments and rehabilitation programs.
- **Assessment:** Tactile discrimination is assessed through various tests and experiments that involve tasks like two-point

discrimination (determining the minimum distance between two points touched on the skin), texture discrimination, and shape recognition.

Pain

Pain is a complex and subjective sensory and emotional experience that serves as a warning mechanism for the body, signaling potential or actual tissue damage or injury. It is a crucial part of the body's defense system, as it alerts an individual to harmful stimuli and encourages behaviors that can help protect against further injury. Here are some key aspects of pain:

Types of Pain

- **Nociceptive pain:** This type of pain results from the activation of nociceptors, specialized sensory receptors that respond to noxious (harmful) stimuli, such as mechanical damage, temperature extremes, or chemical irritation.
- **Neuropathic pain:** Neuropathic pain is caused by damage or dysfunction of the nervous system itself. It often manifests as burning, tingling, or shooting pain and can be chronic.
- **Inflammatory pain:** Inflammation in the body can lead to pain. This type of pain often accompanies conditions like arthritis or tissue injury.

Components of Pain

- **Sensory component:** It includes perception of the location, intensity, and quality of the pain. It helps individuals identify the source of the pain and its characteristics.
- **Emotional component:** Pain also has an emotional aspect, which can include feelings of fear, anxiety, distress, or suffering. The emotional component of pain can vary widely among individuals.
- **Cognitive component:** The perception of pain can be influenced by an individual's thoughts, beliefs, and expectations. Cognitive factors can modulate the pain experience.

Pain Pathways

Pain signals are transmitted through specialized pain pathways in the nervous system. These pathways involve the activation of nociceptors, the transmission of signals to the spinal cord and brain, and the processing of pain in various brain regions, including the somatosensory cortex and the limbic system.

The gate control theory of pain suggests that pain perception can be modulated by nonpainful stimuli, such as rubbing or massaging an injured area, which can "close the gate" and reduce pain perception.

Chronic Pain

Chronic pain is pain that persists beyond the normal time for tissue healing, typically lasting for more than three to six months. Chronic pain can be caused by various factors, including medical conditions, injuries, or neuropathic mechanisms.

Treatment

Pain management and relief can involve a combination of approaches, including medications (e.g., analgesics, anti-inflammatory drugs), physical therapy, behavioral therapy, relaxation techniques, and in some cases, surgical interventions.

Pain Perception

Pain perception can vary among individuals based on genetics, past experiences, psychological factors, and cultural influences. What one person may perceive as painful, another may tolerate differently.

PERIPHERAL NERVOUS SYSTEM; EFFERENT DIVISION

Introduction

As already discussed, peripheral nervous system (PNS) consists of two main divisions:

1. The afferent division
2. The efferent division.

The efferent division of the PNS is responsible for carrying signals from the central nervous system (CNS), which includes the brain and spinal cord, to the rest of the body, primarily to effectors such as muscles and glands. It is involved in transmitting commands from the CNS to initiate motor functions and regulate physiological processes.

The efferent division can be further divided into two main branches: The somatic nervous system and the autonomic nervous system.

Somatic Nervous System)

○ The somatic nervous system controls voluntary muscle movements and is responsible for carrying motor signals from the CNS to skeletal muscles.
○ It allows conscious control over skeletal muscles, enabling activities like walking, talking, and typing.
○ Motor neurons in the somatic nervous system have a single neuron pathway, meaning that they directly innervate skeletal muscles without any intervening ganglia.

Autonomic Nervous System

○ The autonomic nervous system regulates involuntary functions of the body, such as heart rate, digestion, respiration, and glandular activity.
○ It is further divided into two branches: The sympathetic and parasympathetic nervous systems, which often have opposing effects on physiological functions.
○ The sympathetic nervous system is responsible for the "fight or flight" response, increasing heart rate, dilating airways, and redirecting blood flow to muscles during times of stress or danger.
○ The parasympathetic nervous system, on the other hand, promotes "rest and digest"

activities, slowing heart rate, enhancing digestion, and conserving energy.
○ Autonomic motor neurons typically consist of a two-neuron pathway, with a preganglionic neuron synapsing on a ganglionic neuron located in an autonomic ganglion before reaching the effector organ or tissue.

Autonomic Control Centers

○ The ANS functions through specialized nuclei in the brainstem and spinal cord.
○ Key brain regions involved include the medulla oblongata, pons, and hypothalamus.

Autonomic Reflexes

The ANS controls various autonomic reflexes, which are automatic, subconscious responses to specific stimuli. Examples include:
○ **Baroreceptor reflex:** Regulates blood pressure.
○ **Pupillary reflex:** Adjusts pupil size in response to light.
○ **Gastrocolic reflex:** Promotes movement in the digestive tract after eating.

Autonomic Pathways

○ Autonomic signals follow a two-neuron pathway, with a preganglionic neuron synapsing on a ganglionic neuron located in an autonomic ganglion before reaching the effector organ.
○ Postganglionic neurons extend from the ganglia to target organs.
○ Ganglia are clusters of nerve cell bodies.

Functions and Clinical Relevance

○ The ANS regulates a wide range of bodily functions, including heart rate, blood pressure, respiratory rate, digestion, and body temperature.
○ Dysregulation of the ANS can lead to various medical conditions, including

dysautonomia, orthostatic hypotension, and autonomic neuropathy.

○ Understanding the ANS is essential for diagnosing and managing conditions related to autonomic dysfunction.

○ Medications can target the ANS to modify its function.

○ Sympathomimetic drugs mimic sympathetic effects, while sympatholytic drugs block sympathetic responses.

○ Parasympathomimetic drugs mimic parasympathetic effects, and anticholinergic drugs block parasympathetic responses.

Dual Innervation

Dual innervation, also known as dual autonomic innervation, refers to the phenomenon where most of the organs and tissues in the body receive input from both branches of the autonomic nervous system (ANS): the sympathetic nervous system (SNS) and the parasympathetic nervous system (PNS). This dual input allows for fine-tuned control over physiological functions and helps maintain homeostasis.

Here are the key aspects of dual innervation:

Sympathetic and Parasympathetic Nervous Systems:

The SNS and PNS are the two main branches of the autonomic nervous system, each having distinct roles and functions.

The SNS is often associated with the "fight or flight" response, while the PNS is associated with the "rest and digest" response.

Opposing Actions

In many cases, the SNS and PNS have opposing effects on target organs and tissues. For example:

○ The SNS increases heart rate, while the PNS decreases it.

○ The SNS dilates airways for improved oxygen intake, while the PNS constricts them to conserve energy.

○ The SNS inhibits digestion, while the PNS enhances it.

Balance and Homeostasis

○ Dual innervation allows the body to maintain a dynamic balance between sympathetic and parasympathetic influences.

○ The appropriate balance between these two systems is crucial for adapting to changing conditions and ensuring that physiological functions remain within the desired range.

Cooperative and Competitive Effects

○ In some cases, the SNS and PNS may cooperate to produce a combined effect. For example, both systems may act to increase salivary gland secretion during eating.

○ In other cases, they may have competitive effects, where one system's influence predominates. The balance of activity depends on the specific physiological context and the relative strength of the inputs.

Examples of Dual Innervation

Heart: The heart receives dual innervation, with the SNS increasing heart rate and the PNS decreasing it. The balance between these influences helps regulate heart rate under various conditions.

Digestive system: Most digestive organs, such as the stomach and intestines, receive dual innervation. The SNS inhibits digestive processes, while the PNS enhances them during rest and digestion.

Eye: The pupil of the eye is controlled by dual innervation. The SNS dilates the pupil, while the PNS constricts it.

Autonomic Tone

Autonomic tone refers to the baseline level of activity from both the SNS and PNS, even in the absence of external stimuli. This tone ensures that organ systems are ready to respond appropriately to changing demands.

The Adrenal Glands

The adrenal glands, which are located on top of each kidney, play essential roles in the endocrine system and the body's response to stress. There are two parts to the adrenal gland, each with distinct functions:

1. Adrenal Cortex

○ The adrenal cortex is the outer layer of the adrenal gland and is responsible for producing several steroid hormones, including glucocorticoids, mineralocorticoids, and small amounts of sex hormones.

○ **Glucocorticoids (e.g., cortisol):** These hormones are involved in regulating metabolism, immune function, and the body's response to stress. They help increase blood sugar levels, reduce inflammation, and regulate the sleep-wake cycle.

○ **Mineralocorticoids (e.g., aldosterone):** These hormones help control electrolyte and fluid balance in the body. Aldosterone, for example, promotes the reabsorption of sodium and the excretion of potassium by the kidneys, which helps maintain blood pressure and fluid balance.

○ **Sex hormones:** The adrenal cortex also produces small amounts of androgens (male sex hormones) and estrogens (female sex hormones). These hormones play a role in secondary sexual characteristics and can affect sexual function.

2. Adrenal Medulla

○ The adrenal medulla is the inner part of the adrenal gland and is responsible for producing catecholamines, primarily adrenaline (epinephrine) and noradrenaline (norepinephrine).

○ **Adrenaline (epinephrine) and noradrenaline (norepinephrine):** These hormones are involved in the "fight or flight" response to stress. When the body perceives a threat or stressor, the adrenal medulla releases these hormones into the bloodstream, leading to various physiological responses, including increased heart rate, increased blood pressure, and increased energy availability. These responses prepare the body to respond quickly to a perceived danger.

The role of the adrenal glands can be summarized as follows:

○ **Stress response:** The adrenal glands are crucial components of the body's stress response system. When the body encounters a stressful situation, the adrenal medulla releases adrenaline and noradrenaline, which prepare the body for a rapid and vigorous response.

○ **Metabolic regulation:** The adrenal cortex, specifically cortisol, plays a key role in regulating metabolism. It helps mobilize energy stores, regulate blood sugar levels, and modulate the body's response to inflammation and immune challenges.

○ **Fluid and electrolyte balance:** The adrenal cortex, through aldosterone, helps regulate electrolyte balance by controlling sodium and potassium levels in the body, thereby influencing blood pressure and fluid balance.

○ **Sex hormone production:** While the primary production of sex hormones occurs in the gonads (testes and ovaries), the adrenal cortex produces small amounts of androgens and estrogens, which can have secondary effects on sexual development and function.

Acetylcholine Receptors

Acetylcholine (ACh) receptors, often referred to as cholinergic receptors, are specialized proteins found on the surface of cells that can bind with the neurotransmitter acetylcholine. These receptors play a crucial role in transmitting signals within the nervous system and at neuromuscular junctions.

There are two main types of ACh receptors: nicotinic and muscarinic.

1. Nicotinic Receptors

Nicotinic receptors are ligand-gated ion channels, meaning they allow the passage of ions (e.g., sodium, potassium) when acetylcholine binds to them. They are found at various locations in the body, including:

Neuromuscular junctions: Nicotinic receptors are critical for transmitting signals from motor neurons to muscle cells, leading to muscle contraction. The binding of acetylcholine to nicotinic receptors at the neuromuscular junction initiates muscle action potentials.

Autonomic ganglia: These receptors are also present in autonomic ganglia, where they mediate the transmission of signals between preganglionic and postganglionic neurons in the sympathetic and parasympathetic divisions of the autonomic nervous system.

2. Muscarinic Receptors

Muscarinic receptors are G protein-coupled receptors (GPCRs), which means they activate intracellular signaling pathways upon binding acetylcholine.

They are primarily found in the central nervous system (CNS) and on the effector organs of the parasympathetic nervous system, such as the heart, smooth muscle, and glands.

Muscarinic receptor activation can have diverse effects depending on the specific tissue or organ:

○ In the heart, activation of muscarinic receptors slows down the heart rate (bradycardia).

○ In smooth muscle, muscarinic receptor activation can lead to constriction of airways (bronchoconstriction) or increased

gastrointestinal motility. In glands, it can stimulate secretion.

Functions of ACh Receptors

ACh receptors play a fundamental role in neurotransmission, allowing nerve cells to communicate with other nerve cells or with target cells, such as muscles and glands.

Activation of ACh receptors initiates a series of events that lead to changes in the membrane potential of the target cell, ultimately affecting its function.

The specific effects of ACh receptor activation depend on the receptor subtype and the location of the receptor.

The autonomic nervous system (ANS) is regulated by a combination of factors and mechanisms that help maintain its balance and respond to changing physiological demands.

The primary factors and regulators that influence the ANS are:

1. Central Control from the Brain

○ The ANS is under the control of various brain regions, including the medulla oblongata, pons, and hypothalamus, which serve as central control centers.

○ These brain regions receive sensory information and feedback from the body and make adjustments to ANS activity accordingly.

○ The hypothalamus, in particular, plays a central role in regulating ANS function by integrating signals related to stress, emotions, and homeostasis.

2. Feedback Mechanisms

○ The ANS operates via feedback mechanisms that allow it to respond to changes in the body's internal and external environment.

○ For example, baroreceptors in blood vessels monitor blood pressure and send signals to the brainstem to adjust heart rate and blood vessel constriction or dilation to maintain blood pressure within a normal range.

3. Hormonal Regulation

○ Hormones, such as epinephrine (adrenaline) and norepinephrine, play a significant role in regulating ANS activity during stress responses.
The adrenal medulla releases these hormones into the bloodstream in response to stress or perceived threats, and they activate the sympathetic branch of the ANS.

4. Autonomic Tone

○ Autonomic tone refers to the baseline level of activity in both the sympathetic and parasympathetic branches of the ANS, even in the absence of external stimuli.
○ The balance between sympathetic and parasympathetic tone influences the overall activity of the ANS and helps maintain homeostasis.

5. Sensory Input and Reflexes

○ Sensory receptors throughout the body continuously provide information to the CNS about internal and external conditions.
○ Reflexes, such as the baroreceptor reflex and pupillary reflex, allow for rapid, automatic adjustments in ANS activity in response to specific sensory inputs.

6. Pharmacological Agents

○ Medications can directly influence ANS activity. For example, sympathomimetic drugs mimic the effects of the sympathetic nervous system, while parasympathomimetic drugs mimic the effects of the parasympathetic nervous system.

7. Emotions and Psychological State

○ Emotional and psychological factors can significantly affect ANS activity. Stress, anxiety, and relaxation techniques can all modulate autonomic responses.

8. Circadian Rhythms

○ The ANS also follows daily circadian rhythms, which influence patterns of activity, including changes in heart rate, blood pressure, and body temperature.

Somatic Nervous System

The somatic nervous system (SNS) is one of the two major divisions of the peripheral nervous system (PNS), with the other being the autonomic nervous system (ANS). The SNS is responsible for controlling voluntary motor functions and relaying sensory information to the central nervous system (CNS), which includes the brain and spinal cord.

The key features and functions of the somatic nervous system are:

Voluntary Muscle Control

The primary function of the SNS is to control voluntary muscle movements in the body. These movements include actions like walking, talking, typing, and picking up objects.

Motor neurons in the SNS transmit signals from the CNS to skeletal muscles, which are under conscious control. These motor neurons form neuromuscular junctions with muscle fibers, allowing for muscle contraction in response to nerve impulses.

Single-Neuron Pathway

The SNS operates using a single-neuron pathway, meaning there is only one motor neuron between the CNS and the target muscle.

The cell body of the motor neuron is located in the spinal cord, and its axon extends to the muscle it innervates.

Sensory Input

The SNS also plays a role in transmitting sensory information from the body's sensory receptors (e.g., skin, joints, muscles) to the CNS.

Sensory neurons in the PNS send signals to the CNS about various sensory experiences, such as touch, temperature, pain, and proprioception (awareness of body position).

Reflexes

Reflex actions, such as the knee-jerk reflex, are quick and involuntary responses to sensory stimuli. They involve the SNS and are processed in the spinal cord without direct involvement of the brain. Reflexes serve as rapid protective responses to potentially harmful stimuli.

Conscious Perception

Sensory information processed by the SNS is consciously perceived by an individual. For example, you can feel the sensation of touching a hot object or the pressure of a firm handshake because of the SNS.

Cranial Nerves

Some cranial nerves, such as the facial nerve (VII), trigeminal nerve (V), and hypoglossal nerve (XII), are involved in controlling voluntary motor functions of the face, head, and neck and are considered part of the SNS.

Motor Cortex

The motor cortex in the brain is a crucial region for controlling voluntary movements. It sends signals to the SNS to initiate and coordinate muscle contractions.

Autonomic Nervous System

The autonomic nervous system (ANS) is regulated by a combination of factors and mechanisms that help maintain its balance and respond to changing physiological demands. Here are the primary factors and regulators that influence the ANS:

Central Control from the Brain

The ANS is under the control of various brain regions, including the medulla oblongata, pons, and hypothalamus, which serve as central control centers. These brain regions receive sensory information and feedback from the body and make adjustments to ANS activity accordingly. The hypothalamus, in particular, plays a central role in regulating ANS function by integrating signals related to stress, emotions, and homeostasis.

Feedback Mechanisms

The ANS operates via feedback mechanisms that allow it to respond to changes in the body's internal and external environment.

For example, baroreceptors in blood vessels monitor blood pressure and send signals to the brainstem to adjust heart rate and blood vessel constriction or dilation to maintain blood pressure within a normal range.

Hormonal Regulation

Hormones, such as epinephrine (adrenaline) and norepinephrine, play a significant role in regulating ANS activity during stress responses.

The adrenal medulla releases these hormones into the bloodstream in response to stress or perceived threats, and they activate the sympathetic branch of the ANS.

Autonomic Tone

Autonomic tone refers to the baseline level of activity in both the sympathetic and parasympathetic branches of the ANS, even in the absence of external stimuli.

The balance between sympathetic and parasympathetic tone influences the overall activity of the ANS and helps maintain homeostasis.

Sensory Input and Reflexes

Sensory receptors throughout the body continuously provide information to the CNS about internal and external conditions.

Reflexes, such as the baroreceptor reflex and pupillary reflex, allow for rapid, automatic adjustments in ANS activity in response to specific sensory inputs.

Pharmacological Agents

Medications can directly influence ANS activity. For example, sympathomimetic drugs mimic the effects of the sympathetic nervous system, while parasympathomimetic drugs mimic the effects of the parasympathetic nervous system.

Emotions and Psychological State

Emotional and psychological factors can significantly affect ANS activity. Stress, anxiety, and relaxation techniques can all modulate autonomic responses.

Circadian Rhythms

The ANS also follows daily circadian rhythms, which influence patterns of activity, including changes in heart rate, blood pressure, and body temperature.

Electrochemical Events in a Synapse

Electrochemical events in a synapse **(Fig. 1.3)** refer to the complex processes involving the transmission of signals (neurotransmission) from one neuron to another or from a neuron to a target cell, such as a muscle cell or another neuron. These events involve both electrical and chemical signaling and are critical for communication within the nervous system.

Here's an overview of the electrochemical events that occur in a synapse:

Action Potential Propagation

The process begins with an action potential, which is an electrical signal that travels along the length of a neuron's axon. When the action potential reaches the axon terminal (synaptic terminal), it triggers the release of neurotransmitters into the synapse.

Neurotransmitter Release

Within the axon terminal, there are synaptic vesicles containing neurotransmitters, such as serotonin, dopamine, acetylcholine, or glutamate, depending on the type of synapse. The arrival of the action potential at the axon terminal causes voltage-gated calcium channels to open, allowing calcium ions (Ca^{2+}) to enter the axon terminal. The influx of calcium ions triggers the fusion of synaptic vesicles with the presynaptic membrane, releasing neurotransmitters into the synaptic cleft (the small gap between the presynaptic neuron and the postsynaptic neuron or target cell).

Neurotransmitter Binding

Neurotransmitters diffuse across the synaptic cleft and bind to receptors on the postsynaptic membrane. These receptors are often ligand-gated ion channels. The binding of neurotransmitters to their receptors causes a conformational change in the receptor protein, leading to the opening or closing of ion channels.

Postsynaptic Response

Depending on the type of neurotransmitter and receptor, the postsynaptic cell's response may vary.

Excitatory neurotransmitters, such as glutamate, typically open ion channels that allow the influx of positively charged ions (usually sodium ions). This depolarizes the postsynaptic membrane and may trigger an action potential.

Inhibitory neurotransmitters, such as gamma-aminobutyric acid (GABA), often open ion channels that allow the influx of negatively charged ions (usually chloride ions). This hyperpolarizes the postsynaptic membrane, making it less likely for an action potential to occur.

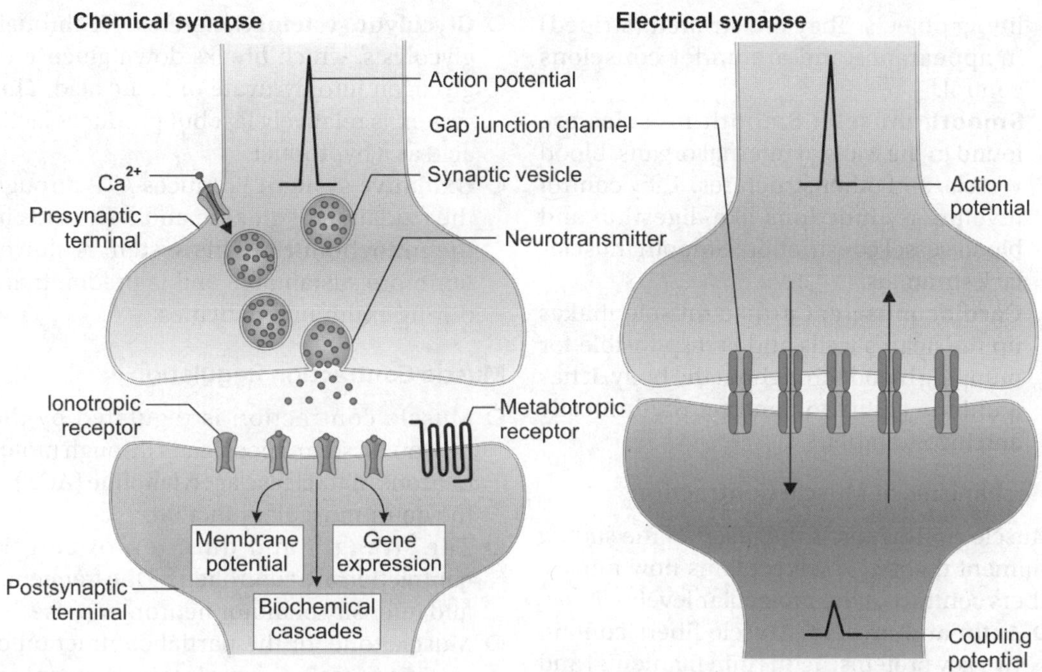

Fig. 1.3: Chemical and electrical synapses.

Postsynaptic Potential

The change in membrane potential in the postsynaptic cell due to the neurotransmitter binding is known as a postsynaptic potential (PSP). Excitatory postsynaptic potentials (EPSPs) make the postsynaptic cell more likely to generate an action potential, while inhibitory postsynaptic potentials (IPSPs) make it less likely.

Integration and Signal Propagation

The postsynaptic potentials generated at various synapses on the postsynaptic cell are integrated at the axon hillock (the trigger zone). If the combined effect reaches the threshold for an action potential, one is generated and travels down the axon.

Neurotransmitter Clearance

To terminate the signal, neurotransmitters are removed from the synaptic cleft through reuptake into the presynaptic neuron, enzymatic degradation, or diffusion away from the synapse.

MUSCLE PHYSIOLOGY

Muscle physiology is the study of how muscles function, contract, and produce force. Muscles are essential for various bodily functions, including movement, maintaining posture, generating heat, and facilitating circulation. Understanding muscle physiology involves examining the mechanisms of muscle contraction, energy metabolism, and the factors that regulate muscle activity.

Types of Muscles

There are three main types of muscles in the human body:

1. **Skeletal muscle:** Skeletal muscles are attached to bones and allow for voluntary movements, such as walking, running, and

lifting objects. They are striated (striped) in appearance and are under conscious control.

2. **Smooth muscle:** Smooth muscles are found in the walls of internal organs, blood vessels, and other structures. They control involuntary functions like digestion and blood vessel constriction. Smooth muscles lack striations.

3. **Cardiac muscle:** Cardiac muscle makes up the heart's walls and is responsible for pumping blood throughout the body. It has a unique ability to contract rhythmically and involuntarily.

Mechanisms of Muscle Contraction

Muscle contraction is the result of the sliding filament theory, which explains how muscle fibers contract at the molecular level:

○ **Actin and myosin:** Muscle fibers contain two key proteins: actin (thin filaments) and myosin (thick filaments). Myosin heads interact with actin to generate force.

○ **Cross-bridge formation:** Myosin heads form cross-bridges with actin when calcium ions (Ca^{2+}) are released from the sarcoplasmic reticulum (SR) in response to an action potential.

○ **Power stroke:** Energy from ATP is used to generate a power stroke, causing the myosin heads to pivot and pull the actin filaments toward the center of the sarcomere (the basic unit of muscle contraction).

○ **Relaxation:** When Ca^{2+} levels decrease, the cross-bridges detach, and the muscle relaxes.

Energy Metabolism in Muscle

Muscle contraction requires energy in the form of adenosine triphosphate (ATP). Different energy pathways contribute to ATP production during muscle activity:

○ **Phosphagen system:** Provides rapid but limited ATP through the breakdown of creatine phosphate.

○ **Glycolytic system:** Generates ATP through glycolysis, which breaks down glucose or glycogen into pyruvate or lactic acid. This system is relatively fast but produces lactic acid as a byproduct.

○ **Oxidative system:** Produces ATP through the oxidation of glucose and fatty acids in the mitochondria. This system is slower but more sustainable and is predominant during endurance activities.

Muscle Contraction Regulation

○ Muscle contraction is regulated by the nervous system, specifically through motor neurons that release acetylcholine (ACh) at the neuromuscular junction.

○ The strength and duration of muscle contraction are controlled by the frequency and intensity of motor neuron impulses.

○ Muscle tone, or the partial contraction of resting muscles, is maintained by spinal reflexes and helps stabilize posture.

Muscle Adaptations

Muscles can adapt to exercise and training through processes such as hypertrophy (increase in muscle size), increased mitochondrial density (for better oxidative capacity), and improved neuromuscular coordination.

Fatigue and Recovery

○ Muscle fatigue occurs when ATP is depleted, lactic acid accumulates, and neurotransmitter release decreases.

○ Recovery involves replenishing ATP, removing metabolic waste, and repairing muscle tissue.

Skeletal Muscle Mechanics

Skeletal muscle mechanics refers to the study of how skeletal muscles function in terms of force production, contraction, and movement. Skeletal muscles are responsible for voluntary movements in the body, such as walking, running, lifting, and many other activities. Understanding the mechanics of skeletal muscle is essential in fields like biomechanics, sports science, and physical therapy.

Important aspects of muscle mechanics are:

Muscle Structure

○ Skeletal muscles are composed of individual muscle fibers, each containing myofibrils, which are the contractile units of the muscle.
○ Myofibrils consist of repeating units called sarcomeres, which are the fundamental structures responsible for muscle contraction.
○ Sarcomeres contain thick filaments (myosin) and thin filaments (actin), which slide past each other during contraction.

Muscle Contraction

○ Muscle contraction occurs when sarcomeres shorten as the myosin heads interact with the actin filaments. This sliding filament theory of muscle contraction explains the molecular basis of muscle force generation.
○ The release of calcium ions (Ca^{2+}) from the sarcoplasmic reticulum triggers muscle contraction by allowing myosin and actin to interact.

Force Generation

○ Muscle force is generated through the recruitment of motor units. A motor unit consists of a motor neuron and all the muscle fibers it innervates.
○ The strength of muscle contraction is modulated by the number of motor units recruited and the frequency of motor neuron firing.
○ Muscle force is influenced by factors such as muscle length, cross-sectional area, and the angle of muscle attachment to bones.

Muscle Length-Tension Relationship

○ The length at which a muscle operates affects its force-generating capacity. Muscles generate the most force when they are at their optimal length (neither too stretched nor too shortened).
○ This relationship is important in tasks like lifting weights, where the muscle's length affects its ability to generate force.

Velocity of Muscle Contraction

○ Muscles can contract at different velocities depending on the load they are lifting. Heavier loads lead to slower contractions, while lighter loads allow for faster contractions.
○ This relationship is described by the force-velocity curve, which demonstrates how force and velocity are inversely related during muscle contractions.

Energy Metabolism

○ Muscle contractions require energy in the form of adenosine triphosphate (ATP). ATP is produced through various metabolic pathways, including the phosphagen system, glycolysis, and oxidative phosphorylation.
○ The choice of metabolic pathway depends on the intensity and duration of muscle activity.

Fatigue

○ Muscle fatigue occurs when a muscle's ability to generate force decreases during prolonged or intense activity.
○ Fatigue can result from factors such as ATP depletion, lactic acid accumulation, and the build-up of metabolites.

Muscle Stretch and Reflexes

The stretch reflex is an involuntary response that occurs when a muscle is rapidly stretched. It helps maintain muscle length and posture by causing the muscle to contract in response to a stretch stimulus.

Muscle Types

Skeletal muscles can be categorized into different fiber types, such as:
- Slow-twitch (Type I)
- Fast-twitch (Type II) fibers, which have varying contractile properties and fatigue characteristics.

Skeletal Muscle Metabolism

Skeletal muscle metabolism refers to the biochemical processes that occur within skeletal muscle tissue to produce energy, maintain muscle function, and support physical activity. Skeletal muscles are the muscles responsible for voluntary movements in the body, such as walking, running, and lifting weights. To support these activities, muscle cells require a continuous supply of energy in the form of adenosine triphosphate (ATP).

1. Energy Sources

Skeletal muscles primarily use three sources of energy for ATP production:
i. **Phosphocreatine (PCr):** Phosphocreatine is a high-energy phosphate molecule stored within muscle cells. During short bursts of intense activity, PCr is rapidly broken down to provide ATP.
ii. **Glycolysis:** Glycolysis is a metabolic pathway that converts glucose or glycogen (stored form of glucose) into ATP. It is a relatively fast process and is used during moderate-intensity exercise.
iii. **Oxidative phosphorylation:** This process occurs in the mitochondria and relies on the oxidation of glucose, fatty acids, and other substrates to produce ATP. It is the primary energy source for prolonged, endurance-type activities.

2. Muscle Fiber Types

Skeletal muscles contain different types of muscle fibers, each with distinct metabolic characteristics:
- **Type I (slow-twitch):** Type I fibers are highly oxidative and rich in mitochondria. They primarily use oxidative phosphorylation for ATP production and are well-suited for endurance activities.
- **Type IIa (fast-twitch oxidative):** Type IIa fibers are fast-contracting and have a moderate level of oxidative capacity. They can use both glycolysis and oxidative phosphorylation and are suitable for activities requiring both strength and endurance.
- **Type IIb (fast-twitch glycolytic):** Type IIb fibers are fast-contracting and rely on glycolysis for ATP production. They fatigue quickly but are used for rapid, powerful movements.

3. Oxygen Consumption

- Oxygen consumption is a critical factor in skeletal muscle metabolism. Oxygen is required for oxidative phosphorylation, which is the most efficient ATP-producing pathway.
- The amount of oxygen consumed during exercise is used as a measure of exercise intensity and energy demand.

4. Lactate Production

- During intense exercise, glycolysis can produce lactate as a by product. Lactate accumulation can lead to muscle fatigue and discomfort.
- Contrary to previous beliefs, lactate is not the cause of muscle soreness but rather a by product of energy metabolism.

5. Fuel Utilization

- The choice of energy substrate (e.g., glucose, fatty acids) depends on exercise intensity and duration. Lower-intensity activities rely more on fatty acids, while higher-intensity activities prefer glucose and glycogen.

○ Carbohydrate availability, as well as training status, can influence fuel utilization.

6. Recovery and Repair

○ After exercise, muscle metabolism shifts toward repair and recovery. Nutrients, particularly protein and amino acids, are essential for muscle repair and growth.

○ Adequate hydration and nutrition are vital for optimizing recovery and muscle adaptation.

7. Hormonal Regulation

Hormones such as insulin, glucagon, adrenaline, and cortisol play a role in regulating skeletal muscle metabolism, particularly in controlling glucose uptake and glycogen storage.

Control of Skeletal Muscle

The control of skeletal muscle involves a complex interplay between the nervous system and muscle tissue, resulting in voluntary and coordinated movements. The process begins with the brain's decision to move a specific muscle and ends with the contraction of muscle fibers.

Control of skeletal muscle mechanism is discussed below:

1. Brain and Central Nervous System (CNS)

The control of skeletal muscles begins in the brain, specifically in the motor areas of the cerebral cortex. These regions are responsible for planning and initiating voluntary movements. The primary motor cortex, located in the frontal lobe, plays a crucial role in the initiation of muscle contractions. It sends signals to specific muscles to generate movement.

2. Motor Neurons

Motor neurons are specialized nerve cells that transmit signals from the central nervous system to skeletal muscle fibers. They are the intermediaries between the brain's instructions and muscle contractions. Lower motor neurons, which are part of the peripheral nervous system, directly innervate (connect to) muscle fibers.

3. Neuromuscular Junction:

The neuromuscular junction is the point of communication between motor neurons and skeletal muscle fibers. When a motor neuron receives a signal from the brain to contract a muscle, it releases the neurotransmitter acetylcholine (ACh) into the neuromuscular junction.

4. Muscle Contraction

The release of acetylcholine at the neuromuscular junction triggers a series of events within the muscle fiber. This includes the depolarization of the muscle cell membrane (sarcolemma) and the release of calcium ions (Ca^{2+}) from the sarcoplasmic reticulum. Calcium ions enable the sliding of actin and myosin filaments within the muscle fibers, leading to muscle contraction.

5. Control by Motor Units

Motor neurons innervate multiple muscle fibers, forming functional units called motor units. The size and number of motor units recruited determine the force and precision of muscle contractions. Fine motor control requires the recruitment of small motor units with fewer muscle fibers. Activities like lifting heavy weights recruit larger motor units with more muscle fibers.

6. Role of Proprioception

Proprioception refers to the body's ability to sense its position and movement in space. Sensory receptors called proprioceptors provide feedback to the brain about muscle length, tension, and joint position. This feedback helps the central nervous system adjust muscle contraction to maintain balance, coordination, and precise movements.

7. Feedback Loops

Sensory feedback from proprioceptors, along with visual and vestibular input, continuously informs the CNS about the body's position and movement. The CNS adjusts muscle activity based on this feedback to maintain equilibrium and execute coordinated movements.

8. Voluntary Control

Skeletal muscles are under voluntary control, meaning that individuals can consciously initiate and modulate muscle contractions to perform specific tasks.

9. Reflexes

In addition to voluntary control, skeletal muscles can also respond to reflexes, which are involuntary responses to specific stimuli. Reflexes are mediated by the spinal cord or brainstem and can bypass conscious control for rapid protective actions.

Muscle Spindles

Muscle spindles are specialized sensory receptors found within skeletal muscles. They play a crucial role in the regulation of muscle length, the detection of changes in muscle length, and the initiation of reflexes to prevent muscle overstretching. Muscle spindles are a key component of the proprioceptive system, which provides information to the central nervous system (CNS) about the body's position, movement, and muscle status.

The key features and functions of muscle spindles are:

Structure of Muscle Spindles

- Muscle spindles are spindle-shaped structures composed of specialized muscle fibers called intrafusal muscle fibers. These intrafusal fibers are surrounded by a connective tissue capsule.
- Two types of intrafusal muscle fibers exist within muscle spindles—nuclear bag fibers and nuclear chain fibers. These two types differ in their arrangement and function.
- Muscle spindles are typically located within the muscle belly, parallel to the regular muscle fibers (extrafusal muscle fibers).

Function of Muscle Spindles

- Muscle spindles serve as stretch receptors, constantly monitoring changes in muscle length.
- When a muscle undergoes stretch (lengthening) due to external forces or muscle contraction, the muscle spindles within that muscle also stretch.
- As muscle spindles stretch, they generate electrical impulses or action potentials, which are transmitted to the central nervous system (CNS) via sensory neurons (afferent neurons). These sensory neurons are called type Ia (primary) and type II (secondary) sensory neurons.

Role in Reflexes

- The information provided by muscle spindles is used by the CNS to regulate muscle tone, maintain posture, and coordinate movements.
- Muscle spindle input is essential for the stretch reflex, which is an automatic and rapid reflex response to muscle stretch.
- When a muscle is stretched, the muscle spindle activates type Ia sensory neurons, which in turn excite alpha motor neurons in the spinal cord.
- Activation of alpha motor neurons leads to the contraction of the stretched muscle, opposing further lengthening and helping to maintain muscle tone and joint stability.
- The stretch reflex is a protective mechanism that prevents sudden, uncontrolled muscle

lengthening, such as during a sudden external force applied to a muscle.

Role in Proprioception

○ Muscle spindles provide crucial proprioceptive information to the CNS. Proprioception is the body's ability to sense its position and movement in space.
○ Proprioceptive information from muscle spindles, along with information from other sensory receptors (e.g., Golgi tendon organs and joint receptors), helps the CNS maintain accurate body awareness and coordinate complex movements.

Golgi Tendon Organs

Golgi tendon organs (GTOs), also known as Golgi tendon receptors or Golgi organs, are specialized sensory receptors located within the tendons of skeletal muscles near their attachment to muscles. These sensory structures play a crucial role in providing feedback to the central nervous system (CNS) about the amount of tension or force generated within a muscle-tendon unit.

Here are the key features and functions of Golgi tendon organs:

Structure of Golgi Tendon Organs

○ Golgi tendon organs consist of bundles of collagen fibers that are intertwined with the muscle fibers and embedded within the tendon.
○ Sensory nerve endings, known as nerve endings of type Ib afferent neurons, wrap around and penetrate the collagen fibers within the Golgi tendon organ.

Function of Golgi Tendon Organs

○ Golgi tendon organs serve as tension or force sensors within the musculotendinous unit.
○ When a muscle contracts, it generates force, which is transmitted to the tendon to produce tension. This tension is detected by the Golgi tendon organ.
○ As tension in the tendon increases during muscle contraction, the collagen fibers within the Golgi tendon organ are stretched, leading to the activation of the sensory nerve endings (type Ib afferent neurons) within the organ.

Role in Reflexes

○ The primary function of Golgi tendon organs is to initiate the Golgi tendon reflex, also known as the inverse myotatic reflex.
○ When tension in the tendon exceeds a certain threshold, Golgi tendon organs activate type Ib afferent neurons, which transmit inhibitory signals to the alpha motor neurons of the same muscle.
○ The inhibitory signals temporarily reduce the excitability of the alpha motor neurons, leading to a decrease in muscle contraction force.
○ The Golgi tendon reflex is a protective mechanism that prevents excessive force generation in the muscle and tendon, reducing the risk of muscle or tendon damage.

Protection Against Overload

○ Golgi tendon organs play a vital role in preventing muscle and tendon injury due to excessive force or overload.
○ For example, during heavy lifting or when a muscle is subjected to an excessive load, the Golgi tendon organs sense the increased tension and initiate the reflexive inhibition of muscle contraction, preventing further force generation that could potentially lead to muscle or tendon damage.

Role in Motor Control and Coordination

○ Golgi tendon organs contribute to motor control and coordination by providing the CNS with information about muscle tension and force production.
○ This proprioceptive feedback helps in fine-tuning muscle contractions, maintaining

appropriate muscle tone, and coordinating movements.

Smooth Muscle

Smooth muscle is one of the three types of muscle tissue found in the human body, alongside skeletal muscle and cardiac muscle. It is characterized by its smooth, nonstriated appearance under a microscope and is responsible for various involuntary movements and functions within the body.

Overview of the functional anatomy and functions of smooth muscle is as under:

Functional Anatomy of Smooth Muscle

○ **Cell structure:** Smooth muscle cells, also known as smooth muscle fibers or myocytes, have a spindle-shaped appearance. Unlike skeletal muscle, they lack the striated (striped) appearance due to the absence of organized sarcomeres. Smooth muscle cells are uninucleated (contain one nucleus) and shorter than skeletal muscle fibers.

○ **Arrangement:** Smooth muscle is found in various organs and structures throughout the body, including the walls of blood vessels (vascular smooth muscle), the digestive tract (gastrointestinal smooth muscle), the respiratory tract (bronchial smooth muscle), the urinary tract (urethral and bladder smooth muscle), and the reproductive system (uterine smooth muscle).

○ **Involuntary control:** Unlike skeletal muscle, which is under voluntary control, smooth muscle is primarily under involuntary control. It responds to autonomic nervous system signals, hormones, and local factors to regulate its contraction and relaxation.

○ **Mechanism of contraction:** Smooth muscle contracts in a coordinated manner but lacks the organized sarcomere structure seen in skeletal muscle. Instead, actin and myosin filaments are scattered throughout the cytoplasm of smooth muscle cells. Contraction is initiated by calcium ions (Ca^{2+}), which enter the cytoplasm and activate the contractile proteins.

Functions of Smooth Muscle

○ **Blood vessel regulation:** Vascular smooth muscle controls the diameter of blood vessels, regulating blood pressure and blood flow. Constriction (vasoconstriction) narrows the vessel, while relaxation (vasodilation) widens it.

○ **Digestive system:** Smooth muscle in the digestive tract, including the esophagus, stomach, intestines, and other organs, facilitates the mixing and movement of food and the propulsion of contents through the digestive system (peristalsis).

○ **Respiratory system:** Smooth muscle in the bronchioles of the respiratory tract helps regulate airway diameter, allowing for the control of airflow into the lungs.

○ **Urinary system:** Smooth muscle in the walls of the urinary bladder contracts during voiding (micturition), expelling urine from the bladder.

○ **Reproductive system:** Uterine smooth muscle contracts during labor, facilitating childbirth. It also plays a role in menstrual regulation.

○ **Eye:** The iris of the eye contains smooth muscle fibers that control the size of the pupil, regulating the amount of light entering the eye.

○ **Skin:** Arrector pili muscles, which are small bands of smooth muscle attached to hair follicles, contract to create "goosebumps" in response to cold or emotional stimuli.

○ **Glands:** Smooth muscle in the walls of some glands, such as sweat glands, can help propel secretions.

○ **Sphincters:** Smooth muscle forms sphincters in various locations in the body, controlling the passage of materials. For example, the lower esophageal sphincter prevents stomach acid from entering the esophagus.

Multiunit Smooth Muscle

Multiunit smooth muscle is one of the two main types of smooth muscle found in the human body, with the other being single-unit smooth muscle. Multiunit smooth muscle differs from single-unit smooth muscle in its structural and functional characteristics.

Structural Characteristics

○ **Organization:** Multiunit smooth muscle is composed of individual, discrete smooth muscle fibers or cells that are not electrically coupled to one another. Each muscle fiber functions independently.

○ **Nerve supply:** Multiunit smooth muscle is typically richly innervated by autonomic nerve fibers (sympathetic and parasympathetic). Each muscle fiber receives input from its own nerve ending, allowing for precise control over contraction.

○ **Location:** Multiunit smooth muscle is found in various structures and organs throughout the body, where fine control and precision of muscle function are required.

Functional Characteristics

○ **Contraction:** Multiunit smooth muscle contracts in response to neural stimulation, hormones, or local factors. Each individual muscle fiber contracts independently of neighboring fibers.

○ **Control:** Contractions of multiunit smooth muscle are highly controlled and graded, allowing for fine-tuned adjustments in muscle activity. This type of smooth muscle can produce relatively strong contractions when needed.

Examples of Multiunit Smooth Muscle Locations

○ **Eye:** The ciliary muscle, which controls the shape of the lens for focusing on objects at different distances, is composed of multiunit smooth muscle fibers. Contraction of the ciliary muscle changes the lens shape for accommodation (focusing).

○ **Blood vessels:** Some blood vessels, especially smaller arteries and arterioles in specific tissues like the iris of the eye and the male reproductive system (such as the muscles controlling erection and ejaculation), contain multiunit smooth muscle. These muscles help regulate blood flow and tissue perfusion in a highly controlled manner.

○ **Respiratory system:** The bronchioles of the respiratory system contain multiunit smooth muscle, allowing for precise control of airway diameter and resistance.

○ **Female reproductive system:** The uterus contains multiunit smooth muscle in the form of the myometrium. Contractions of the myometrial muscle fibers are essential during childbirth and can also occur during menstruation.

Single-Unit Smooth Muscle

Single-unit smooth muscle, also known as unitary or visceral smooth muscle, is one of the two primary types of smooth muscle found in the human body, with the other being multiunit smooth muscle. Single-unit smooth muscle differs in its structural and functional characteristics. Here's an overview of single-unit smooth muscle:

Structural Characteristics

○ **Organization:** Single-unit smooth muscle is composed of interconnected, closely packed smooth muscle cells or fibers that are electrically coupled to one another. These cells contract as a coordinated unit.

○ **Nerve supply:** Single-unit smooth muscle is typically innervated by autonomic nerve fibers (sympathetic and parasympathetic). Neural input can influence the entire muscle network, affecting all cells simultaneously.

○ **Location:** Single-unit smooth muscle is found in the walls of various hollow organs and structures throughout the body, where rhythmic and coordinated contractions are required for functions like peristalsis and regulation of organ activity.

Functional Characteristics

○ **Contraction:** Single-unit smooth muscle cells contract as a synchronized unit, meaning that when one cell contracts, adjacent cells are stimulated to contract as well. This coordinated contraction allows for efficient and synchronized movement of substances within hollow organs.

○ **Control:** Contractions of single-unit smooth muscle are typically involuntary and controlled by neural signals, hormones, or local factors. The coordinated contractions are well-suited for functions such as moving food through the digestive tract, propelling urine through the urinary system, and regulating blood flow through organs.

Examples of Single-Unit Smooth Muscle Locations

○ **Digestive system:** Single-unit smooth muscle is abundant in the walls of the gastrointestinal tract, including the esophagus, stomach, small and large intestines, and the walls of blood vessels within the digestive organs. Contraction of these muscles facilitates the mixing and propulsion of food and helps regulate blood flow for digestion.

○ **Urinary system:** The walls of the ureters, which transport urine from the kidneys to the bladder, contain single-unit smooth muscle that propels urine through peristaltic contractions. The detrusor muscle in the urinary bladder is another example, aiding in the expulsion of urine during voiding.

○ **Reproductive system:** Single-unit smooth muscle is present in the walls of the uterus. During labor and delivery, the uterine muscle contracts as a coordinated unit, facilitating contractions that push the baby through the birth canal.

○ **Respiratory system:** The bronchi and bronchioles of the respiratory system contain single-unit smooth muscle that helps regulate airflow during breathing.

○ **Blood vessels:** Small blood vessels, particularly arterioles and small arteries, contain single-unit smooth muscle that can contract or relax to control blood flow and blood pressure.

CARDIAC PHYSIOLOGY

Cardiovascular System and Heart

The primary function of the cardiovascular system is indeed transport, specifically the transportation of essential substances throughout the body. This intricate system of the heart, blood vessels, and blood serves several vital functions related to the circulation of blood and the delivery of crucial substances to various tissues and organs.

Functions of CVS

○ **Transport of oxygen:** The cardiovascular system carries oxygen from the lungs to all the cells in the body. Oxygen is essential for cellular respiration, where cells use oxygen to generate energy (in the form of adenosine triphosphate or ATP).

- **Transport of nutrients:** Nutrients from the food we consume, such as glucose, amino acids, and fatty acids, are transported via the bloodstream to cells throughout the body. These nutrients provide the necessary energy and building blocks for cell function and growth.
- **Removal of waste products:** The cardiovascular system helps remove metabolic waste products, including carbon dioxide (CO_2) and urea, from cells and tissues. Carbon dioxide is transported back to the lungs for elimination during exhalation, while urea is filtered by the kidneys and excreted in urine.
- **Transport of hormones:** Hormones produced by various glands (e.g., the endocrine system) are released into the bloodstream and transported to target tissues and organs. Hormones are essential for regulating a wide range of physiological processes, including metabolism, growth, and reproduction.
- **Immune response:** Blood contains white blood cells (leukocytes) that play a critical role in the body's immune response. They help defend against infections, pathogens, and foreign invaders by traveling to sites of infection and participating in immune reactions.
- **Temperature regulation:** The circulation of blood helps regulate body temperature. Blood vessels can dilate (widen) to release heat and constrict to conserve heat, assisting the body in maintaining a stable core temperature.
- **Maintenance of blood pressure:** The cardiovascular system helps regulate blood pressure to ensure proper blood flow to all tissues. Specialized sensors (baroreceptors) monitor blood pressure and signal adjustments to maintain adequate perfusion.
- **Clotting and hemostasis:** Platelets in the blood and clotting factors work together to form blood clots when blood vessels are injured. This process, known as hemostasis, prevents excessive bleeding and promotes wound healing.
- **Fluid balance:** The cardiovascular system plays a role in maintaining fluid balance within the body. It helps distribute fluid between blood vessels and tissues while preventing excessive fluid accumulation in tissues (edema).
- **Delivery of oxygen to muscles during exercise:** During physical activity, the cardiovascular system responds to increased oxygen demand by delivering more blood to the muscles and increasing heart rate to meet the body's needs.

Heart as a Pump

The heart functions as a powerful muscular pump that plays a central role in the circulatory system. Its primary function is to propel blood throughout the body, ensuring that oxygen, nutrients, and other essential substances are delivered to cells and tissues, while waste products like carbon dioxide are removed.

Structure of the Heart

- The human heart is a muscular organ located in the chest cavity between the lungs.
- It is roughly the size of a closed fist and consists of four chambers: two atria (the left atrium and right atrium) and two ventricles (the left ventricle and right ventricle).
- The heart is enclosed within a protective sac called the pericardium and is composed of specialized cardiac muscle tissue.

Function of the Heart as a Pump

- **Atria contraction:** The heart's pumping action begins with the contraction of the atria. When the atria contract (atrial systole), blood is pushed from the atria into the ventricles below.

○ **Ventricles contraction:** The more forceful contraction of the ventricles (ventricular systole) follows. When the ventricles contract, the atrioventricular (AV) valves (the tricuspid valve on the right side and the bicuspid or mitral valve on the left side) close to prevent blood from flowing back into the atria.

○ **Ejection of blood:** As the ventricles contract, they generate sufficient pressure to open the semilunar valves (the pulmonary valve in the right ventricle and the aortic valve in the left ventricle). This allows blood to be ejected into the pulmonary artery (right ventricle) and the aorta (left ventricle).

○ **Circulation:** Blood is then pumped into the pulmonary circulation (to the lungs) from the right ventricle and into the systemic circulation (to the body) from the left ventricle.

  ○ In the lungs, blood receives oxygen and releases carbon dioxide.

  ○ In the systemic circulation, oxygenated blood supplies nutrients, oxygen, and other substances to tissues and organs while picking up waste products.

○ **Relaxation and refilling:** Following ventricular contraction (ventricular systole), the ventricles relax (ventricular diastole). During this phase, the atria also relax (atrial diastole). Blood from the veins returns to the atria and fills them, ready to be pushed into the ventricles in the next cardiac cycle.

Heart Rate and Regulation

○ The rate at which the heart pumps (heart rate) is regulated by the autonomic nervous system, specifically through the actions of the sympathetic and parasympathetic branches.

○ Hormones such as epinephrine (adrenaline) can also influence heart rate and the force of contraction.

Blood Pressure

○ The heart's pumping action generates blood pressure, which is necessary for the flow of blood through the arteries and capillaries.

○ Blood pressure is measured in terms of systolic pressure (during ventricular contraction) and diastolic pressure (during ventricular relaxation).

Heart is a Double Pump

The heart functions as a double pump because it pumps blood through two separate circulatory circuits in the body—the pulmonary circulation and the systemic circulation.

○ **Pulmonary circulation:** The right side of the heart is responsible for pulmonary circulation. Deoxygenated blood from the body returns to the right atrium, is pumped into the right ventricle, and then is pumped to the lungs via the pulmonary artery. In the lungs, blood picks up oxygen and releases carbon dioxide before returning to the left side of the heart.

○ **Systemic circulation:** The left side of the heart is responsible for systemic circulation. Oxygen-rich blood from the lungs enters the left atrium, is pumped into the left ventricle, and then is pumped into the aorta, which carries it to all parts of the body. In the systemic circulation, oxygen and nutrients are delivered to cells, and waste products are collected for removal.

Heart Wall: 3 Layered

The heart wall consists of three distinct layers, each with its own function and composition:

1. **Epicardium:** The outermost layer of the heart wall is called the epicardium.

It is a thin, protective layer consisting of connective tissue and adipose tissue (fat). The epicardium is also known as the visceral pericardium because it covers the heart's surface and is continuous with the inner layer of the pericardial sac.

2. **Myocardium:** The middle layer is the myocardium, and it comprises the bulk of the heart's wall. This layer is primarily composed of cardiac muscle tissue (myocardial cells) that contracts rhythmically to pump blood. The myocardium's thickness varies in different regions of the heart to accommodate its pumping functions.

3. **Endocardium:** The innermost layer of the heart wall is the endocardium. It consists of a thin layer of endothelial cells that line the chambers of the heart and form the heart valves. The endocardium is in direct contact with the blood in the heart's chambers and provides a smooth surface to minimize friction.

Pericardial Sac

The pericardial sac, also known simply as the pericardium, is a double-walled, membranous sac that surrounds and encloses the heart. Its primary function is to protect the heart and provide a lubricated environment that allows the heart to beat and move within the chest cavity without friction.

The pericardium consists of two layers:

1. **Fibrous pericardium:** This is the tough, outer layer of the pericardium. It is composed of dense, fibrous connective tissue and serves as a protective layer for the heart. The fibrous pericardium also anchors the heart within the mediastinum, which is the central region of the chest between the lungs.

2. **Serous pericardium:** The serous pericardium is a double-layered membrane located beneath the fibrous pericardium. It consists of two layers:

   a. **Parietal layer:** The parietal layer of the serous pericardium lines the inner surface of the fibrous pericardium. It is attached to the fibrous pericardium and helps stabilize the position of the heart within the chest cavity.

   b. **Visceral layer (epicardium):** The visceral layer of the serous pericardium, also known as the epicardium, is the innermost layer. It is in direct contact with the heart muscle (myocardium) and covers the heart's surface. The visceral layer is continuous with the outermost layer of the heart wall.

Between the parietal and visceral layers of the serous pericardium is a thin fluid-filled space called the pericardial cavity. This cavity contains a small amount of serous fluid, known as pericardial fluid, which serves several important functions:

○ **Lubrication:** The serous fluid acts as a lubricant that reduces friction between the layers of the serous pericardium, allowing the heart to beat and move smoothly within the pericardial sac.

○ **Shock absorption:** The fluid-filled pericardial cavity also provides a cushioning effect, protecting the heart from external mechanical forces and shocks.

○ **Maintaining position:** The pericardial fluid helps maintain the heart's position within the chest, preventing excessive movement and displacement.

Electrical Activity of Heart

The electrical activity of the heart is a complex and highly regulated process that controls the heart's rhythm and contraction. It is essential for maintaining blood circulation and overall cardiovascular function.

Here's an overview of the key aspects of the electrical activity of the heart:

1. Generation of Electrical Signals

○ The heart's electrical activity begins with the generation of electrical signals by specialized cardiac muscle cells known as pacemaker cells.

○ The primary pacemaker of the heart is the sinoatrial (SA) node, located in the right atrium. The SA node generates electrical impulses at a regular rate, initiating each heartbeat.

2. Conduction Pathway

○ Once generated, electrical impulses travel along a specific pathway through the heart, ensuring that the chambers contract in a coordinated and synchronized manner.

○ The electrical impulses move from the SA node to the atria, causing atrial contraction (atrial systole).

○ They then pass through the atrioventricular (AV) node, a specialized region between the atria and ventricles that briefly delays the impulse. This delay allows the ventricles to fill with blood before contracting.

○ After the delay at the AV node, the impulses are conducted down the bundle of His, which divides into right and left bundle branches.

○ The impulse travels through Purkinje fibers, which distribute it throughout the ventricles, causing ventricular contraction (ventricular systole).

3. Electrocardiogram (ECG or EKG)

An electrocardiogram (ECG or EKG) is a diagnostic tool used to record the heart's electrical activity. It provides a visual representation of the electrical signals generated by the heart. The ECG shows characteristic waves and intervals, including the P wave (atrial depolarization), the QRS complex (ventricular depolarization), and the T wave (ventricular repolarization).

4. Cardiac Cycle

The cardiac cycle is the sequence of events that occurs during one complete heartbeat. It includes both electrical and mechanical events. The electrical events correspond to depolarization and repolarization of the atria and ventricles, while the mechanical events involve atrial and ventricular contraction and relaxation.

5. Heart Rate and Rhythm

○ Heart rate refers to the number of heart beats per minute (bpm). It is regulated by the autonomic nervous system and can vary in response to physiological demands.

○ Normal heart rhythm is known as sinus rhythm, which originates from the SA node. Irregular rhythms, such as atrial fibrillation or ventricular tachycardia, can indicate underlying heart conditions.

6. Regulation of Electrical Activity

○ The autonomic nervous system, particularly the sympathetic and parasympathetic branches, regulates the heart's electrical activity. Sympathetic stimulation increases heart rate and contractility, while parasympathetic stimulation (via the vagus nerve) slows heart rate.

○ Electrolyte imbalances, medications, and various medical conditions can also influence the heart's electrical activity.

Autorhythmic Cells

Autorhythmic cells, also known as pacemaker cells, are specialized cardiac muscle cells that spontaneously generate electrical impulses in the heart. These cells play a crucial role in initiating and controlling the heart's rhythm by serving as the primary source of electrical signals that trigger each heartbeat.

Here are key characteristics and functions of autorhythmic cells:

1. Spontaneous Electrical Activity

Autorhythmic cells have the unique ability to generate electrical impulses without external stimulation. These impulses initiate the heartbeat. The spontaneous electrical activity of autorhythmic cells is essential for maintaining the heart's rhythm and ensuring that the heart contracts rhythmically and reliably.

2. Location

Autorhythmic cells are primarily located in specific regions of the heart where they serve as the pacemaker for the heart's electrical activity.

The most important group of autorhythmic cells is found in the sinoatrial (SA) node, located in the right atrium near the entrance of the superior vena cava. The SA node is often referred to as the "natural pacemaker" of the heart because it generates the fastest electrical impulses.

3. Initiation of Heartbeat

The SA node generates electrical impulses at a regular rate (typically around 60–100 times per minute) that initiate each heartbeat.

These impulses spread through the atria, causing atrial contraction (atrial systole).

4. Conduction of Electrical Signals

Autorhythmic cells are interconnected with other regions of the heart, allowing the electrical impulses they generate to propagate efficiently.

The impulses generated by the SA node travel through specialized pathways, including the atria, atrioventricular (AV) node, bundle of His, and Purkinje fibers, to reach the ventricles.

The conduction system ensures that the atria contract before the ventricles, facilitating effective blood pumping.

5. Regulation of Heart Rate

While autorhythmic cells generate impulses spontaneously, their rate of firing can be influenced by the autonomic nervous system.

Sympathetic stimulation increases the rate of firing of autorhythmic cells, leading to an increase in heart rate (a "fight or flight" response).

Parasympathetic (vagal) stimulation decreases the rate of firing of autorhythmic cells, resulting in a decrease in heart rate (a "rest and digest" response).

6. Importance for Heart Function

The proper functioning of autorhythmic cells is crucial for maintaining heart rate, rhythm, and coordination between the atria and ventricles.

Disruptions in the activity of these cells can lead to arrhythmias (irregular heart rhythms) and other cardiac conditions.

The key features of these cells are:
- Specialized cells that initiate and conduct APs
- Display pacemaker activity (no resting potential, changes in potential due to voltage-gated Na^+, K^+ and Ca^{2+} channels)
  - Decreased flow of K^+ out and increased inward flow of Na^+ through "funny" channels results in slow depolarization
  - Near threshold, voltage-gated transient Ca^{2+} channels open and bring membrane to threshold (Ca^{2+} flows in)
  - At threshold voltage-gated long-lasting Ca^{2+} channels open, more Ca^{2+} flows in (this is the AP)
  - At peak of depolarization, voltage-gated K^+ channels open and repolarization occurs
- Locations
  - SA node (sinoatrial)
    - ➤ Right atrium

- ➤ Fastest rate of auto-rhythmicity, it is the pacemaker of the heart (under usual conditions initiates APs)
- ➤ Interatrial pathway extends to left atrium (spreads AP, atria contract)
- ➤ Internodal pathway extends to next node
- ○ AV node (atrioventricular)
  - ➤ Electrical connection between atria and ventricles
  - ➤ Signal slightly delayed (0.1 sec) to allow atria to finish contracting—more efficient blood pumping
- ○ **AV bundle (bundle of His):** Branch into ventricles
- ○ **Purkinje fibers:** Branch throughout ventricular myocardium (ventricles contract)

Cardiac Cycle

The cardiac cycle is the sequence of events that occurs during one complete heartbeat. It involves the contraction and relaxation of the heart's chambers (atria and ventricles) to pump blood through the circulatory system. The cardiac cycle is divided into two main phases—systole and diastole.

Here's an overview of the key events and phases of the cardiac cycle:

Atrial Contraction (Atrial Systole)

- ○ The cardiac cycle begins with atrial contraction, also known as atrial systole.
- ○ During this phase, both atria contract simultaneously, pushing blood into the relaxed ventricles.
- ○ Atrial contraction accounts for the final 20–30% of ventricular filling.

Isovolumetric Contraction (Ventricular Systole)

Ventricular systole begins shortly after atrial systole. It consists of two phases:

1. **Isovolumetric contraction:** In this phase, the ventricles contract forcefully, causing a rapid increase in pressure. The atrioventricular (AV) valves (mitral and tricuspid valves) close to prevent backflow of blood into the atria. However, the semilunar valves (aortic and pulmonary valves) remain closed initially, so no blood is ejected from the ventricles yet. This phase is called "isovolumetric" because the ventricular volume remains constant.
2. **Ejection phase:** After ventricular pressure exceeds arterial pressure, the semilunar valves open, and blood is ejected from the ventricles into the aorta and pulmonary artery. This marks the beginning of the ejection phase of ventricular systole.

Ventricular Relaxation (Early Diastole)

After the ejection phase, the ventricles begin to relax, and ventricular pressure decreases. The semilunar valves close to prevent the backflow of blood from the arteries into the ventricles.

Isovolumetric Relaxation (Late Diastole)

- ○ As ventricular pressure continues to fall, it eventually becomes lower than atrial pressure.
- ○ The AV valves remain closed during this phase, preventing blood from flowing back into the atria.
- ○ The period of isovolumetric relaxation ends when the atrial pressure exceeds ventricular pressure, causing the AV valves to open.

Atrial Filling (Atrial Diastole)

Atrial diastole occurs when the atria are relaxed and filling with blood. As the AV valves open, blood flows passively from the atria into the ventricles.

The cardiac cycle then repeats with the next heartbeat. The duration of each phase can vary depending on heart rate, cardiac output, and other factors. It is important to note that the left and right sides of the heart undergo these phases simultaneously, although the pressures may differ between the two sides due to their respective roles in the pulmonary and systemic circulations.

Cardiac Output

Cardiac output (CO) is the volume of blood pumped by each ventricle in one minute (left and right normally equal).

CO = heart rate (beats/min) × stroke volume (mL/beat)

❍ Typically, about 5 L/min at rest (entire blood volume)

❍ Can increase to 20–25 L/min

Difference between CO at rest and maximum CO is cardiac reserve.

Cardiac reserve refers to the ability of the heart to increase its output of blood (cardiac output) in response to increased demand, such as during physical activity or in response to stress. It represents the difference between a person's resting cardiac output and the maximum cardiac output the heart can achieve. Cardiac reserve is an important concept in cardiovascular physiology because it reflects the heart's capacity to adapt to changing conditions and meet the body's increased need for oxygen and nutrients.

Resting Cardiac Output

At rest, the human heart typically pumps a certain amount of blood per minute, known as the resting cardiac output. This resting cardiac output varies from person to person but is generally around 4–5 liters per minute in adults.

Maximum Cardiac Output

During periods of increased demand, such as during exercise, the heart can increase its pumping capacity to provide more oxygen and nutrients to the body's tissues. This maximum cardiac output is significantly higher than the resting cardiac output and can reach levels of 20 liters per minute or more in highly trained athletes.

Factors Affecting Cardiac Reserve

Several factors influence a person's cardiac reserve, including the individual's cardiovascular fitness, heart rate, stroke volume, and overall cardiac function. Regular aerobic exercise and conditioning can enhance cardiac reserve by improving the heart's efficiency and its ability to respond to increased demands.

Measurement

Cardiac reserve is often expressed as a ratio or percentage, comparing the maximum cardiac output to the resting cardiac output. For example, a person with a resting cardiac output of 5 liters per minute and a maximum cardiac output of 20 liters per minute has a cardiac reserve of 300% {[(20 − 5)/5] × 100%}.

Clinical Significance

Cardiac reserve is an important concept in cardiology and exercise physiology. It can help assess an individual's cardiovascular health and capacity to engage in physical activity. A reduced cardiac reserve may be indicative of cardiovascular disease or limitations in physical performance.

Implications for Disease

Conditions such as heart failure, coronary artery disease, and valvular heart disease can impair the heart's ability to increase cardiac output, leading to a reduced cardiac reserve. In such cases, the heart may struggle to meet the body's increased oxygen demands during exertion or stress.

Factors Influencing Heart Rate (HR)

Heart rate (HR) is the number of times the heart beats per minute and is influenced by a combination of intrinsic and extrinsic factors. Understanding these factors is essential for comprehending the regulation of heart rate and how it can vary under different conditions.

Here are the primary factors that influence heart rate:

Autonomic Nervous System (ANS)

The autonomic nervous system, which consists of the sympathetic and parasympathetic divisions, plays a central role in regulating heart rate.

The sympathetic division ("fight or flight") increases heart rate by releasing norepinephrine, which stimulates beta-adrenergic receptors in the heart, increasing heart rate.

The parasympathetic division ("rest and digest") decreases heart rate by releasing acetylcholine, which binds to muscarinic receptors in the heart, slowing down the heart rate.

Neural Factors

Emotional and psychological factors, such as stress, anxiety, excitement, and fear, can influence heart rate. For example, stress and anxiety can activate the sympathetic nervous system, increasing heart rate (tachycardia).

Hormones

Hormones can affect heart rate. For example, epinephrine (adrenaline), released during the "fight or flight" response, increases heart rate. Thyroid hormones, such as thyroxine, can also influence heart rate by affecting the heart's sensitivity to catecholamines.

Temperature

Both extreme heat and cold can influence heart rate. High temperatures can cause an increase in heart rate as the body tries to dissipate heat, while very cold temperatures can lead to vasoconstriction and a higher heart rate to maintain blood pressure.

Physical Activity and Exercise

Physical activity, especially aerobic exercise, increases heart rate to meet the increased oxygen and nutrient demands of muscles. The intensity, duration, and type of exercise can all affect heart rate. For example, high-intensity interval training (HIIT) can rapidly increase heart rate, while gentle yoga may result in a lower heart rate.

Age

Age is a significant factor influencing heart rate. In general, heart rate tends to decrease with age. Newborns and infants have higher resting heart rates than adults, and heart rate gradually decreases during childhood and adolescence.

Medications and Drugs

Various medications and substances can impact heart rate. For example, stimulants like caffeine and nicotine can increase heart rate, while certain medications used to treat hypertension or arrhythmias can either increase or decrease heart rate.

Blood Pressure

Changes in blood pressure can influence heart rate. For instance, a drop in blood pressure due to hemorrhage or dehydration can increase heart rate as a compensatory mechanism to maintain blood flow.

Medical Conditions

Certain medical conditions, such as arrhythmias, heart disease, fever, and hyperthyroidism, can cause abnormal changes in heart rate.

Sleep

Heart rate typically decreases during sleep, especially during deep, slow-wave sleep (non-REM sleep), and increases upon awakening.

Homeostatic Imbalances

It can result in heart failure (heart can not keep up with demands of body).

Two main reasons of homeostatic imbalance are:

1. Damage from heart attack or impaired circulation to cardiac muscle
2. Prolonged pumping against increased afterload (stenotic semilunar valve or chronically elevated blood pressure)

- Contractility of heart is decreased
  - SV decreased for a given EDV (Frank-Starling curve shifts down to right)
  - Body compensates with increased sympathetic activity and retaining salt and water to expand blood volume and increase EDV
- Eventually body cannot compensate causing
  - **Backward failure:** Blood pools in venous system (congestive heart failure)
  - **Forward failure:** Inadequate supplies to tissues
  - **Left:** Sided failure worse
  - **Backward:** Fluid accumulates in lungs (pulmonary edema), forward—kidney function depressed and they retain even more water and salt

Atherosclerosis and its Effects on the Heart

Atherosclerosis is a condition characterized by the build up of fatty deposits, cholesterol, calcium, and other substances within the arteries. Over time, these deposits can lead to the narrowing and hardening of the arteries, which can have significant effects on the heart and overall cardiovascular health.

Here's an overview of how atherosclerosis affects the heart:

- **Reduced blood flow:** As atherosclerosis progresses, the arteries become narrower due to the buildup of plaque. This narrowing reduces the flow of oxygen-rich blood to the heart muscle, a condition known as coronary artery disease (CAD) or coronary heart disease (CHD). Reduced blood flow to the heart can lead to various symptoms and complications.
- **Angina:** Angina is chest pain or discomfort that occurs when the heart muscle does not receive enough oxygen-rich blood. It is a common symptom of atherosclerosis in the coronary arteries. Angina can manifest as chest pressure, pain, or discomfort and may also be felt in the arms, neck, jaw, shoulder, or back.
- **Heart attack (myocardial infarction):** If an atherosclerotic plaque ruptures or a blood clot forms within a narrowed coronary artery, it can completely block blood flow to a portion of the heart muscle. This results in a heart attack, which can cause permanent damage to the heart and may be life-threatening.
- **Arrhythmias:** Atherosclerosis can disrupt the normal electrical signals in the heart, leading to irregular heart rhythms or arrhythmias. These irregular heartbeats can have serious consequences and may result in palpitations, dizziness, fainting, or even sudden cardiac death.
- **Heart failure:** Chronic, severe atherosclerosis can weaken the heart muscle over time, reducing its ability to pump blood effectively. This condition is known as heart failure, and it can lead to symptoms such as shortness of breath, fatigue, fluid retention, and swelling in the legs and ankles.
- **Stroke:** Atherosclerosis can affect arteries throughout the body, including those supplying blood to the brain. If an atherosclerotic plaque in a cerebral artery ruptures or a clot forms and blocks blood flow to the brain, it can result in a stroke. Depending on the location and severity of the stroke, it can lead to various neurological deficits.

○ **Peripheral artery disease (PAD):** Atherosclerosis can also affect arteries in other parts of the body, such as the legs. When arteries in the legs become narrowed or blocked, it can cause symptoms like leg pain, numbness, and difficulty walking. This condition is known as peripheral artery disease.

○ Transient ischemia causes angina pectoris (chest pain), usually during physical or emotional stress, and may be due to accumulation of lactic acid as heart makes ATP anaerobically.

Risk Factors

○ Genetics
○ Obesity
○ Old age
○ Smoking
○ High blood pressure
○ Diabetes
○ Lack of exercise
○ Nervous tension
○ High blood cholesterol levels

BLOOD VESSELS AND BLOOD PRESSURE

Basics

○ Exchanges between blood and tissue cells take place through the interstitial fluid.
○ All organs receive fresh blood.
○ The amount to each organ is adjusted based on the need.
○ The blood is constantly "reconditioned", so its composition is relatively constant.
○ Reconditioning organs receive a high proportion of cardiac output (digestive system, kidneys).

Organization "Vascular Tree"

Various components of vascular tree are:
○ Arteries (carries blood from heart toward tissues)
○ Arterioles (adjusts blood flow to tissues)
○ Capillaries (exchanges made)
○ Venules (carries blood to veins)
○ Veins (carries blood from tissues toward heart)

Flow rate (volume of blood passing through a particular segment of vascular tree per unit time) is directly proportional to a pressure gradient and inversely proportional to resistance (hindrance to flow from friction)
○ Vessel radius—smaller vessels → more resistance
○ Viscosity of blood—thicker blood → more resistance
○ Length of vessel —longer vessel → more resistance

Arteries

○ Help in fast transport
○ Pressure reservoir
○ Walls contain endothelial lining surrounded by smooth muscle and connective tissue fibers (collagen and elastin), which allow walls to stretch to contain pumped blood
○ When the heart is relaxing, the arteries recoil and keep the blood flowing
○ Arterial pressure fluctuates

Arterioles

○ Major resistance vessels (small radii)
○ Radii adjusted by smooth muscle in vasoconstriction and vasodilation (narrowing and enlarging)
○ Normally partially constricted (vascular tone) due to myogenic activity and sympathetic innervation
○ Metabolic factors causing vasodilation are:
  ○ Decreased O_2
  ○ Increased CO_2
  ○ Increased acid (from CO_2 and lactic acid)
  ○ Increased K^+ (APs outpacing Na^+-K^+ pump in brain or skeletal muscle)

- ○ Increased osmolarity (more solutes formed during the times of elevated metabolism)
  - ○ Release of adenosine (in cardiac muscle)
  - ○ Release of prostaglandins (not well understood)
- ○ Physical influences are:
  - ○ Application of heat (vasodilation) or cold (vasoconstriction)
  - ○ Myogenic responses to stretch (vasoactive substances probably contribute)
  - ○ Tone increases in response to increased stretch (resists stretch)—important to keep flow to tissues constant as MAP changes (pressure autoregulation)
  - ○ Tone decreases in response to decreased stretch—important in restoring flow to previously deprived tissue (reactive hyperemia)
- ○ MAP = CO × total peripheral resistance
- ○ NE at alpha receptors causes vasoconstriction
- ○ Epinephrine (E) at beta receptors causes vasodilation (heart, skeletal muscles)
- ○ Other hormones
  - ○ **Vasopressin:** Important in fluid balance, vasoconstrictor
  - ○ **Angiotensin II:** Important in fluid balance, vasoconstrictor

Capillaries

- ○ Responsible for exchanges between plasma and interstitial fluid (solute exchange mainly by diffusion)
- ○ Thin walled, narrow vessels
- ○ Highly branched
- ○ Blood flows slowly through individual vessels
- ○ Lipid soluble substances pass through cells (O_2, CO_2)
- ○ Water soluble substances pass through pores (ions, glucose, amino acids)
- ○ Degree of "leakiness" may change due to actin-myosin in capillary cells

Precapillary Sphincters

- ○ Rings of smooth muscle can block flow through capillaries in less active tissues.
- ○ Important in the distribution of fluids between plasma and interstitial fluid.
- ○ Fluid (not proteins) pushed out through pores at the arteriolar end (ultrafiltration).
- ○ Fluid reabsorbed at the venular end.
- ○ Ultrafiltration occurs in open capillaries, and reabsorption in closed capillaries.
- ○ Extra fluid picked up by lymph vessels (initial lymphatics) in capillary beds.
- ○ Large valve like openings allow in fluid and any leaked proteins (lymph).

Veins

- ○ Transport back to heart
- ○ Blood reservoir
- ○ Stretchable with little recoil
- ○ Venous storage decreases effective centimeters volume and can be altered based on need

Factors Influencing Venous Return

- ○ **Sympathetic activity**: Vasoconstriction drives more blood toward the heart.
- ○ **Skeletal muscle** activity: Acts as pump.
- ○ **Valves:** One-way valves every few centimeters allow flow toward the heart only.
- ○ **Respiratory activity:** Acts as a pump due to decreased pressure in the thoracic cavity.
- ○ **Cardiac suction:** Blood "sucked in" as ventricles relax.

Blood Pressure

- ○ MAP is a main driving force
- ○ High enough to get blood to tissues
- ○ Blood pressure is the force exerted by blood on the vessel walls, depends on blood volume and distensibility of the vessel.
- ○ Systolic pressure is the maximum pressure during systole (should be <120 mm Hg)

- Diastolic pressure is the pressure during diastole (should be <80 mm Hg)
- Systolic-diastolic = pulse pressure (the pressure felt in arteries near the body surface)
- Mean arterial pressure is the main driving force for blood flow to tissues
- MAP = diastolic pressure + 1/3 pulse pressure

Short-term Regulation (Seconds)
Baroreceptor Reflex

- Pressure sensors in the carotid sinus and aortic arch sense changes in MAP and pulse pressure. The rate of firing increases with increasing pressure, and decreases with decreasing pressure.
- The integrating center is the cardiovascular control center in medulla of brainstem.

Long-term Regulation (Minutes to Days)
- Adjustments in total blood volume via salt/water balance—urinary system and thirst (volume receptors in the left atrium, osmoreceptors in hypothalamus)
- Other contributing factors:
  - **Chemoreceptors in carotid and aortic arteries:** Sense low O_2 and high acid
  - **Cerebral cortex:** Hypothalamic pathway influences emotional/behavioral responses
  - **Exercise:** May be unidentified "exercise centers"
  - **Hypothalamic temperature regulation:** Overrides baroreceptor reflex for skin vessels
  - Vasoactive substances from endothelial cells
  - Neurotransmitter effects in brain (poorly understood)

Hypertension

- BP above 140/90
- Cause identified in about 10% of cases (secondary hypertension): Include athero-sclerosis, endocrine disorders, nervous system defects
- Primary hypertension causes may include:
  - Kidney salt regulation
  - Excessive salt intake
  - Diet low in fruit, vegetables, dairy (low in K^+ and Ca^{2+})
  - Defects in Na^+-K^+ pumps
  - Abnormal local vasoactive substances
  - Excess vasopressin
- Stresses heart and blood vessels to cause
  - Congestive heart failure from increased afterload
  - Rupture of vessels—stroke, heart attack
  - Damage to vessels may cause accumulation of lipids and lead to atherosclerosis
  - Kidney failure due to damaged vessels
  - Loss of vision from damaged vessels

Hypotension

- BP below 100/60
- Transient as in standing up—gravity decreases venous return and in some people emotional stress decreases sympathetic activity (may be adaptive)
- When blood flow to tissues is inadequate, its called circulatory shock
- Causes
  - Loss of blood volume (hemorrhage, diarrhea)
  - Weakened heart
  - Vasodilation (septic or anaphylactic)
  - Loss of sympathetic tone (extreme pain as in crushing injury)
- May become irreversible

BLOOD

Some Basic Facts

Blood forms 8% of body weight, 5–5.5 L

It is a connective tissue and has two components:

1. **Formed elements:** Red blood cells (erythrocytes), white blood cells (leukocytes) and platelets **(Fig. 1.4)**
2. Matrix is plasma

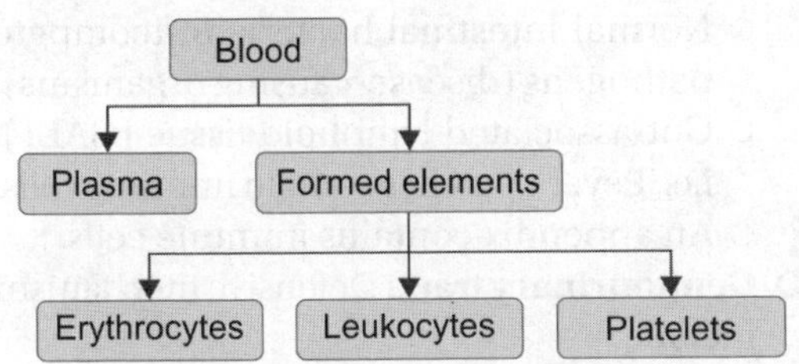

Fig. 1.4: Blood and its components.

Plasma

- It is 90% water.
- It contains proteins, ions, buffers, respiratory gases, nutrients, wastes, hormones
- The proteins are functionally important part of the plasma as they help in establishing osmotic pressure.
- They are of three types:
  1. **Albumin:** Binds substances for transport
  2. **Globulin:** Binds substances for transport, blood clotting, inactive precursors, antibodies.
  3. **Fibrinogen:** Blood clotting

Formed Elements

1. Erythrocytes (Red blood cells)

- Red blood cells carry oxygen
- They contain a protein known as **hemoglobin,** which has the following functions:
  - Carries most of O_2 (4 O_2/molecule)
  - Carries some CO_2
  - Helps buffer blood
- No nucleus or organelles
- Contains glycolytic enzymes for making ATP
- Contain carbonic anhydrase, which converts CO_2 to its transported form (HCO_3, bicarbonate)

Erythropoiesis (Production of RBCs)

- RBCs live about 120 days, and most old, fragile cells die in splenic capillaries.
- It occurs in red bone marrow (in adults—sternum, vertebrae, ends of long bones, ribs, base of skull).
- Contains undifferentiated cells that give rise to all blood cells (pluripotent stem cells).
- Controlled by hormone erythropoietin which is released by kidneys in response to decreased O_2.
- As the RBCs mature, they eject nucleus/organelles.
- The process takes days to weeks, depending on how many cells are needed.

2. Leukocytes (White Blood Cells)

- They help in body defense.
- They are originally made in red marrow in response to stimulating factors.
- These cells are found in blood and tissues.

3. Platelets

- They are cell fragments produced from megakaryocytes in red marrow
- Live about 10 days
- Produced in response to the hormone thrombopoietin (control unknown)
- Can be stored in spleen
- No nucleus, but do have organelles

Hemostasis (Stoppage of Blood Flow)

The various steps of hemostasis are:

- **Vasoconstriction:** Blood flow through a break is minimized by vasoconstriction (vascular response and sympathetically induced)
- **Formation of platelet plug that seals break**
  - Platelets stick to exposed collagen of damaged connective tissue
  - Platelets release chemicals like ADP and thromboxane A_2 that cause more platelets to become "sticky" and build up
  - Normal endothelium releases prostacyclin, which inhibits platelet

aggregation (plug does not spread beyond damaged area)

○ Actin-myosin complex in platelets contracts and strengthens plug

○ Plug releases vasoconstrictors (serotonin, epinephrine, thromboxane A_2)

○ **Blood clotting needed to plug larger holes**

○ Clotting cascade initiated by exposure of plasma precursors to damaged vessel

○ Series of reactions resulting in clotting

○ **Thrombin converts fibrinogen to fibrin, which forms meshwork that traps RBCs.**

○ **Thrombin also activates factor XIII, which stabilizes meshwork.**

○ **Clot retraction:** Platelets contract and squeeze serum from the clot.

○ **Long-term healing begins as fibroblasts from connective tissue form a scar.**

○ **As healing occurs plasmin dissolves the clot (clot retraction).**

BODY DEFENSES

External Defenses

These forms the first line of defense and include:

○ Skin

○ Mucous membrane and associated structures.

Skin (integument): It acts as a:

○ **Physical barrier:** Keratinocytes form a barrier and also influence immune cells.

○ **Skin-associated lymphoid tissue (SALT):** Contains specialized immune cells.

○ **Chemical barrier:** Secretions of sweat and oil (sebaceous) glands are toxic to bacteria.

Mucous Membranes and Associated Structures (Line Cavities Open to the Outside of the Body)

○ **Digestive tract:** Defensive mechanism of digestive tract include:

○ Salivary enzymes kill bacteria.

○ Acid in the stomach kills bacteria.

○ Secretions contain antibodies.

○ Normal intestinal bacteria outcompete pathogens (disease-causing organisms).

○ Gut-associated lymphoid tissue (GALT), i.e., Peyer's patches contain immune cells.

○ An appendix contains immune cells.

○ **Genitourinary tract:** Defensive mechanism include:

○ Acidic urine

○ Acidic vaginal secretions

○ Sticky mucus in the genitourinary tract traps pathogens and has antibodies

Respiratory tract: Defensive mechanism include:

○ Large particles get filtered by hair in nasal passages

○ Tonsils and adenoids contain immune cells

○ Sticky mucus traps pathogens in airways

○ Cilia sweep mucus upward (swallowed, or coughing, sneezing or expectorating removes it from the body)

○ Antibodies secreted in mucus

○ Alveolar (air sac) macrophages engulf pathogens

Defense Cells

The defense cells/tissues of the body

○ White blood cells

○ Lymphoid tissue

○ Interferons

○ Natural killer cells

○ T-cells

○ Innate lymphoid cells (ILC)

White Blood Cells (WBCs)

○ **Neutrophils:** Highly mobile phagocytes.

○ **Eosinophils:** Secrete chemicals that kill parasitic worms, involved in allergic reactions.

○ **Basophils:** Release histamine and heparin (inflammatory response) involved in allergic reactions.

○ **Lymphocytes:** Can reproduce outside bone marrow (in lymphoid tissues like lymph nodes).

- ○ **B lymphocytes:** Secrete antibodies and probably mature in bone marrow
- ○ **T lymphocytes:** Destroy virus-infected and cancer cells, mature in thymus
- ○ **Monocytes:** Become macrophages—large phagocytes in tissues. Most are in tissues and some circulate in the blood.

Lymphoid Tissue

- ○ Lymphoid tissue is a critical immune system component
- ○ Plays a crucial role in protecting the body against infections and diseases.
- ○ It primarily comprises specialized cells and organs that work together to recognize and eliminate foreign invaders, such as bacteria, viruses, and other pathogens.
- ○ Lymphoid tissue is rich in lymphocytes, which are white blood cells that are central to the immune system.
- ○ Lymph nodes, spleen, thymus, tonsils, adenoids, appendix, SALT and GALT are examples of lymphoid tissue.

Interferons

- ○ They are released by virus-infected cells, triggering the production of virus-blocking enzymes in nearby cells.
- ○ Enhances the role of phagocytes and other immune cells on virus-infected and cancer cells.

Natural Killer Cells

They are similar to lymphocyte, lyse virus-infected cells and cancer cells.

T Cells and their Types

- ○ **Cytotoxic T cells (killer cells or CD8 cells):** Destroy virus-infected, cancer or transplanted cells either by direct killing by releasing perforin to poke holes and lyse cell or by indirect by signaling for apoptosis (programmed cell death).

- ○ **Helper T cells (CD4):** Secrete cytokines that regulate nearly all aspects of an immune response, including B cell growth factor, T cell growth factor (interleukin 2), chemotaxins or macrophage-migration inhibiting factor keeps macrophages in the area and makes them more powerful.
- ○ **Suppressor T cells:** They do not require antigen-presenting cells (APC) for their activation. They limit the responses of other immune cells to reproduce more slowly than other immune cells and shut down immune responses after they have served their purpose. Cells that blur the boundaries of innate and adaptive immunity.

Innate Lymphoid Cells (ILCs)

These are a group of immune cells that are part of the innate immune system that do not express antigen-specific receptors like antibodies. Instead, they play a crucial role in the immediate response to infections and tissue damage by detecting and responding to specific signals from the host.

There are three main subsets of ILCs:

1. **Group 1 ILCs (ILC1s):** These cells are functionally similar to CD4+ T helper 1 (Th1) cells. They produce pro-inflammatory cytokines like interferon-gamma (IFN-γ) and play a role in defense against intracellular pathogens, such as viruses.

2. **Group 2 ILCs (ILC2s):** ILC2s are involved in the response to parasitic infections, allergies, and tissue repair. They produce cytokines like interleukin-4 (IL-4), IL-5, and IL-13, which promote inflammation and tissue repair.

3. **Group 3 ILCs (ILC3s):** ILC3s are similar in function to Th17 cells. They produce cytokines like IL-17 and IL-22, which play a role in protecting mucosal surfaces, such as

the gastrointestinal tract, against bacterial and fungal infections.

ILCs are found in various tissues throughout the body, including the gut, skin, and lungs. They are crucial for maintaining tissue homeostasis, promoting tissue repair, and contributing to the early defense against infections. Dysregulation of ILC function has been associated with various inflammatory diseases and immune disorders.

Nonspecific Defenses (General Defenses or Innate Immunity)

- Responses that defend against any invader or abnormal material.
- Triggered by general molecular patterns associated with pathogens or other dangers.

Inflammation (Inflammatory Response)

It is designed to bring phagocytes and plasma proteins to an injured area in order to:
- Destroy/inactivate invaders
- Clean up debris
- Prepare for healing
- Characteristics include redness, heat, swelling, pain and loss of function.

The steps of inflammation are depicted in **Flowchart 2.2.**

Flowchart 2.2: Steps of inflammation.

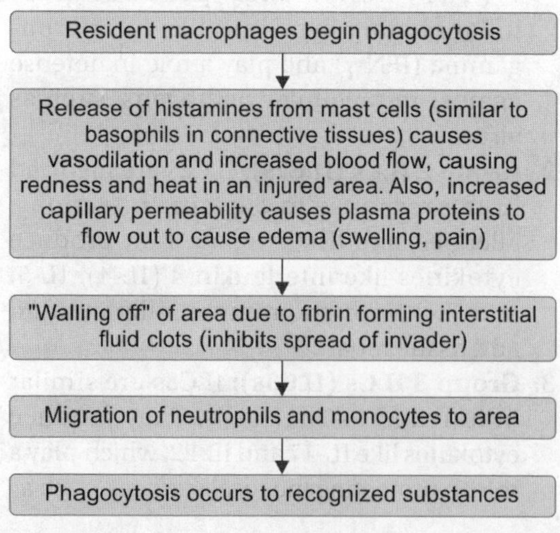

Immunity

- **Specific immune responses (adaptive immunity):** Act on particular invaders:
  - B lymphocytes specialize in recognizing free-existing invaders like bacteria, bacterial toxins, some viruses (antibody-mediated or humoral immunity).
  - T lymphocytes specialize in killing virus-infected and cancer cells (cell-mediated immunity).
  - During maturation each B and T cell becomes capable of responding to a particular invader (only one specific kind of invade for each individual cell) and the invaders to which we can respond to is genetically determined.
  - Antigen recognition—large, complex molecule that the immune system can respond to usually proteins, or large polysaccharides that may be on cell surface or individual molecules secreted by the pathogen.
  - Self-antigens are plasma membrane glycoproteins.
    - ➤ Major histocompatibility complex (MHC) is a group of genes that determines which MHC glycoproteins an individual has.
    - ➤ Lymphocytes do not harm these cells under normal conditions.
- **Antibody-mediated immunity**
  - B cells display antibodies, also called gamma globulins or immunoglobulins (Ig), on their surfaces and secrete them.
  - When a B cell clone is exposed to the right antigen, the cells reproduce and
    - ➤ Some become plasma cells, which secrete antibodies.
    - ➤ Some become memory cells, which launch a more powerful attack if the body is exposed to that antigen again (secondary response).
  - Antibodies enhance the immune response

- ➤ **Neutralization:** Bind to free-floating antigens and stop them from causing harm.
- ➤ Most powerful activator of the complement system (so enhances inflammation).
- ➤ Act as an opsonin, enhancing phagocytosis.
- ➤ Cause agglutination of cells with antigen.
- ➤ Stimulate killer cells to lyse bacteria (similar to natural killer cells but require antibodies).
  - Active immunity occurs when an individual's B cells make antibodies, e.g., infections, vaccines.
  - Passive immunity is when antibodies come from an immune donor, e.g., breast milk, snake bite/rabies/tetanus shots
- **Cell-mediated immunity**
  - Macrophage phagocytises antigen and places it on its surface.
  - Appropriate type of T cell binds and is activated to reproduce and differentiate.
  - T cells require both non-self and self-antigen to bind and destroy a cell.

RESPIRATORY SYSTEM

Basics

- **Pulmonary ventilation:** Breathing
- **External respiration:** Gas exchange between the blood and alveoli (air sacs)
- **Gas transport:** Blood transports gases to tissues (CV system)
- **Internal respiration:** Gas exchange between the blood and tissues (CV/tissues)
- **Cellular respiration:** Use of O_2 to produce ATP (cells)

Functions of Respiratory System

- To obtain O_2, eliminate CO_2

- Nonrespiratory functions:
  - Route for water and heat loss
  - Enhance venous return
  - Acid-base balance (CO_2)
  - Vocalization
  - Defense against inhaled invaders
  - Sense of smell
  - Alters blood composition

Functional Anatomy of the Respiratory System

Trachea (Windpipe)

- The trachea is a tubular structure composed of rings of cartilage.
- It connects the larynx to the bronchial tree and allows air passage.
- The tracheal walls contain ciliated cells and mucous glands that help filter and clear mucus and foreign particles.

Bronchial Tree

- The trachea divides into the right and left primary bronchi, each leading to a lung.
- The bronchi further divide into smaller bronchioles, eventually leading to alveoli.
- This branching network allows air to reach every part of the lungs for gas exchange.

Lungs

- The two lungs are the primary respiratory organs.
- They are enclosed by the pleura, a double-layered membrane that provides lubrication and maintains lung expansion.
- The lungs are divided into lobes: The right has three lobes, while the left has two.

Alveoli

- Alveoli are tiny, sac-like structures within the lungs where gas exchange occurs.
- Oxygen from inhaled air diffuses across the alveolar-capillary membrane into the bloodstream.

○ Carbon dioxide, produced by cellular metabolism, diffuses from the bloodstream into the alveoli for removal during exhalation.

○ They have type I cells—simple squamous epithelium and type II cells—secrete surfactant.

Diaphragm and Intercostal Muscles

○ The diaphragm is the primary muscle responsible for breathing.

○ The diaphragm and intercostal muscle contraction expand the chest cavity during inhalation, creating negative pressure that draws air into the lungs.

○ Relaxation of these muscles during exhalation allows for the expulsion of air.

Pleura

○ The pleura consists of two layers: The visceral pleura (covering the lungs) and the parietal pleura (lining the chest cavity).

○ The pleural cavity between these layers contains pleural fluid, reducing friction and enabling smooth lung expansion and contraction.

Control Centers

The respiratory centers in the brainstem, specifically the medulla oblongata and pons, regulate breathing patterns and respond to changes in blood gas levels, ensuring the body maintains adequate oxygen and carbon dioxide levels.

Respiratory Mechanics

In ventilation, air flows down a pressure gradient.

Important Pressures

○ Atmospheric pressure (760 mm Hg at sea level)

○ Intra-alveolar pressure

○ Intrapleural pressure

○ Intrathoracic pressure is within the pleural sac (756 mm Hg at rest)

Mechanism of Respiration (Flowchart 2.3)

Flowchart 2.3: Mechanism of respiration.

> **Lungs will always expand to fill the thoracic cavity**
> (intra-alveolar pressure always equilibrates with atmospheric pressure and greater pressure outward than inward)

> **Inspiration**
> • Inspiratory muscles contract (diaphragm and external intercostals)
> • Volume of the thoracic cavity and lungs increases
> • Intra-alveolar pressure decreases
> • Air flows in

> **Expiration**
> • Inspiratory muscles relax (quiet breathing)
> • Volume of thoracic cavity and lungs decreases
> • Intra-alveolar pressure increases
> • Air flows out

> **Forced expiration**
> [Expiratory muscles contract (abdominal wall muscles and internal intercostals)]

Airway Resistance

It is adjusted to meet the body's needs.

○ In parasympathetic stimulation → bronchoconstriction → increased resistance → decreased airflow.

○ In sympathetic stimulation/epinephrine → bronchodilation → decreased resistance → increased airflow.

○ Local controls act on bronchiolar smooth muscle and on arteriolar smooth muscle.

○ In bronchioles
  ○ Increased CO_2 → bronchodilation → increased airflow.
  ○ Decreased CO_2 → bronchoconstriction → decreased airflow.

○ In arterioles
  ○ Decreased O_2 → vasoconstriction → decreased blood flow.
  ○ Increased O_2 → vasodilation → increased blood flow.

Elastic Behavior of Lungs

○ Healthy lungs recoil after stretching and are compliant (easy to inflate).

- Two main factors involved in this are elastic fibers and **alveolar** surface tension.
  - Elastin fibers in lung connective tissue.
  - Alveolar surface tension.
    - ➤ Water molecules lining alveoli attract each other, creating surface tension.
    - ➤ Surfactant decreases surface tension (without it lungs would collapse).
    - ➤ Surfactant also increases compliance and reduces work needed to breathe.
    - ➤ Surfactant may also enhance phagocytosis.
- In healthy lungs, breathing requires little energy
  - 3% of total energy at rest
  - 5% during exercise
  - Up to 30% at rest with obstructive lung disease.

Gas Exchange

Gases diffuse down partial pressure gradients (pressure exerted by a particular gas in a mixture of gases or dissolved in a body fluid)

- Alveolar PO_2 is lower than atmospheric PO_2 and alveolar PCO_2 is higher than atmospheric PCO_2
  - Water vapor in lungs dilutes gases.
  - Newly inspired air mixes with old air (15% new air with inspiration).
- CO_2 requires a smaller gradient for efficient transfer because it is more soluble (usually about equal amounts of O_2/CO_2 exchanged).
- At lungs
  - PO_2 is always higher in alveoli, $O_2 \rightarrow$ blood.
  - PCO_2 is always higher in blood, $CO_2 \rightarrow$ alveoli.
- At tissues
  - PO_2 is always higher in blood, $O_2 \rightarrow$ tissues.
  - PCO_2 is always higher in tissues, $CO_2 \rightarrow$ blood.
- Other factors influence the rate of gas transfer.

- **During exercise:** More pulmonary capillaries open, increasing the surface area for exchanges. Also, greater stretching of alveolar membranes increases surface area and thins membrane (decreased distance for diffusion)
- Disease thickens membrane and increases distance for diffusion (pulmonary edema, pulmonary fibrosis, pneumonia)

Hb-O_2 Dissociation Curve

- Plateau portion means that blood can carry nearly maximum amounts of O_2 at varying PO_2 levels (safety margin on low O_2 environments).
- Steep portion means that small decreases in PO_2 at active tissues allow more O_2 to be released.
- The curve shifts to the right in active tissues (more O_2 is released at active tissues at a given PO_2).
  - Bohr effect—increased PCO_2
  - Increased acid (from increased CO_2 and lactic acid)
  - Increased temperature
  - Increased 2,3-bisphosphoglycerate (BPG), produced inside RBCs in increasing amounts when HbO_2 levels below normal

Control of Respiration

Medullary Respiratory Center

- Pattern probably established by pacemaker activity in rostral ventromedial medulla (Pre-Bot zinger complex).
- Dorsal respiratory group (DRG) responsible for quiet breathing.
  - Inspiratory neurons terminate on motor neurons in spinal cord, which supply inspiratory muscles.
  - Quiet expiration begins when neurons stop firing.
- Ventral respiratory group (VRG) is important when demands for ventilation increase.

- Not active in quiet breathing.
- Stimulate motor neurons supplying expiratory muscles.

Pons Respiratory Centers

- Pneumotaxic and apneustic centers "fine tune" medullary centers to produce smooth inspirations and expirations.
- **Hering-Breuer reflex**
  - Pulmonary stretch receptors in airways are activated at large tidal volumes to inhibit inspiratory neurons.
  - Influencing factors:
    - ➤ Central chemoreceptors in medulla sense increased PCO_2 (via increased H^+ in CSF) and signal respiratory centers to increase ventilation.
    - ➤ Peripheral chemoreceptors known as carotid bodies and aortic bodies sense increased H^+ and signal to increase ventilation.
  - PO_2 important only at very low O_2 levels.
  - Peripheral chemoreceptors signal to increase ventilation during exercise.
  - Proprioceptors in muscles and joints send stimulating signals to respiratory center.
  - Increase in body temperature
  - Epinephrine
  - Input from cerebral cortex

Other Factors

- Reflexes like coughing/sneezing
- Pain
- Emotion

URINARY SYSTEM

Basic Functions

- Water balance and osmolarity
- Electrolyte (ion) balance
- Maintain plasma volume, long-term regulation of blood pressure
- Acid/base balance
- Excrete wastes (urea, uric acid, creatinine) and other materials

- Secrete erythropoietin
- Secrete renin (Na^+ balance)
- Converts vitamin D to its active form

Renal Anatomy

Nephron is the functional unit of the kidney.

Glomerulus

- Tuft of capillaries that filters blood.
- Renal artery branches to form afferent and efferent arteriole for each nephron.
- Efferent arteriole divides to form peritubular capillaries (supply renal tissue with blood).

Tubules

- Glomerular capsule surrounds glomerulus and collects filtrate.
- Proximal convoluted tubule (PCT).
- Loop of Henle.
- Distal convoluted tubule (DCT).
- Collecting duct/tubule—drains fluid from several nephrons to the renal pelvis.

Juxtaglomerular Apparatus

- Regulates kidney function.
- **Macula densa:** Specialized cells of DCT as it passes by the glomerulus.
- Granular cells (juxtaglomerular cells or JG cells) are specialized smooth muscle cells of arterioles.

Types of Nephrons

- **Cortical:** Lie mainly in cortex (80%).
- **Juxtamedullary:** Loops dip to end of medulla (important in urine concentration/conserving water).
- Vasa recta are blood vessels that run near the long loop

Renal Processes

The three important renal processes are:
1. Glomerular filtration
2. Tubular reabsorption
3. Tubular secretion

Glomerular Filtration

- About 20% of plasma entering the glomerulus is filtered.
- Entire plasma volume filtered 65 times/day.
- Nonselective process.
- Filtered substances pass through highly permeable filtration membrane.
- Glomerular capillaries are 100x more permeable than other capillaries.
- Basement membrane (collagen for strength and glycoproteins with a negative charge that repels plasma proteins).
- An inner layer of the glomerular capsule contains podocytes wrap around capillaries and form filtration slits.
- Glomerular capillary blood pressure forces fluid through filtration membrane and is higher than in other capillaries.
- Diameter of afferent arteriole larger than efferent arteriole, blood dams up, and filtration occurs throughout the glomerulus.

Glomerular Filtration Rate (GFR)

- GFR = K_f × net filtration pressure (K_f = filtration coefficient, collective properties of filtration membrane)
- Autoregulation
  - Allows GFR to remain constant despite changes in BP (vasoconstriction/dilation of afferent arteriole).
  - Myogenic mechanism—arteriolar smooth muscle constricts when stretched, relaxes with decreased pressure.
  - Tubuloglomerular feedback mechanism—macula densa detects changes in rate of filtrate flow or osmotic changes and signals granular cells to release vasoactive substances.
  - Increased flow → vasoconstriction → decreased GFR.
  - Decreased flow → vasodilation → increased GFR.
  - Sufficient in MAP 80–180 mm Hg range.
- Extrinsic sympathetic control

- GFR changed based on need (override autoregulation to regulate BP).
- Baroreceptor reflex
  - Decreased plasma volume → generalized vasoconstriction, including afferent arteriole → decreased GFR → conservation of fluids.
  - Increased BP → vasodilation → increased GFR → eliminate more fluids.

Tubular Reabsorption

- Selective recovery of filtered substances.
- Typically, nephrons reabsorb 99% of the water, 100% of the sugar, and 99.5% of the salt that is filtered.
- Different portions of tubule specialize in particular substances.
- Most substances pass through tubule cells (transepithelial transport).
  - Can be active or passive (if any step is active, reabsorption of that substance is considered active).

Na^+ reabsorption: It occurs via:

- Occurs via Na^+-K^+ ATPase in the basolateral membrane.
  - Creates gradients for diffusion.
  - Tied to reabsorption of other substances (glucose, amino acids, water, Cl^-, urea).
  - Occurs in PCT and loop—automatically reabsorbs most Na^+ (92%).
  - DCT and collecting tubule—hormonal control, reabsorption according to need.
- Renin-angiotensin-aldosterone system: In response to decreased NaCl/decrease ECF volume/decrease BP, macula densa signals granular cells to release renin (an enzyme) Angiotensinogen → Angiotensin I → Angiotensin II in lungs to cause.
  - Vasoconstriction of arterioles.
  - Stimulates thirst
  - Stimulates vasopressin release (H_2O reabsorption).

○ Adrenal cortex releases aldosterone—promotes insertion of more Na^+ channels and Na^+-K^+ pumps into cells of DCT and collecting tubule (Cl^- and H_2O follow Na^+).
○ Atrial natriuretic peptide (ANP) inhibits Na^+ reabsorption. It is released from atria in response to increased stretch from increase ECF/increase BP.

Water Reabsorption
○ Passively reabsorbed throughout most of nephron (not ascending limb of loop).
○ 80% osmotically follows solute reabsorption (water flows through channels into cells or through leaky tight junctions).
○ 20% reabsorbed according to need in DCT and collecting tubule (hormonal control-vasopressin).

Urea Reabsorption
○ Only waste product reabsorbed.
○ As H_2O reabsorbed in PCT, urea becomes more concentrated and then moves down its concentration gradient (50% reabsorbed).

Tubular Secretion
○ Selective transfer of materials from plasma in peritubular capillaries to filtrate.
○ Enhances removal of some substances.
○ Transepithelial transport (opposite of reabsorption).

H^+ Secretion
○ Important in acid/base balance
○ Actively secreted in PCT, DCT and collecting tubules according to need (increase $H^+ \rightarrow$ increased secretion of H^+)
○ Can be coupled to Na^+ reabsorption instead of K^+ (basolateral pump in distal nephron)

K^+ Secretion
○ Reabsorption in PCT is automatic (active).
○ Controlled secretion of K^+ in DCT and collecting tubule.
○ Important in maintaining membrane potential.

Organic Anion and Cation Secretion
○ Special carriers for each in PCT.
○ Prostaglandins and other chemical messengers.
○ Other substances like drugs or pollutants.

Variations in Urine Solute Concentration (Controlling Amount of H_2O Excreted)

Counter-current Mechanism (Medullary Counter-current System)
○ Long loops of juxtamedullary nephrons establish a vertical osmotic gradient in the interstitial fluid of medulla.
○ Vasa recta prevent loss of gradient.
○ Water can be reabsorbed from collecting tubules as it flows through gradient (under control of vasopressin).
○ Establishing the gradient (counter-current multiplication)—by loop.
  ○ Descending limb permeable to H_2O but not Na^+.
  ○ Ascending limb pumps out Na^+ but is impermeable to H_2O
  ○ As Na^+ is pumped out of ascending limb, water leaves descending limb by diffusion leading to gradient of 300–1,200 mosm/L in medulla

Variable H_2O Reabsorption
○ Filtrate in DCT very dilute.
○ Without vasopressin (antidiuretic hormone or ADH, from hypothalamus/posterior pituitary) DCT and collecting duct impermeable to H_2O (H_2O not reabsorbed, urine dilute).
○ When vasopressin present (released as hypothalamus detects increased osmolarity/decreased H_2O) DCT and collecting ducts become permeable to H_2O.
  ○ cAMP second messenger system—results in insertion of H_2O channels in tubule
  ○ Water reabsorbed as it flows through medullary gradient

Counter-current Exchange in Vasa Recta

○ Medullary gradient does not dissipate because of the construction of the blood supply
○ Vasa recta follow loop and exchanges of NaCl and H_2O occur so that the blood equilibrates with the surrounding interstitial fluid

Micturition (Urination)

○ Urethra has two sphincter muscles that prevent leaking of urine.
  1. Internal urethral sphincter made of smooth muscle (involuntary).
  2. External urethral sphincter made of skeletal muscle (voluntary).
○ Micturition reflex occurs when stretch receptors in bladder are activated and parasympathetic fibers are stimulated (occurs at 250–400 mL urine).
○ Parasympathetic stimulation causes bladder to contract, opening internal sphincter and inhibiting motor neurons to external sphincter.
○ A person become conscious to urinate, but can temporarily override reflex until its convenient.

DIGESTIVE SYSTEM

Function

To transfer nutrients, H_2O and electrolytes from food to the body. Food is an energy source and contains the basic building blocks of body tissues.

Digestive Processes

The four main digestive processes are:
1. **Motility:** Muscular contractions that move food through the digestive tract (propulsive) and mix food.
2. **Secretion:** Digestive juices (enzymes, bile, mucus, hormones).
3. **Digestion:** Breaking down large molecules into smaller units.
4. **Absorption:** Substances moved from the digestive tract to blood or lymph.

Receptors and Reflexes of Digestive Tract

Digestive tract contains:
○ Chemoreceptors
○ Mechanoreceptors
○ Osmoreceptors

Stimulation of receptors initiates reflexes. Short reflexes—entirely within intrinsic nerves and long reflexes—also involve ANS.

Mechanism of Digestion

Mouth

○ Mastication (chewing) starts in the mouth to break down food.
○ Salivary glands produce saliva to:
  ○ Begins digestion of carbohydrate with salivary amylase.
  ○ Moistens food with mucus for easy swallowing.
  ○ Lysozyme lyses bacteria.
  ○ Produced in response to stimulation from chemoreceptors and pressure receptors in mouth, or seeing/smelling food.

Pharynx and Esophagus

These are the pathways to the stomach.

Stomach

Three major functions are:
1. Store food and release to duodenum at the appropriate rate.
2. Secrete HCl and enzymes to begin protein digestion (continue carbohydrate digestion with salivary enzymes).
3. Mix food with gastric secretions to make chyme.

Gastric Motility

Four aspects of motility:
1. **Gastric filling**
   ○ Plasticity: Stomach can stretch without increasing tension.
   ○ Receptive relaxation: Eating triggers reflex relaxation.
2. **Gastric storage:** Food stored mainly in body of stomach.

3. **Gastric mixing**
   - Mostly in antrum (thicker muscle layer).
   - Peristaltic contractions.
4. **Gastric emptying**
   - Peristaltic waves push some chyme into duodenum.
   - Influencing factors (stomach and duodenum).
     - ➤ **Amount of chyme:** More chyme increases emptying via direct effect on smooth muscle, intrinsic and extrinsic neurons, hormone gastrin.
     - ➤ Stimuli such as fat, acid, increased osmolarity and distention in duodenum trigger slowing of gastric emptying via neural and hormonal responses.

Gastric Glands and Secretions

Oxyntic Mucosa (Body and Fundus)

- Surface epithelial cells secrete thick alkaline mucus that protects stomach from acid and digestive enzymes.
- Mucous neck cells produce watery, lubricating mucus, also divide rapidly and differentiate into other cell types (entire mucosa replaced every 3 days).
- Parietal cells secrete HCl and intrinsic factor. HCL activates digestive enzymes and produces optimal pH for protein digestion; breaks down connective tissue and muscle; kills bacteria.
- Intrinsic factor allows absorption of vitamin B_{12}.
- Chief cells secrete pepsinogen (inactive so cells would not be digested), which is converted to protein digestive enzyme pepsin.

Pyloric Gland Area (Antrum)

- Secretes mucus and some pepsinogen (not HCl).
- G cells secrete hormone gastrin that stimulates parietal and chief cells and also stimulates growth of mucosa in stomach and small intestine.

Small Intestine

It is a major organ of digestion and absorption

Motility

- Mixes chyme and exposes chyme to absorptive surfaces.
- Slowly moves chyme forward.
- Duodenum segments in response to distention.
- Ileum segments in response to gastrin when chyme is in the stomach (gastroileal reflex).

Enzymes

- Pancreas secretes digestive enzymes and protective alkaline fluid ($NaHCO_3$) into duodenum.
- Proteolytic enzymes are secreted in inactive forms (trypsinogen) that is converted to an active form trypsin, with enterokinase in luminal border of mucosa. Trypsin digests protein and converts other enzymes to active forms chymotrypsinogen → chymotrypsin and procarboxypeptidase → carboxypeptidase.
- Pancreatic amylase (secreted in active form) to convert polysaccharides → disaccharides.
- Pancreatic lipase (active) convert triglycerides → monoglycerides + fatty acids.
- Liver's digestive function is to produce bile that can be stored in gallbladder until needed in the duodenum.
- Bile salts, cholesterol and lecithin are produced by hepatocytes (other fluids come from bile duct cells). Bile salts emulsify fats—break up fat into droplets to expose more surface area for digestion and form micelles that carry nonwater soluble products of fat digestion to absorption sites on the mucosa.
- Small intestine secretes mucus, but digestive enzymes are in epithelial cell membranes (brush border).

Large Intestine

- ❍ It actively absorbs Na^+, H_2O and Cl^- follow.
- ❍ There is no digestion except bacteria digest cellulose for themselves.
- ❍ Bacteria also synthesize vitamin K, which we absorb (important in clotting).
- ❍ Secretes alkaline, lubricating mucus.

Motility

- ❍ **Haustral contraction (similar to segmentation but slower):** Mostly short reflex control.
- ❍ **Mass movements (gastrocolic reflex):** Strong contractions move contents to rectum for storage until defecation reflex occurs (triggered by distention).

Hormones and Other Factors Involved in Digestive Function

- ❍ **Leptin:** Made by fat cells, tells hypothalamus you have enough energy stored and suppresses appetite (molecular satiety signal).
- ❍ **Ghrelin:** Made by stomach, signals hunger and activates reward system.
- ❍ **PYY:** Released by intestines as food moves through (satiety signal).
- ❍ **Fiber:** Insoluble fiber helps food move faster and generate satiety signal sooner and soluble fiber delays stomach emptying making you feel more full.

ENDOCRINE SYSTEM

Basics

- ❍ It acts via hormones or chemical secreted into the blood that acts on target cells elsewhere in the body.
- ❍ Only target cells have receptors for a particular hormone.
- ❍ Function at very low concentrations.
- ❍ Has prolonged effects.
- ❍ Includes neurohormones.
- ❍ Tropic hormones regulate hormone secretion of other glands.

General Functions

- ❍ Regulate metabolism
- ❍ H_2O and electrolyte balance
- ❍ Coping with stress
- ❍ Growth and development
- ❍ Reproduction
- ❍ RBC production
- ❍ Digestion/absorption

Endocrine Disorders

- ❍ Hyposecretion (genetic, dietary, toxins, immune disorder).
- ❍ Hypersecretion (tumors).
- ❍ Abnormality of target cell (lack of receptors or lack of enzymes for reactions).

Responsiveness of Receptors

- ❍ The action of hormones depends on the number of receptors. Hormone influences number of its own receptors, i.e., down-regulation (more hormone → fewer receptors).
- ❍ Other hormones influence receptors of a different hormone (number of receptors or affinity).
  - ○ **Permissiveness:** Enhances the response of another hormone.
  - ○ **Synergism:** Both hormones enhance each other's response.
  - ○ **Antagonism:** Inhibits the response of another hormone.

Middle Pituitary

Contain pineal gland. Pineal gland secrete melatonin.

Melatonin

- ❍ Regulates biological clock cued by light/dark sensed by eyes
- ❍ May also:
  - ○ Induce sleep
  - ○ Inhibit sex hormones
  - ○ Enhance immunity
  - ○ Slow aging (antioxidant)

Hypothalamus and Posterior Pituitary (Neurohypophysis)

Hypothalamus produces hormones that are stored in posterior pituitary

It includes:

Vasopressin (ADH)

○ Conserves H_2O (when osmolarity increased)
○ Vasoconstrictor (when ECF/BP decreased)

Oxytocin

○ Uterine contractions during childbirth with permissive effects of estrogen and triggered by neuroendocrine reflexes (baby's head pushing against cervix).
○ Milk ejection, triggered by baby nursing.

Hypothalamus and Anterior Pituitary (Adenohypophysis)

Anterior pituitary produces hormones and releases them in response to hormones from hypothalamus.
○ Hypothalamus secretes tropic hormones (releasing and inhibiting hormones).
○ Anterior pituitary tropic hormones act on other endocrine glands.

Thyroid-stimulating Hormone (TSH, Thyrotropin)

○ Growth and secretion of thyroid gland.
○ Thyrotropin-releasing hormone (TRH).

Adrenocorticotropic Hormone (ACTH, Adrenocorticotropin)

○ Growth and secretion of adrenal cortex (cortisol).
○ Corticotropin releasing hormone (CRH).

Gonadotropins

○ Secretion of sex hormones by gonads.
○ Gonadotropin releasing hormone (GnRH).

Growth Hormone (GH, Somatotropin)

○ Regulates growth and metabolism.

○ Growth hormone releasing hormone (GHRH) and growth hormone inhibiting hormone (GHIH).
○ Nontropic anterior pituitary hormone: Prolactin (PRL).
  ○ Breast development and milk production in typical female.
  ○ Prolactin releasing factor (PRF) and prolactin-inhibiting hormone (PIH).

Growth Hormone

It stimulates production of IGF-1 (somatomedins) mainly in liver that then act on target cells (most cells) to promote growth of cells in size/number by stimulating protein synthesis and cellular uptake of amino acids and inhibiting protein breakdown.

GH also stimulates the growth of bones in length/thickness.

It conserves glucose (for brain) and use fat stores by increasing blood fatty acids for muscle use. It is triggered by exercise, stress, changes in blood nutrient levels such as increase in amino acids, decrease in fatty acids.

Thyroid Gland

Functions of thyroid gland are:
○ Mix of T_3 and T_4.
○ Acts on most cells.
○ Increases overall metabolic rate.
○ Permissive effects on E and NE.
○ Critical for normal nervous system activity.
○ Critical for growth, increases GH secretion and has permissive effects.

Diseases: Disorders among most common in endocrine system.
○ **Hypothyroidism:** Decreased metabolic rate, cold intolerant, weight, fatigue, slow reflexes.
○ **Hyperthyroidism:** Increased metabolic rate, perspiration, loss of weight, weakness, palpitations, irritability, bulging eyes.

Calcitonin

- ❍ Involved in Ca^{2+} balance.
- ❍ Inhibits breakdown of bone.
- ❍ Protects bones when there's high Ca^{2+} demand (pregnancy, breast feeding).

Adrenal Cortex (Steroid Hormones)

- ❍ **Mineralocorticoids:** Influence mineral balance (e.g., aldosterone).
- ❍ **Sex hormones:** Similar or identical to gonadal hormones.
- ❍ **Glucocorticoids:** Includes cortisol (stress response; makes energy and building blocks available) that cause.
  - ○ Increases blood glucose by inhibits uptake by most tissues, sparing it for brain and promoting gluconeogenesis by liver (amino acids → glucose).
  - ○ Increases blood amino acids and fatty acids by stimulates breakdown of protein and fat.
  - ○ Permissive actions on hormones of adrenal medulla (catecholamines).
  - ○ Important in adaptation to stress.
  - ○ Alters mood and behavior (mechanisms unclear).
  - ○ Anti-inflammatory

Adrenal Medulla

Secretes both nor-epinephrine (NE) and epinephrine (E) (E more important).

Epinephrine: It has sympathetic and metabolic effects.

- ❍ Sympathetic effects
  - ○ Increases heart rate and cardiac output, vasoconstrictor → increases BP.
  - ○ Vasodilation in skeletal muscle and heart.
  - ○ Bronchodilation
  - ○ Also increases alertness, sweating, dilates pupils.
- ❍ Metabolic effects (stress response makes energy and building blocks available).
  - ○ Increases blood glucose by stimulating gluconeogenesis and glycogenolysis in liver, glycogenolysis in skeletal muscle and inhibiting the secretion of insulin and simulates secretion of glucagon.
  - ○ Increases blood fatty acids by the breakdown of fats.
  - ○ Increases overall metabolic rate.

Pancreas

It secretes insulin and glucagon.

Insulin

- ❍ Stores energy as the body absorbs nutrients (absorptive state).
- ❍ Decreases blood glucose by:
  - ○ Glucose → cells (increases transporters).
  - ○ Glycogenesis in liver (glucose → glycogen).
  - ○ Inhibits glycogenolysis and gluconeogenesis in liver.
- ❍ Decreases blood fatty acids.
  - ○ Glucose → adipose tissue to form fatty acids and glycerol.
  - ○ Fatty acids → cells
  - ○ Inhibits lipolysis
- ❍ Decreases blood amino acids.
  - ○ Amino acids → cells and made into proteins
  - ○ Inhibits protein breakdown
- ❍ Diabetes most common endocrine disorder.

Glucagon

- ❍ Maintains levels of blood nutrients (post-absorptive state, opposite of insulin), major effects are on liver.
- ❍ Increases blood glucose:
  - ○ Decreases glycogenesis
  - ○ Increases glycogenolysis and gluconeogenesis.
- ❍ Increases blood fatty acids by:
  - ○ Increases lipolysis
  - ○ Decreases lipid synthesis

Parathyroid

Parathyroid hormone is produced by parathyroid.

Parathyroid Hormone (PTH)

- Involved in Ca^{2+} balance (opposite of calcitonin).
- Increases plasma Ca^{2+} by:
  - Breaks down bone
  - Stimulates reabsorption by kidneys.
- Helps activate vitamin D, which enhances absorption of Ca^{2+} from diet
  Also involved in PO^3 balance
  This helps to balance the calcium to phosphorous ratio in blood.

REPRODUCTIVE SYSTEM

Basics

Functions of Primary Reproductive Organs (Gonads)

- To produce gametes (gametogenesis)
  - Sperm in typical male
  - Ova in typical female
- To secrete sex hormones (androgens and estrogens)
  - Mainly testosterone (male)
  - Mainly estrogen and progesterone (female).
  - Important in the development of secondary sex characteristics (hair distribution, body shape, voice change) as well as major reproductive functions and development.

Essential Reproductive Functions in the Typical Male

- Spermatogenesis
- Delivery of sperm to female

Essential Reproductive Functions in the Typical Female

- Oogenesis
- Receive sperm and transport for fertilization

- Maintain fetus
- Parturition and nourishment of infant

Sex Differentiation

Spermatogenesis

It begins at puberty

- Parts of sperm
  - Head contains DNA and acrosome has enzymes to penetrate egg.
  - Midpiece has mitochondria.
  - Tail is for movement.

Control of Spermatogenesis

- An increase in GnRH from hypothalamus occurs at puberty (probably due to a decrease in melatonin).
- Anterior pituitary hormones secreted (gonadotropins), luteinizing hormone (LH) → testosterone from interstitial cells →mitosis/meiosis of germ cells. Also follicle-stimulating hormone (FSH) stimulates spermiogenesis.

Semen

- Produced by different glands (seminal vesicles, prostate, bulbourethral glands).
- **Seminal vesicles (about 70%)**
  - Fructose for energy.
  - Prostaglandins for smooth muscle contraction in male and female reproductive tracts (transport).
  - Fibrinogen for clotting.
- **Prostate (about 30%)**
  - Alkaline fluid neutralizes acidic female reproductive tract.
  - Enzymes activate clotting.
  - Enzymes break down clot (fibrinolysin).
- **Bulbourethral glands:** Neutralize acidic male urethra.

Oogenesis

It begins during fetal development and is arrested during meiosis.

○ An ovarian cycle occurs due to an increase in GnRH occurs at puberty. The phases of ovarian cycle are:
  ○ **Follicular phase**
    ➤ Luteinizing hormone (LH) → thecal cells make androgen (DHEA).
    ➤ FSH → granulosa cells make estrogen from androgen.
    ➤ Developing follicle makes low levels of estrogen (negative feedback).
    ➤ **Ovulation:** LH surge triggers the release of ovum due to high estrogen levels from developed follicle (positive feedback)
  ○ **Luteal phase**
    ➤ High LH level triggers development of corpus luteum.
    ➤ If pregnancy occurs developing zygote produces human chorionic gonadotropin (hCG) that acts like LH and maintains corpus luteum.

○ Uterine cycle includes proliferative phase, secretory phase and menstrual phase.
  ○ **Proliferative phase:** Estrogen stimulates the growth of endometrium and synthesis of progesterone receptors in the endometrium.
  ○ **Secretory phase:** Progesterone further prepares endometrium (loosens connective tissue, blood vessel growth, secretes glycogen, decreases uterine contractility).
  ○ **Menstrual phase:** Endometrium breaks down due to lack of estrogen and progesterone (because of negative feedback effects of progesterone and LH).

MULTIPLE CHOICE QUESTIONS

1. **What is essential for the absorption of glucose from complex carbohydrates:**
   a. Salivary amylase b. Enterokinase
   c. Na^+K^+ ATPase d. Secretin

2. **Glycerol is one of the digestive products of:**
   a. Carbohydrates b. Fats
   c. Proteins d. Nucleic acids

3. **Hyperkinetic syndromes such as chorea and athetosis are usually associated with pathological changes in:**
   a. Motor areas of cerebral cortex
   b. Anterior hypothalamus
   c. Pathways for recurrent collateral inhibition in the spinal cord
   d. Basal ganglia complex

4. **The concentration of a substance is 2 mg% in the afferent arteriole and 0 mg% in the efferent. The conclusion is that the substance is:**
   a. Secreted in cortical nephron
   b. Absorbed in PCT
   c. Freely filtered in the glomerulus
   d. Impermeable in the loop of Henle

5. **Which of the following statement is true for the glomerulus:**
   a. Efferent arteriole is smaller in diameter
   b. Capillaries are more permeable than most other capillaries in the body
   c. Capillary blood is separated from the glomerular filtrate by the capillary membrane only
   d. Capillary pressure is normally 15–35 mm Hg

6. **The percentage of sensory fibers in a pure motor nerve is:**
   a. 3% b. 10%
   c. 20% d. 25%
   e. 40%

7. **The flocculonodular lobe is directly connected to:**
   a. Red nucleus
   b. Inferior olivary nucleus
   c. Vestibular nucleus
   d. Dentate nucleus

8. **Cryptorchidism means:**
   a. A method of family planning
   b. Disturbances in the menstrual cycle
   c. Delayed puberty
   d. Undescended testis

9. **The difference of pulmonary microcirculation from systemic is:**
   a. Resistance low; pulsatile flow
   b. Resistance low; capillary pressure low
   c. Capillary pressure high; pulsatile flow
   d. None of the above

10. **REM sleep is:**
   a. That point at which the individual becomes aware and alert
   b. Referred to as paradoxical sleep
   c. Characterized by loss of alt muscular activity
   d. Characterized by slow high voltage regular EEG activity

---

Answers:

1. a	2. b	3. d	4. c
5. a	6. e	7. c	8. d
9. b	10. b		

11. **Inulin clearance is:**
    a. 40 mL/min
    b. 55 mL/min
    c. 125 mL/min
    d. 625 mL/min

12. **Testosterone is mainly produced by:**
    a. Sertoli cells
    b. Leydig cells
    c. Seminiferous tubules
    d. Epididymis

13. **This is not a vitamin K-dependent blood clotting factor:**
    a. Factor i
    b. Factor ii
    c. Factor vii
    d. Factor x

14. **EEG rhythm recorded during REM sleep:**
    a. Alpha
    b. Beta
    c. Delta
    d. Theta

15. **The satiety center is located in the following hypothalamic nucleus:**
    a. Supraoptic
    b. Ventromedial
    c. Lateral
    d. Dorsomedial

16. **Cardiac output divided by heart rate is equal to:**
    a. Cardiac index
    b. Mean stroke volume
    c. Cardiac efficiency
    d. Mean arterial pressure

17. **A 3-year-old boy has cystic fibrosis. He is failing to thrive and is producing foul-smelling, pale stools which float. What is the single most appropriate treatment?**
    a. Addition of pancreatic enzymes to the diet
    b. Addition of salivary amylase to the diet
    c. High-protein diet
    d. Low-fat diet
    e. IV antibiotic treatment

18. **Calcitonin produces hypocalcemia by:**
    a. Increased renal Ca^{++} excretion
    b. Decreased bone resorption
    c. Decreased renal ca^{++} absorption
    d. Decreased intestinal ca^{++} absorption

19. **Interstitial fluid has maximum:**
    a. Na^+
    b. K^+
    c. Cl
    d. HCO_3^-

20. **The best screening test for hemophilia is:**
    a. BT
    b. PT
    c. PTT
    d. PCV

21. **A 28-year-old with Bell's palsy complains of hearing all noises at excessively loud volumes. What is the mechanism behind this feature?**
    a. Increased inner hair cell activity
    b. Increased ossicle movement
    c. Increased tympanic membrane movement
    d. Reduced outer hair cell activity
    e. Reduced round window movement

22. **The repolarization of an action potential is associated with all of the following,, *except*:**
    a. Loss of positive charges from inside the cell
    b. Outward diffusion of K^+
    c. Return of the membrane potential toward its resting value
    d. Closure of sodium channels in the cell membrane
    e. Decreased potassium permeability of cell membrane

Answers:

11. c	12. b	13. a	14. b
15. b	16. b	17. a	18. b
19. a	20. c	21. b	22. e

23. **The parietal cell is stimulated by all the following, *except*:**
a. Insulin
b. Gastrin
c. Stretch of stomach wall
d. Histamine

24. **ACTH level is highest during:**
a. Early morning   b. Evening
c. Afternoon   d. Night

25. **The "diuretic" activity of the anterior pituitary can be explained in terms of the actions of:**
a. ACTH
b. TSH
c. Growth hormone
d. All of the above

26. **Thrombus means:**
a. Increase in thrombocyte count
b. Blood clot in a test tube
c. Decreased thrombocyte count
d. Blood clot inside a blood vessel

27. **Tissue hypoxia without alteration of oxygen content of blood occurs in:**
a. Co poisoning
b. Methemoglobinemia
c. Respiratory acidosis
d. Cyanide poisoning

28. **Addition of PUFA in plasma membrane causes:**
a. Increase in fluidity of the membrane
b. Decrease in the fluidity of the membrane
c. No change in fluidity of the membrane
d. Membrane becomes rigid

29. **Tachycardia at the onset of exercise is caused by stimulation of:**
a. Chemoreceptors

b. Baroreceptors
c. Joint proprioceptors
d. Stretch receptors

30. **What is true about serum albumin:**
a. Contributes maximally to plasma oncotic pressure
b. It is anionic
c. Freely filterable in renal filter
d. Not synthesized in liver

31. **A 32-year-old man is running around the park. Which tissue is most sensitive to sympathetically-mediated vasoconstriction?**
a. Brain   b. Genitalia
c. Gut   d. Heart
e. Liver

32. **All are properties of spinal cord reflex, *except*:**
a. Summation   b. Delay
c. Fatigue   d. Memory

33. **The most important substance controlling alveolar ventilation is:**
a. O_2 b. CO_2
c. H_2O
d. None of the above

34. **The part of sarcomere that disappears on muscle contraction:**
a. M line   b. H zone
c. I band   d. A band

35. **Initiation of nerve impulse occurs at axon hillock because:**
a. It has a lower threshold than the rest of the axon
b. It is unmyelinated
c. Neurotransmitter release occurs here
d. None of the above

Answers:
23. a	24. a	25. d	26. d
27. d	28. a	29. c	30. a
31. c	32. d	33. b	34. b
35. a			

36. **Troponin C binds with:**
   a. Actin
   b. ATP
   c. Tropomyosin
   d. Calcium

37. **Hyperosmolar coma is seen in all, *except*:**
   a. Hyperglycemia
   b. Uremia
   c. Increased concentration of plasma proteins
   d. Increase in plasma Na^+ concentration

38. **P-R interval indicates which of the following:**
   a. Av node conduction time
   b. Ventricular repolarization
   c. Atrial depolarization
   d. Both a and c

39. **The commonest neurotransmitter in the synapse outside brain is:**
   a. Acetylcholine
   b. Secretin
   c. CCK
   d. Acetylcholinesterase

40. **Sertoli cells have receptors for:**
   a. Inhibin
   b. LH
   c. FSH
   d. Melatonin

41. **Ejection fraction increases with an increase in:**
   a. End-systolic volume
   b. Peripheral vascular resistance
   c. End-diastolic volume
   d. Venodilation

42. **Ablation of the somatosensory area I of cerebral cortex leads to:**
   a. Total loss of pain sensation
   b. Total loss of touch sensation
   c. Loss of tactile localization and 2-point discrimination
   d. Loss of tactile localization but not of 2-point discrimination

43. **Urinary bilirubin is absent in which type of jaundice:**
   a. Hepatic jaundice
   b. Hemolytic jaundice
   c. Obstructive jaundice
   d. Prehepatic jaundice

44. **The arterial pulse pressure in the femoral artery is normally:**
   a. Slightly less than the pulse pressure in the upper aorta
   b. Greater than the pulse pressure in the upper aorta
   c. Equal to the peak pressure in the upper aorta
   d. One of the above

45. **Vitamin B12 is absorbed primarily in:**
   a. Stomach
   b. Duodenum
   c. Jejunum
   d. Ileum

46. **The hormone increases uterine contractility:**
   a. Vasopressin
   b. LH
   c. FSH
   d. Oxytocin

47. **Insulin is not involved in the glucose transport to the following cell:**
   a. Adipose tissue
   b. Liver
   c. Alveolar epithelial cells
   d. Muscle

48. **A septic 4-day-old boy is hypothermic in the neonatal intensive care unit. Why are neonates particularly susceptible to hypothermia?**
   a. Large amount of subcutaneous fat
   b. Small surface area/weight ratio
   c. Thick skin
   d. Unable to shiver
   e. Use of brown fat

Answers:	36. d	37. c	38. d	39. a
	40. c	41. c	42. c	43. c
	44. c	45. d	46. d	47. c
	48. d			

49. Which of the following reflects glycemic control in diabetics:
   a. HbA
   b. HbA$_2$
   c. HbA$_{1C}$
   d. HbC

50. CO$_2$ affects respiratory center via:
   a. Carotid body
   b. Aortic body
   c. CSF H$^+$ concentration
   d. Inflation and deflation receptors

51. Gated ion channels open or close by:
   a. Alteration in membrane potential
   b. Binding to an internal ligand
   c. Binding to an external ligand
   d. Depending upon the lipid solubility of an ion

52. The part of the eye which transduces blue, green and red light is:
   a. Cornea
   b. Fovea
   c. Periphery of retina
   d. Optic nerve

53. Mouth-to-mouth respiration provides an O$_2$ concentration of:
   a. 16%
   b. 20%
   c. 22%
   d. 24%

54. Which of the following is false regarding sodium-potassium pump?
   a. It is electrogenic
   b. It needs ATP
   c. It is inactivated at 4°C
   d. It is required for generation of action potential

55. Liver bile and gallbladder bile have the respective pH as:
   a. 6.4–7.2 and 8.6–9.4
   b. 8.2–9.0 and 4.2–6
   c. 6–7 and 8–9
   d. 7.8–8.6 and 7.0–7.4

56. CSF pressure in lying down posture is:
   a. 20–50 mm
   b. 50–150 mm
   c. 150–200 mm
   d. 200–300 mm

57. Ventricular filling:
   a. Produces third heart sound in some healthy persons
   b. Depends mainly on a contraction of atria
   c. Begins during isometric ventricular relaxation
   d. Will not occur unless atrial pressure is higher than atmospheric pressure

58. Gastrin is produced by:
   a. Pancreas
   b. Pituitary
   c. Gastric antral cells
   d. All

59. Ca^{2+} binding proteins are involved in excitation-contraction coupling in:
   a. Skeletal muscle
   b. Smooth muscle
   c. Both
   d. Neither

60. The nourishment for the development of spermatozoa is provided by:
   a. Seminiferous tubules
   b. Leydig's cells
   c. Sertoli's cells
   d. Any of the above

61. Turbulent blood flow is caused by:
   a. Decreased velocity of circulation
   b. Decreased hematocrit
   c. Decreased cardiac output
   d. All of the above

62. Principal site of Na$^+$ reabsorption:
   a. PCT
   b. DCT
   c. Thick ascending limb of the loop of Henle
   d. Collecting duct

Answers:

49. c	50. c	51. a	52. b
53. a	54. d	55. d	56. b
57. a	58. d	59. a	60. c
61. b	62. a		

63. Sperms have:
a. 22 autosomes + Y chromosome
b. 22 autosomes + X chromosome
c. 23 pairs of chromosomes
d. 22 autosomes + either X or Y chromosome

64. Effect of pregnancy on respiration is:
a. ↑ Respiratory rate
b. ↑ Tidal volume
c. ↑ Respiratory volume
d. ↑ Total being capacity

65. **Dicoumarol therapy inhibits the synthesis of all the following factors, *except*:**
a. Factor ix
b. Factor ii
c. Factor vii
d. Factor i

66. **A major part of total peripheral resistance is due to:**
a. Medium and small arteries
b. Arterioles
c. Capillaries
d. Venules

67. **Secretion of prolactin is affected by:**
a. Dopamine
b. Serotonin
c. FSH
d. GnRH analog

68. **Where is active Na^+-K^+-$2Cl^-$ pump located:**
a. Proximal tubule
b. Thick ascending limb of the loop of Henle
c. Distal convoluted tubule

69. **A 71-year-old man has a left anterior cerebral artery infarction, causing ischemia to the medial part of the frontal lobe. What single body part** would be expected to have the greatest weakness?
a. Eyebrow
b. Hand
c. Leg
d. Tongue
e. Trunk

70. **Broca's area:**
a. Is for planning and making decisions
b. Contains primary visual cortex
c. Contains somatic sensory area
d. Co-ordinates muscles used in speech production

71. **In renal glycosuria, renal threshold for glucose is:**
a. Low
b. High
c. Same
d. Greatly increased

72. **Anemic hypoxia is due to:**
a. ↓pO_2 in arterial blood
b. ↑pO_2 in arterial blood
c. ↑pO_2 in arterial blood
d. ↓O_2 content in arterial blood

73. **A 43-year-old woman has worse muscle weakness at the end of the day. She is positive for anti-nicotinic acetylcholine receptor antibodies. What is the single most appropriate treatment?**
a. Acetylcholinesterase inhibitor
b. Choline acetyl-transferase activator
c. Neurosecretory vesicle fusion inhibitor
d. Uptake-1 inhibitor
e. Voltage-gated sodium channel blocker

Answers:	63. d	64. b	65. d	66. b
	67. a	68. b	69. c	70. d
	71. a	72. d	73. a	

74. Contraction of which of the following muscles is most important for causing forceful expiration:
a. Internal intercostal
b. Diaphragm and abdominal muscles
c. External intercostal
d. Sternocleidomastoid

75. All of the following hormones mediate their major effects without actually entering the target cell, *except*:
a. Cortisol
b. Insulin
c. Growth hormone
d. Glucagon
e. Parathyroid hormone

76. Obstructive jaundice is caused by:
a. Defective pancreas
b. Impacted-gallstone in the common bile duct
c. Liver deficiency
d. When bile is not removed from the blood

77. A 22-year-old woman is breastfeeding an hour after delivery. During lactation the 'let-down' reflex is stimulated by the action of which hormone?
a. Human placental lactogen
b. Estrogen
c. Oxytocin
d. Prolactin
e. Progesterone

78. Shock always involves:
a. External hemorrhage
b. Internal hemorrhage
c. Central nervous system
d. Decreased tissue perfusion

79. Which structure in the eye is pain-sensitive?
a. Iris
b. Choroid
c. Cornea
c. All of the above

80. The medium with the highest refractive index in the eye is:
a. Cornea
b. Nucleus of the lens
c. Cortex of the lens
d. Aqueous humor

81. Not true about respiratory center:
a. Situated in medulla and pons
b. Sends out regular impulses to inspiratory muscles during quiet respiration
c. Sends out regular impulses to expiratory muscles during quiet respiration
d. Is inhibited during swallowing and vomiting 100

82. The cell membrane of human erythrocyte is more permeable to:
a. Cl^- than K^+
b. K^+ than Na^+
c. K^+ than urea

83. Intraocular fluid:
a. Is reabsorbed by ciliary process
b. Is produced at the canal of Schlemm
c. Helps to maintain corneal curve
d. None of the above

84. In man, the least useful physiological response to low environmental temperature is:
a. Shivering
b. Vasoconstriction
c. Piloerection
d. Release of thyroxine

Answers:	74. b	75. a	76. b	77. c
	78. d	79. d	80. b	81. c
	82. b	83. c	84. c	

85. Lymph capillaries are best characterised by:
a. Less permeable than blood capillaries
b. Have smaller diameter than blood capillaries
c. Have no endothelial lining
d. Have a discontinuous basement membrane

86. The following are seen in REM sleep, *except*:
a. Bruxism
b. Hypotonia
c. Tachycardia
d. Dreams

87. Total alveolar ventilation volume in L/min is:
a. 1.5
b. 3.5
c. 4.2
d. 5

88. In WPW syndrome, a connection exists between atria and:
a. Bundle of his
b. Ventricles
c. AV node
d. Purkinje fibers

89. Maximum blood supply to liver is through:
a. Hepatic artery
b. Portal vein
c. Splenic artery
d. Mesenteric artery

90. Which of the following is an excitatory neurotransmitter:
a. GABA
b. Glycine
c. Melatonin
d. Glutamate

91. Most important stimulus for intestinal secretion:
a. Gastrin
b. Secretin
c. Tactile stimulation
d. VIP

92. Increase in which of the following parameters will shift the O_2 dissociation curve to the left:
a. Temperature
b. $PaCO_2$
c. 2,3-DPG concentration
d. Oxygen affinity of Hb

93. Gap junctions are present in:
a. Choroid plexus
b. Skeletal muscle
c. Renal tubular epithelium
d. Smooth muscle

94. A 78-year-old man with advanced cancer is treated with vincristine, a microtubule inhibitor. During which single stage of mitosis are the tumor cells likely to arrest?
a. Anaphase
b. Cytokinesis
c. Metaphase
d. Prophase
e. Telophase

95. Hydrostatic pressure in glomerular capillary (mm Hg) is:
a. About 45
b. About 10
c. About 5
d. 60

96. Acetylcholine causes, through nicotinic receptors:
a. Decrease in heart rate
b. Contraction of skeletal muscle
c. Secretion of saliva
d. Contraction of pupils

97. Impulses of the taste buds of the tongue come from cerebral cortex through:
a. Internal capsule
b. Thalamus
c. Trochlear nerve
d. Hypoglossal nerve

Answers:	85. d	86. a	87. c	88. b
	89. b	90. d	91. d	92. d
	93. d	94. c	95. d	96. b
	97. b			

98. Functional residual capacity is:
a. Tidal volume + volume inspired forcefully
b. Volume remaining after forceful expiration
c. Volume remaining after normal expiration
d. Tidal volume + volume expired forcefully

99. The following are present in circulating blood, *except*:
a. Fibrinogen
b. Prothrombin
c. Thrombin
d. Albumin

100. In GIT, the longest transit time is seen in:
a. Stomach
b. Jejunum
c. Ileum
d. Colon

101. Incisura in the aortic pressure curve is:
a. Because of increased aortic pressure
b. Associated with third HS
c. Rapid peripheral emptying
d. Backward flow of blood from aorta to ventricle

102. The first reactive change occurring after hemorrhage:
a. Vasoconstriction
b. Tachycardia
c. Raised adrenaline
d. Raised cortisol

103. The part of eye which bends light and protects inner eye is the:
a. Cornea
b. Fovea
c. Pupil
d. Ciliary muscle

104. Plateau phase of plateau type of action potential is mainly caused by:
a. Sustained K^+ efflux
b. Ca^{2+} influx
c. Na^+ influx
d. Na^+-k^+ pump

105. One of the following is not a second messenger:
a. NO
b. cGMP
c. IP3
d. cAMP

106. PR interval is said to be prolonged if it exceeds:
a. 0.2 sec
b. 0.25 sec
c. 0.30 sec
d. 0.35 sec

107. Pepsinogen is activated by the following:
a. Enterokinase
b. Low pH
c. Trypsin
d. Chymotrypsin

108. A hormone that is a derivative of a single amino acid is:
a. Estrogen
b. Epinephrine
c. Thyroxine
d. Progesterone

109. cAMP is a second messenger of all, *except*:
a. FSH
b. Estrogen
c. Glucagon
d. Epinephrine

110. Myasthenia gravis is due to:
a. Old age
b. Nonproduction of ACH
c. Excess destruction of ACH
d. Destruction of ach receptors

111. Testosterone, the male sex hormone, is synthesized in:
a. Interstitial cells
b. Seminiferous tubules
c. Prostate gland
d. Vas deferens

Answers:	98. c	99. c	100. d	101. d
	102. a	103. a	104. b	105. a
	106. a	107. b	108. b	109. b
	110. d	111. a		

112. Fertilization of the ovum normally occurs in:
a. Uterus
b. Cervix of uterus
c. Fallopian tube
d. None of the above
Your answer: not attempted

113. True statement regarding excitation-contraction coupling in smooth muscle is:
a. Presence of troponin is essential
b. Sustained contraction occurs with high calcium concentration
c. Phosphorylation of actin is required for contraction
d. Presence of cellular ca is essential to cause muscle contraction

114. The area responsible for short-term memory is located in:
a. Cerebellum
b. Hypothalamus
c. Thalamus
d. Hippocampus

115. The supraoptic nucleus of the hypothalamus is believed to control the secretion of which of the following hormones?
a. Serotonin
b. Oxytocin
c. Growth hormone
d. Adrenocorticotropic hormone

116. End plate potential is characterized by:
a. Hyperpolarization
b. Normal polarity
c. Depolarization
d. None

117. In dividing cells, the spindle is formed by:
a. Tubulin
b. Ubiquitin
c. Laminin
d. Keratin

118. The transition temperature of the lipid bilayer of a cell membrane is raised by:
a. Saturated fatty acids
b. Cholesterol
c. Hydrocarbons
d. Unsaturated fatty acids

119. Calcitonin is secreted by:
a. Thyroid gland
b. Parathyroid gland
c. Adrenal glands
d. Ovaries

120. Renal plasma flow is:
a. 125 mL/min
b. 700 mL/min
c. 500 mL/min
d. 1,250mL/min

121. The combination of hemoglobin with O_2 in the lungs can be promoted by:
a. Decreasing O_2 concentration in blood
b. Increasing O_2 concentration in blood O_2
c. Increasing CO_2 concentration in blood
d. Introducing CO_2 into the blood

122. Blood flow in carotid body in mL/100g of tissue:
a. 500
b. 1,000
c. 2,000
d. 4,000

123. Fast response action potential is seen in:
a. SA node
b. AV node
c. Ventricular muscle
d. All the above

Answers:	112. c	113. d	114. d	115. b
	116. c	117. a	118. a	119. a
	120. b	121. a	122. c	123. c

124. Tropomyosin:
a. Helps in the fusion of action and myosin
b. Slides over myosin
c. Covers myosin and prevents attachment of actin and myosin
d. Causes calcium release

125. If clearance of a drug is more than GFR, it means that:
a. Drug is reabsorbed in the tubules
b. Drug is secreted in the tubules
c. Drug is excreted in bile
d. Drug is neither secreted nor reabsorbed

126. The hormone secretin is produced in:
a. Pancreas and influences the conversion of glycogen into glucose
b. Adrenal glands and accelerates heart beat
c. Testis and produces male secondary sexual characteristics
d. Small intestine and stimulate pancreas

127. Temporal lobe lesion causes:
a. Homonymous upper quadrantinopia
b. Homonymous lower quadrantanopia
c. Bitemporal hemianopia
d. Binasal hemianopia

128. Δ waves in EEG:
a. Occur in deep sleep
b. Occur at a rate below 3 to 5 cycles / second
c. Strictly occur in the cortex independent of activities of lower regions of the brain
d. All the above

129. Which of the following is true about adrenaline:
a. Converted to norepinephrine by methylation
b. Increases glycogen breakdown in liver and muscle
c. Is a polypeptide
d. Increases triglyceride deposition in adipose tissue

130. Cell type which lacks HLA antigen, is:
a. Monocyte
b. Thrombocyte
c. Neutrophil
d. RBC

131. A 75-year-old man has an anterior spinal artery infarction at the T10 level. What single neurological deficit will he experience?
a. Loss of motor activity on the left, pain on the right, below T10
b. Loss of motor activity, pain and temperature below T10 bilaterally
c. Loss of motor activity, proprioception and vibration below T10 bilaterally
d. Loss of proprioception and vibration below T10 bilaterally
e. Loss of proprioception on the right, pain on the left, below T10

132. Which of the following secretes thromboxane A2?
a. RBCs
b. Neutrophils
c. Platelets
d. WBCs

133. Work during normal respiration is mainly done to overcome:
a. Lung elasticity
b. Respiratory air passages
c. Alveolar air spaces
d. Creating negative pleural pressure

Answers: 124. c   125. b   126. d   127. a
128. a   129. b   130. d   131. b
132. c   133. a

134. During cardiac cycle, aortic valve opens at:
a. Beginning of systole
b. End of diastole
c. End of isovolumetric contraction
d. End of diastasis

135. Vasopressin exerts its action by:
a. Water absorption at the medullary duct
b. Water reabsorption across the collecting duct
c. Water secretion at the loop of Henle
d. Water transport at PCT

136. Hypertension is a common complication of all of the following conditions, *except*:
a. Anaphylaxis
b. Pregnancy
c. Cushing's syndrome
d. Posterior pituitary fossa tumor
e. Pyelonephritis

137. Neuronal degeneration is seen in all, *except*:
a. Crush nerve injury
b. Senescence
c. Fetal development
d. Neuropraxia

138. Regarding Na^+-K^+-ATPase, the true statement is:
a. It is an antiport carrying $3Na^+$ into the cell and $2K^+$ outside the cell
b. Maintains cell volume
c. A symport of $3Na^+$ and $2K^+$ into a cell
d. It is an electrogenic pump maintaining cell positivity

139. The first reflex response to appear as the spinal shock wears off in man is:
a. Tympanic reflex
b. Neck righting reflex
c. Withdrawal reflex
d. Labyrinthine reflex

140. The sigmoid nature of Hb-O_2 dissociation curve is due to:
a. Binding of one O_2 molecule increases the affinity for the next oxygen molecule
b. A-chain has more affinity for O_2 than β-chain
c. B-chain has more affinity for O_2 than β-chain
d. Hemoglobin is acidic in nature

141. Microfilaments are made up of:
a. Calmodulin
b. Myosin
c. Actin
d. Titin

142. The ascending reticular formation:
a. Is located in cerebral hemisphere
b. Has increased activity during sleep
c. Is located in brainstem
d. All

143. Vitamin B12 is absorbed in:
a. Ileum
b. Duodenum
c. Jejunum
d. Stomach

144. Glucose-mediated insulin release is mediated through:
a. Camp
b. ATP-dependent K^+ channels
c. Carrier modulators
d. Receptor phosphorylation

Answers:

134. c	135. b	136. a	137. d
138. b	139. c	140. a	141. c
142. c	143. a	144. b	

145. Dorsal column-medial lemniscus pathway, true is:
a. Carries a sense of temperature to the cortex
b. Carries sense of crude touch and pain to the cortex
c. Carries sensation of fine touch, vibration and proprioception
d. Does not help in detecting movement of different parts

146. The portion of the ear involved in balancing is:
a. Sacculus
b. Cochlea
c. Three semicircular canals with ampullae
d. Utriculus

147. A 52-year-old man with acromegaly secondary to a macroadenoma undergoes visual field assessment. What single visual field defect is most characteristic of this condition?
a. Binasal hemianopia
b. Bitemporal hemianopia
c. Loss of binocular vision
d. Right-sided homonymous hemianopia
e. Right-sided quadrantanopia

148. Organ not involved in ca homeostasis:
a. Skin
b. Kidneys
c. Intestine
d. Lungs

149. Human cell membrane is composed of:
a. Protein molecules
b. Carbohydrate and phospholipid
c. Lipoprotein mainly
d. Amino acid residues

150. Most potent stimulus for secretin secretion is:
a. Dilatation of intestine
b. Protein
c. Fat
d. Acid chyme

151. The inactive trypsin is converted to active trypsin by:
a. HCl
b. Enterokinase
c. Both a and b
d. None of these

152. Which of the following is false regarding sodium-potassium pump?
a. It is electrogenic
b. It needs ATP
c. It is inactivated at 4°C
d. It is required for the generation of action potential

153. The buffering properties of Hb are due to:
a. Histidine residue
b. Glycoprotein nature
c. Iron molecules
d. Weak acidic nature

154. A 54-year-old treated for schizophrenia has uncontrollable, slow, writhing movements of the face and neck. Abnormal signaling by which neurotransmitter mediates these symptoms?
a. 5-HT3
b. Dopamine
c. GABA
d. Glutamate
e. Substance P

155. The low-intensity light during the night is detected by:
a. Cones
b. Rods
c. Both
d. Crystalline lens

Answers:

145. c	146. c	147. b	148. d
149. c	150. d	151. b	152. d
153. a	154. b	155. b	

156. **Tachycardia at the onset of exercise is caused by stimulation of:**
    a. Chemoreceptors
    b. Baroreceptors
    c. Joint proprioceptors
    d. Stretch receptors

157. **The normal pulmonary systolic arterial pressure is .... mm Hg.**
    a. 35
    b. 25
    c. 10

158. **Ca is found in:**
    a. Leukocytes
    b. Erythrocytes
    c. Plasma
    d. Lymphocytes

159. **Blood group antigens are:**
    a. Attached to plasma proteins
    b. Attached to a hemoglobin molecule
    c. Found in saliva of all persons
    d. None

160. **The extrapyramidal system is not directly concerned with:**
    a. Stretch reflexes
    b. Sensation from viscera
    c. Both a and b
    d. None

161. **Glycogen content is lowest in:**
    a. Slow oxidative fibers
    b. Fast glycolytic fibers
    c. Fast oxidative fibers
    d. All the above

162. **Profound hypothermic signs include all, *except*:**
    a. Hypotension
    b. Bradycardia
    c. Slow breathing
    d. Hyperactivity

163. **Normal O_2 tension with decreased O_2 carrying capacity is seen in:**
    a. Histotoxic hypoxia
    b. Anemic hypoxia
    c. Stagnant hypoxia
    d. Hypoxic hypoxia

164. **Glycogenolysis in muscle does not raise blood sugar levels due to the lack of:**
    a. Lactate dehydrogenase
    b. Pyruvate kinase
    c. G-6-phosphatase
    d. Argininosuccinase

165. **Which of the following are part of the limbic system:**
    a. Red nuclei
    b. Amygdaloid nuclei
    c. Posterior commissure
    d. Cingulate cortex

166. **Part of action potential that coincides with an absolute refractory period is:**
    a. Depolarization
    b. Hyperpolarization
    c. Depolarization and 1/3 of repolarization
    d. After repolarization

167. **'Molecular motors' are:**
    a. Myosin and myoglobin
    b. Dynein and kinesin
    c. Calmodulin and g proteins
    d. Troponin

168. **Which of the following membranes has the highest protein content (per gram of tissue):**
    a. Outer mitochondrial membrane
    b. Inner mitochondrial membrane
    c. Plasma membrane
    d. Myelin sheath

Answers: | 156. c | 157. b | 158. b | 159. d |
160. c	161. a	162. d	163. b
164. c	165. b, d	166. c	167. b
168. b			

169. Assuming GFR is 125 mL/min and plasma glucose level is 100 mg%, the amount of glucose filtered by a glomerular membrane in 10 min would be:
a. 125 mg
b. 1.25 g
c. 2 g
d. 2.5 g

170. Colonic bacteria, on digestion of dietary fibers, produce:
a. Free radicals
b. Sucrose
c. Butyrate
d. Glycerol

171. Sweating as a result of exertion is mediated through:
a. Adrenal hormones
b. Sympathetic adrenergic nerve
c. Sympathetic cholinergic nerve
d. Parasympathetic cholinergic nerve

172. The nuclear bag portion of the muscle spindle is innervated by:
a. Type I fiber
b. Type II fiber
c. Both
d. None

173. The function of iris is to:
a. Move the lens forwards and backwards
b. Alter the diameter of the pupil
c. Close the eyelids
d. Secrete aqueous humor

174. The oxygen dissociation curve shifts to the right in all, *except*:
a. High altitude
b. Diabetic ketoacidosis
c. Anemia
d. Blood transfusion

175. Crude touch sensations are carried by:
a. Lateral spinothalamic tract
b. Ventral spinothalamic tract
c. Posterior column tract
d. Spinocerebellar tract

176. An 83-year-old man has a new ischemic stroke. He can follow three-step commands, but his speech is limited and does not make sense. Which area is most affected?
a. Arcuate fasciculus
b. Broca's area
c. Midbrain
d. Primary auditory cortex
e. Wernicke's area

177. Phagocytosis in the CNS is done by:
a. Astrocytes
b. Schwann cells
c. Microglia
d. Oligodendrogliocytes

178. A 67-year-old patient is unwell with sepsis. What single autonomic transmitter is most crucial for the maintenance of systemic vasoconstriction?
a. Acetylcholine
b. Dopamine
c. Nitric oxide
d. Noradrenaline
e. Serotonin

179. The membranous labyrinth is called a stat acoustic organ because it is concerned with:
a. Hearing
b. Balancing
c. Both
d. Sound production

180. All are features of panhypopituitarism, *except*:
a. Infertility
b. Pigmentation
c. Loss of secondary sexual characters
d. Cold intolerance

Answers:

169. b	170. c	171. c	172. a
173. b	174. d	175. c	176. b
177. c	178. d	179. c	180. b

181. The satiety center is in:
a. Dorsomedial nucleus of hypothalamus
b. Ventromedial nucleus of hypothalamus
c. Lateral hypothalamic area
d. Perifornical organ

182. Urge for micturition is felt when the bladder contains:
a. 100–200 cc urine
b. 200–300 cc urine
c. 500–700 cc urine
d. 700–800 cc urine

183. The arterial pulse pressure in the femoral artery is normally:
a. Slightly less than the pulse pressure in the upper aorta
b. Greater than the pulse pressure in the upper aorta
c. Equal to the peak pressure in the upper aorta
d. One of the above

184. Broca's area is present in:
a. Superior temporal gyrus
b. Precentral gyrus
c. Postcentral gyrus
d. Inferior frontal gyrus

185. The total blood protein in 100 mL of blood is about:
a. 7.3 g
b. 23 g
c. 45 g
d. 23 mg

186. Ventilation-perfusion ratio is maximum at:
a. Apex of lung
b. Base of lung
c. Middle of the lung
d. Posterior lobe of lung

187. The main excitatory neurotransmitter in the central nervous system is:
a. Glycine
b. Acetylcholine
c. Aspartate
d. Glutamate

188. The main driving force for counter-current multiplier system is:
a. Reabsorption of Na^+ in thick ascending limb
b. Medullary hyperosmolality
c. Action of ADH on aquaporin channels
d. Urea recycling

189. Which of the following is not a function of no?
a. Kills cancer cells
b. Vasoconstriction
c. Relaxation of vascular smooth muscles
d. Deficiency may cause clinical hypertension

190. Hypothalamus regulates all, *except*:
a. Food intake
b. Temperature
c. Hypophysis
d. Anticipatory rise in heart rate

191. Regional arterial resistance of mesentery and renal vessels is reduced by:
a. Dopamine
b. Dobutamine
c. Noradrenaline
d. Isoprenaline

192. Chyme in the small intestine is propelled forward by:
a. Haustration
b. Segmentation
c. MMC
d. Peristalsis

Answers:	181. b	182. a	183. c	184. d
	185. a	186. a	187. b	188. a
	189. b	190. d	191. a	192. d

193. The EEG waves are called:
a. Delta waves
b. Berger's rhythm
c. REM rhythm
d. Neurogenic rhythm

194. Destruction of the lateral nucleus of the hypothalamus leads to:
a. Aphagia
b. Hyperphagia
c. Satiety
d. Somnolence

195. The substance essential for the transfer of fatty acids across the mitochondrial membrane:
a. Creatine
b. Creatinine
c. Carnitine
d. Co-enzymeA

196. Chronaxie is minimum in:
a. Large myelinated nerve fiber
b. Skeletal muscle fiber
c. Unmyelinated nerve fiber
d. Cardiac muscle

197. Arneth count is:
a. Counting the lymphocytes
b. Counting the lobes of neutrophil
c. Counting the granules in eosinophil
d. WBC counting in bone marrow

198. The jugular venous:
a. Pulse cannot be seen in people with normal heart
b. Pressure is typically raised in right ventricular failure
c. Pulse is not exaggerated in patients suffering from tricuspid incompetence

199. The frequency of alpha waves in EEG is:
a. 8–12 cycles/sec
b. 15–25 cycles/sec
c. 2–5 cycles/sec
d. None of the above

200. Normal average sperm count in semen is:
a. 5 million/cumm
b. 50 million/mL
c. 100 million/cumm
d. 100 million/mL

201. The type of nerve fiber that has a conduction velocity of approximately 1 meter per second:
a. Type A alpha
b. Type A beta
c. Type A delta
d. Type C

202. EEG with spike and dome pattern is characteristic of:
a. Jacksonian epilepsy
b. Grandmal epilepsy
c. Petitmal epilepsy
d. Temporal lobe epilepsy

203. Circadian rhythm is controlled by:
a. Arcuate nucleus
b. Suprachiasmatic nucleus
c. Optic chiasma
d. Globus pallidus

204. Circadian rhythm is controlled by:
a. Suprachiasmatic nucleus of hypothalamus
b. Posteroventral nucleus of thalamus
c. Dentate nucleus of cerebellum
d. Pineal gland

205. Cushing's syndrome is characterized by:
a. Eosinophilia
b. Hypercalcemia
c. Nitrogen retention
d. Poor wound healing

206. False regarding IgG:
a. Pentamer with J chain
b. No additional chain
c. Only γ-chains as heavy chain
d. Performs complement fixation

Answers:

193. b	194. a	195. c	196. a
197. b	198. b	199. a	200. d
201. d	202. c	203. b	204. d
205. d	206. a		

207. **Which of the following is the correct activation order after stimulation of Purkinje fibers?**
    a. Endocardium, epicardium (uppermost part of), septum
    b. Endocardium, septum, epicardium
    c. Epicardium, endocardium, septum
    d. Epicardium, septum, endocardium

208. **A 55-year-old man is brought to the emergency room by his son in a stuporous and bounded condition. Physical examination reveals BP 120/70 and pulse 90 (supine); BP 90/50, and pulse 120 (standing). Serum chemistries are: Na^+= 141 mEq/L Cl = 87 mEq/L K^+= 2.9 mEq/L $HCO3$ = 42 mEq/L arterial pH = 7.53 $pCO2$ = 50 mm Hg the disease process that best accounts for this problem:**
    a. Ethylene glycol poisoning
    b. Chronic obstructive pulmonary disease
    c. Congestive heart failure
    d. Lactic acidosis
    e. Vomiting
    f. Chronic renal failure

209. **Which of these are not lung capacities:**
    a. Inspiratory capacity
    b. TLC
    c. MVV
    d. FRC

210. **Which of the following is a test for inner ear deafness:**
    a. Finger nose test
    b. Weber's test
    c. Rinne's test
    d. Both b and c

211. **In moderate exercise, stimulation of respiration is due to stimulation of:**
    a. J receptors
    b. Joint proprioceptors
    c. Lung receptors
    d. Medullary centers

212. **During isotonic contraction:**
    a. I band remains constant
    b. A band changes in length
    c. Z line approach each other
    d. H zone remains constant

213. **All the statements are true regarding cortisol, *except*:**
    a. It increases blood sugar level
    b. Hyposecretion of it produces Cushing's syndrome
    c. Increases blood volume
    d. It shows anti-inflammatory action

214. **A 71-year-old man has a left anterior cerebral artery infarction, causing ischemia in the medial part of the frontal lobe. What single body part would be expected to have the greatest weakness?**
    a. Eyebrow
    b. Hand
    c. Leg
    d. Tongue
    e. Trunk

215. **The maximum amount of each substance that can be transported in one minute by the kidney tubules is called:**
    a. Transport maximum
    b. Tubular maximum
    c. Secretion maximum
    d. Diodrast clearance

Answers: 207. a   208. e   209. c   210. d
         211. b   212. c   213. b   214. c
         215. b

216. Combination of hemoglobin with O_2 in the lungs can be promoted by:
a. Decreasing O_2 concentration in blood
b. Increasing O_2 concentration in blood
c. Increasing CO_2 concentration in blood
d. Introducing CO_2 into the blood

217. In vitro coagulation is initiated by the following factor:
a. VII
b. XII
c. XI
d. X

218. Nerve fibers involved in proprioception:
a. Type A fiber
b. Type B fiber
c. Type C fiber
d. Type IV fiber
e. J fiber

219. Renal threshold is less than the calculated value in practice because:
a. Different nephrons have different TM
b. Depends on renal blood flow
c. Depends on GFR
d. Depends on blood pressure

220. Reticulocytes are stained with:
a. Brilliant cresyl blue
b. Sudan black
c. Indigo Carmine
d. None

221. The fovea centralis of the eye:
a. Contains only rods
b. Is the region of highest visual acuity
c. Has lowest light threshold

222. Meiosis occurs in human males in:
a. Epididymis
b. Seminiferous tubules
c. Vas deferens
d. Seminal vesicle

223. Left ventricular systole corresponds to:
a. Auricular diastole
b. Auricular systole
c. ST wave of ECG
d. P wave of ECG

224. Compared to blood, CSF has all the following, *except*:
a. Lower calcium
b. Lower sodium
c. Lower chloride
d. Lower cells

225. Which of the following is seen in obstructive jaundice:
a. Excess of urobilinogen
b. Excess of unconjugated serum bilirubin
c. Excess of bile salts in the urine
d. All of the above

226. The increase in vascular permeability responsible for 'wheal' formation in triple response is due to:
a. Serotonin
b. Acetylcholine
c. Histamine
d. Adrenaline

227. The internal ear is responsible for:
a. Fixation of gaze
b. Sensing changes in atmospheric pressure
c. Maintaining a gravitational balance of the body at rest
d. Both a and c

228. Cortisol:
a. Secretion increases following gross injury
b. Favors protein synthesis
c. Enhance effects of antigen-antibody reactions
d. Tends to lower blood pressure

Answers: 216. a   217. b   218. a   219. a
220. a   221. b   222. b   223. a
224. c   225. c   226. c   227. d
228. a

229. The excretion of estrogen and progesterone is through:
a. Bile
b. Sweat
c. Urine
d. Feces

230. Which of the following transmitter substances always or almost always tend to inhibit the postsynaptic neuron?
a. Gaba
b. Dopamine
c. Norepinephrine

231. Actin combines with myosin to form actomyosin in the presence of:
a. Ca^{2+} and Mg^{2+}
b. Mg^{2+} and ATP
c. Ca^{2+} and ATP
d. Ca^{2+} and K^+

232. All are true regarding thyroid hormone, *except*:
a. T4 has a maximum plasma concentration
b. T3 is more active than T4
c. T3 is more avidly bound to nuclear receptors than T4
d. T4 has a shorter half-life than T3

233. In a normal adult, the ratio of physiological and anatomical dead space is:
a. 2:01
b. 1:03
c. 1:01
d. 3:01

234. Gap junctions:
a. Not present in cardiac muscle
b. Are present but of little functional importance in case of cardiac muscle
c. Are present and are important in the initiation of a pathway for the rapid spread of excitation from one cardiac muscle fiber to another
d. Are not present in smooth muscle

235. The cones in the eye:
a. Are responsible for dim light vision
b. Are much more sensitive to light than the rods
c. Have higher visual acuity than rods
d. Have impaired function in the absence of vitamin A

236. A true statement about calmodulin is that it is:
a. A plasma binding protein for calcium
b. An intracellular calcium-binding protein
c. Involved in intestinal absorption of calcium
d. None of the above

237. Hemoglobin is a buffer because of its:
a. Histidine residue
b. Glycoprotein nature
c. Weak acidic nature
d. Iron molecule

238. All are effects of testosterone, *except*:
a. Hematopoiesis
b. Ca retention
c. Increase in BMR
d. Increase in quantity of bone matrix
e. None

239. Growth hormone increases all of the following, *except*:
a. Blood glucose concentration
b. Blood-free fatty acid concentration
c. Protein synthesis
d. Storage of proteins in cells

240. Pressure on carotid sinus causes:
a. Hyperpnea
b. Dyspnea
c. Tachycardia
d. Reflex bradycardia

Answers:	229. c	230. a	231. a	232. d
	233. c	234. c	235. b	236. b
	237. a	238. e	239. d	240. d

241. A 27-year-old woman attends an antenatal clinic at 32 weeks of gestation, complaining of gradually increasing shortness of breath through pregnancy. Although you feel it is important to exclude serious pathology, you know this could be a normal symptom of advancing pregnancy. Which of the following contributors to lung volume and capacity occurs in a normal pregnancy?
a. Chest compliance increases
b. Expiratory reserve volume increases
c. Residual volume decreases
d. Tidal volume decreases by up to 40%

242. Restrictive lung disease shows:
a. ↑FEV1/FVC; ↓compliance of lung tissue
b. ↓FEV1/FVC; ↓compliance of lung tissue
c. ↑FRC; ↑ compliance of lung tissue
d. ↑TLC; ↓RV

243. The plateau phase of cardiac action potential is due to:
a. Opening of K^+ channels
b. Opening of Na^+ channels
c. Opening of slow Ca^{++} channels
d. Closure of Na^+ channels

244. Which of the following statements about the action of the somatomedins is not true:
a. Inhibit protein synthesis
b. Promote the growth of the bone and cartilage
c. Stimulate the secretion of hormones by pancreatic islet cells
d. None of the above

245. Impulses generated in the taste buds of the tongue reach the cerebral cortex via:
a. Thalamus
b. Internal capsule
c. Trochlear nerve
d. Hypoglossal nerve

246. A reflex action:
a. May be carried out by skeletal, smooth and cardiac muscles as well as by glands
b. Pathway is: efferent → spinal cord → brain → afferent
c. Pathway is: spinal cord → brain → afferent → efferent → target tissue
d. Pathway is: receptor → spinal cord → brain → efferent

247. Hormones secreted from the adrenal medulla are:
a. Glucagon   b. Cortisol
c. Norepinephrine   d. Aldosterone

248. Increased γ-efferent discharge is seen in all, *except*:
a. Anxiety
b. Jendrassik's maneuver
c. Rapid shallow breathing
d. Stimulation of skin

249. Which is not responsible for urine concentration?
a. Aldosterone
b. Angiotensin-II
c. Vasopressin
d. Epinephrine

250. Patients with anemia tend to have:
a. Decrease in cardiac output
b. Low oxygen tension in the arterial blood
c. Pallor of the mucous membrane
d. All of the above

Answers: 241. c   242. a   243. c   244. c
               245. a   246. a   247. d   248. c
               249. d   250. c

251. Motor area of Brodmann is area:
- a. 1
- b. 4
- c. 5
- d. 7

252. All are steps in a contraction of skeletal muscle, *except*:
- a. Discharge of motor neuron
- b. Ca^{2+} release from the sarcoplasmic reticulum
- c. Binding of Ca^{2+} to troponin C
- d. Release of Ca^{2+} from troponin C

253. A 41-year-old woman has anxiety, a tremor, goiter and exophthalmos. Against which single enzyme is drug treatment targeted?
- a. 1-α-hydroxylase
- b. 5-α-reductase
- c. Aromatase
- d. Thyroid peroxidase

254. All inhibit pain transmission, *except*:
- a. Morphine
- b. Enkephalin
- c. Substance p
- d. Beta-endorphin

255. Chymotrypsin acts upon:
- a. Starch in duodenum
- b. Proteins in stomach
- c. Proteins in duodenum in alkaline medium
- d. Proteins in duodenum in acidic medium

256. Resting membrane potential develops mainly due to:
- a. K^+ efflux
- b. Cl^- influx
- c. Ca^{2+} influx
- d. Na^+ efflux

257. The most potent respiratory stimulant is:
- a. Oxygen
- b. CO_2
- c. K^+
- d. H^+

258. The primary contractile pattern of small intestine during digestive period is:
- a. Segmentation
- b. Peristalsis
- c. Retropulsion
- d. Pendular movements

259. Gastrin regulates gastric acid secretion at:
- a. Gastric cardia
- b. Antrum
- c. Pyloric canal
- d. First part of duodenum

260. Severe diarrhea leads to:
- a. A decreased K^+ contents of the body fluid
- b. Alkalosis
- c. Increased Na^+ contents in the body
- d. None of the above

261. FIGLU excretion in the urine is an index of the deficiency of:
- a. Thiamine
- b. Niacin
- c. Pyridoxine
- d. Folate

262. When under certain conditions, the p50 value of hemoglobin rises, the affinity of the pigment for combining with O_2 will:
- a. Remain the same
- b. Fall
- c. Rise
- d. First rise, then fall

Answers:

251. b	252. d	253. d	254. c
255. c	256. a	257. b	258. a
259. b	260. a	261. d	262. b

263. Bohr effect is:
a. Effect of Zn on carbonic anhydrase activity
b. Effect of pCO_2 on oxyhemoglobin dissociation
c. HCO_3- leaving the RBC in exchange for Cl
d. H^+ leaving RBC for each CO_2 that enters

264. The modality that is lost on the ipsilateral side in Brown-Sequard syndrome is:
a. Pain
b. Temperature
c. Crude touch
d. Proprioception

265. The bitter taste is mediated by the action of:
a. Guanyl cyclase
b. G protein
c. Tyrosine kinase
d. Epithelial Na channels

266. The part of the eye which transduces blue, green and red light is:
a. Cornea
b. Fovea
c. Periphery of retina
d. Optic nerve

267. What is the most important event in trivial injury:
a. Blood coagulation
b. Formation of platelet plug
c. Vascular spasm
d. Formation of thromboplastin

268. A 32-year-old man has poor libido. Gynecomastia is evident on examination. His partner has previously had a child with another partner. What is the single most appropriate investigation to perform?
a. Serum estrogen
b. Serum prolactin
c. Serum testosterone
d. Ultrasound testes

269. Filtration of protein across cerebral capillaries is prevented by:
a. Foot process of astrocytes
b. Fibrous tissue
c. Low BP
d. High CSF pressure

270. A 72-year-old diabetic man has suffered a right-sided stroke affecting his subthalamic nucleus. What clinical feature may he demonstrate?
a. Excessive left-side movement
b. Excessive right-side movement
c. Reduced movement bilaterally
d. Reduced left-side movement

271. Massage and application of liniments relieve pain due to:
a. Stimulation of endogenous analgesia system
b. Release of endorphins by the first-order neuron in the brainstem
c. Release of glutamate and substance p in the spinal cord
d. Inhibition by large myelinated afferent fibers

272. All are absorbed in DCT, *except*:
a. Water
b. Potassium
c. Chloride
d. Sodium

Answers:

263. b	264. d	265. b	266. b
267. b	268. b	269. a	270. b
271. d	272. b		

273. All of the following increase renin secretion, *except*:
a. Decreased amount of Na⁺ in DCT
b. Decreased amount of Na⁺ in PCT
c. Narrowing of afferent arterioles
d. Renal ischemia

274. A 45-year-old man has stable congestive cardiac failure. His resting heart rate is 102 bpm. What single factor mediates his tachycardia?
a. Decreased angiotensin-II
b. Decreased atrial natriuretic peptide
c. Increased aldosterone
d. Increased sympathetic tone

275. All influence hemoglobin dissociation curve, *except*:
a. CO_2 tension
b. Temperature
c. 2,3-DPG level
d. Chloride concentration

276. EPSP is due to:
a. Na⁺ efflux
b. K⁺ influx
c. Na⁺ influx
d. Ca⁺⁺ influx

277. A large greasy, smelly stool usually indicates failure of digestion of:
a. Carbohydrates
b. Fats
c. Proteins
d. Peptones

278. All the following reflexes are multi synaptic, *except*:
a. Cord righting reflex
b. Withdrawal reflex
c. Stretch reflex
d. Golgi tendon reflex

279. Antibodies against sperm develop:
a. After infection
b. After vasectomy
c. After orchidectomy
d. After trauma

280. Net ATP molecules generated during the conversion of glycogen to lactate:
a. 2
b. 14
c. 36
d. 38

281. Parkinsonism is due to the lesion of:
a. Corticostriate fibers
b. Thalamocortical fibers
c. Nigrostriatal fibers
d. Rubrothalamocortical fibers

282. Decompression sickness occurs in:
a. Diver
b. Pilot
c. Diver and pilot
d. Diver, pilot and mountaineer

283. Increase in which of the following parameters will shift the O_2 dissociation curve to the left:
a. Temperature
b. $PaCO_2$
c. 2,3-DPG concentration
d. Oxygen affinity of Hb

284. CO_2 affects the respiratory center via:
a. CSF H⁺ concentration
b. Carotid body
c. Aortic body
d. All of the above

285. Flocculonodular lobe of the cerebellum is concerned with:
a. Equilibrium
b. Co-ordination
c. Baroreception
d. Chemoreception

286. The vomiting center is situated in:
a. Hypothalamus
b. Amygdala
c. Pons
d. Medulla

Answers:

273. b	274. d	275. d	276. c
277. b	278. c	279. b	280. a
281. c	282. c	283. d	284. d
285. a	286. d		

287. Insulin increases glucose entry into:
a. Skeletal muscle
b. Intestine
c. Renal tubular cells
d. Cortical neuron

288. A 78-year-old man with advanced cancer is treated with vincristine, a microtubule inhibitor. During which single stage of mitosis are the tumor cells likely to arrest?
a. Anaphase
b. Cytokinesis
c. Metaphase
d. Prophase

289. Which one is not found in semen:
a. Testosterone
b. Fructose
c. Citric acid
d. Ascorbic acid

290. Osteoclasts are inhibited by:
a. Parathormone
b. 1,25-dihydroxy cholecalciferol
c. Calcitonin
d. Tumor necrosis factor

291. Alkali-resistant Hb is:
a. HbA
b. HbA_{1c}
c. HbS
d. HbF

292. Thyroxine and tri-iodothyronine are transported in plasma bound to several different proteins, which do not include:
a. Thyroglobulin
b. Thyroxine binding globulin (TBG)
c. Albumin
d. Thyroxine binding prealbumin

293. Conduction of which type of nerve fiber is blocked maximally by pressure?
a. C
b. A
c. B
d. D

294. Blood flow in liver in mL/min is:
a. 800
b. 1,200
c. 1,500
d. 1,800

295. Maximum peripheral resistance is offered by:
a. Blood capillaries
b. Arteries
c. Arterioles
d. Venules

296. Not true about capillaries:
a. Greatest cross-sectional area
b. Contains less blood than veins
c. Contains 25% of blood volume
d. Have a single layer of cells bounding the lumen

297. The swallowing center is situated in:
a. Midbrain
b. Pons
c. Medulla
d. Cerebellum

Answers:	287. a	288. c	289. a	290. c
	291. d	292. a	293. b	294. c
	295. c	296. c	297. c	

SECTION 2

Biochemistry

Section Outline

Chapter 3: Biochemistry

3 Biochemistry

CARBOHYDRATES

Carbohydrates are organic compounds that are vital in providing energy for the human body.

They are classified into three main types: monosaccharides, disaccharides, and polysaccharides.

1. **Monosaccharides:** These are the simplest form of carbohydrates and cannot be further hydrolyzed. Common examples include glucose, fructose, and galactose. Key properties of monosaccharides are:
   - They have a single sugar unit.
   - They are usually sweet-tasting.
   - They are the building blocks for other carbohydrates.
   - They are quickly absorbed and used as an immediate energy source.
2. **Disaccharides:** Disaccharides are formed when two monosaccharide units join together. Examples include sucrose, lactose, and maltose. Important points about disaccharides are:
   - They require specific enzymes to break them down into monosaccharides.
   - They are commonly found in foods and provide a source of energy.
   - They can have different sweetness levels based on their composition.
3. **Polysaccharides:** Polysaccharides are complex carbohydrates composed of long chains of monosaccharide units. Starch and glycogen are examples of polysaccharides.

Key properties of polysaccharides include:
- They serve as storage forms of glucose in plants (starch) and animals (glycogen).
- They are insoluble in water.
- They provide a sustained release of energy due to their complex structure.
- They play a crucial role in regulating blood sugar levels.

Properties of Carbohydrates

- **Solubility:** Most monosaccharides and disaccharides are water-soluble due to their hydrophilic nature. However, some polysaccharides like cellulose are insoluble in water.
- **Sweetness:** Many carbohydrates, especially monosaccharides and some disaccharides, exhibit a sweet taste.
- **Reducing or nonreducing:** Carbohydrates with a free aldehyde or ketone group are reducing sugars and can undergo oxidation reactions. Nonreducing sugars lack these functional groups.
- **Molecular weight:** Carbohydrates can range in molecular weight from small monosaccharides to large polysaccharides.
- **Stability:** Carbohydrates can undergo hydrolysis under acidic or enzymatic conditions, resulting in the breakdown of glycosidic bonds.

Isomerism in Carbohydrates

- **Structural isomerism:** Carbohydrates can exhibit structural isomerism based on the arrangement of their carbon skeletons. For example, glucose and fructose are structural isomers.

○ **Stereoisomerism:** Carbohydrates can also exhibit stereoisomerism due to the presence of chiral carbons. The two main types of stereoisomerism in carbohydrates are:

1. **Enantiomerism:** Enantiomers are non-superimposable mirror images of each other.
   Example: D-glucose and L-glucose.
2. **Diastereomerism:** Diastereomers are stereoisomers that are not mirror images.
   Example: Glucose and galactose.

Glycosidic bonds: In carbohydrates, monosaccharides can join together through glycosidic bonds (covalent bond) to form disaccharides, oligosaccharides, and polysaccharides.

This reaction occurs between the hydroxyl (OH) group of one monosaccharide and the anomeric carbon of another monosaccharide.

Example of glycosidic bonds:

○ **Lactose:** β-1,4-glycosidic bond between glucose and galactose.
○ **Sucrose (table sugar):** α-1,2-glycosidic bond between glucose and fructose.
○ **Starch and glycogen:** Primarily α-1,4-glycosidic bonds.
○ **Cellulose:** β-1,4-glycosidic bonds.

Polysaccharides: Are complex carbohydrates composed of long chains of monosaccharide units joined together by glycosidic bonds.

They serve various functions in organisms, including energy storage, structural support, and cell signaling.

Examples of polysaccharides:

○ **Starch:** Starch is the primary energy storage polysaccharide in plants. It is made up of glucose units joined by α-1,4-glycosidic bonds. Starch exists in two forms: (1) amylose: a linear chain of glucose molecules, (2) amylopectin: a branched chain of glucose molecules. It is commonly found in staple foods like potatoes, rice, and wheat.

○ **Glycogen:** Glycogen is the main energy storage polysaccharide in animals and humans. It is similar to amylopectin in structure but has more extensive branching. Glycogen is stored primarily in the liver and muscles and serves as a readily available source of glucose when energy is needed.

○ **Cellulose:** Cellulose is a structural polysaccharide that forms the cell walls of plants. It is composed of glucose units linked by β-1,4-glycosidic bonds. Unlike starch and glycogen, cellulose cannot be digested by most animals due to the lack of specific enzymes to break the β-glycosidic bonds. However, it serves as an important dietary fiber, aiding in digestion and promoting bowel regularity.

○ **Chitin:** Chitin is a polysaccharide found in the exoskeletons of arthropods (such as insects and crustaceans) and the cell walls of fungi. It is composed of N-acetylglucosamine units joined by β-1,4-glycosidic bonds. Chitin provides strength and rigidity to the structures it forms.

○ **Heparin:** Heparin is a complex polysaccharide found in the body that acts as an anticoagulant. It consists of repeating units of glucuronic acid and N-acetylglucosamine linked by glycosidic bonds. Heparin prevents blood clotting by inhibiting the clotting factors in the blood.

Metabolic pathways: Are interconnected series of chemical reactions that occur within cells to convert nutrients into energy, generate building blocks for macromolecules, and perform other essential cellular functions.

These pathways can be broadly categorized into three main types: catabolic, anabolic, and amphibolic.

1. **Catabolic pathways:** Catabolic pathways involve the breakdown of complex molecules into simpler ones, releasing energy in the process. One of the key catabolic pathways is cellular respiration, which occurs in three stages: glycolysis, the Krebs cycle (or citric acid cycle), and oxidative phosphorylation.
2. **Anabolic pathways:** Anabolic pathways are involved in the synthesis of complex molecules from simpler ones, requiring energy input. One notable anabolic pathway is protein synthesis, which involves transcription and translation. Anabolic pathways also include processes such as gluconeogenesis, where glucose is synthesized from noncarbohydrate sources, and fatty acid synthesis, which creates fatty acids from acetyl-CoA.
3. **Amphibolic pathways:** Amphibolic pathways are those that have both catabolic and anabolic functions. For example, the citric acid cycle (Krebs cycle) is not only involved in catabolism by generating energy-rich molecules like NADH and $FADH_2$ but also provides precursor molecules for anabolic pathways.

Different Metabolic Pathways Related to Carbohydrate Metabolism

1. **Glycolysis/Embden-Meyerhof-Parnas pathway (EMP):**
   ○ Takes place in the cytoplasm of the cell.
   ○ Glucose is oxidized to pyruvate or lactate.
   ○ Under anaerobic condition, lactic acid is the end product and in aerobic condition, pyruvate is the end product.
   ○ Total ATP formed: 10 ATP
   ○ ATP consumption: 2 ATP consumed
   ○ Net ATP gain: 8 ATP
2. **Pyruvate decarboxylation:**
   ○ Occurs in the mitochondria.
   ○ Pyruvate is converted into acetyl-CoA.
3. **Citric acid cycle/TCA cycle (Krebs cycle):**
   ○ Takes place in the mitochondria.

○ Acetyl-CoA enters the cycle and undergoes a series of reactions, producing energy-rich molecules.
○ Aerobic and amphibolic pathway
○ Common metabolic pathway for carbohydrates, proteins and lipids.

TCA cycle inhibitors:
○ **Fluoroacetate:** Aconitase enzyme inhibitor.
○ **Arsenite:** Alpha-ketoglutarate dehydrogenase enzyme inhibitor.
○ **Malonate:** Succinate dehydrogenase enzyme inhibitor (competitive inhibition).

4. **Electron transport chain (ETC):**
   ○ Occurs in the inner mitochondrial membrane.
   ○ Electrons from energy-rich molecules are transferred along the chain, generating a proton gradient.
   ○ **ATP generation:** Around 28–32 ATP produced (varies).
   ○ **ATP consumption:** None directly consumed.

   Glycogen storage diseases is shown in Table 3.1.
5. **Glycogenesis:**
   ○ Process of converting excess glucose into glycogen for storage.
   ○ Occurs in the liver and muscles.
6. **Glycogenolysis:**
   ○ Breakdown of glycogen into glucose for energy release.
   ○ Occurs in the liver and muscles.
7. **Gluconeogenesis:**
   ○ Formation of glucose from non-carbohydrate sources (such as amino acids or glycerol).
   ○ Occurs mainly in the liver.
8. **Hexose monophosphate (HMP) pathway/pentose Phosphate pathway or the phosphogluconate pathway:**
   Alternative metabolic pathway parallel to glycolysis.

Table 3.1: Glycogen storage diseases.

Glycogen storage disease	Alternate names	Enzyme deficiency
Glycogen storage disease type I	Von Gierke's disease	Glucose-6-phosphatase deficiency
Glycogen storage disease type II	Pompe disease	Acid maltase (alpha-glucosidase) deficiency
Glycogen storage disease type III	Cori disease	Debranching enzyme (amylo-1,6-glucosidase) deficiency
Glycogen storage disease type IV	Andersen disease	Glycogen branching enzyme deficiency
Glycogen storage disease type V	McArdle disease	Muscle glycogen phosphorylase deficiency
Glycogen storage disease type VI	Hers disease	Liver glycogen phosphorylase deficiency
Glycogen storage disease type VII	Tarui disease	Muscle phosphofructokinase deficiency
Glycogen storage disease type IX	Phosphorylase b kinase deficiency disease	Phosphorylase kinase deficiency
Glycogen storage disease type X	Danon disease	Lysosome-associated membrane protein 2 (LAMP2) deficiency

○ Glucose-6-phosphate (G6P) is the starting point of the HMP pathway.

○ The pathway produces NADPH, a reducing agent crucial for biosynthetic reactions and cellular defense against oxidative stress.

○ NADPH is generated through a series of reactions involving the enzyme glucose-6-phosphate dehydrogenase (G6PD).

○ The HMP pathway generates ribose-5-phosphate (R5P), a precursor for nucleotide synthesis.

○ R5P is essential for DNA, RNA, and coenzyme synthesis.

○ The HMP pathway is active in tissues with high biosynthetic demands and plays a vital role in red blood cells, liver, and adipose tissue.

○ The HMP pathway also produces important intermediates like erythrose-4-phosphate and fructose-6-phosphate, contributing to other metabolic pathways.

Overall, the HMP pathway plays a crucial role in providing NADPH for cellular redox reactions and generating important intermediates required for biosynthesis.

Role of Vitamins in Carbohydrate Metabolism

Vitamins play essential roles as cofactors and coenzymes in various metabolic pathways of carbohydrate metabolism. Here are some vitamins and their involvement in these pathways:

1. **Thiamine (vitamin B_1):**
   ○ Required for the conversion of pyruvate to acetyl-CoA in the citric acid cycle.
   ○ Acts as a cofactor for enzymes involved in decarboxylation reactions.

2. **Riboflavin (vitamin B_2):**
   ○ Necessary for the conversion of glucose to pyruvate during glycolysis.
   ○ Participates in redox reactions by serving as a component of flavin adenine dinucleotide (FAD) and flavin mononucleotide (FMN) coenzymes.

3. **Niacin (vitamin B$_3$)**
   ○ Essential for the breakdown of glucose and other nutrients to produce ATP.
   ○ Functions as a precursor for coenzymes NAD$^+$ and NADP$^+$ involved in redox reactions.
4. **Pantothenic acid (vitamin B$_5$):**
   ○ Required for the synthesis of coenzyme A (CoA), a vital molecule in carbohydrate metabolism.
   ○ Facilitates the oxidation of glucose during the citric acid cycle.
5. **Pyridoxine (vitamin B$_6$):**
   ○ Plays a role in glycogen metabolism by participating in glycogen phosphorylase activity.
   ○ Assists in the conversion of amino acids to glucose through gluconeogenesis.
6. **Biotin (vitamin B$_7$):**
   ○ Acts as a cofactor for several carboxylase enzymes involved in gluconeogenesis.
   ○ Required for the utilization of glucose and fatty acids as energy sources.
7. **Cobalamin (vitamin B$_{12}$):**
   ○ Assists in the conversion of methyl malonyl-CoA to succinyl-CoA during carbohydrate metabolism.
   ○ Plays a role in the synthesis of nucleotides and red blood cells.

These vitamins are crucial for the proper functioning of enzymes and metabolic pathways involved in carbohydrate metabolism, enabling the body to efficiently utilize and generate energy from carbohydrates.

Estimation of Blood Glucose

Enzymatic Methods

1. **Glucose oxidase peroxidase (GOD-POD) method:**
   ○ Specifically react with glucose and produce a measurable signal.
   ○ **Principle:** Glucose oxidase catalyzes the oxidation of glucose to produce gluconic acid and hydrogen peroxide. Hydrogen peroxide is converted to water molecule and oxygen by peroxidase enzyme, in presence of oxygen acceptor which itself converted into a colored compound that can be measured by colorimetric or electrochemical method.
2. **Hexokinase method (reference method):**
   ○ Enzymatic methods provide accurate and precise measurements of blood glucose levels (true glucose).
   ○ These methods are commonly used in clinical laboratories for routine glucose testing.

Nonenzymatic Methods

○ Alkaline copper reduction methods
○ Ortho-toluidine method

Principle: Nonenzymatic methods use chemical reactions that directly or indirectly measure glucose levels without the involvement of enzymes.

Nonenzymatic methods are often based on colorimetric or spectrophotometric reactions and can provide rapid results.

However, they may have lower specificity and sensitivity compared to enzymatic methods.

○ **Fasting plasma glucose (FPG) test:**
   ○ Measures blood glucose levels after an overnight fast (usually 8–12 hours).
   ○ Commonly used to diagnose diabetes and monitor glucose control.
   ○ Normal fasting glucose levels typically range from 70–100 mg/dL.
○ **Random plasma glucose (RPG) test:**
   ○ Measures blood glucose levels at any time during the day, regardless of the time of the last meal.
   ○ Useful for diagnosing severe hyperglycemia.
   ○ Normal random glucose levels should be below 140 mg/dL.
○ **Oral glucose tolerance test (OGTT)/ glucose tolerance test (GTT):**

- GTT is a diagnostic test used to assess how the body metabolizes glucose.
- The test involves fasting overnight, followed by consuming a glucose-rich drink (75 g of anhydrous glucose in 200–300 mL of water).
- Blood samples are taken at regular intervals (e.g., 1 hour, 2 hours) to measure blood glucose levels.
- The interpretation of GTT is based on the blood glucose values at different time points.
- Used to diagnose gestational diabetes and assess impaired glucose tolerance.

Interpretation of Blood Glucose Levels

- **Normal fasting glucose:** FPG levels below 100 mg/dL are considered normal.
- **Impaired fasting glucose (prediabetes):** FPG levels between 100–125 mg/dL indicate impaired fasting glucose, a prediabetic state.
- **Diabetes:**
  - FPG levels equal to or above 126 mg/dL on two separate occasions suggest diabetes.
  - RPG levels above 200 mg/dL with classic symptoms (polydipsia, polyphagia, and polyhydria) also indicate diabetes.

Glucose Tolerance Test Interpretation

- **Normal glucose tolerance:** FPG levels below 100 mg/dL and 2-hour OGTT levels below 140 mg/dL indicate normal glucose tolerance.
- **Impaired glucose tolerance (prediabetes):** 2-hour OGTT levels between 140–199 mg/dL suggest impaired glucose tolerance, a prediabetic state.
- **Diabetes:** 2-hour OGTT levels equal to or above 200 mg/dL on two separate occasions indicate diabetes.

Hypoglycemia

Hypoglycemia refers to abnormally low blood glucose levels, typically below 70 mg/dL.

Causes of Hypoglycemia

- Excessive insulin or other blood glucose-lowering medications.
- Delayed or missed meals.
- Intense physical activity without adequate carbohydrate intake.
- Alcohol consumption without accompanying food.
- Certain medical conditions affecting the liver, pancreas, or adrenal glands.
- Malnutrition or eating disorders.

Hyperglycemia

Hyperglycemia refers to high blood glucose levels, typically above 130 mg/dL (fasting) or 180 mg/dL (postprandial).

Causes of Hyperglycemia

- Diabetes mellitus (both type 1 and type 2).
- Inadequate or insufficient use of insulin or oral antidiabetic medications.
- Overconsumption of carbohydrates or sugary foods.
- Lack of physical activity.
- Stress, illness, or infections.
- Certain medications (e.g., corticosteroids)

Glycosylated hemoglobin/(HbA1c) is a form of hemoglobin that reflects average blood glucose levels over a period of approximately 2–3 months.

- **Normal reference range:**
  - The normal reference range: below 5.7%.
  - Prediabetes is diagnosed: 5.7–6.4%.
  - Diabetes mellitus: 6.5% or higher.
- **Clinical utility:**
  - HbA1c is widely used as a diagnostic tool for diabetes mellitus.
  - It provides an indication of long-term blood glucose control, reflecting average blood glucose levels over several months.
  - HbA1c can help monitor the effectiveness of diabetes management and treatment strategies.
  - It is a convenient and standardized measure that does not require fasting.

- **Significance:**
  - Elevated HbA1c levels indicate poor blood glucose control and an increased risk of complications associated with diabetes.
  - Long-term exposure to high blood glucose levels can lead to complications affecting various organs, including the eyes, kidneys, nerves, and cardiovascular system.
  - Lowering HbA1c through lifestyle modifications and medication interventions can help reduce the risk of diabetes-related complications.
  - HbA1c levels are used as a target for glycemic control in diabetes management guidelines.

LIPIDS

Simple Lipids

Simple lipids are esters of fatty acids and various alcohols.

They can be further classified into three subcategories:

1. **Fats (triglycerides):** They are formed by esterification of three fatty acids with glycerol. Examples include butter, olive oil, and animal fats.
2. **Waxes:** Waxes are esters of fatty acids with high molecular weight alcohols. They serve as protective coatings for plants and animals. Beeswax and carnauba wax are examples.
3. **Sterols:** Sterols are a type of simple lipid with a characteristic structure. Cholesterol is a prominent example and is found in animal cell membranes.

Compound Lipids

Compound lipids are formed by the combination of simple lipids with other chemical groups.

They can be further classified into three subcategories:

1. **Phospholipids:** Phospholipids consist of a glycerol molecule, two fatty acids, a phosphate group, and an alcohol. They are crucial components of cell membranes. Examples include phosphatidylcholine and phosphatidylserine.
2. **Glycolipids:** Glycolipids contains a carbohydrate moiety along with a lipid. They are involved in cell recognition and adhesion. Cerebrosides and gangliosides are examples.
3. **Lipoproteins:** Lipoproteins are complex compounds formed by the combination of lipids and proteins. They transport lipids in the bloodstream. Examples include high-density lipoprotein (HDL) and low-density lipoprotein (LDL).

Derived Lipids

Derived lipids are derived from simple or compound lipids through various chemical reactions. Examples include:

- **Fatty acids:** Fatty acids can be derived from the hydrolysis of triglycerides or phospholipids.
- **Eicosanoids:** Eicosanoids are derived from arachidonic acid, a fatty acid. They include prostaglandins, leukotrienes, and thromboxanes.
- **Steroid hormones:** Steroid hormones such as cortisol and estrogen are derived from cholesterol.

AMINO ACIDS AND PROTEIN

Amino acid chemistry: Amino acids are the building blocks of proteins and play a crucial role in various biological processes.

Structure of Amino Acids

- Amino acids consist of a central carbon atom (α-carbon) bonded to four groups: an amino group ($-NH_2$), a carboxyl group ($-COOH$), a hydrogen atom ($-H$), and a variable side chain (R group).

- The side chain varies among different amino acids, giving each amino acid its unique properties.

Properties of Amino Acids

- Amino acids are amphoteric, meaning they can act as both acids (due to the carboxyl group) and bases (due to the amino group).
- They have a zwitterionic form at physiological pH, where the amino group is positively charged and the carboxyl group is negatively charged.
- Amino acids are optically active due to the presence of a chiral α-carbon, except for glycine, which has a hydrogen atom as its R group.

Classification of Amino Acids

Amino acids are classified into several categories based on the properties of their side chains. The main categories include:

Based on Polarity

- **Nonpolar (hydrophobic) amino acids:** These amino acids have nonpolar side chains that are hydrophobic and do not interact with water.
  Examples: Alanine, valine, leucine, isoleucine, methionine, phenylalanine, tryptophan, proline.
- **Polar (hydrophilic) amino acids:** These amino acids have polar side chains that can form hydrogen bonds and interact with water.
  Examples: Serine, threonine, tyrosine, cysteine, asparagine, glutamine.

Based on Charge

- **Positively charged (basic) amino acids:** These amino acids have positively charged side chains at physiological pH.
  Examples: Lysine, arginine, histidine.
- **Negatively charged (acidic) amino acids:** These amino acids have negatively charged side chains at physiological pH.
  Examples: Aspartic acid, glutamic acid.

Based on Nutritional Requirements: Essential and Nonessential Amino Acids

- Essential amino acids cannot be synthesized by the human body and must be obtained from the diet. There are nine essential amino acids: Phenylalanine, valine, threonine, tryptophan, isoleucine, methionine, leucine, lysine, and histidine.
- Nonessential amino acids can be synthesized by the body.

Functions of Amino Acids

Amino acids have various biological functions:

- **Protein synthesis:** Amino acids are assembled into polypeptide chains during protein synthesis.
- **Enzyme catalysis:** Amino acids play critical roles as enzyme catalysts.
- **Cell signaling:** Some amino acids function as neurotransmitters or signaling molecules.
- **Structural support:** Amino acids contribute to the structural integrity of tissues such as collagen and keratin.
- **Energy production:** Amino acids can be metabolized for energy when needed.

Clinical Significance

Imbalances or deficiencies in amino acids can have significant clinical implications:

- **Inborn errors of metabolism:** Genetic defects in amino acid metabolism can lead to disorders such as phenylketonuria (PKU) and maple syrup urine disease.
- **Protein-energy malnutrition:** Inadequate protein intake can result in protein-energy malnutrition, leading to growth impairments and compromised immune function.

○ **Amino acid analysis:** Amino acid analysis is performed to diagnose and monitor certain metabolic disorders and nutritional deficiencies.

Proteins Structure Organization

1. **Primary structure:**
   ○ Primary structure refers to the linear sequence of amino acids in a protein.
   ○ The sequence is determined by the DNA sequence of the corresponding gene.
   Example: The primary structure of insulin consists of 51 amino acids.
2. **Secondary structure:**
   ○ Secondary structure refers to the local folding patterns within a protein.
   ○ The two most common secondary structures are alpha helix and beta-sheet.
   Example: Hemoglobin
3. **Tertiary structure:**
   ○ Tertiary structure refers to the three-dimensional arrangement of a protein's secondary structural elements.
   ○ It is stabilized by various interactions, including hydrogen bonds, disulfide bonds, hydrophobic interactions, and electrostatic interactions.
   Example: The tertiary structure of enzymes determines their active sites and catalytic functions.
4. **Quaternary structure:**
   ○ Quaternary structure refers to the arrangement of multiple protein subunits to form a functional protein complex.
   ○ Subunits may be identical or different.
   Example: Hemoglobin is a tetramer consisting of two alpha and two beta subunits.

Protein Folding

○ Protein folding is the process by which a protein assumes its functional three-dimensional structure.

○ The interactions between amino acid residues guide it.
Example: The folding of the prion protein is crucial for its normal cellular function.

Protein Denaturation

○ Denaturation refers to the disruption of a protein's native structure, leading to loss of function.
○ It can be caused by extreme temperature, pH changes, or exposure to certain chemicals.
Example: Cooking an egg causes denaturation of the proteins, changing the texture and appearance.

Protein Function

○ Protein function is determined by its structure and organization.
○ Proteins can have diverse functions such as enzymatic activity, structural support, transport, and signaling.
Example: Antibodies are proteins that recognize and bind to specific antigens, playing a role in immune response.

Protein Conformational Changes

○ Conformational changes refer to alterations in a protein's three-dimensional structure.
○ They are often associated with changes in protein function or regulation.
Example: In muscle contraction, conformational changes in the protein myosin generate the sliding movement of actin and myosin filaments.

NUCLEIC ACID AND NUCLEOTIDES

Nucleic Acid

Nucleic acids are essential biomolecules that carry and transmit genetic information in living organisms. They are crucial in various biological processes, including protein synthesis and heredity.

Definition

- Nucleic acids are macromolecules composed of nucleotide monomers.
- They are classified into deoxyribonucleic acid (DNA) and ribonucleic acid (RNA).

Structure

- Nucleotides are the building blocks of nucleic acids.
- Each nucleotide consists of a sugar molecule (ribose in RNA, deoxyribose in DNA), a phosphate group, and a nitrogenous base (adenine, guanine, cytosine, or thymine/uracil).

DNA Structure

- DNA is a double-stranded helical structure resembling a twisted ladder (double helix).
- It consists of two complementary strands held together by hydrogen bonds between the nitrogenous bases.
- Adenine pairs with thymine (A-T) and guanine pairs with cytosine (G-C).

RNA Structure

- RNA is a single-stranded molecule that can fold into various secondary structures.
- It contains ribose sugar instead of deoxyribose and uracil instead of thymine.

Functions of DNA

- DNA carries and stores genetic information in the form of genes.
- It is involved in protein synthesis through the process of transcription and translation.

Functions of RNA

- RNA plays a role in protein synthesis by carrying the genetic information from DNA to ribosomes.
- It can also have regulatory functions, such as microRNA and small interfering RNA.

Laboratory Techniques for Nucleic Acid Analysis

- Polymerase chain reaction (PCR) is used for amplifying specific DNA sequences.
- Gel electrophoresis separates DNA or RNA fragments based on their size and charge.
- DNA sequencing determines the exact sequence of nucleotides in a DNA molecule.

Nucleic Acid Disorders

Genetic disorders, such as sickle cell anemia and cystic fibrosis, result from mutations in the nucleic acid sequence.

MOLECULAR TECHNIQUES

Importance and applications of molecular techniques in diagnosing diseases and monitoring treatment responses.

Nucleic Acid Extraction

- Methods for extracting DNA and RNA from various biological samples.
- Principles of sample preparation, lysis, and purification.
- Common extraction techniques such as phenol-chloroform extraction, column-based purification, and magnetic bead-based methods.

Polymerase Chain Reaction (PCR)

Principle and Steps Involved in PCR

Principle

- PCR is a widely used molecular technique that allows for the amplification of specific DNA sequences.
- It is based on the natural process of DNA replication and utilizes a heat-stable DNA polymerase enzyme.

Steps Involved in PCR

Denaturation

- The PCR reaction starts with denaturation, where the DNA template is heated to a high temperature (typically 94–98°C).
- High temperature breaks the hydrogen bonds between the DNA strands, separating them into single strands.

Annealing

- After denaturation, the temperature is lowered to allow the primers to anneal or bind to their complementary sequences on the DNA template.
- The annealing temperature is typically between 50 and 65°C and is specific to the primers used.

Extension

- Once the primers are bound, the temperature is raised to the optimal temperature for DNA polymerase activity (usually around 72°C).
- The DNA polymerase enzyme synthesizes new DNA strands by extending from the primers, using the original DNA strands as templates.

Cycling

- The denaturation, annealing, and extension steps are repeated multiple times in a process called cycling.
- Each cycle doubles the amount of DNA, resulting in exponential amplification of the targeted DNA sequence.

Final Extension

After the desired number of cycles, a final extension step is performed at a slightly higher temperature (usually 72°C) to ensure the completion of any remaining DNA synthesis.

Final Hold

- The reaction is then held at a low temperature (around 4–10°C) to keep the DNA stable until further analysis or storage.
- PCR allows for the amplification of specific DNA sequences, making it a powerful tool in various applications such as genetic testing, forensics, and molecular research.

Types of PCR

- Conventional PCR
- Real-time PCR
- Reverse transcription PCR (RT-PCR)

Applications of PCR

- In genetic testing
- Viral load quantification
- Identification of pathogens.

Gel Electrophoresis

- Principle of gel electrophoresis for separating DNA and RNA fragments.
- Agarose gel and polyacrylamide gel electrophoresis.
- Visualization of DNA/RNA bands using dyes or fluorescent probes.

DNA Sequencing

Overview of DNA sequencing methods, including Sanger sequencing and next-generation sequencing (NGS).

Applications of DNA Sequencing

- In genetic testing
- Personalized medicine
- Studying genetic variations

Restriction Enzyme Analysis

- Introduction to restriction enzymes and their role in DNA analysis.
- Restriction fragment length polymorphism (RFLP) analysis and its applications in genetic fingerprinting and identification.

Hybridization Techniques

Principles of hybridization, including Southern blotting and fluorescence in situ hybridization (FISH).

Applications of Hybridization Techniques

- In gene mapping
- Genetic disorders
- Cancer diagnostics

Microarray Technology

- Introduction to DNA microarrays and gene expression profiling.
- Designing microarray experiments and data analysis.
- Role of microarrays in studying gene expression patterns and identifying disease biomarkers.

Gene Editing Techniques: Like CRISPR-Cas9

Applications of Gene Editing

- Gene therapy
- Genetic engineering
- Studying gene functions

Molecular Diagnostics

- Role of molecular techniques in diagnosing infectious diseases, genetic disorders, and cancer.
- Integration of molecular diagnostics with other laboratory tests for comprehensive patient assessment.

ENZYMES

Enzymes are biological catalysts that accelerate chemical reactions in living organisms.

- They are typically proteins with specific three-dimensional structures.
- Enzymes play a crucial role in various physiological processes.

Enzyme Classification

- Enzymes are classified into six main groups based on the type of reaction they catalyze:

- **Oxidoreductases:** Catalyze redox reactions.
- **Transferases:** Transfer functional groups between molecules.
- **Hydrolases:** Catalyze hydrolysis reactions.
- **Lyases:** Catalyze the addition or removal of groups from molecules.
- **Isomerases:** Catalyze isomerization reactions.
- **Ligases:** Catalyze the joining of two molecules using ATP.

Enzyme Structure

- Enzymes have a specific three-dimensional structure, including active sites.
- Active sites are regions where substrate molecules bind and undergo chemical reactions.
- Enzymes are highly specific to their substrates due to the complementary shape and chemical properties of the active site.

Enzyme Kinetics

- Enzyme kinetics study the rate of enzyme-catalyzed reactions.
- Factors influencing enzyme activity include temperature, pH, substrate concentration, and enzyme concentration.
- Enzyme activity is often measured by the rate of product formation or substrate consumption.

Enzyme Inhibition

- Enzyme activity can be regulated by inhibitors.
- Competitive inhibitors compete with the substrate for binding to the active site.
- Noncompetitive inhibitors bind to a different site, altering the enzyme's structure and reducing its activity.

Enzyme Regulation

- Enzyme activity can be regulated through various mechanisms, such as: (a) Allosteric regulation: Binding of regulatory molecules to nonactive site regions. (b) Covalent modification: Addition or removal of chemical groups to alter enzyme activity. (c) Enzyme induction and repression: Control of enzyme synthesis based on cellular needs.

Enzymes in Clinical Diagnosis (Clinical Enzymology)

Involves the measurement and interpretation of enzyme activities in patient samples for diagnostic purposes.

○ Enzymes are released into the bloodstream during tissue damage, inflammation, or organ dysfunction.
○ Abnormal enzyme levels can indicate the presence, severity, or progression of various diseases.

Commonly Assayed Enzymes

Alanine Aminotransferase (ALT)

○ Present in liver cells and used to assess liver function.
○ Elevated levels indicate liver damage or disease, such as hepatitis.

Aspartate Aminotransferase (AST)

○ Found in various tissues, including the liver, heart, and muscles.
○ Elevated levels may indicate liver or heart damage.

Alkaline Phosphatase (ALP)

○ Found in the liver, bone, and other tissues.
○ Elevated levels may indicate liver or bone disorders, such as liver disease or bone abnormalities.

Creatine Kinase (CK)

○ Found in muscles, including cardiac and skeletal muscles.

○ Elevated levels indicate muscle damage or injury, such as myocardial infarction or muscular dystrophy.

Amylase

○ Produced by the pancreas and salivary glands.
○ Elevated levels may indicate pancreatic disorders, such as pancreatitis.

Lipase

○ Produced by the pancreas and involved in fat digestion.
○ Elevated levels may indicate pancreatic disorders, such as pancreatitis.

Cardiac Enzymes

Cardiac enzymes are a group of enzymes that are released into the bloodstream following damage to the heart muscle. These enzymes play a crucial role in the diagnosis and monitoring of cardiac conditions, particularly acute myocardial infarction (heart attack).

By measuring the levels of specific cardiac enzymes, healthcare professionals can assess the extent of cardiac damage and evaluate the effectiveness of treatment.

Commonly Assayed Cardiac Enzymes

Troponin

○ Troponin I and troponin T are specific markers for cardiac muscle damage.
○ Troponin levels start to rise within 3–4 hours of myocardial infarction and peak within 24–48 hours.
○ Elevated troponin levels indicate myocardial injury.

Creatine Kinase-MB (CK-MB)

○ CK-MB is an isoform of creatine kinase found primarily in the heart.
○ Elevated CK-MB levels suggest myocardial damage, particularly in the early stages of a heart attack.

○ CK-MB levels rise within 3–6 hours after onset, peak at 12–24 hours, and return to baseline within 48–72 hours.

Myoglobin

○ Myoglobin is an early marker of cardiac injury.
○ Elevated myoglobin levels can be detected within 1–3 hours after the onset of myocardial infarction.
○ Myoglobin levels peak within 6–9 hours and return to normal within 24–36 hours.

Lactate Dehydrogenase (LDH)

○ LDH is an enzyme found in various tissues, including the heart.
○ Elevated LDH levels may indicate cardiac muscle damage, but it is not specific to the heart.
○ LDH levels rise within 24–48 hours of myocardial infarction and may remain elevated for 10–14 days.

Clinical Utility and Interpretation

○ Cardiac enzyme measurements are essential in the diagnosis of acute myocardial infarction.
○ Elevated levels of troponin, CK-MB, myoglobin, and LDH in the appropriate clinical context support the diagnosis of a heart attack.
○ Serial measurements of cardiac enzymes can provide valuable information about the timing and progression of cardiac injury.
○ Cardiac enzyme levels are also useful in risk stratification and determining the prognosis of patients with cardiovascular disease.

BODY FLUIDS

Pleural Fluid Examination

Pleural fluid is a clear, serous fluid that fills the pleural cavity surrounding the lungs.

Analyzing the biochemical composition of pleural fluid can provide valuable diagnostic information for various respiratory and systemic conditions.

Collection of Pleural Fluid

○ Pleural fluid is obtained through a procedure called thoracentesis or pleural tap.
○ The fluid is collected using a sterile needle and syringe inserted into the pleural cavity.
○ It is essential to collect an adequate amount of fluid for accurate analysis.

Biochemical Parameters

○ **Protein levels:** Total protein concentration in pleural fluid is measured.
○ **Lactate dehydrogenase (LDH):** LDH is an enzyme that indicates tissue damage or inflammation.
○ **Glucose levels:** Glucose levels are compared to blood glucose levels and provide insights into metabolic activity.
○ **pH:** Pleural fluid pH is measured to assess acidity or alkalinity.

Interpretation of Biochemical Parameters

○ **Increased protein levels:** Seen in conditions like infection, malignancy, and inflammation.
○ **Increased LDH levels:** Indicate tissue damage, infection, or malignancy.
○ **Decreased glucose levels:** May suggest infection or malignancy.
○ **Abnormal pH levels:** Acidic pH may indicate infection, while alkaline pH may suggest esophageal rupture.

Additional Tests

○ **Microscopic examination:** Presence of cells (e.g., neutrophils, lymphocytes) and microorganisms.
○ **Gram stain and culture:** To identify bacterial or fungal infections.
○ **Cytology:** Examination of pleural fluid cells for the presence of cancer cells.

Clinical Significance

- Biochemical pleural fluid examination helps diagnose and differentiate various pleural diseases.
- It aids in identifying infections, such as bacterial or fungal pleuritis.
- Malignant pleural effusions can be detected through abnormal protein and LDH levels.
- Monitoring pleural fluid parameters helps assess treatment response.

Synovial Fluid Examination

Synovial fluid is a clear, viscous fluid found within joint cavities. Its analysis provides valuable information for the diagnosis and management of joint-related conditions.

Collection of Synovial Fluid

- Synovial fluid is collected using aseptic technique via joint aspiration.
- The most commonly aspirated joints include the knee, shoulder, and hip.
- A small amount of fluid (1–2 mL) is obtained using a syringe and needle.

Physical Examination

- Physical examination involves assessing the macroscopic appearance of the synovial fluid.
- Normal synovial fluid is clear and viscous, resembling egg white.
- Abnormal findings include turbidity, color changes, and presence of clots or debris.

Biochemical Analysis

Biochemical analysis helps assess the metabolic and inflammatory status of the joint.

Parameters Measured Include

- **Total protein:** Elevated levels may indicate inflammation or joint pathology.
- **Glucose:** Decreased levels may indicate infection or inflammatory conditions.
- **Lactate dehydrogenase (LDH):** Elevated levels may suggest joint inflammation or injury.
- **Rheumatoid factor (RF):** Presence may indicate rheumatoid arthritis.
- **Crystals:** Presence of urate or calcium pyrophosphate crystals can aid in diagnosing gout or pseudogout, respectively.

Microscopic Examination

- Microscopic examination involves the examination of synovial fluid cells and particles.
- Cell types observed include:
  - **Neutrophils:** Increased neutrophils indicate joint inflammation or infection.
  - **Lymphocytes:** Increased lymphocytes may suggest chronic inflammation or autoimmune disorders.
  - **Macrophages:** Presence may indicate chronic inflammation or joint degeneration.
  - **Red blood cells:** Increased red blood cells can indicate joint trauma or bleeding.

Microbiological Examination

- Microbiological examination is performed to identify the presence of microorganisms.
- Gram stain, culture, and sensitivity testing are commonly performed.
- Positive results indicate joint infection.

Crystal Analysis

- Crystals observed in synovial fluid can provide diagnostic information.
- Polarized light microscopy is used to identify crystals such as monosodium urate (gout) or calcium pyrophosphate (pseudogout).

ORGAN FUNCTION TESTS

Gastric Function Tests

Diagnostic tests used to evaluate the functioning of the stomach and assess various aspects of gastric secretion and digestion.

Gastric Acid Analysis

- Gastric acid analysis measures the quantity and quality of gastric acid secretion.
- **Indications:** Evaluation of acid-related disorders such as gastric ulcers, gastritis, or gastric hypersecretion.
- **Procedure:** Gastric fluid is aspirated via a nasogastric tube, and acid content is measured using pH determination or acid titration methods.

Pepsinogen Levels

- Pepsinogen levels assess the production of pepsin, an enzyme involved in protein digestion.
- **Indications:** Diagnosis of gastric mucosal damage, chronic gastritis, or monitoring response to treatment.
- **Procedure:** Blood samples are collected, and pepsinogen levels are measured using immunoassay techniques.

Gastrin Levels

- Gastrin levels evaluate the secretion of gastrin, a hormone that stimulates gastric acid secretion.
- **Indications:** Diagnosis of gastrinomas (gastrin-secreting tumors), evaluation of gastric acid regulation disorders.
- **Procedure:** Blood samples are collected, and gastrin levels are measured using immunoassay techniques.

Intrinsic Factor Antibodies

- Intrinsic factor antibodies test assesses the presence of antibodies against intrinsic factor, a protein required for vitamin B_{12} absorption.
- **Indications:** Diagnosis of pernicious anemia or autoimmune gastritis.
- **Procedure:** Blood samples are collected, and the presence of antibodies is detected using immunoassay methods.

Fecal Pancreatic Elastase

- Fecal pancreatic elastase test measures the activity of pancreatic elastase, an enzyme involved in fat digestion.
- **Indications:** Evaluation of exocrine pancreatic insufficiency.
- **Procedure:** Stool samples are collected, and the level of fecal pancreatic elastase is measured using enzyme-linked immunosorbent assay (ELISA).

Gastric Emptying Study

- Gastric emptying study assesses the rate at which the stomach empties its contents.
- **Indications:** Evaluation of gastroparesis (delayed gastric emptying) or dumping syndrome (rapid gastric emptying).
- **Procedure:** Radiographic or nuclear medicine techniques are used to track the movement of a test meal through the stomach.

Urea Breath Test

- Urea breath test detects the presence of *Helicobacter pylori (H. pylori)*, a bacterium associated with gastric ulcers and gastritis.
- **Indications:** Diagnosis of *H. pylori* infection and monitoring treatment response.
- **Procedure:** The patient ingests a solution containing labeled urea, and exhaled breath samples are collected and analyzed for labeled carbon dioxide.

Fasting Serum Gastrin

- Fasting serum gastrin levels evaluate the baseline level of gastrin in the blood.
- **Indications:** Assessment of gastric acid regulation disorders or suspected gastrinoma.
- **Procedure:** Blood samples are collected after an overnight fast, and fasting serum gastrin levels are measured using immunoassay techniques.

Pancreatic Function Tests

- Biochemical tests are essential tools used in clinical laboratories to evaluate pancreatic function. These tests are used to assess pancreatic exocrine and endocrine functions, along with their interpretations and clinical significance.

Pancreatic Exocrine Function Tests

- **Fecal elastase-1 test:** Measures elastase-1 levels in feces to assess pancreatic exocrine insufficiency.
- **Serum amylase and lipase:** Elevated levels indicate pancreatic inflammation, such as acute pancreatitis.

Pancreatic Endocrine Function Tests

- **Fasting blood glucose:** Measures blood glucose levels after an overnight fast to evaluate pancreatic insulin secretion and glucose regulation.
- **Oral glucose tolerance test (OGTT):** Assesses the ability of the pancreas to release insulin in response to glucose ingestion.
- **Glycated hemoglobin (HbA1c):** Reflects long-term glucose control and is used for monitoring diabetes mellitus.

Interpretations and Clinical Significance

- Fecal elastase-1 <200 µg/g indicates pancreatic exocrine insufficiency.
- Elevated serum amylase and lipase levels suggest acute pancreatitis.
- Impaired fasting glucose or impaired glucose tolerance indicates prediabetes.
- Fasting blood glucose >126 mg/dL or HbA1c ≥6.5% indicates diabetes mellitus.
- Abnormal OGTT results may indicate impaired glucose tolerance or diabetes.

Additional Tests for Pancreatic Function Evaluation

- **Secretin stimulation test:** Measures pancreatic secretions in response to secretin administration.

- **C-peptide and insulin levels:** Assess pancreatic beta cell function and insulin production.

Clinical Conditions Associated with Pancreatic Dysfunction

- **Acute and chronic pancreatitis:** Inflammation of the pancreas affecting exocrine and endocrine functions.
- **Diabetes mellitus:** Insufficient insulin production or impaired insulin function.
- **Cystic fibrosis:** Genetic disorder affecting exocrine pancreatic function.

Liver Function Tests (LFTs)

Provides valuable information about liver diseases, liver damage, and overall liver function.

Alanine Aminotransferase (ALT)

- ALT is an enzyme found primarily in liver cells.
- Increased ALT levels indicate liver cell damage or injury.
- Commonly used to diagnose and monitor liver diseases such as hepatitis.

Aspartate Aminotransferase (AST)

- AST is an enzyme found in the liver, heart, muscles, and other organs.
- Elevated AST levels indicate liver cell damage, but it is less specific to the liver than ALT.
- AST levels may also increase in conditions affecting the heart or muscles.

Alkaline Phosphatase (ALP)

- ALP is an enzyme found in the liver, bones, intestines, and other tissues.
- Elevated ALP levels suggest liver or bone disorders.
- Used to diagnose liver diseases such as hepatitis, cholestasis, and liver tumors.

Total Bilirubin

○ Bilirubin is a yellow pigment produced from the breakdown of red blood cells.
○ Elevated levels of total bilirubin indicate liver dysfunction, such as hepatitis or bile flow obstruction.

Gamma-glutamyl Transferase (GGT)

○ GGT is an enzyme found in the liver, bile ducts, and other tissues.
○ Elevated GGT levels suggest liver or biliary tract disorders, including alcohol abuse.

Albumin

○ Albumin is a protein produced by the liver.
○ Decreased albumin levels indicate liver dysfunction or malnutrition.

Total Protein

○ Total protein includes albumin and other proteins in the blood.
○ Abnormal total protein levels may indicate liver diseases, kidney diseases, or malnutrition.

Prothrombin Time (PT) and International Normalized Ratio (INR)

○ PT and INR measure the blood's ability to clot.
○ Prolonged PT and increased INR suggest impaired liver function.

Hepatitis Serology

○ Serological tests detect antibodies or antigens associated with different hepatitis viruses.
○ Useful in diagnosing and monitoring viral hepatitis infections.

Imaging Studies

Imaging techniques like ultrasound, CT scan, or MRI can provide additional information about liver structure and function.

Renal Function Tests

Renal function tests are laboratory tests used to assess the functioning of the kidneys and detect any abnormalities in kidney function.

Blood Urea Nitrogen (BUN)

○ BUN measures the amount of urea nitrogen in the blood.
○ Urea is a waste product formed in the liver from the breakdown of proteins.
○ Elevated BUN levels indicate impaired kidney function or dehydration.

Serum Creatinine

○ Serum creatinine measures the level of creatinine in the blood.
○ Creatinine is a waste product produced by muscle metabolism.
○ Increased serum creatinine levels indicate impaired kidney function.

Glomerular Filtration Rate (GFR)

○ GFR is a calculated value that estimates the rate at which blood is filtered by the kidneys.
○ It is considered the best indicator of overall kidney function.
○ A decrease in GFR suggests impaired kidney function.

Urinalysis

○ Urinalysis is a routine test that evaluates the physical, chemical, and microscopic properties of urine.
○ It helps detect urinary tract infections, kidney stones, and other kidney disorders.
○ Parameters assessed include color, pH, specific gravity, presence of protein, glucose, blood cells, and bacteria.

Urine Albumin

○ Urine albumin measures the amount of albumin, a protein, in the urine.

○ Increased levels of urine albumin indicate kidney damage or dysfunction.

○ It is a sensitive marker for early detection of kidney disease.

Urine Creatinine Clearance

○ Creatinine clearance measures the amount of creatinine cleared from the blood by the kidneys.

○ It provides an estimate of the GFR and helps assess kidney function.

○ The test requires a 24-hour urine collection along with a blood sample.

Electrolyte Levels

○ Electrolyte levels, such as sodium, potassium, and bicarbonate, are measured in blood.

○ Imbalances in electrolyte levels can indicate kidney dysfunction.

○ Electrolyte levels help assess acid–base balance and overall renal function.

Renal Imaging

○ Renal imaging techniques: Ultrasound, CT scan, or MRI, provide detailed images (structure and anatomy) of the kidneys.

○ Useful for identifying kidney stones, tumors, or structural abnormalities.

Estimation of Serum Calcium

Estimation of serum calcium is an important diagnostic test that provides valuable information about the body's calcium balance and helps in the evaluation of various medical conditions.

Principle of Serum Calcium Estimation

Serum calcium estimation is based on the principle of complex formation between calcium ions and specific chelating agents.

The most common method used is the colorimetric method, where the intensity of color developed is proportional to the concentration of calcium ions in the serum sample.

Methods of Serum Calcium Estimation

○ **O-cresolphthalein complexone (OCPC) method:** This method uses OCPC as a chelating agent that forms a complex with calcium ions. The complex formed exhibits a color change, which can be measured spectrophotometrically at a specific wavelength. The absorbance of the colored complex is proportional to the calcium concentration in the sample.

○ **Arsenazo III method:** Arsenazo III is a chelating agent that forms a colored complex with calcium ions. The complex absorbs light at a specific wavelength, and the absorbance is measured to determine the calcium concentration. This method is widely used for its accuracy and sensitivity.

○ **Ion-selective electrode (ISE) method:** This method utilizes a calcium ion-selective electrode that generates an electrical potential proportional to the concentration of calcium ions in the sample. The potential is measured and converted into calcium concentration using a calibration curve. ISE methods offer rapid results and high precision.

Factors Affecting Serum Calcium Levels

○ Serum calcium levels are influenced by various factors, including hormonal regulation, dietary intake, vitamin D metabolism, and certain medical conditions.

○ Abnormalities in these factors can lead to hypo- or hypercalcemia, which may require further investigation and management.

Estimation of Serum Phosphorus

Serum phosphorus is an essential electrolyte and important for assessing mineral metabolism and diagnosing and monitoring certain medical conditions.

Principle of Serum Phosphorus Estimation

○ The estimation of serum phosphorus is based on the principle of colorimetry.
○ Phosphorus reacts with ammonium molybdate under acidic conditions to form a yellow phosphomolybdate complex.
○ The intensity of the color formed is directly proportional to the concentration of phosphorus in the sample.

Sample Collection and Handling

It is important to handle the sample carefully to avoid hemolysis, as it can release intracellular phosphorus and affect the accuracy of the results.

Methods for Serum Phosphorus Estimation

○ **Spectrophotometric method**: The most commonly used method for serum phosphorus estimation is the spectrophotometric method. It involves the use of a spectrophotometer to measure the absorbance of the colored complex formed between phosphorus and ammonium molybdate.
○ **Enzymatic method:** This method utilizes enzymes that selectively hydrolyze organic phosphates, releasing inorganic phosphate, which can then be measured using a colorimetric assay.
○ **Ion-selective electrode method:** This method utilizes an ion-selective electrode that directly measures the concentration of phosphate ions in the sample.

Interference and Precautions

○ Hemolysis can lead to falsely elevated serum phosphorus levels due to the release of intracellular phosphorus from red blood cells.
○ Lipemia and bilirubinemia can interfere with the colorimetric reaction and cause inaccurate results. Lipid and bilirubin removal methods may be required in such cases.
○ Proper calibration and quality control measures should be followed to ensure accurate and reliable results.

Reference Range and Clinical Significance

○ The reference range for serum phosphorus levels in adults: 2.5–4.5 mg/dL.
○ Abnormal serum phosphorus levels can be indicative of various medical conditions, such as renal disorders, metabolic bone diseases, hormonal imbalances, and nutritional deficiencies.

Estimation of Serum Electrolytes

The measurement of serum electrolytes, such as sodium (Na^+), potassium (K^+), and chloride (Cl^-), is crucial in diagnosing and monitoring electrolyte imbalances and related disorders.

Sodium Estimation

○ **Principle:** Sodium ions are measured using ion-selective electrodes (ISE) based on the Nernst equation.
○ **Methods:** Flame photometry, ion-selective electrode (ISE) methods, and indirect colorimetric methods can be used.
○ Flame photometry measures the emission of light by excited sodium atoms in a flame.
○ ISE methods use a specific electrode that selectively responds to sodium ions.
○ Indirect colorimetric methods involve the reaction of sodium ions with specific reagents, producing a color change that can be measured.

Potassium Estimation

○ **Principle:** Potassium ions are measured using ISE methods based on the Nernst equation.
○ **Methods:** Flame photometry, ISE methods, and indirect colorimetric methods are commonly employed.
○ Flame photometry measures the emission of light by excited potassium atoms in a flame.

- ISE methods use a specific electrode that selectively responds to potassium ions.
- Indirect colorimetric methods involve the reaction of potassium ions with specific reagents, producing a color change that can be measured.

Chloride Estimation

- **Principle:** Chloride ions are measured using ion-selective electrodes (ISE) based on the Nernst equation.
- **Methods:** ISE methods and indirect colorimetric methods are commonly used.
- ISE methods use a specific electrode that selectively responds to chloride ions.
- Indirect colorimetric methods involve the reaction of chloride ions with specific reagents, producing a color change that can be measured.

Quality Control and Interpretation

- Quality control measures, including calibration, use of controls, and adherence to standard operating procedures, are essential to ensure accurate and reliable results.
- Results are interpreted in comparison to reference ranges and in conjunction with clinical signs and symptoms.
- Abnormalities in sodium, potassium, or chloride levels may indicate electrolyte imbalances, dehydration, kidney disorders, or other medical conditions.

Reference Ranges and Clinical Interpretation

Serum Sodium (Na+)

- **Reference range:** 135–145 mmol/L
- Clinical Interpretation
  - **Hyponatremia (low sodium levels)**
    - ➤ **Causes:** Drinking too much water, kidney disorders, adrenal insufficiency, or certain medications. Symptoms may include weakness, confusion, seizures, and nausea.

- **Hypernatremia (high sodium levels)**
  - ➤ **Causes:** Excessive sodium intake, dehydration, diabetes insipidus, or certain medications. Symptoms may include excessive thirst, dry mouth, restlessness, and confusion.

Serum Potassium (K+)

- **Reference range:** 3.5–5.0 mmol/L
- **Clinical interpretation**
  - **Hypokalemia (low potassium levels)**
    - ➤ **Causes:** Excessive potassium loss (e.g., diarrhea, vomiting), kidney disorders, certain medications, or inadequate dietary intake. Symptoms may include muscle weakness, fatigue, irregular heartbeat, and constipation.
  - **Hyperkalemia (high potassium levels)**
    - ➤ **Causes:** Kidney dysfunction, certain medications, trauma, or excessive potassium intake. Symptoms may include muscle weakness, palpitations, numbness, and tingling sensations.

Serum Chloride (Cl−)

- **Reference range:** 98–107 mmol/L
- **Clinical interpretation:**
  - Hypochloremia (low chloride levels)
    - ➤ **Causes:** Excessive sweating, vomiting, kidney disorders, or certain medications. Symptoms may include muscle cramps, weakness, metabolic alkalosis, and fluid imbalances.
  - **Hyperchloremia (high chloride levels)**
    - ➤ **Causes:** Dehydration, kidney dysfunction, metabolic acidosis, or certain medications. Symptoms may include excessive thirst, lethargy, increased blood pressure, and edema.

Proteinuria and Microalbuminuria

Proteinuria and microalbuminuria are important indicators of kidney function and can be detected through laboratory analysis.

Principles of Proteinuria and Microalbuminuria

Proteinuria refers to the presence of excess protein in the urine, indicating potential kidney dysfunction.

Microalbuminuria is the detection of small amounts of albumin in the urine and is considered an early marker of kidney damage.

Methods for Proteinuria and Microalbuminuria Detection

Proteinuria can be detected using qualitative and quantitative methods:

○ **Qualitative methods:** Dipstick tests that detect protein using chemical reagents.

○ **Quantitative methods:** Measurement of protein concentration in urine using laboratory techniques, such as the Bradford assay or immunoturbidimetry.

Microalbuminuria can be assessed through albumin-to-creatinine ratio (ACR) or albumin excretion rate (AER) measurements.

○ **ACR:** The ratio of albumin to creatinine in a random urine sample.

○ **AER:** Measurement of the total amount of albumin excreted in a 24-hour urine collection.

Reference Range

The reference range for proteinuria varies depending on the method used for analysis.

In a healthy individual, the normal range for proteinuria is typically <150 mg/24 hours or <20 mg/dL.

For microalbuminuria, the ACR reference range is 30–300 mg/g or 3–30 mg/mmol in a random urine sample.

Significance of Proteinuria and Microalbuminuria

Persistent proteinuria or increased levels of microalbuminuria can indicate kidney damage or dysfunction.

Proteinuria may be associated with various conditions, including renal diseases, hypertension, diabetes mellitus, and urinary tract infections.

Microalbuminuria is often an early sign of diabetic nephropathy, a complication of diabetes leading to kidney damage.

Renal Clearance Tests

Renal clearance tests are important diagnostic tools used to assess kidney function.

Principles of Renal Clearance Tests

○ Renal clearance refers to the volume of plasma from which a substance is completely removed by the kidneys per unit of time.

○ Clearance tests involve measuring the clearance of specific substances to assess kidney function.

○ The principle is based on the fact that the clearance of a substance depends on its filtration, reabsorption, and secretion by the kidneys.

Methods of Renal Clearance Tests

○ Commonly used substances for renal clearance tests include creatinine, inulin, and radioactive markers.

○ Clearance is calculated using the formula: Clearance = (urine concentration × urine flow rate)/plasma concentration.

○ The urine and blood samples are collected, and the concentrations of the substance of interest are measured.

○ Urine flow rate is determined by measuring the volume of urine over a specific period.

Interpretation of Renal Clearance Tests

○ Renal clearance tests provide an estimation of glomerular filtration rate (GFR), which is a measure of kidney function.

○ GFR reflects the rate at which the kidneys filter blood to remove waste products and excess substances.

○ Reduced clearance values indicate decreased kidney function, while normal or increased values suggest normal or hyperfiltration, respectively.

Reference Ranges for Renal Clearance Tests

○ The normal reference range for GFR varies depending on age, sex, and body size.
○ In adults, the normal GFR is typically around 90–120 mL/min/1.73m^2.
○ Reference ranges may differ slightly between laboratories due to variations in measurement methods.

Urea Clearance Test

○ Urea is a waste product resulting from protein metabolism.
○ Urea clearance tests are used to evaluate kidney function and assess the urea nitrogen excretion rate.
○ The principle and methods of urea clearance tests are similar to other renal clearance tests.
○ The reference range for urea clearance varies, but a GFR of 70–120 mL/min is considered normal.

Uric Acid Estimation

Uric acid is a metabolic waste product formed from the breakdown of purines in the body. Elevated levels of uric acid can lead to conditions such as gout and kidney stones.

Principle of Uric Acid Estimation

○ Uric acid estimation is based on the enzymatic method, which involves the oxidation of uric acid by the enzyme uricase.
○ Uricase catalyzes the reaction of uric acid with oxygen, forming allantoin and hydrogen peroxide.
○ The hydrogen peroxide produced in the reaction is measured spectrophotometrically.

Methods of Uric Acid Estimation

Colorimetric Method

○ In this method, a colorimetric reaction is used to measure the concentration of uric acid.

○ Uric acid reacts with specific reagents, producing a colored compound that can be measured using a spectrophotometer.

Enzymatic Method

○ This method utilizes the enzyme uricase to specifically catalyze the reaction of uric acid.
○ The reaction produces a product that can be quantified using spectrophotometric techniques.

Clinical Significance

○ Uric acid estimation is commonly used to diagnose and monitor conditions such as gout, kidney stones, and certain types of kidney disease.
○ High levels of uric acid in the blood (hyperuricemia) can indicate increased production or decreased excretion of uric acid, leading to various health issues.
○ Low levels of uric acid can be observed in conditions such as Wilson's disease or during treatment with certain medications.

Factors Affecting Uric Acid Levels

Diet: Consumption of purine-rich foods like organ meats, seafood, and alcohol can increase uric acid levels.

Medications: Certain medications like diuretics and aspirin can influence uric acid levels.

Medical conditions: Conditions such as obesity, hypertension, and metabolic syndrome can affect uric acid metabolism.

Arterial Blood Gas (ABG) Testing

Arterial blood sample collection and arterial blood gas (ABG) testing are crucial procedures performed in clinical settings to assess the oxygenation, acid–base balance, and ventilation status of patients. This chapter provides an overview of arterial blood sample collection techniques, the components of an ABG test, and the interpretation of ABG results.

Arterial Blood Sample Collection

- Arterial blood samples are collected directly from an artery, typically the radial artery in the wrist or the femoral artery in the groin.
- The procedure requires aseptic technique and specialized arterial blood gas syringes.
- The sample collection site is cleaned, and a local anesthetic may be used to minimize discomfort.
- The blood sample is collected using a syringe with heparin to prevent clotting.
- After collection, the sample is immediately placed on ice and transported to the laboratory for analysis.

Components of an ABG Test

- An ABG test measures several parameters, including:
  - **pH:** Measures the acidity or alkalinity of blood.
  - **Partial pressure of oxygen (PaO_2):** Reflects the amount of oxygen dissolved in arterial blood.
  - **Partial pressure of carbon dioxide ($PaCO_2$):** Reflects the amount of carbon dioxide dissolved in arterial blood.
  - **Bicarbonate (HCO_3^-):** Reflects the metabolic component of acid–base balance.
  - **Oxygen saturation (SaO_2):** Measures the percentage of hemoglobin saturated with oxygen.

Interpretation of ABG Results

- ABG results are interpreted in conjunction with the patient's clinical condition and other laboratory findings.
- The pH value indicates the acid–base balance. A pH below 7.35 indicates acidosis, while a pH above 7.45 indicates alkalosis.
- PaO_2 reflects oxygenation status, and low levels may indicate respiratory or circulatory impairment.
- $PaCO_2$ reflects ventilation status. High levels suggest respiratory acidosis, while low levels suggest respiratory alkalosis.
- HCO_3^- reflects metabolic acid–base balance. High levels indicate metabolic alkalosis, while low levels indicate metabolic acidosis.
- SaO_2 provides information about the efficiency of oxygen delivery to tissues.

Thyroid Function Test

Thyroid function tests are important diagnostic tools used to assess the functioning of the thyroid gland.

Thyroid Hormones

- The thyroid gland produces two primary hormones: triiodothyronine (T3) and thyroxine (T4).
- T3 and T4 play crucial roles in regulating metabolism, growth, and development.

Thyroid-stimulating Hormone (TSH)

- TSH, also known as thyrotropin, is produced by the pituitary gland.
- TSH stimulates the thyroid gland to release T3 and T4.
- TSH levels are inversely proportional to T3 and T4 levels in the blood.

Principles of Thyroid Function Tests

- Thyroid function tests measure the levels of TSH, T3, and T4 in the blood to evaluate thyroid function.
- These tests help diagnose thyroid disorders, monitor treatment effectiveness, and assess thyroid hormone balance.

Methods of Thyroid Function Testing

- **Radioimmunoassay (RIA):** It involves the use of radioactive isotopes to detect and quantify hormone levels. RIA is highly sensitive and specific.

○ **Enzyme linked immunosorbent assay (ELISA):** It uses enzyme-labeled antibodies to measure hormone levels. ELISA is widely used due to its simplicity and cost-effectiveness.

○ **Chemiluminescent immunoassay (CLIA):** It utilizes light-emitting reactions to measure hormone levels. CLIA offers high sensitivity and a wide dynamic range.

○ **Immunofluorescence assay (IFA):** It uses fluorescent-labeled antibodies to detect hormone levels. IFA provides rapid results and is suitable for small sample sizes.

Thyroid Function Test Panels

○ Thyroid function tests are commonly performed together to provide a comprehensive assessment of thyroid function.

○ Panels may include TSH, T3, T4, free T3 (FT3), free T4 (FT4), and thyroid autoantibodies.

Reference Ranges

○ Reference ranges for thyroid function tests may vary slightly among laboratories.

○ Normal reference ranges for TSH, T3, and T4 depend on factors such as age, sex, and pregnancy status.

Interpretation of Results

○ Abnormal results can indicate thyroid dysfunction:

   ○ **Hypothyroidism:** Elevated TSH and reduced T3 and T4 levels.

   ○ **Hyperthyroidism:** Reduced TSH and elevated T3 and T4 levels.

   ○ **Thyroid autoimmunity:** Presence of thyroid autoantibodies.

VITAMINS

Vitamins are essential organic compounds required in small amounts for the proper functioning of the body.

Classification of Vitamins

○ **Vitamins are classified into two categories:** Fat-soluble vitamins and water-soluble vitamins.

○ Fat-soluble vitamins include vitamins A, D, E and K, stored in the body's fat tissues.

○ Water-soluble vitamins include vitamin C and the B-complex vitamins (B_1, B_2, B_3, B_5, B_6, B_7, B_9, and B_{12}), which are not stored in large amounts and are eliminated through urine.

Types of Vitamins

○ Vitamin A (retinol) is essential for vision, immune function, and cell growth.

○ Vitamin D (calciferol) is important for bone health and calcium absorption.

○ Vitamin E (tocopherol) acts as an antioxidant, protecting cells from damage.

○ Vitamin K (phylloquinone) plays a role in blood clotting.

○ Vitamin C (ascorbic acid) is involved in collagen synthesis and acts as an antioxidant.

○ B-complex vitamins have various functions, including energy production, nerve function, and red blood cell formation.

Deficiency and Toxicity Disorders

○ Deficiency disorders result from insufficient vitamin intake or poor absorption.

○ Vitamin deficiencies can lead to conditions such as night blindness (vitamin A deficiency), rickets (vitamin D deficiency), scurvy (vitamin C deficiency), and beriberi (vitamin B_1 deficiency).

○ Toxicity disorders occur when excessive amounts of vitamins are consumed.

○ Vitamin toxicity can lead to symptoms such as nausea, diarrhea, and, in severe cases, organ damage.

Principles and Methods of Analysis

○ Various methods are used to analyze vitamin levels, including spectrophotometry, high-performance liquid chromatography (HPLC), and immunoassays.

MULTIPLE CHOICE QUESTIONS

1. **Which type of carbohydrate cannot be further hydrolyzed?**
   a. Monosaccharides
   b. Disaccharides
   c. Polysaccharides
   d. None of the above

2. **Which of the following is an example of a monosaccharide?**
   a. Sucrose
   b. Lactose
   c. Glucose
   d. Maltose

3. **What is the main function of polysaccharides?**
   a. Providing immediate energy
   b. Serving as building blocks for other carbohydrates
   c. Regulating blood sugar levels
   d. Serving as storage forms of glucose

4. **Disaccharides require specific enzymes to break them down into:**
   a. Monosaccharides
   b. Polysaccharides
   c. Lipids
   d. Proteins

5. **Which type of carbohydrate is commonly found in plants and animals as a storage form of glucose?**
   a. Monosaccharides
   b. Disaccharides
   c. Starch
   d. Glycogen

6. **Carbohydrates are a major source of energy for the body. True or False?**

7. **Carbohydrate analysis is performed in which laboratory discipline?**
   a. Hematology
   b. Microbiology
   c. Clinical biochemistry
   d. Histopathology

8. **Which carbohydrate is commonly found in fruits, vegetables, grains, and legumes?**
   a. Monosaccharides
   b. Disaccharides
   c. Polysaccharides
   d. All of the above

9. **Carbohydrates can be involved in the pathogenesis of which condition?**
   a. Cardiovascular diseases
   b. Respiratory infections
   c. Metabolic disorders
   d. Bone fractures

10. **What type of carbohydrate is commonly measured in glucose estimation tests?**
    a. Monosaccharides
    b. Disaccharides
    c. Polysaccharides
    d. None of the above

11. **Which property determines whether a carbohydrate is reducing or non-reducing?**
    a. Solubility
    b. Sweetness
    c. Molecular weight
    d. Presence of free aldehyde or ketone group

Answers:

1. a	2. c	3. d	4. a
5. d	6. True	7. c	8. c
9. c	10. a	11. d	

12. **Which type of isomerism is observed between glucose and fructose?**
    a. Structural isomerism
    b. Enantiomerism
    c. Diastereomerism
    d. None of the above

13. **Which carbohydrate is insoluble in water?**
    a. Glucose
    b. Sucrose
    c. Lactose
    d. Cellulose

14. **Which type of isomerism is observed between D-glucose and L-glucose?**
    a. Structural isomerism
    b. Enantiomerism
    c. Diastereomerism
    d. None of the above

15. **Which enzyme is responsible for the breakdown of starch into smaller glucose units?**
    a. Protease
    b. Lipase
    c. Amylase
    d. Sucrase

16. **Which carbohydrate is known as "blood sugar" and serves as a primary energy source for the body?**
    a. Fructose
    b. Glucose
    c. Galactose
    d. Maltose

17. **Which of the following carbohydrates is a nonreducing sugar?**
    a. Trihelos
    b. Lactose
    c. Maltose
    d. All of the above

18. **Which type of carbohydrate is commonly found in the exoskeleton of insects and crustaceans?**
    a. Starch
    b. Cellulose
    c. Chitin
    d. Glycogen

19. **Which property of carbohydrates allows them to form hydrogen bonds with water molecules?**
    a. Solubility
    b. Sweetness
    c. Reducing nature
    d. Stereochemistry

20. **Which carbohydrate is commonly used as an energy storage molecule in plants?**
    a. Glycogen
    b. Starch
    c. Cellulose
    d. Lactose

21. **Which type of isomerism is observed between glucose and mannose?**
    a. Structural isomerism
    b. Enantiomerism
    c. Diastereomerism
    d. Geometric isomerism

22. **Which carbohydrate is commonly used in the laboratory as a carbon and energy source for microbial growth?**
    a. Glucose
    b. Fructose
    c. Lactose
    d. Maltose

23. **Which carbohydrate is a component of nucleic acids, such as DNA and RNA?**
    a. Glucose
    b. Ribose
    c. Fructose
    d. Sucrose

24. **Which enzyme is responsible for the hydrolysis of lactose into glucose and galactose?**
    a. Lipase
    b. Protease
    c. Lactase
    d. Amylase

25. **Which type of carbohydrate is commonly found in honey?**
    a. Glucose
    b. Fructose
    c. Maltose
    d. Sucrose

Answers:

12. a	13. d	14. b	15. c
16. b	17. a	18. c	19. a
20. b	21. c	22. a	23. b
24. c	25. b		

26. **Which carbohydrate is used as an intravenous source of energy for patients in the hospital?**
    a. Glucose
    b. Fructose
    c. Maltose
    d. Lactose

27. **Which carbohydrate is commonly used as a thickening agent in food products?**
    a. Starch
    b. Glycogen
    c. Cellulose
    d. Chitin

28. **Which type of isomerism is observed between glucose and galactose?**
    a. Structural isomerism
    b. Enantiomerism
    c. Diastereomerism
    d. Geometric isomerism

29. **Which carbohydrate is the main component of dietary fiber and aids in digestion and bowel movements?**
    a. Starch
    b. Glycogen
    c. Cellulose
    d. Chitin

30. **Which carbohydrate is commonly used as energy source in sports drinks and energy gels?**
    a. Glucose
    b. Fructose
    c. Lactose
    d. Sucrose

31. **Which property of carbohydrates allows them to form complex three-dimensional structures?**
    a. Solubility
    b. Sweetness
    c. Reducing nature
    d. Stereochemistry

32. **Which carbohydrate is commonly used in the intravenous infusion for the patients of dehydration?**
    a. Glucose
    b. Fructose
    c. Lactose
    d. Maltose

33. **A glycosidic bond is a type of bond that forms between:**
    a. Two amino acids
    b. Two monosaccharides
    c. Two nucleotides
    d. Fatty acids and glycerol

34. **Glycosidic bonds are formed through a condensation reaction, resulting in the elimination of:**
    a. Water
    b. Carbon dioxide
    c. Oxygen
    d. Hydrogen

35. **Sucrose is formed by the glycosidic bond between:**
    a. Glucose and fructose
    b. Glucose and galactose
    c. Glucose and glucose
    d. Fructose and fructose

36. **Lactose is an example of a disaccharide formed by the glycosidic bond between:**
    a. Glucose and fructose
    b. Glucose and galactose
    c. Glucose and glucose
    d. Fructose and fructose

37. **Which of the following is a polysaccharide formed by glycosidic bonds?**
    a. Maltose
    b. Sucrose
    c. Cellulose
    d. Lactose

38. **The glycosidic bond in cellulose is primarily composed of:**
    a. α-1,4-glycosidic bond
    b. β-1,4-glycosidic bond
    c. α-1,6-glycosidic bond
    d. β-1,6-glycosidic bond

Answers:

26. a	27. a	28. c	29. c
30. a	31. d	32. a	33. b
34. a	35. a	36. b	37. c
38. b			

39. Which of the following is an example of a glycosidic bond in a disaccharide?
a. Peptide bond in lactose
b. Ester bond in maltose
c. Glycosidic bond in sucrose
d. Phosphodiester bond in cellulose

40. The glycosidic bond in maltose is formed by the linkage between:
a. Two glucose molecules
b. Glucose and galactose
c. Glucose and fructose
d. Glucose and mannose

41. Which polysaccharide serves as the primary energy storage form in plants?
a. Starch   b. Glycogen
c. Cellulose   d. Chitin

42. Glycosidic bond in sucrose is:
a. α-1,4-glycosidic bonds
b. β-1,4-glycosidic bonds
c. α-1,β-2-glycosidic bonds
d. β-1,6-glycosidic bonds

43. Which of the following is a structural polysaccharide?
a. Starch   b. Glycogen
c. Cellulose   d. Heparin

44. Chitin is primarily found in:
a. Plant cell walls
b. Animal exoskeletons
c. Bacterial cell walls
d. Fungal cell walls

45. Heparin is known for its:
a. Role in energy storage
b. Structural support function
c. Anticoagulant properties
d. Role in cell signaling

46. Which metabolic pathway breaks down glucose into pyruvate?
a. Glycolysis
b. Gluconeogenesis
c. Citric acid cycle
d. Pentose phosphate pathway

47. Which vitamin is essential for the conversion of pyruvate to acetyl-CoA?
a. Vitamin B_1 (thiamine)
b. Vitamin B_2 (riboflavin)
c. Vitamin B_3 (niacin)
d. Vitamin B_5 (pantothenic acid)

48. The conversion of pyruvate to lactate occurs during:
a. Glycolysis
b. Gluconeogenesis
c. Citric acid cycle
d. Pentose phosphate pathway

49. The primary function of the citric acid cycle is to:
a. Generate NADH and $FADH_2$
b. Produce ATP directly
c. Convert pyruvate to glucose
d. Synthesize glycogen

50. Which enzyme is responsible for the conversion of glucose-6-phosphate to fructose-6-phosphate?
a. Glucose-6-phosphatase
b. Hexokinase
c. Phosphofructokinase-1
d. Pyruvate kinase

51. In which cellular compartment does the citric acid cycle occur?
a. Nucleus
b. Mitochondria
c. Cytoplasm
d. Endoplasmic reticulum

Answers: 39. c   40. a   41. a   42. c
43. c   44. b   45. c   46. a
47. a   48. a   49. a   50. c
51. b

52. The major end product of glycolysis is:
a. Acetyl-CoA
b. Lactate
c. Pyruvate
d. Oxaloacetate

53. Which metabolic pathway is responsible for the synthesis of glucose from noncarbohydrate precursors?
a. Glycolysis
b. Gluconeogenesis
c. Citric acid cycle
d. Pentose phosphate pathway

54. How many ATP molecules are produced directly from one molecule of glucose during glycolysis?
a. 1 ATP
b. 2 ATP
c. 4 ATP
d. 8 ATP

55. The enzyme hexokinase is inhibited by:
a. Fructose-6-phosphate
b. ATP
c. Glucose-6-phosphate
d. Pyruvate

56. The key regulatory enzyme of the citric acid cycle is:
a. Citrate synthase
b. Isocitrate dehydrogenase
c. Succinyl-CoA synthetase
d. Malate dehydrogenase

57. Which metabolic pathway is involved in the production of NADPH?
a. Glycolysis
b. Gluconeogenesis
c. Pentose phosphate pathway
d. Citric acid cycle

58. Which of the following vitamins is required for the synthesis of coenzyme A?
a. Vitamin B_1 (thiamine)
b. Vitamin B_2 (riboflavin)
c. Vitamin B_5 (pantothenic acid)
d. Vitamin B_6 (pyridoxine)

59. The net ATP yield from the complete oxidation of one molecule of glucose is approximately:
a. 2 ATP
b. 4 ATP
c. 30-32 ATP
d. 38 ATP

60. Which enzyme is responsible for the rate-limiting step of glycolysis?
a. Glucose-6-phosphatase
b. Hexokinase
c. Phosphofructokinase-1
d. Pyruvate kinase

61. The primary role of the pentose phosphate pathway is to:
a. Generate ATP directly
b. Produce glucose from pyruvate
c. Produce NADPH and pentose sugars
d. Convert glucose-6-phosphate to fructose-6-phosphate

62. The enzyme responsible for converting glucose-6-phosphate to ribose-5-phosphate in the Pentose pentose phosphate pathway is:
a. Glucose-6-phosphatase
b. Hexokinase
c. Transketolase
d. Transaldolase

Answers:	52. c	53. b	54. b	55. c
	56. b	57. c	58. c	59. c
	60. c	61. c	62. c	

63. **Which metabolic pathway primarily occurs in the liver and kidneys?**
    a. Glycolysis
    b. Gluconeogenesis
    c. Citric acid cycle
    d. Pentose phosphate pathway

64. **Which molecule acts as an allosteric activator of phosphofructokinase-1 in glycolysis?**
    a. ATP
    b. ADP
    c. Fructose-6-phosphate
    d. Pyruvate

65. **The conversion of glucose-6-phosphate to glucose during gluconeogenesis occurs primarily in which organ?**
    a. Liver
    b. Pancreas
    c. Kidneys
    d. Adrenal glands

66. **The tricarboxylic acid (TCA) cycle is also known as:**
    a. Glycolysis
    b. Krebs cycle
    c. Calvin cycle
    d. Pentose phosphate pathway

67. **Where does the TCA cycle occur in eukaryotic cells?**
    a. Cytoplasm
    b. Mitochondria
    c. Nucleus
    d. Endoplasmic reticulum

68. **The TCA cycle is a series of enzymatic reactions that occur in:**
    a. Cytosol
    b. Ribosomes
    c. Mitochondrial matrix
    d. Golgi apparatus

69. **Which molecule enters the TCA cycle to initiate the cycle?**
    a. Acetyl-CoA
    b. Glucose
    c. Pyruvate
    d. ATP

70. **The TCA cycle produces which of the following as a byproduct?**
    a. Carbon dioxide (CO_2)
    b. Oxygen (O_2)
    c. Water (H_2O)
    d. Glucose

71. **How many rounds of the TCA cycle are required to completely oxidize one molecule of glucose?**
    a. 1
    b. 2
    c. 3
    d. 4

72. **The TCA cycle generates energy in the form of:**
    a. NADH
    b. $FADH_2$
    c. ATP
    d. All of the above

73. **Which of the following enzymes is NOT involved in the TCA cycle?**
    a. Citrate synthase
    b. Isocitrate dehydrogenase
    c. Pyruvate kinase
    d. Malate dehydrogenase

74. **How many ATP molecules are directly produced through substrate-level phosphorylation during one round of the TCA cycle?**
    a. 1
    b. 2
    c. 3
    d. 4

75. **The end products of the TCA cycle are:**
    a. Glucose and ATP
    b. Pyruvate and NADH
    c. Carbon dioxide, NADH, and ATP
    d. Lactic acid and FAD

Answers:
63. a	64. b	65. a	66. b
67. b	68. c	69. a	70. a
71. d	72. d	73. c	74. a
75. c			

76. Glycolysis is the metabolic pathway that converts glucose into:
a. Pyruvate
b. Acetyl-CoA
c. Fructose-1,6-bisphosphate
d. Lactate

77. How many molecules of ATP are consumed during the energy investment phase of glycolysis?
a. 1 ATP
b. 2 ATP
c. 3 ATP
d. 4 ATP

78. The end product of glycolysis under anaerobic conditions is:
a. Acetyl-CoA
b. Pyruvate
c. Lactate
d. Fructose-1,6-bisphosphate

79. During glycolysis, glucose is initially converted to:
a. Fructose-6-phosphate
b. Glucose-6-phosphate
c. 3-phosphoglycerate
d. 2-phosphoglycerate

80. Which enzyme is responsible for the conversion of fructose-1,6-bisphosphate to glyceraldehyde-3-phosphate?
a. Aldolase
b. Phosphofructokinase-1
c. Hexokinase
d. Pyruvate kinase

81. Which of the following statements is true regarding glycogenesis?
a. It is the breakdown of glycogen into glucose molecules.
b. It occurs primarily in the liver.
c. It requires the enzyme glucose-6-phosphatase.
d. It is an energy-releasing process.

82. Glycogen is primarily stored in which two tissues?
a. Liver and muscles
b. Kidneys and brain
c. Adipose tissue and pancreas
d. Heart and lungs

83. The process of glycogenolysis involves:
a. Conversion of glucose to glycogen.
b. Formation of glucose from non-carbohydrate sources.
c. Breakdown of glycogen into glucose molecules.
d. Conversion of glucose to pyruvate.

84. Which enzyme is responsible for glycogenolysis?
a. Glucose-6-phosphatase
b. Glycogen synthase
c. Glycogen phosphorylase
d. Phosphofructokinase

85. Glycogen phosphorylase catalyzes the removal of glucose units from glycogen by:
a. Phosphorylation
b. Hydrolysis
c. Dehydration synthesis
d. Oxidation

86. Which hormone stimulates glycogenolysis?
a. Insulin
b. Glucagon
c. Estrogen
d. Thyroxine

87. During glycogenesis, glucose molecules are added to glycogen chains by the enzyme:
a. Glucose-6-phosphatase
b. Glycogen synthase
c. Glycogen phosphorylase
d. Phosphofructokinase

Answers:

76. a	**77.** b	**78.** c	**79.** b
80. a	**81.** b	**82.** a	**83.** c
84. c	**85.** a	**86.** b	**87.** b

88. Which of the following is an end product of glycogenolysis?
a. Pyruvate b. Glucose
c. Acetyl-CoA d. Fructose

89. Glycogenolysis is stimulated during:
a. Fasting state
b. Postprandial state
c. Resting state
d. Exercise

90. The conversion of glucose-6-phosphate to glucose is essential for which organ?
a. Liver
b. Kidney
c. Pancreas
d. Adrenal gland

91. The pentose phosphate pathway (PPP) is an alternative metabolic pathway to:
a. Glycolysis
b. Krebs cycle
c. Gluconeogenesis
d. Electron transport chain

92. The primary function of the PPP is to:
a. Generate ATP for energy production
b. Produce NADH for oxidative phosphorylation
c. Generate NADPH for biosynthetic reactions and defense against oxidative stress
d. Convert pyruvate to lactate

93. Which enzyme is responsible for the first committed step of the PPP?
a. Glucose-6-phosphatase
b. Glucose-6-phosphate dehydrogenase (G6PD)
c. Phosphofructokinase-1
d. Pyruvate dehydrogenase

94. The PPP generates which important molecule for nucleotide synthesis?
a. Glucose-6-phosphate
b. Fructose-6-phosphate
c. Ribose-5-phosphate
d. Glyceraldehyde-3-phosphate

95. The PPP is especially active in tissues with high biosynthetic demands, such as:
a. Muscle tissue
b. Adipose tissue
c. Liver tissue
d. Cardiac tissue

96. The PPP is an important source of:
a. ATP b. NADH
c. NADPH d. Pyruvate

97. Which of the following is a product of the oxidative phase of the PPP?
a. Ribulose-5-phosphate
b. Glucose-6-phosphate
c. Sedoheptulose-7-phosphate
d. Xylulose-5-phosphate

98. The PPP generates reducing power in the form of:
a. NADH b. $FADH_2$
c. NADPH d. ATP

99. In which cellular compartment does the PPP occur?
a. Cytosol
b. Mitochondria
c. Endoplasmic reticulum
d. Golgi apparatus

100. The PPP is regulated by the ratio of:
a. ATP/ADP
b. $NADH/NAD^+$
c. $NADPH/NADP^+$
d. Glucose/fructose

Answers:

88. b	89. a	90. a	91. a
92. c	93. b	94. c	95. c
96. c	97. a	98. c	99. a
100. c			

101. Gluconeogenesis is the process of:
a. Breaking down glucose into pyruvate
b. Converting non carbohydrate sources into glucose
c. Synthesizing glycogen from glucose
d. Generating energy from glycolysis

102. The primary site of gluconeogenesis in the body is:
a. Liver
b. Pancreas
c. Adipose tissue
d. Kidneys

103. Which of the following is NOT a precursor for gluconeogenesis?
a. Lactate
b. Pyruvate
c. Amino acids
d. Fatty acids

104. The key enzyme involved in the rate-limiting step of gluconeogenesis is:
a. Hexokinase
b. Phosphofructokinase-1
c. Glucose-6-phosphatase
d. Pyruvate kinase

105. During gluconeogenesis, pyruvate is converted to:
a. Acetyl-CoA
b. Oxaloacetate
c. Succinyl-CoA
d. Malate

106. Which of the following hormones inhibits gluconeogenesis?
a. Insulin
b. Glucagon
c. Cortisol
d. Epinephrine

107. The primary source of carbon atoms for gluconeogenesis is derived from:
a. Fatty acids
b. Amino acids
c. Nucleotides
d. Ketone bodies

108. Gluconeogenesis is most active during:
a. Fasting state
b. Postprandial state
c. Exercise
d. Sleep

109. All enzymes are involved in gluconeogenesis, *except* one:
a. Phospho Enol Pyruvate Carboxy Kinase (PEPCK)
b. Fructose-1,6-bisphosphatase (FB-Pase)
c. Glucose-6-phosphatase (G6Pase)
d. Pyruvate kinase (PK)

110. Gluconeogenesis is an energetically:
a. Anabolic process
b. Catabolic process
c. Equally anabolic and catabolic
d. None of the above

111. Which of the following is NOT a characteristic feature of glycogen storage diseases (GSDs)?
a. Deficiency of enzymes involved in glycogen metabolism
b. Accumulation of glycogen in various tissues
c. Autosomal recessive inheritance pattern
d. Excessive breakdown of fatty acids

112. In GSD Type I (von Gierke's disease), the deficient enzyme is:
a. Glucose-6-phosphatase
b. Glucokinase
c. Branching enzyme
d. Phosphorylase kinase

113. Which of the following is a clinical manifestation of GSD Type II (Pompe disease)?
a. Hepatomegaly (enlarged liver)
b. Cardiomyopathy (heart muscle disease)
c. Muscle weakness and respiratory difficulties
d. All of the above

Answers:
101. b   102. a   103. d   104. c
105. b   106. a   107. b   108. a
109. d   110. a   111. d   112. a
113. d

114. **GSD Type III (Cori's disease) is characterized by a deficiency of which enzyme?**
    a. Amylo-1,6-glucosidase
    b. Phosphorylase kinase
    c. Debranching enzyme
    d. Lysosomal α-glucosidase

115. **Which of the following GSDs is associated with muscle cramps and myoglobinuria (dark urine)?**
    a. GSD Type IV (Andersen's disease)
    b. GSD Type V (McArdle's disease)
    c. GSD Type VI (Hers disease)
    d. GSD Type VII (Tarui disease)

116. **In the normal metabolic pathway of carbohydrate, the enzyme phosphoglucomutase converts glucose-1-phosphate to:**
    a. Fructose-1,6-bisphosphate
    b. Glucose-6-phosphate
    c. Glucose-1,6-bisphosphate
    d. Fructose-6-phosphate

117. **Which of the following enzymes is involved in the final step of glycolysis, converting phosphoenolpyruvate to pyruvate?**
    a. Aldolase
    b. Pyruvate kinase
    c. Phosphoglycerate kinase
    d. Hexokinase

118. **Fructose intolerance is a disorder characterized by the inability to metabolize fructose properly. Which enzyme is deficient in fructose intolerance?**
    a. Fructokinase
    b. Glucose-6-phosphatase
    c. Fructose-1-phosphate aldolase
    d. Aldolase B

119. **Fructose intolerance leads to the accumulation of which metabolite in the liver?**
    a. Glucose
    b. Galactose
    c. Fructose-6-phosphate
    d. Fructose-1-phosphate

120. **The deficiency of which enzyme in fructose intolerance disrupts the conversion of fructose-1-phosphate to glyceraldehyde and dihydroxyacetone phosphate?**
    a. Aldolase B
    b. Glucokinase
    c. Glucose-6-phosphatase
    d. Fructokinase

121. **Which of the following symptoms is commonly associated with fructose intolerance?**
    a. Hypoglycemia
    b. Hyperglycemia
    c. Hyperbilirubinemia
    d. Hypobetalipoproteinemia

122. **Fructose intolerance can be diagnosed by which of the following tests?**
    a. Glucose tolerance test
    b. Lactose intolerance test
    c. Fructose tolerance test
    d. Ketone bodies test

123. **Fructose is primarily metabolized in which organ?**
    a. Liver
    b. Pancreas
    c. Kidneys
    d. Small intestine

Answers: 114. c   115. b   116. b   117. b
118. d   119. d   120. a   121. a
122. c   123. a

124. Which of the following substances is an alternative energy source used to bypass the blocked fructose metabolism in fructose intolerance?
a. Galactose
b. Lactose
c. Sorbitol
d. Glucose

125. Fructose intolerance is an autosomal recessive genetic disorder. This means that:
a. Both parents must be affected for the child to have the disorder.
b. Only the mother needs to be affected for the child to have the disorder.
c. Only the father needs to be affected for the child to have the disorder.
d. It occurs randomly without inheritance.

126. Which of the following sweeteners should be avoided in individuals with fructose intolerance?
a. Sucrose
b. Stevia
c. Aspartame
d. Xylitol

127. Treatment for fructose intolerance includes:
a. Complete avoidance of fructose and sucrose.
b. Increasing dietary intake of fructose.
c. Taking high doses of fructose-1-phosphate.
d. Regular insulin injections.

128. Lactose intolerance is caused by the deficiency of which enzyme?
a. Lactase
b. Sucrase
c. Maltase
d. Amylase

129. What is the primary carbohydrate found in milk?
a. Glucose
b. Fructose
c. Sucrose
d. Lactose

130. Which metabolic pathway is impaired in individuals with lactose intolerance?
a. Glycolysis
b. Krebs cycle
c. Pentose phosphate pathway
d. Lactose metabolism

131. In lactose intolerance, undigested lactose in the gut is fermented by bacteria, leading to the production of:
a. Glucose
b. Fructose
c. Galactose
d. Lactic acid

132. Lactose intolerance is most commonly due to:
a. Genetic factors
b. Environmental factors
c. Poor diet
d. Infection

133. Which of the following symptoms is commonly associated with lactose intolerance?
a. Abdominal bloating
b. Diarrhea
c. Flatulence
d. All of the above

134. How is lactose intolerance typically diagnosed?
a. Lactose tolerance test
b. Blood glucose test
c. Stool analysis
d. Urine analysis

135. What is the treatment for lactose intolerance?
a. Avoiding lactose-containing foods
b. Enzyme replacement therapy
c. Dietary supplements
d. All of the above

Answers:

124. d	125. a	126. a	127. a
128. a	129. d	130. d	131. d
132. a	133. d	134. a	135. a

136. Which of the following dairy products is usually well-tolerated by individuals with lactose intolerance?
a. Milk
b. Cheese
c. Ice cream
d. Yogurt

137. Galactosemia is a metabolic disorder characterized by the inability to metabolize:
a. Glucose
b. Galactose
c. Fructose
d. Sucrose

138. In individuals with galactosemia, there is a deficiency of the enzyme:
a. Lactase
b. Glucokinase
c. Galactose-1-phosphate uridylyl-transferase
d. Hexokinase

139. Galactose-1-phosphate uridylyltransferase is responsible for converting galactose-1-phosphate to:
a. Galactose-6-phosphate
b. Galactose-1,6-bisphosphate
c. Glucose-6-phosphate
d. Glucose-1-phosphate

140. Accumulation of galactose-1-phosphate in galactosemia can lead to:
a. Liver dysfunction
b. Kidney dysfunction
c. Brain dysfunction
d. All of the above

141. The affected pathway in galactosemia is directly related to the metabolism of:
a. Starch
b. Glycogen
c. Lactose
d. Cellulose

142. Which of the following is a common symptom of galactosemia in infants?
a. Jaundice
b. Lethargy
c. Poor weight gain
d. All of the above

143. Galactosemia can be diagnosed by measuring the levels of:
a. Glucose in the blood
b. Galactose in the blood
c. Lactose in the urine
d. Fructose in the urine

144. The main treatment for galactosemia involves:
a. Galactose-restricted diet
b. High galactose intake
c. Vitamin supplementation
d. Enzyme replacement therapy

145. Galactosemia is an inherited genetic disorder that follows which pattern of inheritance?
a. Autosomal dominant
b. Autosomal recessive
c. X-linked dominant
d. X-linked recessive

146. Untreated galactosemia can lead to long-term complications, such as:
a. Mental retardation
b. Liver cirrhosis
c. Cataracts
d. All of the above

147. G-6PD deficiency is a disorder related to which metabolic pathway?
a. Glycolysis
b. Krebs cycle
c. Hexose monophosphate (HMP) pathway
d. Gluconeogenesis

Answers:	136. d	137. b	138. c	139. a
	140. d	141. c	142. d	143. b
	144. a	145. b	146. d	147. c

148. G-6PD deficiency primarily affects which component of the HMP pathway?
a. Glucose-6-phosphate dehydrogenase (G6PD) enzyme
b. Ribose-5-phosphate (R5P) production
c. NADPH generation
d. Erythrose-4-phosphate synthesis

149. Which of the following is a characteristic feature of G-6PD deficiency?
a. Enhanced red blood cell production
b. Increased resistance to oxidative stress
c. Impaired NADPH production
d. Accelerated glucose metabolism

150. The reduced production of NADPH in G-6PD deficiency leads to:
a. Enhanced cellular energy production
b. Increased susceptibility to oxidative damage
c. Accelerated glycolysis
d. Elevated levels of glycogen

151. Which of the following triggers can lead to hemolysis in individuals with G-6PD deficiency?
a. Vitamin B_{12} deficiency
b. Excessive carbohydrate intake
c. Exposure to certain drugs or infections
d. High-altitude environments

152. Which hormone is responsible for regulating blood glucose levels?
a. Insulin
b. Glucagon
c. Thyroxine
d. Estrogen

153. What is the normal fasting blood glucose range in milligrams per deciliter (mg/dL)?
a. 70–99 mg/dL
b. 100–125 mg/dL
c. 126–150 mg/dL
d. 150–200 mg/dL

154. Elevated blood glucose levels are indicative of which condition?
a. Hypoglycemia
b. Diabetes mellitus
c. Hyperthyroidism
d. Anemia

155. Which of the following is a diagnostic test for diabetes mellitus?
a. Blood urea nitrogen (BUN) test
b. Electrocardiogram (ECG)
c. Glucose tolerance test (GTT)
d. Complete blood count (CBC)

156. How many hours of fasting are required before performing a fasting blood glucose test?
a. 2 hours
b. 4 hours
c. 8 hours
d. 12 hours

157. A fasting blood glucose level of 140 mg/dL is indicative of:
a. Hypoglycemia
b. Normal blood glucose
c. Impaired fasting glucose
d. Diabetes mellitus

158. The oral glucose tolerance test (OGTT) is commonly used to diagnose:
a. Hypothyroidism
b. Hyperlipidemia
c. Gestational diabetes
d. Vitamin deficiency

Answers: 148. a   149. c   150. b   151. c

152. a   153. a   154. b   155. c

156. c   157. d   158. c

159. Which of the following is/are the cause/s of Hyponatremia?
a. Severe and chronic vomiting
b. Kidney disorders
c. Adrenal insufficiency
d. All of the above

160. During an oral glucose tolerance test, blood glucose levels are measured at which time points?
a. 0 hour, 1 hour, 2 hours
b. 1 hour, 2 hours, 3 hours
c. 2 hours, 4 hours, 6 hours
d. 4 hours, 8 hours, 12 hours

161. Impaired glucose tolerance (IGT) is characterized by:
a. Fasting blood glucose >126 mg/dL
b. Fasting blood glucose 100–125 mg/dL
c. 2 hours blood glucose levels of 140–199 mg/dL
d. Normal blood glucose levels

162. A 2-hour postprandial blood glucose level above _____ mg/dL is considered abnormal.
a. 100 mg/dL   b. 126 mg/dL
c. 140 mg/dL   d. 200 mg/dL

163. Which of the following factors can affect blood glucose levels?
a. Stress
b. Exercise
c. Medications
d. All of the above

164. Which method is commonly used to estimate blood glucose levels in the laboratory?
a. Enzymatic method
b. Colorimetric method
c. Spectrophotometric method
d. Hemoglobin A1c assay

165. Hemoglobin A1c (HbA1c) reflects average blood glucose levels over a period of approximately:
a. 1 week   b. 1 month
c. 3 months   d. 6 months

166. An HbA1c level of 7% or higher is indicative of:
a. Normal blood glucose control
b. Prediabetes
c. Poor blood glucose control in diabetes
d. Hypoglycemia

167. The normal range for HbA1c is typically:
a. <5%
b. Below 5.7%
c. 7–9%
d. >9%

168. What is the purpose of performing a glucose tolerance test?
a. To assess insulin resistance
b. To diagnose gestational diabetes
c. To evaluate diabetes management
d. All of the above

169. Which of the following statements is true regarding gestational diabetes?
a. It occurs only in women with a family history of diabetes.
b. It resolves after childbirth.
c. It is diagnosed based on a fasting blood glucose test.
d. It does not require any dietary modifications.

170. The primary treatment for gestational diabetes is:
a. Insulin therapy
b. Oral antidiabetic medications
c. Diet and exercise
d. No treatment is necessary

Answers:	159. d	160. a	161. c	162. c
	163. d	164. a	165. c	166. c
	167. b	168. d	169. b	170. c

171. Which of the following is an example of a simple lipid?
a. Phospholipid
b. Cholesterol
c. Triglyceride
d. Lipoprotein

172. Waxes are examples of which type of lipid?
a. Simple lipid
b. Compound lipid
c. Derived lipid
d. Sterol

173. What is the main function of phospholipids?
a. Energy storage
b. Cell recognition
c. Transport of lipids
d. The structural component of cell membranes

174. Which of the following is a compound lipid?
a. Triglyceride
b. Cholesterol
c. Glycolipid
d. Sterol

175. Which category of lipids is involved in cell recognition and adhesion?
a. Fats
b. Phospholipids
c. Glycolipids
d. Sterols

176. Prostaglandins are derived from which type of lipid?
a. Fatty acids
b. Triglycerides
c. Cholesterol
d. Waxes

177. What is the function of lipoproteins?
a. Energy storage
b. Cell recognition
c. Lipid transport
d. Hormone synthesis

178. Which lipid is a precursor for the synthesis of steroid hormones?
a. Triglyceride
b. Phospholipid
c. Cholesterol
d. Glycolipid

179. Cerebrosides and gangliosides are examples of which type of lipid?
a. Fats
b. Phospholipids
c. Glycolipids
d. Sterols

180. Which type of lipid is found in animal cell membranes?
a. Fats
b. Phospholipids
c. Glycolipids
d. Sterols

181. What is the primary function of triglycerides?
a. Energy storage
b. Cell recognition
c. Structural component of cell membranes
d. Hormone synthesis

182. Which lipid is a key component of lipoproteins?
a. Fatty acids
b. Triglycerides
c. Phospholipids
d. Cholesterol

183. Which lipid category forms protective coatings on the surface of plants and animals?
a. Fats
b. Phospholipids
c. Waxes
d. Sterols

184. What is the main function of glycolipids?
a. Energy storage
b. Cell adhesion
c. Hormone synthesis
d. Blood clotting

Answers:

171. c	172. a	173. d	174. c
175. c	176. a	177. c	178. c
179. c	180. d	181. a	182. d
183. c	184. b		

185. **Which lipid is involved in the transport of dietary lipids in the bloodstream?**
    a. Fats
    b. Phospholipids
    c. Glycolipids
    d. Lipoproteins

186. **Triglycerides are classified as:**
    a. Simple lipids
    b. Compound lipids
    c. Derived lipids
    d. None of the above

187. **Phospholipids are major components of:**
    a. Cell membranes
    b. Adipose tissue
    c. Waxes
    d. Steroids

188. **Glycolipids are involved in:**
    a. Energy storage
    b. Blood clotting
    c. Cell recognition
    d. Hormone synthesis

189. **Lipoproteins are complexes of:**
    a. Fatty acids and carbohydrates
    b. Fatty acids and proteins
    c. Fatty acids and nucleic acids
    d. Fatty acids and vitamins

190. **Steroids are characterized by:**
    a. A four-ring structure
    b. A long-chain fatty acid structure
    c. A carbohydrate moiety
    d. A phosphate group

191. **Terpenes are derived from the condensation of:**
    a. Fatty acids
    b. Amino acids
    c. Isoprene units
    d. Nucleotides

192. **Eicosanoids are derived from:**
    a. Triglycerides
    b. Phospholipids
    c. Polyunsaturated fatty acids
    d. Glycolipids

193. **Amino acids are the building blocks of:**
    a. Carbohydrates
    b. Proteins
    c. Lipids
    d. Nucleic acids

194. **Amino acids contain which functional groups?**
    a. Amino and hydroxyl groups
    b. Amino and carboxyl groups
    c. Carboxyl and hydroxyl groups
    d. Carboxyl and phosphate groups

195. **How many common amino acids are found in proteins?**
    a. 10   b. 15
    c. 20   d. 25

196. **Nonpolar amino acids are:**
    a. Hydrophobic
    b. Hydrophilic
    c. Positively charged
    d. Negatively charged

197. **Essential amino acids:**
    a. Can be synthesized by the body
    b. Must be obtained through the diet
    c. Are only found in animal proteins
    d. Have no biological function

198. **Which group of amino acids carries a positive charge at physiological pH?**
    a. Nonpolar amino acids
    b. Polar amino acids
    c. Basic amino acids
    d. Acidic amino acids

Answers:

185. d	186. a	187. a	188. c
189. b	190. a	191. c	192. c
193. b	194. b	195. c	196. a
197. b	198. c		

199. The side chains of acidic amino acids carry a:
a. Positive charge
b. Negative charge
c. Hydrophobic group
d. Hydrophilic group

200. Amino acids participate in the catalytic activity of:
a. Carbohydrates
b. Proteins
c. Lipids
d. Nucleic acids

201. Which amino acid is known as the "building block of life"?
a. Glycine
b. Alanine
c. Proline
d. Tryptophan

202. Which amino acid serves as a precursor for the synthesis of serotonin?
a. Aspartate
b. Serine
c. Tryptophan
d. Glutamine

203. Which type of amino acids cluster in the protein core?
a. Nonpolar amino acids
b. Polar amino acids
c. Acidic amino acids
d. Basic amino acids

204. Amino acids are joined together through:
a. Glycosidic bonds
b. Peptide bonds
c. Ester bonds
d. Phosphodiester bonds

205. Which amino acid is involved in collagen formation?
a. Leucine
b. Arginine
c. Proline
d. Glutamate

206. How many nonpolar amino acids are there?
a. 5
b. 10
c. 15
d. 20

207. Amino acids are amphoteric, meaning they can:
a. Act as acids and bases
b. Absorb light
c. Form hydrogen bonds
d. Undergo hydrolysis

208. The amino acid sequence of a protein is also known as its:
a. Secondary structure
b. Tertiary structure
c. Quaternary structure
d. Primary structure

209. Which amino acid is responsible for disulfide bond formation?
a. Cysteine
b. Methionine
c. Tyrosine
d. Histidine

210. Amino acids are classified based on the properties of their:
a. Carboxyl group
b. Amino group
c. Side chains
d. Peptide bonds

211. The synthesis of new proteins from amino acids is called:
a. Glycolysis
b. Gluconeogenesis
c. Protein folding
d. Translation

212. Amino acids play a role in:
a. DNA replication
b. Cell division
c. Energy production
d. All of the above

Answers:
199. b	200. b	201. a	202. c
203. a	204. b	205. c	206. d
207. a	208. d	209. a	210. c
211. d	212. d		

213. **The primary structure of a protein is determined by:**
    a. Tertiary interactions
    b. Secondary structure
    c. DNA sequence
    d. Quaternary structure

214. **The secondary structure of a protein includes:**
    a. Folding into a three-dimensional shape
    b. The linear sequence of amino acids
    c. Alpha helix and beta-sheet
    d. Multiple protein subunits

215. **Hydrogen bonds, disulfide bonds, and hydrophobic interactions contribute to the:**
    a. Primary structure of proteins
    b. Secondary structure of proteins
    c. Tertiary structure of proteins
    d. Quaternary structure of proteins

216. **Hemoglobin is an example of a protein with:**
    a. Primary structure only
    b. Secondary structure only
    c. Tertiary structure only
    d. Quaternary structure

217. **Protein denaturation can be caused by:**
    a. Temperature changes
    b. pH changes
    c. Exposure to chemicals
    d. All of the above

218. **Antibodies are proteins involved in:**
    a. Muscle contraction
    b. Blood clotting
    c. Immune response
    d. Oxygen transport

219. **Protein conformational changes are associated with:**
    a. Changes in protein function
    b. Changes in protein structure
    c. Changes in DNA sequence
    d. Changes in cellular location

220. **The folding of a protein into its functional three-dimensional structure is called:**
    a. Protein denaturation
    b. Protein synthesis
    c. Protein folding
    d. Protein degradation

221. **The quaternary structure of a protein involves:**
    a. Folding into a three-dimensional shape
    b. The linear sequence of amino acids
    c. Multiple protein subunits
    d. Hydrogen bond interactions

222. **Protein function is determined by:**
    a. DNA sequence
    b. Protein folding
    c. Protein structure and organization
    d. Protein denaturation

223. **Which of the following is a nucleic acid?**
    a. Lipids
    b. Carbohydrates
    c. Proteins
    d. DNA

224. **Nucleotides are composed of:**
    a. Amino acids
    b. Sugar, phosphate, and nitrogenous base
    c. Fatty acids and glycerol
    d. Monosaccharides

Answers: 213. c   214. c   215. c   216. d
         217. d   218. c   219. b   220. c
         221. c   222. c   223. d   224. b

225. The sugar molecule in DNA is:
a. Ribose
b. Glucose
c. Deoxyribose
d. Fructose

226. The complementary base pairing in DNA is:
a. A-T, C-G
b. A-G, T-C
c. A-C, G-T
d. A-U, C-G

227. RNA contains which nitrogenous base instead of thymine?
a. Adenine
b. Guanine
c. Uracil
d. Cytosine

228. DNA is involved in:
a. Protein synthesis
b. Cell division
c. Lipid metabolism
d. Carbohydrate digestion

229. Polymerase chain reaction (PCR) is used for:
a. Amplifying DNA sequences
b. Separating DNA fragments
c. Determining protein structure
d. Analyzing lipid composition

230. Gel electrophoresis separates DNA fragments based on:
a. Size and charge
b. Hydrophobicity
c. Molecular weight
d. Optical density

231. DNA sequencing is used to determine:
a. Protein structure
b. RNA function
c. DNA sequence
d. Lipid composition

232. Genetic disorders can result from:
a. Mutations in nucleic acid sequence
b. Enzyme deficiencies
c. Protein folding abnormalities
d. Carbohydrate metabolism disorders

233. What is the purpose of denaturation in PCR?
a. DNA amplification
b. Primer annealing
c. DNA template separation
d. DNA synthesis

234. At what temperature does annealing occur in PCR?
a. 37°C
b. 50–65°C
c. 72°C
d. 94–98°C

235. Which enzyme is responsible for DNA synthesis in PCR?
a. Ligase
b. Helicase
c. DNA polymerase
d. RNA polymerase

236. How does PCR achieve exponential amplification of DNA?
a. Through denaturation of DNA
b. Through multiple cycles of denaturation, annealing, and extension
c. By adding more primers
d. By using RNA as a template

237. What is the purpose of the final extension step in PCR?
a. To complete DNA synthesis
b. To separate DNA strands
c. To anneal primers
d. To denature DNA

238. Which technique is used to amplify specific DNA sequences?
a. Gel electrophoresis
b. PCR
c. DNA sequencing
d. Southern blotting

Answers:

225. c	226. a	227. c	228. a
229. a	230. a	231. c	232. a
233. c	234. b	235. c	236. b
237. a	238. b		

239. What is the purpose of DNA extraction in molecular techniques?
a. To amplify DNA
b. To separate DNA fragments
c. To purify DNA from biological samples
d. To visualize DNA bands

240. Which technique is used to visualize DNA bands in gel electrophoresis?
a. PCR
b. DNA sequencing
c. Western blotting
d. Staining with dyes or fluorescent probes

241. What is the principle behind Sanger sequencing?
a. Amplification of DNA fragments
b. Separation of DNA fragments based on size
c. Incorporation of chain-terminating dideoxynucleotides
d. Hybridization of DNA probes to target sequences

242. What is the purpose of hybridization techniques in molecular biology?
a. Amplification of DNA
b. Identification of DNA fragments
c. Analysis of gene expression
d. Visualization of proteins

243. Which technology allows the simultaneous analysis of gene expression for thousands of genes?
a. Microarray
b. PCR
c. DNA sequencing
d. Gel electrophoresis

244. Which gene editing technique utilizes CRISPR-Cas9?
a. Sanger sequencing
b. Microarray
c. PCR
d. Gene therapy

245. Molecular diagnostics is commonly used for:
a. Diagnosis of infectious diseases
b. Protein purification
c. Cell culture techniques
d. Blood typing

246. Which technique is used for genetic fingerprinting?
a. PCR
b. DNA sequencing
c. Restriction enzyme analysis
d. Microarray

247. What is the primary role of molecular techniques in medical laboratory technology?
a. Gene therapy
b. Protein purification
c. Diagnosis and monitoring of diseases
d. Blood transfusion

248. Enzymes are classified into six main groups based on:
a. Protein structure
b. Substrate specificity
c. Reaction type
d. Cellular location

249. The region of an enzyme where the substrate binds is called:
a. Active site
b. Allosteric site
c. Catalytic site
d. Regulatory site

Answers: 239. c   240. d   241. c   242. c
243. a   244. d   245. a   246. c
247. c   248. c   249. a

250. Enzyme kinetics study the:
a. Structure of enzymes
b. Rate of enzyme-catalyzed reactions
c. Substrate specificity of enzymes
d. Cellular location of enzymes

251. Competitive inhibitors:
a. Bind to the active site of enzymes
b. Bind to a different site than the active site
c. Increase enzyme activity
d. Have no effect on enzyme activity

252. Enzyme activity can be regulated through:
a. Allosteric regulation
b. Covalent modification
c. Enzyme induction and repression
d. All of the above

253. Enzyme markers in clinical diagnosis can indicate:
a. Organ damage or dysfunction
b. Enzyme synthesis
c. Substrate concentration
d. Enzyme structure

254. Enzymes are:
a. Nucleic acids
b. Carbohydrates
c. Proteins
d. Lipids

255. Enzymes function by:
a. Increasing activation energy
b. Lowering activation energy
c. Increasing substrate concentration
d. Binding to products

256. The active site of an enzyme:
a. Binds to the substrate
b. Inhibits the enzyme's activity
c. Contains cofactors
d. Is composed of lipids

257. The enzyme tyrosinase activated by:
a. Iron
b. Copper
c. Zinc
d. Potassium

258. The Michaelis constant (Km) represents:
a. Maximum velocity of the reaction
b. Rate of product formation
c. Enzyme concentration
d. Substrate concentration at half Vmax

259. Enzyme activity is influenced by:
a. Temperature and pH
b. Substrate concentration
c. Enzyme concentration
d. All of the above

260. Competitive inhibition occurs when:
a. Inhibitor binds to a different site on the enzyme
b. Inhibitor binds only to the enzyme-substrate complex
c. Inhibitor competes with the substrate for binding to the active site
d. Inhibitor prevents product formation

261. Enzyme assays are used in diagnostics to:
a. Measure enzyme concentration in tissues
b. Monitor disease progression
c. Assess patient's diet
d. Determine genetic mutations

Answers:

250. b	251. a	252. d	253. a
254. c	255. b	256. a	257. b
258. d	259. d	260. c	261. b

262. **The maximum number of substrate molecules converted per enzyme active site per second is represented by:**
   a. Km
   b. Vmax
   c. kcat
   d. Turnover number

263. **Enzyme denaturation can occur due to:**
   a. Extreme pH
   b. High temperature
   c. Presence of inhibitors
   d. All of the above

264. **Which enzyme is primarily used to assess liver function?**
   a. ALT   b. CK
   c. ALP   d. AST

265. **Elevated levels of CK indicate:**
   a. Liver dysfunction
   b. Muscle damage
   c. Pancreatic disorders
   d. Bone abnormalities

266. **Which enzyme is involved in fat digestion?**
   a. ALT   b. CK
   c. Lipase   d. Amylase

267. **Enzyme assays involve measuring:**
   a. Enzyme concentration
   b. Enzyme activity
   c. Enzyme size
   d. Enzyme structure

268. **Serial measurements of enzyme activity are useful for:**
   a. Monitoring disease progression
   b. Assessing age-related changes
   c. Determining gender-related differences
   d. Evaluating medication effects

269. **Troponin is a specific marker for:**
   a. Liver damage
   b. Kidney dysfunction
   c. Cardiac muscle damage
   d. Pancreatic disorders

270. **CK-MB is an isoform of:**
   a. Troponin
   b. Myoglobin
   c. Creatine kinase
   d. Lactate dehydrogenase

271. **Myoglobin levels in the blood rise:**
   a. Immediately after myocardial infarction
   b. After 24 hours of myocardial infarction
   c. After 48 hours of myocardial infarction
   d. After 72 hours of myocardial infarction

272. **LDH levels in myocardial infarction typically:**
   a. Peak within 3–6 hours
   b. Peak within 12–24 hours
   c. Peak within 24–48 hours
   d. Peak within 72 hours

273. **Which cardiac enzyme shows the earliest rise following myocardial injury?**
   a. Troponin
   b. Creatine kinase-MB
   c. Myoglobin
   d. Alanine aminotransferase

274. **When do troponin levels typically peak after the onset of myocardial infarction?**
   a. Within 1–3 hours
   b. Within 4–6 hours
   c. Within 12–24 hours
   d. Within 48–72 hours

Answers:	262. c	263. d	264. a	265. b
	266. c	267. b	268. a	269. c
	270. c	271. a	272. c	273. c
	274. c			

275. The normal color of urine is:
a. Red
b. Green
c. Pale yellow to amber
d. Clear

276. Proteinuria is the presence of:
a. Glucose in urine
b. Protein in urine
c. Ketones in urine
d. Blood in urine

277. A urine pH of 4.0 indicates:
a. Acidic urine
b. Alkaline urine
c. Normal urine pH
d. No urine pH value exists

278. Hematuria refers to the presence of:
a. Glucose in urine
b. Protein in urine
c. Blood in urine
d. Ketones in urine

279. The normal range of urine pH is:
a. 1.5–3.0
b. 4.6–8.0
c. 8.0–10.0
d. 10.0–12.0

280. Elevated protein levels in urine may indicate:
a. Diabetes
b. Kidney damage
c. Liver disease
d. Urinary tract infection

281. Ketones in urine are commonly seen in:
a. Hypertension
b. Malnutrition
c. Diabetes
d. Urinary tract infection

282. The presence of red blood cells (RBCs) in urine may indicate:
a. Liver disease
b. Kidney stones
c. Urinary tract infection
d. Diabetes

283. Which test is used to determine the acidity or alkalinity of urine?
a. Protein test
b. Glucose test
c. pH test
d. Ketone test

284. An elevated level of glucose in urine may indicate:
a. Kidney dysfunction
b. Uncontrolled diabetes
c. Urinary tract infection
d. Liver disease

285. Which component of urine can be evaluated using a refractometer?
a. Protein
b. pH
c. Specific gravity
d. Glucose

286. Increased red blood cells in urine sediment may indicate:
a. Urinary tract bleeding
b. Kidney dysfunction
c. Liver disease
d. Urinary tract infection

287. Which biochemical test is used to detect glucose in urine?
a. Biuret test
b. Hay's test
c. Glucose oxidase test
d. Nitroprusside reaction

288. Which biochemical test is used to detect protein in urine?
a. Heat coagulation test
b. Hay's test
c. Glucose oxidase test
d. Nitroprusside reaction

Answers:

275. c	276. b	277. a	278. c
279. b	280. b	281. c	282. b
283. c	284. b	285. c	286. a
287. c	288. a		

289. **The detection of ketone bodies in urine may indicate:**
 a. Diabetic ketoacidosis
 b. Liver dysfunction
 c. Kidney inflammation
 d. Urinary tract infection

290. **Bile salts in urine are suggestive of:**
 a. Impaired liver function
 b. Glucose metabolism disorders
 c. Kidney damage
 d. Proteinuria

291. **Bile pigments in urine may indicate:**
 a. Impaired liver function
 b. Renal glycosuria
 c. Fasting states
 d. Urinary tract infection

292. **CSF is produced primarily in which of the following structures?**
 a. Brain ventricles
 b. Spinal cord
 c. Meninges
 d. Cerebral cortex

293. **The normal volume of CSF in adults is approximately:**
 a. 50–100 mL
 b. 150–200 mL
 c. 250–300 mL
 d. 350–400 mL

294. **Which of the following is the most common method for collecting CSF?**
 a. Lumbar puncture
 b. Venepuncture
 c. Arterial puncture
 d. Thoracentesis

295. **Which enzyme is typically measured in CSF to assess central nervous system (CNS) damage?**
 a. Amylase
 b. Lactate dehydrogenase (LDH)
 c. Creatine kinase (CK)
 d. Alanine aminotransferase (ALT)

296. **What is the normal glucose level in CSF compared to blood glucose?**
 a. Higher
 b. Lower
 c. Equal
 d. Variable

297. **Increased protein levels in CSF may indicate:**
 a. Infection
 b. Hemorrhage
 c. CNS tumor
 d. All of the above

298. **Which of the following is a marker for blood-brain barrier disruption?**
 a. Glucose
 b. Protein
 c. Red blood cells
 d. White blood cells

299. **CSF lactate levels are elevated in conditions associated with:**
 a. Bacterial meningitis
 b. Viral meningitis
 c. Multiple sclerosis
 d. Guillain-Barré syndrome

300. **Which of the following tests is used to detect intrathecal antibody synthesis?**
 a. Oligoclonal banding
 b. Polymerase chain reaction (PCR)
 c. Gram stain
 d. India ink preparation

301. **What is the primary purpose of CSF cytology?**
 a. Detecting the presence of tumor cells
 b. Assessing glucose levels
 c. Identifying bacterial pathogens
 d. Evaluating blood-brain barrier integrity

Answers: 289. a 290. a 291. a 292. a
293. a 294. a 295. b 296. b
297. d 298. b 299. a 300. a
301. a

302. Which of the following CSF findings is characteristic of bacterial meningitis?
a. Elevated glucose
b. Decreased protein
c. Lymphocytic pleocytosis
d. Neutrophilic pleocytosis

303. The presence of xanthochromia in CSF indicates:
a. Hemorrhage
b. Infection
c. Elevated protein levels
d. Normal CSF

304. Which of the following CSF components is typically measured to assess CNS inflammation?
a. Neutrophils
b. Red blood cells
c. White blood cells
d. Platelets

305. CSF oligoclonal bands are associated with which condition?
a. Multiple sclerosis
b. Bacterial meningitis
c. Viral encephalitis
d. Guillain-Barré syndrome

306. CSF lactate levels are measured to evaluate:
a. Liver function
b. Kidney function
c. Metabolic acidosis
d. CNS ischemia

307. Which CSF finding is characteristic of subarachnoid hemorrhage?
a. Xanthochromia
b. Elevated glucose
c. Lymphocytic pleocytosis
d. Decreased protein

308. The presence of which cells in CSF is indicative of CNS infection?
a. Neutrophils
b. Lymphocytes
c. Monocytes
d. Eosinophils

309. CSF analysis is not routinely performed for which of the following conditions?
a. Meningitis
b. Encephalitis
c. Stroke
d. Alzheimer's disease

310. What is the normal range for CSF protein levels in adults?
a. 10–20 mg/dL
b. 15–50 mg/dL
c. 60–80 mg/dL
d. 90–100 mg/dL

311. Which of the following CSF findings is characteristic of viral meningitis?
a. Elevated protein
b. Lymphocytic pleocytosis
c. Neutrophilic pleocytosis
d. Xanthochromia

312. Which test is used to detect the presence of oligoclonal bands in CSF?
a. Gram stain
b. Polymerase chain reaction (PCR)
c. Western blot
d. Immunofixation electrophoresis

313. Elevated CSF pressure may indicate:
a. Head injury
b. Infections
c. CNS tumor
d. All of the above

Answers:

302. d	303. a	304. c	305. a
306. d	307. a	308. a	309. c
310. b	311. b	312. d	313. d

314. Which of the following CSF findings is characteristic of Guillain-Barré syndrome?
   a. Elevated glucose
   b. Elevated protein with normal WBC counts
   c. Neutrophilic pleocytosis
   d. Xanthochromia

315. CSF glucose levels are decreased in which condition?
   a. Bacterial meningitis
   b. Viral meningitis
   c. Multiple sclerosis
   d. Encephalitis

316. CSF analysis is performed to diagnose which of the following conditions?
   a. CNS tumors
   b. Spinal cord injury
   c. Meningitis
   d. All of the above

317. Which of the following CSF findings is used to differentiate between traumatic tap and subarachnoid hemorrhage?
   a. Xanthochromia
   b. Elevated protein
   c. Neutrophilic pleocytosis
   d. Decreased glucose

318. The normal range for CSF glucose levels is approximately:
   a. 20–40 mg/dL   b. 40–70 mg/dL
   c. 80–100 mg/dL   d. 110–130mg/dL

319. CSF lactate levels are primarily affected by:
   a. Glucose concentration
   b. Protein concentration
   c. Anaerobic metabolism
   d. Cerebral blood flow

320. What is the meaning of xanthochromia in CSF?
   a. Elevated protein
   b. Lymphocytic pleocytosis
   c. Presence of bilirubin in CSF
   d. Neutrophilic pleocytosis

321. The primary function of CSF is to:
   a. Provide cushioning and support to the brain and spinal cord
   b. Transport nutrients to the CNS
   c. Remove metabolic waste products from the CNS
   d. All of the above

322. Pleural fluid is collected through a procedure called:
   a. Thoracentesis
   b. Pleural biopsy
   c. Bronchoscopy
   d. Pulmonary function test

323. The enzyme that indicates tissue damage or inflammation in pleural fluid is:
   a. Amylase
   b. Lipase
   c. Lactate dehydrogenase (LDH)
   d. Alkaline phosphatase

324. Increased protein levels in pleural fluid are associated with:
   a. Infection
   b. Malignancy
   c. Inflammation
   d. All of the above

325. Decreased glucose levels in the pleural fluid may suggest:
   a. Infection
   b. Malignancy
   c. Normal findings
   d. Diabetes mellitus

Answers: 314. **b**   315. **a**   316. **d**   317. **a**
318. **b**   319. **c**   320. **c**   321. **d**
322. **a**   323. **c**   324. **d**   325. **a**

326. Pleural fluid pH is measured to assess:
a. Protein concentration
b. Glucose levels
c. Acidity or alkalinity
d. Cell count

327. Neutrophils and lymphocytes are observed in pleural fluid during:
a. Normal findings
b. Bacterial infection
c. Fungal infection
d. Head injury

328. Gram stain and culture of pleural fluid help to identify:
a. Enzyme levels
b. pH levels
c. Bacterial or fungal infections
d. Glucose levels

329. Cytology of pleural fluid is performed to detect:
a. Enzyme levels
b. pH levels
c. Protein concentration
d. Cancer cells

330. The biochemical pleural fluid examination helps in diagnosing:
a. Respiratory infections only
b. Malignant pleural effusions only
c. Pleural diseases and differentiating causes
d. Pulmonary embolism

331. The pleural fluid examination is not useful for detecting:
a. Infections
b. Malignancy
c. Metabolic disorders
d. Pulmonary embolism

332. The gastric acid analysis is performed to assess:
a. Pepsinogen levels
b. Gastrin levels
c. Pancreatic elastase
d. Gastric acid secretion

333. The main indication for measuring pepsinogen levels is:
a. Gastritis
b. Pernicious anemia
c. Gastrinoma
d. Gastroparesis

334. Gastrin levels are measured to evaluate:
a. Gastric emptying
b. Pepsinogen production
c. Gastrin-secreting tumors
d. Pancreatic elastase activity

335. Intrinsic factor antibodies test is used to diagnose:
a. Pernicious anemia
b. Gastroparesis
c. Gastritis
d. Pancreatic insufficiency

336. A fecal pancreatic elastase test is performed to evaluate:
a. Gastric acid secretion
b. *H. pylori* infection
c. Exocrine pancreatic function
d. Gastrin levels

337. A gastric emptying study is performed to assess:
a. Vitamin B_{12} absorption
b. Gastric motility
c. Gastric acid secretion
d. *H. pylori* infection

Answers:

326. c	327. b	328. c	329. d
330. c	331. d	332. d	333. a
334. c	335. a	336. c	337. b

338. **The urea breath test is used to diagnose:**
    a. Gastritis
    b. Pernicious anemia
    c. *H. pylori* infection
    d. Pancreatic insufficiency

339. **Fasting serum gastrin levels are measured to assess:**
    a. Gastric emptying
    b. Pancreatic elastase activity
    c. Gastric acid regulation
    d. *H. pylori* infection

340. **The fecal elastase-1 test is used to evaluate:**
    a. Pancreatic exocrine function
    b. Pancreatic endocrine function
    c. Pancreatic lipase levels
    d. Pancreatic amylase levels

341. **Elevated serum amylase and lipase levels indicate:**
    a. Pancreatic exocrine insufficiency
    b. Prediabetes
    c. Acute pancreatitis
    d. Cystic fibrosis

342. **The fasting blood glucose test is used to assess:**
    a. Pancreatic exocrine function
    b. Pancreatic endocrine function
    c. Pancreatic lipase levels
    d. Pancreatic elastase-1 levels

343. **The oral glucose tolerance test evaluates:**
    a. Pancreatic exocrine function
    b. Pancreatic endocrine function
    c. Pancreatic lipase levels
    d. Pancreatic elastase-1 levels

344. **Glycated hemoglobin (HbA1c) reflects:**
    a. Short-term glucose control
    b. Liver function
    c. Pancreatic exocrine function
    d. Long-term glucose control

345. **Fecal elastase-1 levels <200 µg/g indicate:**
    a. Pancreatic exocrine insufficiency
    b. Pancreatic endocrine dysfunction
    c. Acute pancreatitis
    d. Cystic fibrosis

346. **Impaired oral glucose tolerance test may indicate:**
    a. Prediabetes
    b. Acute pancreatitis
    c. Cystic fibrosis
    d. Diabetes mellitus

347. **The secretin stimulation test measures:**
    a. Pancreatic lipase levels
    b. Pancreatic elastase-1 levels
    c. Pancreatic secretions
    d. Blood glucose levels

348. **C-peptide and insulin levels assess:**
    a. Pancreatic exocrine function
    b. Pancreatic endocrine function
    c. Pancreatic lipase levels
    d. Pancreatic elastase-1 levels

349. **Acute and chronic pancreatitis affect both:**
    a. Pancreatic exocrine and endocrine functions
    b. Liver and kidney functions
    c. Lung and heart functions
    d. Intestinal and stomach functions

Answers: 338. c   339. c   340. a   341. c
342. b   343. b   344. d   345. a
346. a   347. c   348. b   349. a

350. Which enzyme is primarily found in liver cells?
a. Alanine aminotransferase (ALT)
b. Aspartate aminotransferase (AST)
c. Alkaline phosphatase (ALP)
d. Gamma-glutamyl transferase (GGT)

351. Elevated levels of ALT indicate:
a. Heart disease
b. Kidney dysfunction
c. Liver cell damage
d. Bone disorders

352. Alkaline phosphatase is found in the:
a. Liver only
b. Kidneys only
c. Bones and liver
d. Intestines and liver

353. Bilirubin is a pigment produced from the breakdown of:
a. Red blood cells
b. White blood cells
c. Platelets
d. Plasma proteins

354. Increased GGT levels may indicate:
a. Liver disorders
b. Kidney dysfunction
c. Heart disease
d. Muscle damage

355. Albumin is a protein produced by the:
a. Liver
b. Kidneys
c. Heart
d. Lungs

356. Prolonged PT and increased INR suggest:
a. Impaired liver function
b. Kidney dysfunction
c. Heart disease
d. Lung disorders

357. Hepatitis serology tests detect:
a. Antibodies or antigens associated with hepatitis viruses
b. Enzyme levels in the liver
c. Prothrombin time
d. Red blood cell count

358. LFTs are used to assess the health and function of the:
a. Liver
b. Kidneys
c. Heart
d. Lungs

359. BUN measures the level of:
a. Glucose in the blood
b. Urea nitrogen in the blood
c. Creatinine in the blood
d. Albumin in the blood

360. Serum creatinine is a waste product of:
a. Liver metabolism
b. Muscle metabolism
c. Kidney metabolism
d. Pancreatic metabolism

361. Glomerular filtration rate estimates:
a. Blood pressure
b. Oxygen saturation
c. Blood filtering by the kidneys
d. Blood glucose levels

362. Urinalysis assesses:
a. Blood pressure
b. Kidney size
c. Urine color and pH
d. Lung function

363. Elevated urine albumin levels indicate:
a. Lung disease
b. Heart disease
c. Kidney damage
d. Liver dysfunction

Answers:	350. a	351. c	352. c	353. a
	354. a	355. a	356. a	357. a
	358. a	359. b	360. b	361. c
	362. c	363. c		

364. Creatinine clearance estimates:
a. Glomerular filtration rate
b. Urine specific gravity
c. Hemoglobin levels
d. Red blood cell count

365. Electrolyte levels help assess:
a. Liver function
b. Lung function
c. Kidney function
d. Heart function

366. Renal imaging techniques provide detailed images of:
a. Liver
b. Lungs
c. Kidneys
d. Heart

367. Serum calcium estimation is based on the principle of:
a. Complex formation
b. Oxidation-reduction
c. Enzyme activity
d. Antibody-antigen reaction

368. The most common method for serum calcium estimation is based on:
a. O-Cresolphthalein complexone (OCPC)
b. Nephelometry
c. Immunoturbidimetry
d. Chemiimmunoassay

369. Which chelating agent is commonly used in the OCPC method?
a. EDTA
b. Arsenazo III
c. OCPC
d. Thymol

370. The principle of the Arsenazo III method involves the formation of a complex between calcium ions and:
a. EDTA
b. OCPC
c. Arsenazo III
d. Thymol

371. The ion-selective electrode (ISE) method measures calcium concentration based on:
a. Absorbance of a colored complex
b. Electrical potential
c. Antibody-antigen reaction
d. Enzyme activity

372. Which method offers rapid results and high precision for serum calcium estimation?
a. OCPC method
b. Arsenazo III method
c. ISE method
d. Nephelometry

373. For serum calcium estimation, blood samples are collected in tubes:
a. With anticoagulants
b. Containing EDTA
c. Without anticoagulants
d. Containing heparin

374. Serum calcium estimation is important for evaluating the body's:
a. Iron balance
b. Glucose metabolism
c. Bone metabolism
d. Lipid profile

375. Hypocalcemia refers to:
a. Serum calcium of <8.5 mg/dL
b. Serum calcium of >10.5 mg/dL
c. Serum potassium levels <3.5 mEq/L
d. Serum potassium levels <5.5 mEq/L

Answers:	364. a	365. c	366. c	367. a
	368. a	369. c	370. c	371. b
	372. c	373. c	374. c	375. a

376. Hypercalcemia refers to:
a. Serum calcium of <8.5 mg/dL
b. Serum calcium of >10.5 mg/dL
c. Serum potassium levels <3.5 mEq/L
d. Serum potassium levels <5.5 mEq/L

377. Serum phosphorus estimation is based on the principle of:
a. Colorimetry   b. Fluorescence
c. Electrophoresis   d. Ionization

378. The color formed during serum phosphorus estimation is:
a. Blue   b. Yellow
c. Green   d. Red

379. The most commonly used method for serum phosphorus estimation is:
a. Spectrophotometric method
b. Enzymatic method
c. Ion-selective electrode method
d. Chromatographic method

380. The serum is obtained by:
a. Centrifugation
b. Filtration
c. Distillation
d. Dialysis

381. Hemolysis can affect serum phosphorus estimation by:
a. Decreasing phosphorus levels
b. Increasing phosphorus levels
c. No effect on phosphorus levels
d. Changing the color of the complex

382. Lipemia and bilirubinemia can interfere with serum phosphorus estimation by:
a. Increasing absorbance
b. Decreasing absorbance
c. No effect on absorbance
d. Causing turbidity

383. The reference range for serum phosphorus in adults is typically:
a. 0.5–1.5 mg/dL
b. 1.5–3.0 mg/dL
c. 2.5–4.5 mg/dL
d. 4.5–6.0 mg/dL

384. Abnormal serum phosphorus levels may indicate:
a. Renal disorders
b. Metabolic bone diseases
c. Hormonal imbalances
d. All of the above

385. The spectrophotometric method for serum phosphorus estimation involves:
a. Direct measurement of phosphate ions
b. Hydrolysis of organic phosphates
c. Formation of a colored complex
d. Separation of lipids and bilirubin

386. The most appropriate sample for serum phosphorus estimation is:
a. Plasma
b. Whole blood
c. Serum
d. Urine

387. The estimation of sodium is based on:
a. Flame photometry
b. Indirect colorimetric methods
c. Ion-selective electrodes
d. All of the above

388. Potassium estimation can be performed using:
a. Flame photometry
b. Ion-selective electrodes
c. Indirect colorimetric methods
d. All of the above

Answers:

376. b	377. a	378. b	379. a
380. a	381. b	382. d	383. c
384. d	385. c	386. c	387. d
388. d			

389. Chloride estimation is based on:
a. Flame photometry
b. Ion-selective electrodes
c. Indirect colorimetric methods
d. None of the above

390. The principle behind ion-selective electrodes is:
a. Nernst equation
b. Avogadro's law
c. Boyle's law
d. Law of conservation of mass

391. Flame photometry measures the:
a. Absorption of light
b. Emission of light
c. Reflection of light
d. Refraction of light

392. Which electrolyte estimation method involves a color change reaction?
a. Flame photometry
b. Ion-selective electrodes
c. Indirect colorimetric methods
d. None of the above

393. Quality control measures for electrolyte estimation include:
a. Calibration
b. Use of controls
c. Adherence to standard operating procedures
d. All of the above

394. Abnormalities in sodium levels may indicate:
a. Dehydration
b. Kidney disorders
c. Electrolyte imbalances
d. All of the above

395. Potassium estimation is based on the measurement of:
a. Absorption of light
b. Emission of light
c. Potentiometric changes
d. Color change reactions

396. Which equation is used in ion-selective electrode measurements?
a. Nernst equation
b. Avogadro's law
c. Boyle's law
d. Law of conservation of mass

397. Proteinuria refers to:
a. Presence of glucose in the urine
b. Presence of excess protein in the urine
c. Presence of excess red blood cells in the urine
d. Presence of bacteria in the urine

398. Microalbuminuria is:
a. Detection of more than 300 mg per day of albumin in the urine
b. Detection of 30–300 mg per day albumin in the urine
c. Detection of more than 150 mg per day glucose in the urine
d. Detection of red blood cells in the urine

399. Which of the following methods can be used for the qualitative detection of proteinuria?
a. Bradford assay
b. Immunoturbidimetry
c. Dipstick test
d. Albumin-to-creatinine ratio

Answers: 389. b   390. a   391. b   392. c
393. d   394. d   395. c   396. a
397. b   398. b   399. c

400. The reference range for proteinuria in a 24-hour urine sample is typically:
a. <30 mg/24 hours
b. <150 mg/24 hours
c. <300 mg/24 hours
d. <500 mg/24 hours

401. The albumin-to-creatinine ratio (ACR) is used for the detection of:
a. Proteinuria
b. Glucose in the urine
c. Microalbuminuria
d. Red blood cells in the urine

402. Which of the following is a quantitative method for detecting proteinuria?
a. Dipstick test
b. Bradford assay
c. Immunoturbidimetry
d. Random urine sample

403. The normal reference range for microalbuminuria in the albumin-to-creatinine ratio is:
a. 1–10 mg/g
b. 30–300 mg/g
c. 100–1000 mg/g
d. 1000–5000 mg/g

404. Proteinuria can be associated with:
a. Hypertension
b. Diabetes mellitus
c. Renal diseases
d. All of the above

405. Microalbuminuria is an early sign of:
a. Diabetic nephropathy
b. Liver cirrhosis
c. Lung cancer
d. Thyroid dysfunction

406. The principle of renal clearance tests is based on:
a. Filtration, reabsorption, and secretion by the kidneys
b. Absorption and metabolism by the liver
c. Diffusion across cell membranes
d. Hormonal regulation

407. Which substance is commonly used for renal clearance tests?
a. Glucose
b. Urea
c. Sodium
d. Creatinine

408. How is renal clearance calculated?
a. Urine volume × plasma concentration
b. Urine concentration × urine flow rate/plasma concentration
c. Plasma concentration × urine flow rate
d. Plasma volume × urine concentration

409. Glomerular filtration rate (GFR) reflects:
a. Kidney blood flow
b. Kidney tubular function
c. Rate of urine production
d. Rate of waste excretion

410. The normal reference range for GFR in adults is approximately:
a. 30–50 mL/min
b. 60–90 mL/min
c. 90–120 mL/min
d. 150–200 mL/min

Answers:

400. b	401. c	402. c	403. b
404. d	405. a	406. a	407. d
408. b	409. d	410. c	

411. **Normal synovial fluid appears:**
   a. Turbid
   b. Red
   c. Clear and viscous
   d. Yellow-green

412. **Which parameter is measured to assess joint inflammation?**
   a. Total protein
   b. Glucose
   c. Hemoglobin
   d. Uric acid

413. **Rheumatoid factor (RF) presence may indicate:**
   a. Osteoarthritis
   b. Gout
   c. Rheumatoid arthritis
   d. Lupus erythematosus

414. **Increased neutrophils in synovial fluid indicate:**
   a. Infection
   b. Autoimmune disorder
   c. Trauma
   d. Gout

415. **Microbiological examination of synovial fluid is performed to:**
   a. Assess glucose levels
   b. Identify crystals
   c. Detect microorganisms
   d. Determine protein levels

416. **Crystal analysis in synovial fluid is performed using:**
   a. Polarized light microscopy
   b. Gram stain
   c. Culture
   d. Enzyme-linked immunosorbent assay (ELISA)

417. **The presence of monosodium urate crystals is indicative of:**
   a. Gout
   b. Rheumatoid arthritis
   c. Osteoarthritis
   d. Systemic lupus erythematosus

418. **Which cell type is increased in chronic inflammation?**
   a. Neutrophils
   b. Lymphocytes
   c. Macrophages
   d. Eosinophils

419. **Uric acid is a metabolic waste product of:**
   a. Carbohydrate metabolism
   b. Lipid metabolism
   c. Protein metabolism
   d. Nucleic acid metabolism

420. **Uric acid estimation is based on the:**
   a. Enzymatic method
   b. Chromatographic method
   c. Microscopic method
   d. Immunological method

421. **The enzyme used in the enzymatic method of uric acid estimation is:**
   a. Uricase
   b. Amylase
   c. Lipase
   d. Protease

422. **The product formed in the reaction of uric acid with uricase is:**
   a. Allantoin
   b. Urea
   c. Uric acid
   d. Hydrogen peroxide

423. **Which method of uric acid estimation involves the use of colorimetric reactions?**
   a. Enzymatic method
   b. Spectrophotometric method
   c. Gravimetric method
   d. Colorimetric method

Answers:	411. c	412. a	413. c	414. a
	415. c	416. a	417. a	418. b
	419. d	420. a	421. a	422. a
	423. d			

424. Blood samples for uric acid estimation are collected in tubes:
a. With anticoagulant
b. Without anticoagulant
c. With EDTA
d. With sodium citrate

425. High levels of uric acid in the blood can indicate:
a. Hypouricemia
b. Wilson's disease
c. Gout
d. Hypertension

426. Uric acid estimation is commonly used to diagnose and monitor:
a. Diabetes mellitus
b. Hypothyroidism
c. Gout
d. Anemia

427. Which of the following factors can influence uric acid levels?
a. Diet
b. Medications
c. Medical conditions
d. All of the above

428. Hyperuricemia refers to:
a. Low uric acid levels
b. High uric acid levels
c. Normal uric acid levels
d. No uric acid production

429. Arterial blood samples are typically collected from:
a. Veins
b. Arteries
c. Capillaries
d. Lymphatic vessels

430. The most common site for arterial blood sample collection is the:
a. Radial artery
b. Brachial artery
c. Femoral artery
d. Dorsalis pedis artery

431. Arterial blood sample collection requires the use of:
a. Standard syringes
b. EDTA tubes
c. Arterial blood gas syringes
d. Vacutainer tubes

432. The purpose of using heparin in arterial blood sample collection is to:
a. Prevent clotting
b. Preserve sample stability
c. Enhance oxygenation
d. Facilitate sample transport

433. Which parameter reflects the acidity or alkalinity of blood?
a. pH
b. PaO_2
c. $PaCO_2$
d. HCO_3^-

434. A pH below 7.35 indicates:
a. Acidosis
b. Alkalosis
c. Normal blood pH
d. Blood clotting

435. The PaO_2 value in ABG reflects:
a. Oxygenation status
b. Ventilation status
c. Metabolic balance
d. Acid–base balance

436. Elevated $PaCO_2$ levels suggest:
a. Respiratory acidosis
b. Respiratory alkalosis
c. Metabolic acidosis
d. Metabolic alkalosis

Answers:	424. b	425. c	426. c	427. d
	428. b	429. b	430. a	431. c
	432. a	433. a	434. a	435. a
	436. a			

437. HCO$_3^-$ levels indicate:
a. Oxygen saturation
b. Respiratory status
c. Metabolic balance
d. Acid-base balance

438. SaO$_2$ measures:
a. Oxygen saturation
b. Carbon dioxide levels
c. Acidic pH
d. Blood clotting

439. Which hormones are produced by the thyroid gland?
a. Adrenalin and cortisol
b. Triiodothyronine (T3) and thyroxine (T4)
c. Insulin and glucagon
d. Estrogen and progesterone

440. Thyroid-stimulating hormone (TSH) is produced by:
a. Thyroid gland
b. Pituitary gland
c. Adrenal gland
d. Pancreas

441. Which method utilizes radioactive isotopes in thyroid function testing?
a. Radioimmunoassay (RIA)
b. Enzyme-linked immunosorbent assay (ELISA)
c. Chemiluminescent Immunoassay (CLIA)
d. Immunofluorescence assay (IFA)

442. Which thyroid function test method offers high sensitivity and a wide dynamic range?
a. RIA
b. ELISA
c. CLIA
d. IFA

443. Thyroid function test panels may include:
a. TSH only
b. T3 and T4 only
c. TSH, T3, and T4
d. TSH, T3, T4, FT3, FT4, and thyroid autoantibodies

444. Reference ranges for thyroid function tests:
a. Are the same for all individuals
b. Depend on age and sex only
c. Are influenced by pregnancy status
d. Do not vary among laboratories

445. Abnormal thyroid function test results may indicate:
a. Hypothyroidism
b. Hyperthyroidism
c. Thyroid autoimmunity
d. All of the above

446. Which vitamins are classified as fat-soluble?
a. vitamins B complex
b. C and D vitamins
c. A, D, E, and K vitamins
d. C and E vitamins

447. Which vitamin deficiency is associated with night blindness?
a. Vitamin A
b. Vitamin B$_1$
c. Vitamin C
d. Vitamin D

448. Pellagra is caused by the deficiency of:
a. Vitamin A
b. Vitamin B$_1$
c. Vitamin B$_3$
d. Vitamin B$_6$

449. Which vitamin is involved in the formation of red blood cells and neurological function?
a. Vitamin B$_{12}$
b. Vitamin B$_2$
c. Vitamin C
d. Vitamin D

Answers: 437. c   438. a   439. b   440. b
441. a   442. c   443. d   444. c
445. d   446. c   447. a   448. c
449. a

450. The deficiency of which vitamin can lead to scurvy?
- a. Vitamin A
- b. Vitamin B_{12}
- c. Vitamin C
- d. Vitamin K

451. Vitamin D is essential for the absorption of:
- a. Calcium
- b. Iron
- c. Copper
- d. Zinc

452. Which vitamin is known for its antioxidant properties?
- a. Vitamin K
- b. Vitamin C
- c. Vitamin D
- d. Vitamin E

453. Anemia and neurological disorders are associated with the deficiency of:
- a. Vitamin B_6
- b. Vitamin C
- c. Vitamin D
- d. Vitamin E

454. Which vitamin is synthesized by the body with the help of sunlight?
- a. Vitamin A
- b. Vitamin B_{12}
- c. Vitamin C
- d. Vitamin D

455. Vitamin K is important for:
- a. Vision
- b. Blood clotting
- c. Bone health
- d. Immune function

Answers: 450. c   451. a   452. d   453. a
454. d   455. b

Hematology and Blood Banking

Section Outline

Chapter 4: Hematology and Blood Banking

Hematology and Blood Banking

INTRODUCTION TO HEMATOLOGY

Hematology is a branch of science that deals with the study of blood.

It involves the study of blood and blood-forming elements such as red blood cells, white blood cells, platelets and also the disorders related to blood such as anemia, leukemia, and clotting disorders.

Components of Blood

- **Red blood cells (RBCs or erythrocytes):** These cells carry oxygen from the lungs to the rest of the body.
- **White blood cells (WBCs or leukocytes):** They are an integral part of our immune system and play an important role in fighting infections and diseases. The different types of white blood cells are neutrophils, lymphocytes, monocytes, and eosinophils.
- **Platelets (thrombocytes):** These cells help the blood to clot and prevent excessive bleeding.
- **Plasma:** It is a straw-colored liquid component of blood that makes up to 55% of its volume. It carries nutrients, hormones, waste products, and proteins such as clotting factors.
- **Hemoglobin:** This iron-containing protein in red blood cells helps to carry oxygen from the lungs to the rest of the body.
- **Electrolytes:** These are minerals, such as sodium, potassium, and chloride, that are dissolved in the plasma and play an important role in maintaining fluid balance and supporting many of the body's functions.
- **Proteins:** Blood contains various proteins, including clotting factors, immunoglobulins (antibodies), and enzymes.

The main differences between whole blood, serum, and plasma are as follows:

Whole Blood

- Whole blood refers to the blood that is collected directly from a patient or donor without any processing or separation.
- It consists of a mixture of cellular components (red blood cells, white blood cells, and platelets) suspended in a liquid called plasma.
- Whole blood is commonly used for blood transfusions or when all blood components are required, such as in certain laboratory tests.

Serum

- Serum is the liquid portion of blood that remains after coagulation and removal of the clotting factors, mainly fibrinogen, during the clotting process.
- It does not contain RBCs or clotting factors like factor II, V, VII, VIII and IX as they are removed during the clot formation.
- Serum retains the biochemical constituents of plasma, including electrolytes, proteins, hormones, and metabolites.

- Serum is often used for diagnostic tests that require measurement of specific analytes, such as blood glucose, cholesterol, or liver function tests.
- When blood is allowed to stand in a tube with red top or yellow top for one hour, it gets clotted and serum can be separated from it. By moving a thin stick along the side of the tube, the clot retracts and straw colored serum can be separated. If we pour the serum in a separate tube and centrifuge it at 3,000 rpm for 15 min, RBCs separate and settle down and clear serum can be obtained in the tube.

Plasma

- Plasma is the liquid component of blood that remains after whole blood is collected with an anticoagulant and then centrifuged to separate the cells from the liquid.
- Plasma contains all the components of whole blood, including red blood cells, white blood cells, platelets, and clotting factors (such as fibrinogen).
- Plasma is obtained after centrifugating the blood with anticoagulants, e.g., citrated blood at 3,000 RPM for 20 minutes. RBCs settle at the bottom and the plasma can be collected as the supernatant.

Uses of Serum

- **Diagnostic testing:** Serum is widely used in clinical laboratories for diagnostic testing. It is used to measure the levels of various analytes such as glucose, cholesterol, liver enzymes (e.g., alanine aminotransferase, aspartate aminotransferase), kidney function markers (e.g., creatinine), electrolytes (e.g., sodium, potassium), and hormonal markers (e.g., thyroid hormones).
- **Disease monitoring:** Serial measurements of specific serum markers can help monitor the progression or response to treatment of certain diseases. For example, tumor markers like prostate-specific antigen (PSA) or carcinoembryonic antigen (CEA) are measured in serum to monitor cancer progression.
- **Immunological testing:** Serum is used to detect and measure antibodies in various immunoassays, such as enzyme-linked immunosorbent assays (ELISA). It helps diagnose infectious diseases, autoimmune disorders, and assess immunization status.
- **Blood typing:** Serum is crucial for blood typing and cross-matching procedures to determine the compatibility between donor and recipient blood types before blood transfusions.

Uses of Plasma

- **Coagulation studies:** Plasma is used in coagulation tests to evaluate the clotting factors and screen for bleeding disorders. Tests like prothrombin time (PT), activated partial thromboplastin time (aPTT), and international normalized ratio (INR) require plasma.
- **Blood transfusion:** Plasma can be processed to obtain fresh frozen plasma (FFP), which contains clotting factors. FFP is transfused to patients with clotting factor deficiencies or to manage bleeding disorders.
- **Component separation:** Plasma can be further processed to obtain specific blood components such as cryoprecipitate (rich in clotting factors), albumin (used for plasma volume expansion), or platelet concentrates (for platelet transfusions).
- **Drug monitoring:** Plasma is used for therapeutic drug monitoring (TDM) to measure drug levels and adjust dosages for drugs with a narrow therapeutic index. It helps ensure the drug is within the desired therapeutic range and minimizes toxicity or inefficacy.

Table 4.1: Differences between serum and plasma.

	Serum	*Plasma*
Definition	The liquid portion of blood obtained after clotting	The liquid portion of blood obtained by anticoagulation
Formation	Formed after blood coagulates and clot is removed	Obtained by centrifuging whole blood with an anticoagulant
Components	Contains all blood components except clotting factors	Contains all blood components, including clotting factors
Clotting	Lacks clotting factors (fibrinogen, prothrombin, etc.)	Contains clotting factors necessary for coagulation
Usage	Used for testing analytes such as antibodies and enzymes	Used for testing clotting factors, blood gases, and more
Appearance	Clear, yellowish fluid	Straw-colored fluid
Preparation	Blood is allowed to clot and then centrifuged to obtain serum	Blood is anticoagulated, and centrifugation yields plasma

○ **Research:** Plasma is valuable for research purposes, such as investigating biomarkers, studying disease mechanisms, and developing new diagnostic tests or therapies.

The main differences between plasma and serum are depicted in **Table 4.1**.

BLOOD COLLECTION AND ANTICOAGULANTS

Phlebotomy

It is the collection of blood samples to evaluate the health status of a person. A needle is inserted into the vein and sample is collected.

Methods of Blood Collection

○ **Venipuncture:** It is the most common method of blood collection, where a needle is inserted into the vein, preferably in the arm, and a sample of blood is drawn into a tube.

○ **Fingerstick:** In this method, a small needle is used to pierce the skin on the finger and a drop of blood is collected on a special card or in a small tube.

○ **Heel stick:** This method is used to collect blood from newborns, in which small needles are used to prick the heel and collect a small sample of blood in a small tube.

Complications

○ **Failure to obtain blood:** This happens if the vein is missed, or excessive pull is applied to the plunger causing the collapse of the vein.

○ Occurrence of hematoma, thrombosis, thrombophlebitis, abscess, or bleeding.

○ Transmission of infections like hepatitis B or human immunodeficiency virus (HIV) if reusable syringes or needles which are not properly sterilized, are used.

Requirements for Blood Collection

○ **Tourniquets**
○ **Alcohol swabs**
○ **Band aid**
○ **Needles:** Different types of needle used in hematology are listed below:
18G: For blood transfusion.

21 G: Most common needle for venipuncture in adults.

23 G or butterflies: Used when a person's vein is much narrower than average and children.

○ **Syringes:** Sterilized glass syringes or disposable syringes as 2 mL, 5 mL, 10 mL and 20 mL can be used depending upon the type and quantity of sample needed.

○ **Vacutainers:** Vacutainers are used to collect blood by venipuncture. Different vacutainers used are identified by the stopper color/color tops and they have different additives or anticoagulants **(Table 4.2)**. These are:

Table 4.2: Different vacutainers used in hematology.

Color	Additive/anticoagulant	Uses
Red	Serum separator/no additive	Biochemistry studies after serum separation (LFTs, RFTs, hormones, serum electrolytes and blood bank)
Gray	Sodium fluoride	Used for glucose estimation

Contd...

Contd...

	Gel as additive	Biochemistry studies after serum separation (LFTs, RFTs, hormones, serum electrolytes and serum osmolality)
Yellow		
Blue	Citrate	Coagulation studies like PT, APTT, estimation of ESR by Westergren method
Green	Heparin	Osmotic fragility test, Immunophenotyping

Contd...

Contd...

	EDTA	Collection of whole blood for CBC, blood smear examination, hemoglobin estimation, electrophoresis, sickling test, ESR estimation
Lavender		

(For color version, see Plate 1)

Anticoagulants Used in Blood Collection

An anticoagulant must have the following characteristic properties:

- It must not alter the size of a cell.
- It must not cause hemolysis.
- It must minimize platelet aggregation
- It must be readily soluble in water and blood
- It must not disrupt the staining and leukocyte morphology.

The different anticoagulants used are listed in Table 4.3: Anticoagulated blood samples should be tested within 1–2 hours of collection. If this is not possible, the sample can be stored

Table 4.3: Anticoagulants used for blood collection.

Name	Mode of action	Concentration	Main uses	Disadvantages
Ethylene diamine tetra acetic acid (EDTA)	Chelation of calcium	1.5 mg/mL	Complete blood count	Excessive concentration of EDTA will cause shrinkage of RBCs and erroneous PCV, MCV, and MCHC results
Heparin	It interferes with the formation and or activity of thrombin	15 U/mL or 0.1–0.2 mg/mL	Osmotic fragility test	It causes clumping of leukocytes, interferes with staining of leukocytes. It causes blue background in blood smears; expensive
Double oxalate (sodium or potassium and ammonium oxalate in the ratio of 2:3 is used)	0.5 mL/5 mL	Removal of calcium	ESR and hematocrit	Leukocyte morphology is not well preserved, not suitable for smear examination. Cannot be used in blood banks as it causes the calcium to precipitate
Sodium fluoride	1 mg/mL	It inhibits the glycolytic enzymes responsible for the breakdown of glucose in the blood	Glucose estimation	Inhibition of urease, and glycolytic enzymes may interfere with urea and glucose determinations that employ enzyme activity

Contd...

Contd...

Name	Mode of action	Concentration	Main uses	Disadvantages
Tri sodium citrate	0.109 mg/mL	Chelation of calcium	Coagulation studies	It has a tendency to shrink cells

in a refrigerator at 4–6°C for a maximum of 24 hour.

Sequence of Filling the Tubes

The following order of filling of tubes should be followed after the withdrawal of blood from the patient if multiple investigations are ordered, mix all tubes by inverting 6–8 times:

○ **First tube (yellow top):** Blood culture.

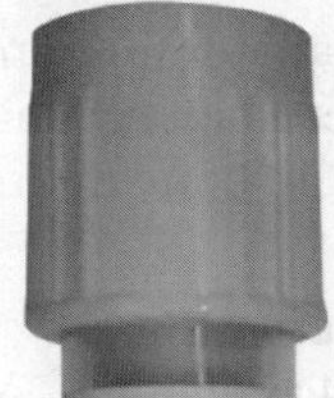

(For color version, see Plate 2)

○ **Second tube—blue top with 3.2% sodium citrate:** Coagulation studies.

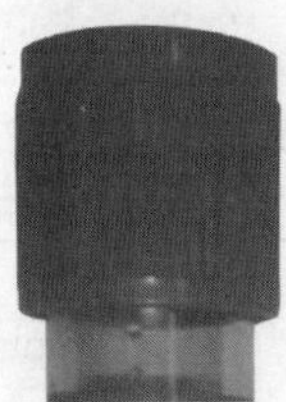

(For color version, see Plate 2)

○ **Third tube—red top without any preservative:** Serum chemistry

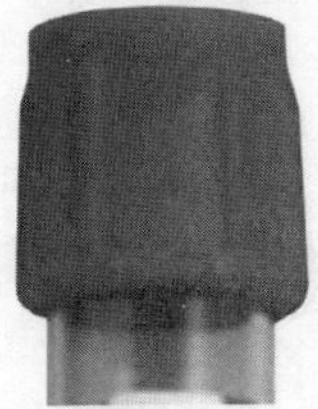

(For color version, see Plate 2)

○ **Fourth tube—green top with sodium heparin:** Osmotic fragility test, immunophenotyping

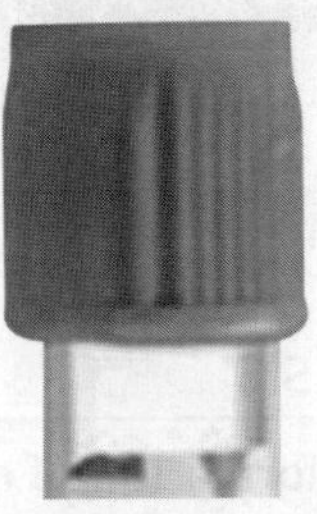

(For color version, see Plate 2)

○ **Fifth tube—lavender top with EDTA:** For collection of whole blood for CBC

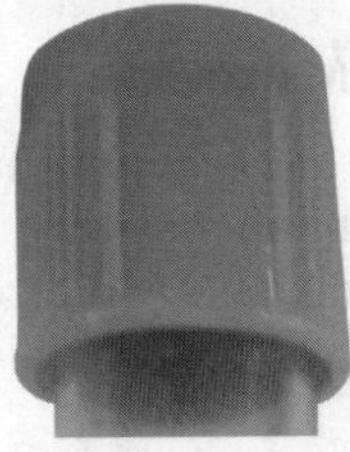

(For color version, see Plate 2)

○ **Sixth tube—gray top with sodium fluoride as a preservative:** Glucose estimation

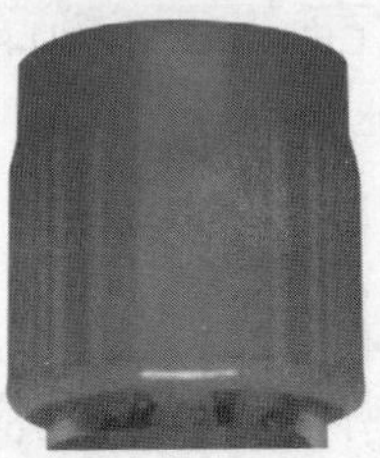

(For color version, see Plate 2)

Table 4.4: Hematopoiesis sites and stages.

Stage of life	Stage	Site
3rd week of intrauterine life	Mesoblastic	Yolk sac
3rd month	Hepatic	Liver, spleen, lymph node, thymus
4th month and after	Myeloid	Bone marrow (pelvis, vertebra, skull, ribs, sternum, long bones)

Table 4.5: Types of bone marrow.

Type of BM	Composition	Seen in
Red/active BM	Hematopoietic tissue	Children
Yellow/inactive BM	Fat cells	Elderly/old age

HEMATOPOIESIS

The process of formation of cellular components of blood is known as hematopoiesis. It is a physiological phenomenon with different principal sites of formation as shown in **Table 4.4**.

Types of Bone Marrow

BM is primarily of two types **(Table 4.5)**:
1. Red (active) bone marrow
2. Yellow (inactive) bone marrow

Process of Hematopoiesis

All the blood cell components are derived from pleuripotent hematopoietic stem cells (PHSC), present in bone marrow as depicted in **Figure 4.1**.

Properties of stem cells
- Express CD34 antigen
- Have a capacity of self-renewal
- Resemble lymphocytes morphologically.

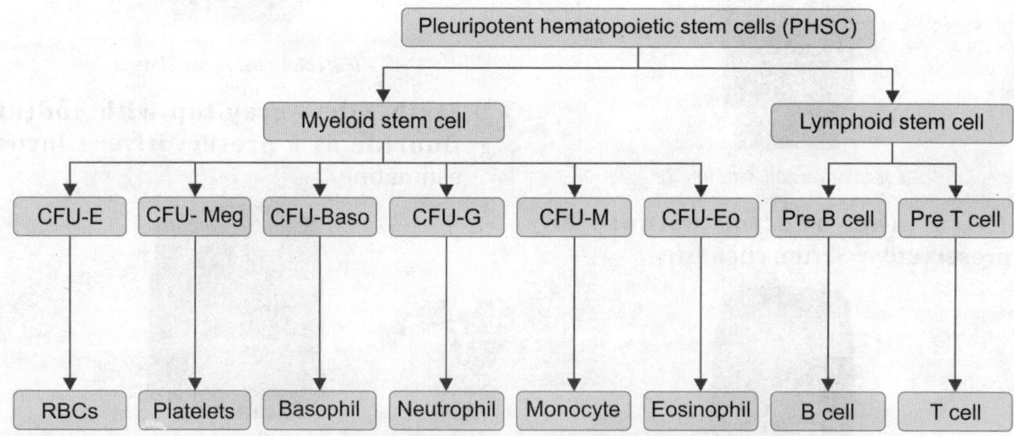

Fig. 4.1: Process of hematopoiesis.

(CFU-E: colony stimulating factor—erythroid; CFU-Meg: colony stimulating factor—megakaryocyte; CSF-Baso: colony stimulating factor—basophil; CSF-G: colony stimulating factor—granulocyte; CSF-M: colony stimulating factor—monocyte; CSF-Eo: colony stimulating factor—eosinophil)

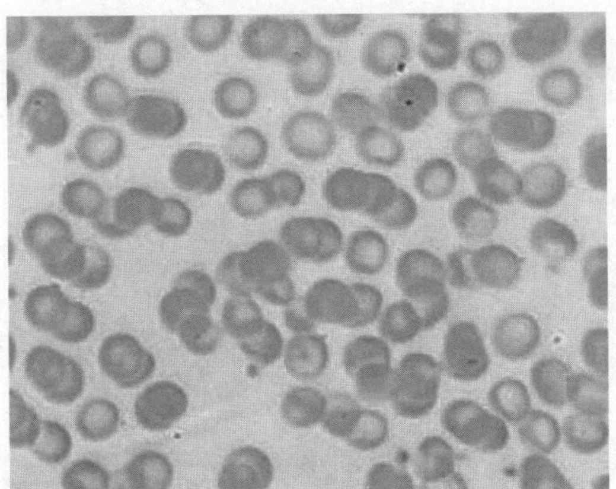

Fig. 4.2: Red blood cells (RBCs) in the blood smear.
(For color version, see Plate 2)

Extramedullary Hematopoiesis

It is the process of formation and activation of blood components outside the bone marrow such as spleen, liver, lymph node. It is seen in certain infections and diseases like leukemias, lymphomas, myeloproliferative neoplasm, etc.

Erythropoiesis

Red Blood Cells (Fig. 4.2)

The process of formation of red blood cells is known as erythropoiesis.

Stages of Erythropoiesis

Refer **Table 4.6**.

Granulopoiesis

White Blood Cells

The process of formation of white blood cells (WBCs) is known as granulopoiesis.

Types of WBCS

○ Granulocytes (called so because of the presence of granules in cytoplasm). It includes:
  ○ Neutrophils
  ○ Eosinophils
  ○ Basophils
○ Agranulocytes (called so because of the absence or few granules in cytoplasm). It includes:
  ○ Lymphocytes (small and large)
  ○ Monocytes

Each of the cell of WBCs series is explained in detail below:

Neutrophils (Fig. 4.3)

Stages of maturation of a neutrophil are depicted in **Table 4.7**.
Function: It plays an important role in acute inflammation.

Eosinophil

The following are the characteristic features of eosinophil **(Fig. 4.4)**:
Size: 15–16 um

Stage	Type of erythroblast	Size (u)	Nucleus (N) and cytoplasm (C)
	Table 4.6: Stages of erythropoiesis.		
1	Proerythroblast	15–20	Large nucleus with immature chromatin, usually single nucleolus, cytoplasm is blue in color
2	Early/Basophilic erythroblast	12–16	Chromatin is fine with barely visible nucleolus, deep blue colored cytoplasm
3	Intermediate/Polychromatophilic	12–15	Coarse chromatin with polychromatic cytoplasm
4	Late/Orthochromatic erythroblast	8–12	Pyknotic, small, dense, blue colored N with polychromatic cytoplasm
5	Reticulocyte	8–10	There is no nucleus, cytoplasm is polychromatic with remnants of RNA
6	Mature RBC/erythrocyte (as shown in **Fig. 4.2**)	7–9	No nucleus, cytoplasm is pink in color with central 1/3rd pallor

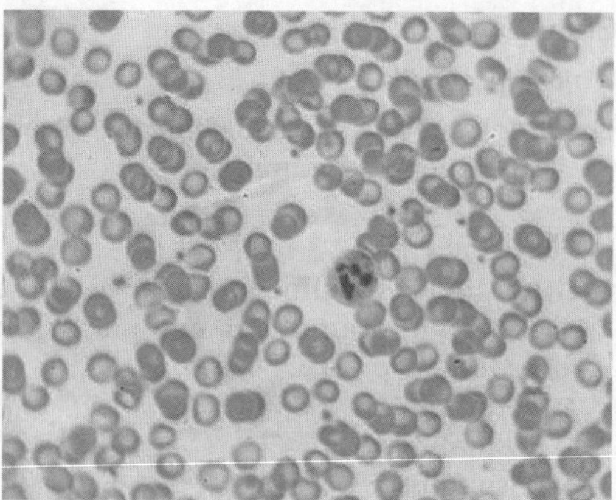

Fig. 4.3: A bilobed neutrophil in the center of the blood smear.

(For color version, see Plate 2)

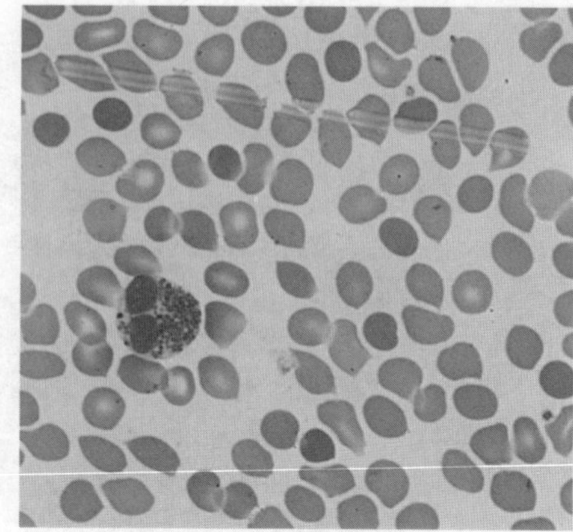

Fig. 4.4: Bilobed eosinophil in the center of the blood smear.

(For color version, see Plate 2)

Table 4.7: Stages of maturation of a neutrophil.

Stage	Cell	Size (u)	Nucleus and cytoplasm
1	Myeloblast	15–20	Fine chromatin, 2–3 nucleoli, large nucleus with scant light blue cytoplasm
2	Promyelocyte	16–20	Nucleus is slightly eccentric, show azurophilic granules in cytoplasm
3	Myelocyte	14–18	Condensed chromatin, nucleoli disappear. There is predominance of specific granules
4	Metamyelocyte	14–18	Kidney shaped/indented nucleus, faint pink cytoplasm
5	Band form	14–16	Band/U-shaped nucleus, clumped chromatin, pink cytoplasm
6	Mature neutrophil	14–15	2–5 lobed nucleus joined by chromatin strands, pink cytoplasm and blue granules **(Fig. 4.3)**

Nucleus: 2–3 lobed

Cytoplasm: Cytoplasm is of pink color with large, bright orange red granules packed in cytoplasm.

It plays an important role in allergic and parasitic infections.

Basophil

Size: 9–12 um.

Presence of large, coarse, deep purple-colored granules cover the nucleus making it difficult to appreciate the nucleus and cytoplasm.

Monocyte

The morphological features of monocyte are **(Fig. 4.5)**:

Size: 15–20 um, largest of all the leukocytes.

Nucleus: Kidney shaped with fine chromatin.

Cytoplasm: Abundant, ground glass cytoplasm with presence of vacuolations in cytoplasm.

Small Lymphocyte

Size: 7–8 um.

Nucleus: Large nucleus with blue-colored clumped chromatin.

Cytoplasm: Thin rim of light blue cytoplasm.

Large Lymphocyte

The morphological features of a large lymphocyte are as under **(Fig. 4.6)**.

Size: 10–15 um

Nucleus: Oval to round shaped

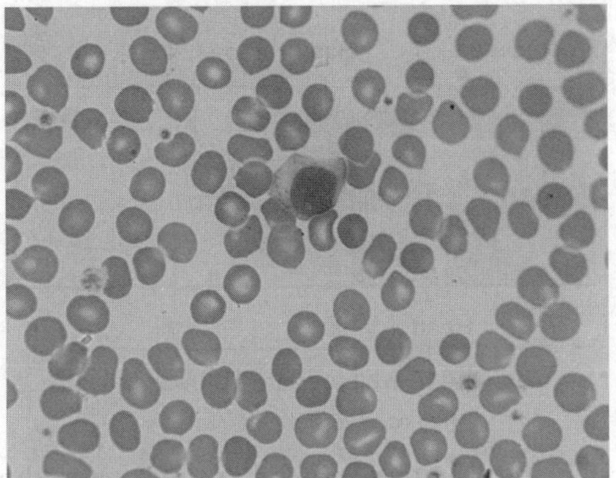

Fig. 4.5: Monocyte in the center of the blood smear.

(For color version, see Plate 3)

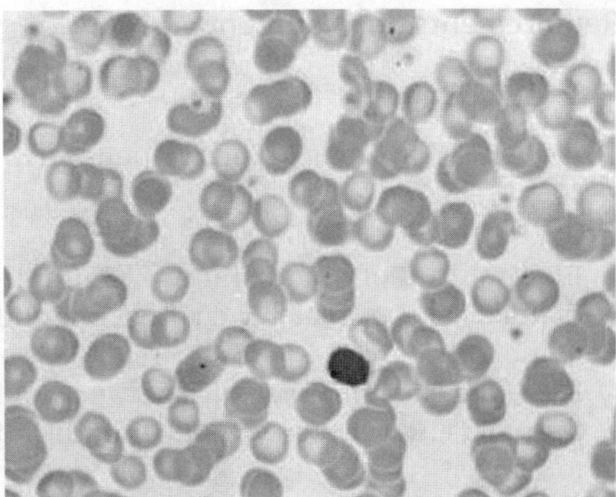

Fig. 4.6: Large lymphocyte in the center of the blood smear.

(For color version, see Plate 3)

Cytoplasm: Abundant pale blue cytoplasm with few azurophilic granules.

Thrombopoiesis

Platelets

The process of formation of platelets is called as thrombopoiesis.

The morphologically identifiable stages of thrombopoiesis are:

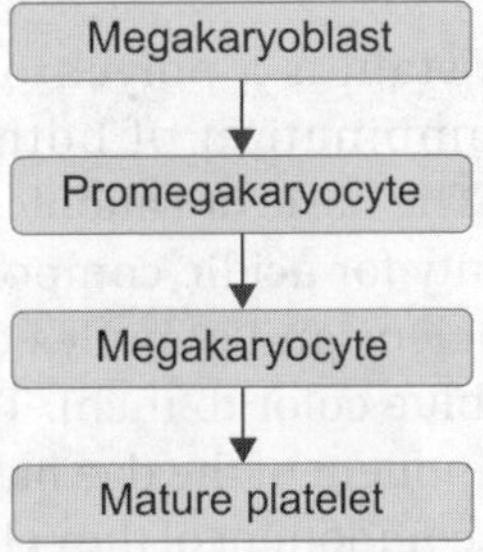

These are small, 1–3 um blood cells, purple in color.

They play an important role in blood clotting.

BLOOD SMEAR PREPARATION AND STAINING

Blood smear is a specimen that is prepared by spreading a drop of blood on a clear glass slide followed by staining for examination under a microscope.

Uses of Peripheral Blood Smear

The uses of peripheral blood smear are listed below:

- ❍ Evaluation of anemia
- ❍ Evaluation of platelet count
- ❍ To do TLC, DLC
- ❍ Identification of abnormal cells/blast
- ❍ To identify Inclusions like basophilic stippling, Howell-Jolly bodies, Cabot ring, etc.
- ❍ To identify parasites like malaria, microfilaria, etc.

Methods of Preparation of Blood Smear

There are five types of blood smears:

1. The wedge smear
2. The cover glass smear
3. The spun smear
4. Buffy coat smear
5. Thick blood smears for blood parasites

Preparation by Blood Smear by Wedge Method

It is the most common, convenient as well as easy method that is used for blood smear preparation.

Requirements of Equipment

○ Spreaders
○ Clean glass slides
○ Blood capillary tube or micropipette 10 μL

Steps

○ Place a drop of blood, about 2–3 mm in diameter approximately 1 cm from one end of the slide.
○ Place the slide on a flat surface, and hold the other end between your left thumb and forefinger.
○ Hold the spreader with your right hand with its smooth clean edge on the specimen slide, just in front of the blood drop.
○ Hold the spreader slide at a 30–45° angle, and draw it back against the drop of blood.
○ Allow the blood to spread almost to the edges of the slide and make the smear with the gentle, free and forward movement of your right hand.
○ Label one edge with patient name, laboratory ID and date.
○ The slides should be rapidly air dried by waving in the air.

Precautions

Some of the precautions to be taken during the slide preparation are:
○ The glass slide should be clean and grease free.
○ Put a drop of blood appropriate size as if a drop is too large, then the smear will be thick and if the drop is too small, then it will be too thin smear.
○ The edge of the spreader should be smooth
○ The spreader should be at an angle of 30 degree while preparing the smear.
○ The movement of the spreader should be forward and free.

Characteristics of a Good Blood Smear

○ Good smear should be tongue shaped with head, body and tail as shown in **Figure 4.7**.

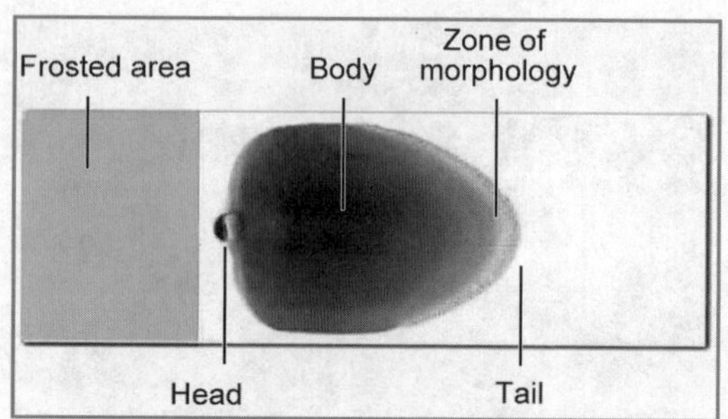

Fig. 4.7: A well prepared blood smear.
(For color version, see Plate 3)

○ It should not cover the entire area of the slide.
○ It should have both thick and thin areas with gradual transition.
○ It should not contain any lines or holes.
○ It should not contain any striations.

Staining of the Blood Smear

Leishman Stain

This stain is named after its inventor William Boog Leishman, who was the British Pathologist.

Principle of Leishman Stain

Leishman's stain is a polychromatic stain with the combination of both basic and acidic dyes. The basic or cationic component has the affinity for acidic components of the cells like nucleus and granules of basophils and impart blue color to them. The acidic or anionic component of the dye has the affinity for the basic component of the cell and impart pink color like granules of eosinophil or hemoglobin.

The components are depicted in **Table 4.8**.

Precautions for Storing of Stain

○ Keep the prepared stain in dark colored bottle with tight stopper.
○ It should be stored at room temperature in a cool and dark place.

Table 4.8: The components of Leishman stain.

Sl. No.	Component	Nature of the dye	Function
1.	Methanol	—	Fixes smear to the slide
2.	Methylene blue	Cationic/basic	Stains RNA, DNA in blue-grey color
3.	Eosin	Anionic/acidic	Stains hemoglobin, eosin granules orange-red color

○ It should not be exposed to direct sunlight to prevent the deterioration of the stain.

Steps of Staining

○ Air dry the smear and fix it with methyl alcohol for 2–3 minutes.
○ Place the slide on the staining rack placed over the sink.
○ Flood the smear with Leishman stain for 2 minutes.
○ Add double the amount of buffer solution and mix the stain by blowing gently over the slide.
○ Leave the stain on the slide for 10–15 min.
○ A metallic scum/sheen will appear on the surface as depicted in a **Figure 4.8**.
○ Wash off the stain by running water.
○ Wipe the slide from the back side.
○ keep slide on end of the rack, and let dry in air.

Characteristics of a Good Stained Smear

○ It should be of pink color at thinner areas
○ At thicker areas, it should be purple blue

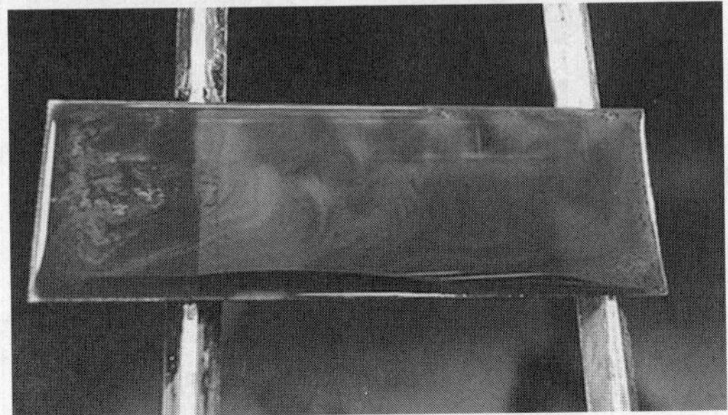

Fig. 4.8: A metallic sheen on the slide.
(For color version, see Plate 3)

○ There should be no precipitates of residual stain on the smear.

Examination of Peripheral Blood Film

A blood smear is examined for the following:
○ **RBCs:** To look for morphology, inclusions, immature form.
○ **WBCs:** To do total leukocyte count (TLC), differential leucocyte count (DLC), to look for abnormal or immature forms.
○ **Platelets:** To do platelet count and look for abnormal forms.
○ To look for parasites like malaria, filaria.

Examination of PBF at:

10X/low power:
○ To assess whether the smear is properly spread and stained.
○ To assess the cell distribution.
○ To find an appropriate area for blood cell examination.
○ To see rouleaux formation or autoagglutination.

40X/high power:
○ To do DLC, TLC.
○ To look for red cell morphology.

100X/Oil immersion:
○ For detailed examination of any abnormal cell.
○ To do platelet count.
○ To look for parasite.

RED BLOOD CELLS AND ITS ABNORMALITIES

Normal morphological characteristics of RBCs are the following:

○ **Size:** 7–9 um
○ **Shape:** Biconcave disc shaped
○ **Staining:** Deep pink at periphery and pale in the center, i.e., central 1/3rd area is pallor
○ Size of a RBC corresponds to the size of a nucleus of a small lymphocyte.
○ Normal RBCs are normocytic (of normal size) and normochromic (normal staining intensity).

Red Cell Abnormalities

RBCs with Abnormal Size/Anisocytosis

Variation in the size of cells is known as anisocytosis.

It is seen in various conditions as listed in **Table 4.9**.

RBCs with Abnormal Staining

Refer **Table 4.10**.

RBCs with Abnormal Shape/Poikilocytosis (Table 4.11)

Increased variation in red cell shape is called poikilocytosis. Red cells with variation in cell shape are known as poikilocyte.

Immature RBCs

Refer **Table 4.12**.

Red Cells with Abnormal Arrangement (Table 4.13)

Abnormal RBCs rearrangement can be in the form of rouleaux or agglutination.

Table 4.9: RBCs with abnormal size.

Abnormal size	Size of a RBC	Seen in
Microcytes	Size of a RBC is smaller than normal	Iron deficiency anemia, thalassemia, anemia of chronic disease
Macrocytes	Size of a RBC is larger than normal	Oval macrocytes are seen in megaloblastic anemia, myelodysplastic syndrome, and in patients being treated with cancer chemotherapy. Round macrocytes are seen in liver disease, alcoholism and hypothyroidism

Table 4.10: RBCs with abnormal staining.

Abnormal staining	Pallor of RBC	Seen in
Hypochromia	Red cells have increased area of central pallor (i.e., containing less hemoglobin)	Iron deficiency, thalassemias, anemia of chronic disease, and sideroblastic anemia
Hyperchromia	Increase in the intensity of red blood cell color	Spherocytes, microspherocytes or macrocytes

Table 4.11: RBCs with abnormal shape.

Cell	Abnormal shape	Seen in
Sickle cell	Narrow and elongated red cells with one or both ends pointed	Sickle cell anemia
Spherocytes	Smaller in size than normal RBCs, intensely stained and round in shape without any central area of pallor	• Hereditary spherocytosis • Autoimmune hemolytic anemia (warm antibody type) • ABO hemolytic disease of newborn
Burr cells/echinocytes	Small sized RBCs with regularly placed small projections on the surface	Uremia
Acanthocytes	Irregularly spaced sharp projections of variable length on surface of RBCs	• Liver disease • Post-splenectomy

Contd...

Contd...

Cell	Abnormal shape	Seen in
Schistocytes	Fragmented RBCs, which take various forms like helmet, crescent, triangle, etc.	• Microangiopathic hemolytic anemia • Cardiac valve prosthesis • Severe burns
Tear drop cells/dacryocytes	RBCs having the shape of tear drops	Myelofibrosis and myelophthisic anemia
Bite cells	A part of RBC is bitten off	G6PD deficiency

Table 4.12: Immature RBCs.

Cell	Morphology	Seen in
Polychromatic RBC	Larger than normal RBCs, diffuse bluish grey and contain remnants of RNA	• Hemolytic anemia • Acute blood loss • Following specific therapy for nutritional anemia
Nucleated RBCs (nRBCs)	RBCs with nucleus	• Hemolytic disease of newborn • Hemolytic anemia • Leukemias • Myelophthisic anemia • Myelofibrosis

Table 4.13: RBCs with abnormal arrangement.

Rearrangement	Cellular morphology	Seen in
Rouleaux formation	Stack of coins	• Multiple myeloma • Waldenström's macroglobulinemia • Hypergammaglobulinemia • Hyperfibrinogenemia
Autoagglutination	Clumping of RBCs in large, irregular groups on blood smear	Cold agglutinin disease

WHITE BLOOD CELLS AND ITS ABNORMALITIES

White blood cells (WBCs) are divided into granulocytes and agranulocytes.

The normal morphology of WBCS has already been explained. This chapter will be explaining the abnormalities in WBCs **(Table 4.14)**.

Some of the abnormalities seen in WBCs are depicted in **Table 4.14.**

Neutrophilia

When an absolute neutrophil count (ANC) is >7,500/µL, it is called neutrophilia or neutrophilic leukocytosis.

Causes

The causes of neutrophilia are listed in **Table 4.15**.

Neutropenia

It is defined as a decrease in absolute neutrophil count (ANC), <2,000/µL.

It is graded into three types:

○ Mild, when ANC is between 2,000–1,000/µL
○ Moderate when ANC is 1,000–500/µL
○ Severe, when ANC is <500/µL

Causes

Causes of neutropenia are listed in **Table 4.16**.

Table 4.14: Abnormalities seen in WBCs.

Abnormal WBC	Morphological details	Seen in
Döhle inclusion bodies	Oval, pale blue colored small inclusions present in the periphery of cytoplasm in neutrophil, comprising of ribosomes and rough endoplasmic reticulum	Bacterial infection/sepsis
Toxic granules	Blue colored darkly stained coarse granules seen in the cytoplasm of neutrophils	Bacterial infection/sepsis
Cytoplasmic vacuolation	Vacuolations are seen in the cytoplasm of leukocyte	Bacterial infection/sepsis
Hypersegmented neutrophils **(Fig. 4.9)**	When >5% of neutrophils have 5 or more lobes (as shown in **Fig. 4.9**)	Vitamin B12 or folate deficiency
Left shift of neutrophils	Immature cells of neutrophil series	Bacterial infection/sepsis
Atypical lymphocytes	Large, irregularly shaped lymphocytes with abundant cytoplasm and irregular nuclei and occasional nucleolus	Viral infections Infectious mononucleosis
Blast **(Fig. 4.10)**	Premature, large (15–25 μm), round to oval cells, with high nuclear cytoplasmic ratio. Nucleus shows one or more nucleoli and nuclear chromatin is immature (as shown in **Fig. 4.10**)	Leukemia

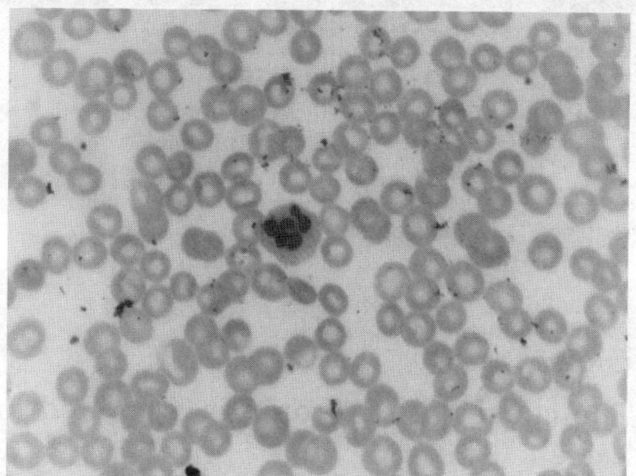

Fig. 4.9: Hypersegmented neutrophil having 6 lobes present in the center of the blood smear.

(For color version, see Plate 3)

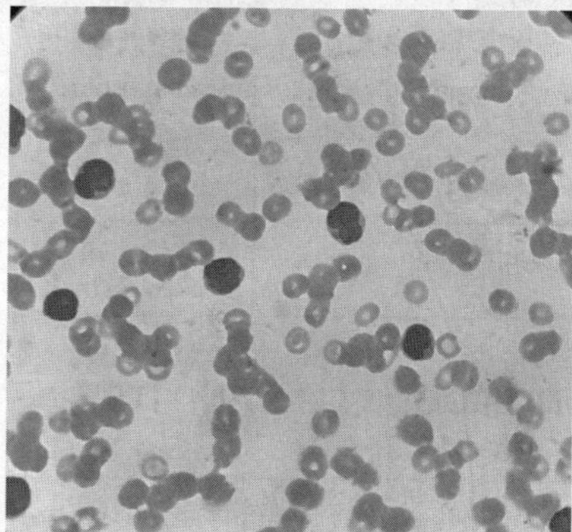

Fig. 4.10: Showing the multiple blasts that are larger in size with high N:C ratio with prominent nucleolus in some of them.

(For color version, see Plate 4)

Table 4.15: Causes of neutrophilia.

Conditions	Example
Acute bacterial infections	Abscess, pneumonia, meningitis, septicemia, acute rheumatic fever, urinary tract infection
Acute blood loss	Trauma, accidents, intra operative
Metabolic disorders	Uremia, acidosis, gout

Contd...

Contd...

Conditions	Example
Tissue injury	Burns, necrosis, myocardial infarction.
Blood disorders	Myeloproliferative disorders, leukemia, etc.
Physiological causes	Exercise, labor, pregnancy, stress.

Table 4.16: Causes of neutropenia.

Conditions	Example
Certain infections	Typhoid, paratyphoid, tuberculosis, influenza, measles, rubella, infectious mononucleosis, malaria, etc.
Drugs	Analgesics, antibiotics, anticancer drugs, antithyroid drugs, anticonvulsant, etc.
Blood related disorders	Megaloblastic anemia, aplastic anemia, myelofibrosis, infiltration of marrow by tumor cells, etc.
Miscellaneous	• Hypersplenism • Exposure to ionizing radiation • Felty syndrome, etc

Eosinophilia

When absolute eosinophil count (AEC) is >600/µL, it is known as eosinophilia. The causes of eosinophilia are listed in **Table 4.17**.

Table 4.17: Causes of eosinophilia.

Conditions	Example
Allergic conditions	Asthma, rhinitis, hay fever, urticaria, etc.
Parasitic infections	Filariasis, trichinosis, echinococcosis
Blood disorders	Hodgkin's disease, chronic myeloproliferative disorders
Miscellaneous	Loeffler's syndrome, tropical eosinophilia, hypereosinophilic syndrome, exposure to radiotherapy, etc.

Basophilia

It is defined as increased number of basophils in blood (>100/µL).

Causes

○ Chronic myeloid leukemia (CML)
○ Polycythemia vera
○ Idiopathic myelofibrosis
○ Basophilic leukemia, etc.

Monocytosis

It is defined as an increase in the absolute monocyte count >1,000/µL.

Some of the causes of monocytosis are listed below.

○ **Infections:** Tuberculosis, subacute bacterial endocarditis, malaria, kala azar
○ Autoimmune disorders.
○ **Hematologic diseases:** Myeloproliferative disorders, monocytic leukemia, Hodgkin's disease.

Lymphocytosis

It is defined as an increase in absolute lymphocyte count above 4,000/µL in adults, >7,200/µL in adolescents, >9,000/µL in children and infants.

Causes of Lymphocytosis

○ **Infections:** Cytomegalovirus, mumps, rubella, varicella, Tuberculosis, parasitic infestation.

○ **Hematological disorders:** Acute lymphoblastic leukemia (ALL), chronic lymphocytic leukemia (CLL), multiple myeloma, lymphoma.

○ **Miscellaneous:** Serum sickness, post-vaccination, drug reactions.

PLATELETS AND ITS DISORDERS

Platelets are produced in bone marrow from megakaryocytes by their cytoplasmic fragmentation.

Life-span of platelets is about 7–10 days. Normal platelet count in peripheral blood is 1.5–4.0 lac/μL.

Functions: Adhesion, release reaction, and aggregation.

Thrombocytopenia

It is defined as the decrease in platelet count.

The causes and consequences of thrombocytopenia are given in **Table 4.18**.

Platelet count in the range of 1,50,000–50,000/μL is generally not associated with bleeding.

Count between 50,000–20,000/μL causes excess bleeding following surgery or mild degree of spontaneous bleeding.

The platelet count below 20,000/μL is usually associated with spontaneous, severe hemorrhage.

Table 4.18: Causes of thrombocytopenia.

Causes of thrombocytopenia	Seen in
1. Increased destruction of platelets	
a. Disorder	• Idiopathic thrombocytopenic purpura (ITP) • Disseminated intravascular coagulopathy (DIC)
b. Infections	• Malaria, dengue, septicemia, subacute bacterial endocarditis, rubella, etc.
c. Drugs	Quinine, heparin, procainamide
d. Miscellaneous	• Massive blood transfusion • Thrombotic thrombocytopenic purpura • Alcohol • Toxemia of pregnancy
2. Increased pooling of platelets in spleen	Hypersplenism
3. Decreased production of platelets in bone marrow	• Aplastic anemia • Bone marrow infiltration by leukemias, lymphomas, myeloma • Megaloblastic anemia • Drugs • Infections • Radiation
4. Defective platelet function	
a. Acquired causes	• Drugs like NSAIDS, antibiotics, aspirin, etc • Myeloproliferative disorders • Uremia
b. Hereditary causes	• Bernard-Soulier syndrome • Glanzmann's thrombasthenia

Thrombocytosis

It is defined as increase in platelet count > 4,00,000/µL.

TOTAL LEUKOCYTE COUNT AND DIFFERENTIAL LEUKOCYTE COUNT

Total leukocyte count (TLC) refers to the total number of WBCs in the blood.

Differential leukocyte count (DLC), also known as a white blood cell differential provides information about the different types of white blood cells (leukocytes) present in a blood sample.

Estimation of TLC

Various methods are available for the measurement which include manual method using a Neubauer's chamber or by an automated electronic cell counter.

Manual Method

Principle: Whole blood on being diluted with WBC fluid hemolyses the RBCs. Nuclei of the nucleated WBCs get stained by the gentian violet dye and can be visualized under the microscope using a Neubauer's chamber.

The manual method for measuring the total leukocyte count (TLC) involves using a hemocytometer and a microscope. Materials needed:

- Hemocytometer set containing WBC pipette and improved Neubauer's chamber with coverslip.
- Diluting fluid (such as Turk's solution).
- WBC pipette (usually calibrated at 1:20 dilution).
- Microscope
- Pipettes
- Timer or stopwatch
- Clean glass slides

Composition of WBC Diluting Fluid

- Glacial acetic acid: 2 mL
- Gentian violet 1%—5-10 drops to stain WBCs
- Water—100 mL

Procedure

- Prepare the diluting fluid:
  - Follow the instructions or guidelines provided with the specific diluting fluid being used.
  - Prepare the diluting fluid by following the recommended dilution ratio and ensure it is properly mixed.
- Clean the Neubauer's chamber:
  - Clean the Neubauer's chamber thoroughly with ethanol or an appropriate cleaning agent to ensure it is free from any debris or contaminants.
  - Place a clean coverslip over the central square grid of the Neubauer's chamber, ensuring that there are no air bubbles trapped underneath.
- Dilute the blood sample:
  - Mix the blood sample well to ensure it is properly homogenized.
  - Using a WBC pipette, draw the blood sample to mark 0.5 on the pipette. Now fill the pipette with Turk's fluid up to the mark 11 by drawing fluid from the bottle. This is 1:20 dilution.
  - Mix the diluted blood sample gently by rotating the pipette to ensure it is well mixed. The white bead in the pipette helps in thorough mixing.
  - Discard one drop of WBC fluid as the fluid up to mark 1 was not mixed with blood.
- Load the Neubauer's chamber:
  - Carefully place a small drop of the diluted blood sample onto the edge of the coverslip of the Neubauer's chamber.
  - Capillary action will draw the diluted blood sample between the coverslip and the Neubauer's chamber, filling the counting chambers.

The Neubauer chamber is a type of hemocytometer used for manual cell counting. The Neubauer chamber has specific size and dimensions. Here are the commonly used dimensions of a Neubauer chamber:

- **Overall dimensions:** The Neubauer chamber typically has an overall size of approximately 20 mm × 20 mm.
- **Grid pattern:** The central area of the Neubauer chamber contains a grid pattern used for cell counting. This grid is further divided into several squares and lines to facilitate counting. The central grid typically covers an area of 1 mm × 1 mm.
- **Counting area:** The central grid of the Neubauer chamber is further divided into 9 large squares, each measuring 1 mm × 1 mm in size. Each of these large squares is divided into smaller squares, making up a total of 25 (5 × 5) small squares.
- **Depth:** The depth of the chamber is typically around 0.1 mm. This allows for proper visualization and counting of cells within the chamber.

1. **Counting:**
   - Allow the blood cells to settle for a specific period of time, usually 5 minutes, to ensure proper settling of cells on the counting grid.
   - Place the Neubauer's chamber on the microscope stage and set the appropriate magnification.
   - Focus the microscope to visualize the cells within the counting area of the Neubauer's chamber that is the 4 large corner square (1 × 1 mm) each.
   - Record the number of white blood cells counted.

2. **Calculation:**
   - Use the formula provided with the specific dilution used to calculate the total leukocyte count based on the number of cells counted.

4* corner squares counted.

- TLC = N × 20/4* × 0.1
    = N × 50

Where 0.1 is the depth of the chamber and dilution is 1 in 20.

N is number of WBCs in 4 large squares.

Nucleated RBCs are not lysed, do not get stained and hence are counted with the WBCs. If nucleated RBCs are more than 4/100 WBCs in the DLC, a correction for nucleated RBCs should be made.

Corrected TLC = TLC × 100/100 + number of nRBCs per 100 WBCs.

Normal Range of TLC

- Adults 4,000–10,000 cells/cumm
- At birth 8,000–28,000 cells/cumm
- Children 6,000–15,000 cells/cumm

Causes of Leukocytosis (Raised White Blood Cell Count >11,000/cumm)

- **Infection:** Bacterial, viral, fungal, or parasitic infections can stimulate the production of white blood cells as part of the immune response.
- **Inflammation:** Inflammatory conditions such as rheumatoid arthritis, inflammatory bowel disease, or tissue injury can lead to an increased white blood cell count.
- **Medications:** Certain medications, such as corticosteroids, can cause leukocytosis as a side effect.
- **Physical or emotional stress:** Stressful conditions, including severe exercise, trauma, or emotional stress, can trigger leukocytosis.
- **Smoking:** Smoking tobacco products can cause an increase in white blood cell count.
- **Leukemia:** Various types of leukemia, a cancer of the blood cells, can lead to significantly elevated white blood cell counts.
- **Other underlying medical conditions:** Certain medical conditions, such as myeloproliferative disorders (e.g.,

polycythemia vera), can result in leukocytosis.

Causes of Leukopenia (Decreased White Blood Cell Count <4,000/cumm)

- **Bone marrow disorders:** Diseases affecting the bone marrow, such as aplastic anemia, myelodysplastic syndrome, or chemotherapy-induced suppression of bone marrow function, can lead to a decrease in white blood cell production.
- **Infections:** Some viral infections like HIV, can cause a decrease in white blood cell count by directly attacking and reducing the number of white blood cells.
- **Autoimmune disorders:** Autoimmune conditions such as systemic lupus erythematosus (SLE) or rheumatoid arthritis can cause leukopenia due to immune system dysregulation.
- **Medications:** Certain medications, such as chemotherapy drugs, immunosuppressants, or certain antibiotics can cause leukopenia as a side effect.
- **Vitamin deficiencies:** Deficiencies in vitamins like vitamin B12 or folate can lead to decreased white blood cell production.
- **Radiation exposure:** Exposure to high levels of radiation can suppress bone marrow function and lead to leukopenia.
- **Sepsis:** Severe infections especially those progressing to sepsis can lead to leukopenia due to an overwhelming immune response.

Automated Method for Cell Counting

Automated electronic cell counters are widely used in clinical laboratories for the rapid and accurate measurement of various blood cell parameters. These instruments utilize different principles to count and characterize blood cells. The two commonly employed principles are impedance-based and optical-based methods:

1. **Impedance-based principle:**
- This principle relies on changes in electrical impedance as cells pass through a small aperture or channel.
- A diluted blood sample is aspirated into the instrument, and the cells flow through a narrow flow cell.
- As each cell passes through the aperture, it causes a change in electrical impedance.
- The impedance changes are detected and measured, and the information is used to determine cell counts and size.
- Different cell types (such as red blood cells, white blood cells, and platelets) have distinct impedance characteristics, allowing the instrument to differentiate and count them.

2. **Optical-based principle:**
- Optical-based methods employ light scattering and absorption properties of cells to determine their characteristics.
- A light source, typically a laser or halogen lamp emits a beam of light that interacts with the cells.
- **Forward scatter:** The intensity of light scattered in the forward direction is measured providing information about cell size.
- **Side scatter:** The intensity of light scattered at larger angles is measured providing information about cell granularity and internal structure.
- **Absorption:** The amount of light absorbed by cells at specific wavelengths is measured, allowing identification of specific cell types based on their optical properties.

The detected light signals are processed and analyzed by the instrument's software to determine cell counts, size and various parameters.

These automated electronic cell counters are capable of processing a large number of samples quickly and providing comprehensive information about different blood cell populations. The instruments are calibrated

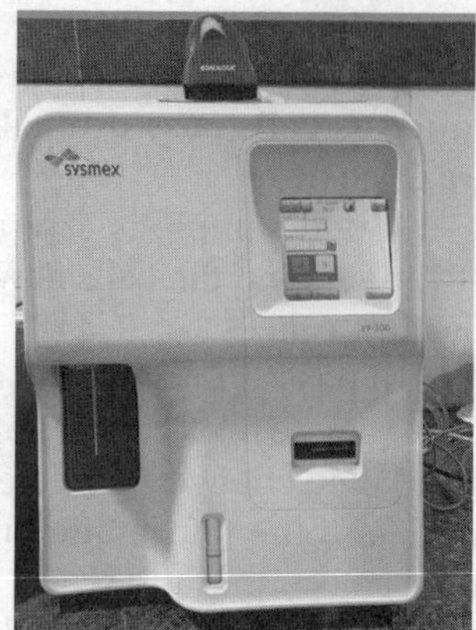

Fig. 4.11: Showing electronic 3-part differential counter.

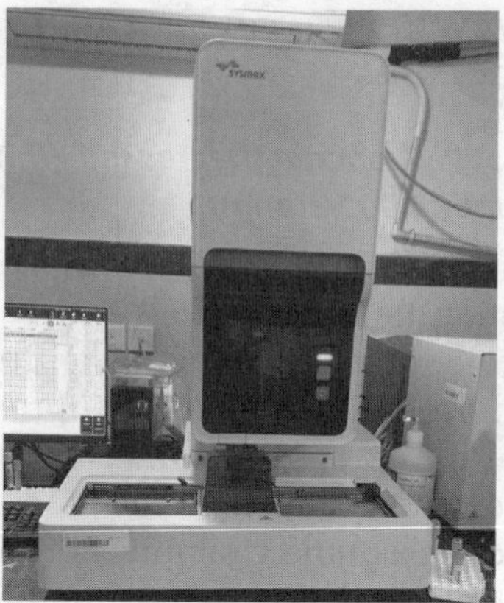

Fig. 4.12: Showing electronic 6-part differential counter.

and validated against reference methods to ensure accuracy and precision in cell counting and characterization.

The differences between 3-part and 6-part cell counters lie in the number of blood cell populations they can identify and the parameters they provide.

3-Part Cell Counter (Fig. 4.11)

○ **Cell populations:** A 3-part cell counter identifies and differentiates three main blood cell populations—red blood cells (RBCs), white blood cells (WBCs) and platelets.
○ **Parameters:** It provides basic parameters such as total RBC count, hemoglobin concentration, hematocrit, total WBC count and platelet count.
○ **WBC differential:** While it can provide a total WBC count, it typically does not provide a detailed breakdown of different WBC subtypes (such as neutrophils, lymphocytes, monocytes, eosinophils and basophils). Instead, it may give a WBC differential as a percentage of granulocytes, lymphocytes and monocytes combined.
○ **Application:** 3-part cell counters are commonly used for routine complete blood counts (CBCs) in clinical settings,

where a basic assessment of blood cell populations is sufficient.

6-Part Cell Counter (Fig. 4.12)

○ **Cell populations:** A 6-part cell counter provides a more detailed differentiation of WBC subtypes, in addition to RBCs and platelets. It can identify and differentiate neutrophils, lymphocytes, monocytes, eosinophils, basophils as well as immature granulocytes.
○ **Parameters:** In addition to the basic parameters provided by a 3-part cell counter, a 6-part cell counter offers more extensive parameters. These may include absolute counts of different WBC subtypes, WBC differentials and additional parameters related to cell size, granularity and maturity.
○ **WBC differential:** A 6-part cell counter provides a detailed breakdown of WBC subtypes, giving percentages and absolute counts for each subtype.
○ **Application:** 6-part cell counters are typically used in specialized settings such as hematology laboratories, where a more comprehensive assessment of blood cell populations is necessary. They are particularly valuable in diagnosing and monitoring hematological disorders.

Table 4.19: Differences between granulocytes and agranulocytes.

	Granulocytes	Agranulocytes
1	Have granules in their cytoplasm.	Agranulocytes lack visible granules in their cytoplasm
2	Based on the staining properties of their granules—three types: neutrophils, eosinophils and basophils.	Two types—lymphocytes and monocytes.
3	Possess lobed nuclei	Non-lobed nuclei—agranulocytes typically have round or slightly indented nuclei
4	Have high phagocytic activity and are involved in engulfing and destroying pathogens or foreign substances.	Play role in adaptive immunity

The differential leukocyte count examines the relative proportions of different types of white blood cells including neutrophils, lymphocytes, monocytes, eosinophils and basophils. These cells are categorized based on their size, shape and staining properties and each type has its own unique functions in the immune system.

Brief overview of the different types of white blood cells and their roles:

❍ **Neutrophils:** Neutrophils are the most abundant type of white blood cell and play a key role in defending against bacterial infections. They are typically the first responders to sites of infection or tissue damage.

❍ **Lymphocytes:** Lymphocytes are involved in immune responses and are responsible for coordinating and regulating the body's immune system. There are two main types of lymphocytes: B cells, which produce antibodies and T cells, which directly attack infected or abnormal cells.

❍ **Monocytes:** Monocytes are large white blood cells that are involved in the immune response. They help remove dead or damaged cells and also act as antigen-presenting cells, which activate other immune cells.

❍ **Eosinophils:** Eosinophils are involved in allergic reactions and defense against parasitic infections. They help regulate inflammation and play a role in modulating the immune response.

❍ **Basophils:** Basophils are the least common type of white blood cell. They release chemical mediators such as histamine during allergic reactions and contribute to the body's inflammatory response.

❍ White blood cells (WBCs) are broadly categorized into two main types: granulocytes and agranulocytes.

❍ Differences between granulocytes and agranulocytes are listed in **Table 4.19**.

Complete Blood Count

A complete blood count (CBC) is a common blood test that provides valuable information about the cellular components of blood. The CBC is typically performed using an automated cell counter or hemogram. Here are the key components and parameters included in a CBC:

Red Blood Cells (RBCs)

○ **Red blood cell count (RBC):** The total number of red blood cells per volume of blood.

○ **Hemoglobin (Hb):** The amount of oxygen-carrying protein in the red blood cells.

○ **Hematocrit (Hct):** The percentage of blood volume occupied by red blood cells.

○ **Mean corpuscular volume (MCV):** The average size of red blood cells.

○ **Mean corpuscular hemoglobin (MCH):** The average amount of hemoglobin per red blood cell.

○ **Mean corpuscular hemoglobin Concentration (MCHC):** The average concentration of hemoglobin in red blood cells.

White Blood Cells (WBCs)

○ **White blood cell count (WBC):** The total number of white blood cells per volume of blood.

○ **Differential white blood cell count:** The percentage and absolute count of different types of white blood cells including neutrophils, lymphocytes, monocytes, eosinophils and basophils.

○ **Neutrophil-to-lymphocyte ratio (NLR):** The ratio of neutrophils to lymphocytes which can be an indicator of inflammation or infection.

Platelets

○ **Platelet count:** The total number of platelets per volume of blood.

○ **Mean platelet volume (MPV):** The average size of platelets.

Additional Parameters

○ **Red cell distribution width (RDW):** A measure of the variation in size of red blood cells.

○ **Platelet distribution width (PDW):** A measure of the variation in size of platelets.

○ **Mean platelet volume-to-platelet count ratio (MPV/PLT):** A ratio that can indicate platelet activation or dysfunction.

These parameters provide valuable insights into various aspects of blood health and can help diagnose and monitor a wide range of conditions including anemia, infections, inflammation and bleeding disorders.

ERYTHROCYTE SEDIMENTATION RATE AND PACKED CELL VOLUME ESTIMATION

ESR, or erythrocyte sedimentation rate is a blood test that measures the rate at which red blood cells settle to the bottom of a test tube over a specific period of time. It is a non-specific marker of inflammation and is often used to help diagnose and monitor certain conditions such as infections, autoimmune diseases and certain types of cancer.

The normal range for ESR can vary depending on the laboratory and the specific method used to perform the test. However, as a general guideline, the normal range for ESR in adults is typically:

○ **For men:** 0–22 millimeters per hour (mm/hr)

○ **For women:** 0–29 mm/hr

Methods of Estimation of ESR

There are several methods for estimating erythrocyte sedimentation rate (ESR). The commonly used methods are:

○ **Westergren method:** The Westergren method is the most widely used method for ESR estimation. It involves collecting blood in a vertical tube, and mixing it with an anticoagulant to prevent clotting. The rate at which red blood cells settle to the bottom of the tube over a period of one hour is measured and reported as the ESR **(Fig. 4.13)**. **Figure 4.14** shows the method of ESR estimation.

○ Westergren's pipette typically has a length of 300 mm (12 inches) and is marked with graduations along its length.

○ The markings on the pipette are usually in millimeters (mm).

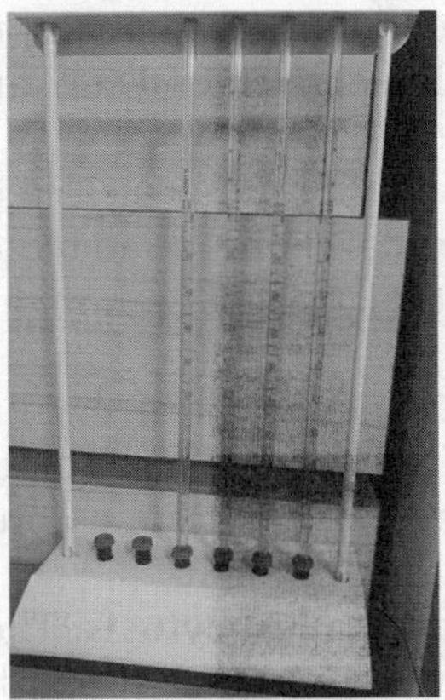

Fig. 4.13: Showing ESR pipettes with the stand.

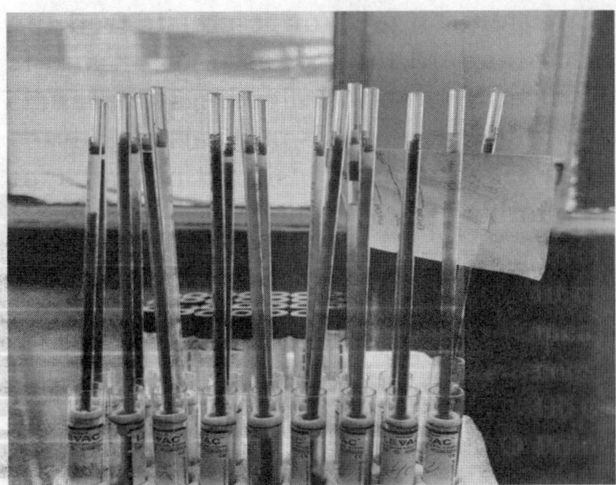

Fig. 4.14: Method of ESR estimation by westergren method.
(For color version, see Plate 4)

○ The pipette is calibrated from the tip (zero mark) to the upper end.

○ The most common scale used on Westergren's pipette is from 0 to 200 mm

○ The pipette is marked at regular intervals, typically every millimeter, allowing for precise measurements of the settling rate of red blood cells during the ESR test.

During the test, the pipette is filled with blood mixed with an anticoagulant, and the column of blood is allowed to settle for a specific time period, usually one hour. After the settling period, the distance between the upper boundary of the settled red blood cells and the uppermost point of the plasma column is measured using the markings on the pipette, providing the ESR value in millimeters per hour (mm/hr).

○ **Wintrobe method:** The Wintrobe method is similar to the Westergren method but uses a shorter tube, usually 100 mm long. The blood is also mixed with an anticoagulant and the rate of red blood cell sedimentation is measured over a period of one hour **(Fig. 4.15)**.

○ **Modified Westergren method:** The modified Westergren method is a variation of the Westergren method that uses a 100 mm long tube but includes a larger bore size. This method is often used in settings where the standard Westergren method is not available.

○ **Microhematocrit method:** The microhematocrit method is a rapid and relatively simple method for estimating ESR. It involves collecting blood in a capillary tube which is then centrifuged to separate the red blood cells from the plasma. The length of the column of red blood cells is measured and reported as the ESR.

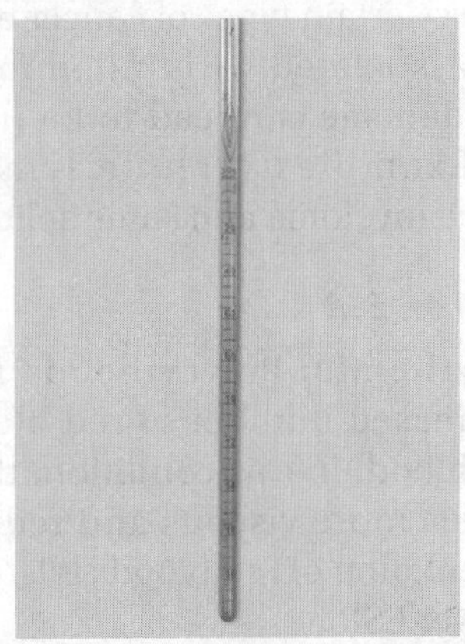

Fig. 4.15: Showing Wintrobe's tube for PCV and ESR.

Westergren method is considered the gold standard for ESR estimation and is preferred in most clinical settings. The results from different methods may vary slightly, so its essential to use consistent methods for monitoring ESR over time.

Factors Causing Raised ESR

- **Inflammation:** ESR is a non-specific marker of inflammation. Any condition associated with inflammation such as infections (e.g., bacterial, viral), autoimmune diseases (e.g., rheumatoid arthritis, lupus) and tissue injury can cause an elevated ESR.
- **Infection:** Certain infections, including bacterial, viral and fungal infections can lead to an increased ESR. This is often seen in conditions like pneumonia, urinary tract infections, tuberculosis and endocarditis.
- **Autoimmune diseases:** Conditions like rheumatoid arthritis, systemic lupus erythematosus, vasculitis and polymyalgia rheumatica can cause chronic inflammation and elevated ESR.
- **Tissue necrosis:** In conditions where there is tissue damage or necrosis, such as in large burns, extensive trauma or some types of cancer, the release of inflammatory mediators can cause an elevated ESR.
- **Cancer:** Certain types of cancer especially those associated with inflammation or tissue damage can lead to an increased ESR. Examples include lymphoma, multiple myeloma and some solid tumors.

Causes of Low ESR

- **Polycythemia:** Polycythemia refers to an increased number of red blood cells in the blood. In this condition, the blood becomes more viscous and reduces the sedimentation of red blood cells, resulting in a lower ESR.
- **Hypofibrinogenemia:** Fibrinogen is a plasma protein involved in clotting. Low levels of fibrinogen can reduce the aggregation of red blood cells and result in a decreased ESR.
- **Sickle cell anemia:** In sickle cell anemia, the abnormal shape of red blood cells can impede their sedimentation, leading to a lower ESR.
- **Congestive heart failure:** In congestive heart failure, the decreased blood flow and decreased plasma protein concentration can cause a lower ESR.
- **Hereditary spherocytosis:** The presence of sphere-shaped RBCs inhibits the rouleaux formation and decreases the ESR.
- **Extreme leukocytosis:** In conditions with extremely high white blood cell counts, such as leukemia or severe infections, the increased viscosity of the blood can reduce red blood cell sedimentation and result in a lower ESR.

PCV, or packed cell volume a, also known as hematocrit, is a blood test that measures the volume of red blood cells (RBCs) as a percentage of the total blood volume. It provides information about the proportion of RBCs in the blood and is used to evaluate anemia, dehydration and other blood disorders.

There are several methods for estimating PCV:

- **Microhematocrit method:** The microhematocrit method is the most commonly used method for PCV estimation. It involves collecting blood in a capillary tube and sealing one end with clay or a specialized sealant. The capillary tube is then placed in a microhematocrit centrifuge, which spins the tube at high speed causing the RBCs to pack at the bottom. After centrifugation, the length of the packed RBCs is measured and reported as the PCV percentage.
- **Automated hematology analyzer:** Modern hematology analyzers often include a module that measures PCV automatically. These analyzers use principles such as

electrical impedance or optical detection to determine the PCV. The blood sample is aspirated into the analyzer and it calculates the PCV based on the proportion of RBCs in the sample.

○ **Manual calculation:** PCV can also be estimated by manually calculating it using the red cell and total blood volume. The red cell volume is obtained by multiplying the RBC count by the mean corpuscular volume (MCV) and the total blood volume is calculated by multiplying the plasma volume by a correction factor. The PCV is then calculated by dividing the red cell volume by the total blood volume and multiplying by 100.

Normal Range of PCV

The normal range for PCV, also known as hematocrit, can vary slightly between men and women. The normal range for PCV in adults is generally:

○ **For men:** 40–54%
○ **For women:** 35–47%
○ **Infants:** 45–60% (cord blood)
○ Wintrobe's tube, also known as a hematocrit tube **(Fig. 4.14)**, is a specialized glass tube used to measure the packed cell volume (PCV) or hematocrit value of blood.
○ The PCV represents the percentage of red blood cells (erythrocytes) in the total volume of blood.
○ Wintrobe's tube is marked with graduations along its length, allowing for the measurement of the height of the packed red blood cells.
○ The tube is typically made of glass and has a length of approximately 110 mm (11 centimeters) and an internal diameter of about 2 mm.
○ The markings on Wintrobe's tube are usually in millimeters (mm) and are engraved or etched onto the glass surface. The tube is marked from the bottom (zero mark) to the upper end. The scale may vary between different manufacturers or versions of the tube, but the most common scale used is from 0 to 100 mm.

To determine the PCV using Wintrobe's tube, blood is drawn into the tube by capillary action or by using a microhematocrit centrifuge. The tube is then sealed at one end and centrifuged to allow the red blood cells to settle at the bottom. After centrifugation, the height of the packed red blood cells is measured using the markings on the tube. The PCV value is calculated by dividing the height of the packed red blood cells by the total height of the column of blood in the tube and multiplying by 100.

Differences between ESR and PCV

○ **Measurement:** ESR measures the rate of sedimentation of red blood cells over time, while PCV measures the proportion of red blood cells in the total blood volume.
○ **Purpose:** ESR is a non-specific marker of inflammation and is used to detect or monitor various conditions associated with inflammation. PCV is primarily used to evaluate anemia, dehydration and blood disorders.
○ **Units:** ESR is reported in mm/hr, while PCV is reported as a percentage.
○ **Influencing factors:** ESR can be influenced by various factors, including plasma proteins and fibrinogen, which increase during inflammation. PCV is influenced by factors affecting red blood cell production and destruction, such as anemia or polycythemia.
○ **Interpretation:** ESR alone does not provide a specific diagnosis but serves as an indicator of inflammation. PCV provides information about the proportion of red blood cells and can help identify conditions like anemia or polycythemia.

Table 4.20: Normal range for ESR.

Age	Westergren method (mm/hour) in 1st hour
Newborn	0–2
Infants	3–13
Children	3–13
Men	0–15
Women	0–20
Elderly men	0–20
Elderly women	0–30

In summary, ESR and PCV are different blood tests that provide information about different aspects of blood composition. ESR reflects the rate of red blood cell sedimentation as an indicator of inflammation, while PCV measures the proportion of red blood cells in the total blood volume and aids in assessing anemia and other blood disorders.

The normal range for ESR (erythrocyte sedimentation rate) and PCV (packed cell volume) can vary depending on factors such as age, sex, and the specific laboratory reference range used.

Normal range for ESR is shown in **Table 4.20**.

METHODS FOR HEMOGLOBIN ESTIMATION

Several methods are commonly used for estimating hemoglobin (Hb) levels in the body. Here are some of the main methods:

○ **Hemoglobinometer/hemoglobinometer strip:** This is a portable device that uses a chemical reaction to estimate Hb levels from a small blood sample. The strip is inserted into the device and the Hb concentration is determined based on the color change produced.

○ **Hematology analyzer:** These automated machines are commonly used in clinical laboratories to perform complete blood counts (CBC). They provide a range of information, including Hb levels. The analyzer uses different techniques, such as spectrophotometry or electrical impedance to measure Hb concentration.

○ **Cyanmethemoglobin method:** This is a laboratory-based method that involves the conversion of hemoglobin to cyanmethemoglobin which can be measured spectrophotometrically. It is considered a reference method for accurate Hb estimation.

○ **Point-of-care testing devices:** These are portable devices designed for use at the patient's bedside or in a non-laboratory setting. They use various technologies, such as photometry or electrical impedance to estimate Hb levels from a small blood sample.

○ **Color scale comparison:** This method involves comparing the color of a blood sample with a standardized color scale. The scale has different color shades corresponding to different Hb concentrations.

○ **Noninvasive methods:** Some emerging technologies aim to estimate Hb levels without the need for a blood sample. These methods include pulse oximetry which measures oxygen saturation in the blood and spectroscopy techniques that analyze light absorption or reflectance to estimate Hb levels.

It is important to note that different methods may have variations in accuracy, precision, and suitability for different settings. The choice of method depends on factors such as the clinical context, available resources and specific requirements of the healthcare setting. For accurate and reliable results, it is generally recommended to use laboratory-based methods or automated hematology analyzers.

Red Blood Cell Parameters

Mean corpuscular volume (MCV), mean corpuscular hemoglobin (MCH) and mean corpuscular hemoglobin concentration (MCHC) are indices used in a complete blood count (CBC) to assess the characteristics of red blood cells. Here's how each index is calculated:

○ **Mean corpuscular volume (MCV):** MCV represents the average volume of red blood cells and is expressed in femtoliters (fL). It is calculated by dividing the total volume of packed red blood cells (hematocrit) by the total number of red blood cells. The formula for MCV is:

MCV = (Hematocrit/Red blood cell count) × 10

Note: MCV is multiplied by 10 to convert from deciliters (dL) to femtoliters (fL).

○ **Mean corpuscular hemoglobin (MCH):** MCH indicates the average amount of hemoglobin in each red blood cell and is expressed in picograms (pg). It is calculated by dividing the total amount of hemoglobin by the total number of red blood cells. The formula for MCH is:

MCH = Hemoglobin/Red blood cell count

○ **Mean corpuscular hemoglobin concentration (MCHC):** MCHC represents the average concentration of hemoglobin within red blood cells and is expressed as a percentage. It is calculated by dividing the total amount of hemoglobin by the hematocrit and then multiplying by 100. The formula for MCHC is:

MCHC = (Hemoglobin/Hematocrit) × 100

It is important to note that these indices provide information about the size (MCV), hemoglobin content (MCH) and hemoglobin concentration (MCHC) of red blood cells. They can help diagnose and classify various types of anemia and other blood disorders.

ANEMIA

○ Anemia is a medical condition characterized by a decrease in the number of red blood cells (RBCs) or a decrease in the amount of hemoglobin in the blood when compared with normal for that age, sex and ethnicity. Also it is functionally defined as insufficient RBC mass to deliver oxygen to peripheral tissues adequately.

○ Parameters such as Hb concentration (g/dL), Hct (%) and RBC concentration (10^{6}/ul) can also be used to establish anemia.

WHO criteria of normal hemoglobin value:

○ Adult male: 13–17 g/dL
○ Adult female (nonpregnant): 12–15 g/dL
○ Adult female (pregnant): 11–14 g/dL
○ Newborn: 13.6–19.6 g/dL
○ Infants, 2–6 months: 9.5–14 g/dL
○ Children, 6 months to 6 years: 11–14 g/dL
○ Children, 6–12 years: 11.5–15.5 g/dL

WHO criteria of anemia:

○ Adult male: <13 g/dL
○ Adult female: <12 g/dL
○ Pregnant women: <11 g/dL

Grading of anemia:

○ **Mild:** Hb from lower limit of normal to 10.0 g/dL
○ **Moderate:** 10.0-7.0 g/dL
○ **Severe:** <7.0 g/dL

Classification of Anemia

Anemia can be classified in various ways based on different criteria, including the underlying cause, the size and appearance of red blood cells and the etiology of the condition. Here are some common classifications of anemia:

Based on the Underlying Cause

○ **Iron-deficiency anemia:** Caused by insufficient iron in the body leading to reduced production of hemoglobin.

○ **Vitamin deficiency anemia:** Caused by a deficiency of specific vitamins essential for RBC production such as vitamin B12 or folate.

○ **Anemia of chronic disease:** Associated with chronic illnesses, infections or inflammatory conditions that disrupt normal red blood cell production or increase their destruction.

○ **Hemolytic anemia:** Resulting from increased destruction of red blood cells often due to inherited conditions, autoimmune disorders or certain medications.

○ **Aplastic anemia:** Occur when the bone marrow fails to produce enough new blood cells.

○ **Sickle cell anemia:** An inherited disorder where the shape of red blood cells is abnormal leading to their breakdown and a reduced lifespan.

Based on the Size and Appearance of Red Blood Cells

○ **Microcytic anemia:** Characterized by small red blood cells, often seen in iron deficiency anemia or certain genetic conditions.

○ **Normocytic anemia:** Involving normal-sized red blood cells which can occur in various types of anemia, including some chronic diseases and early stages of anemia.

○ **Macrocytic anemia:** Involving larger than normal red blood cells, often associated with deficiencies of vitamin B12 or folate.

Based on Etiology

○ **Congenital anemias:** Inherited or present at birth such as sickle cell anemia or thalassemia.

○ **Acquired anemias:** Develop during a person's lifetime due to various factors such as nutritional deficiencies, chronic diseases or certain medications.

The peripheral blood film findings can provide valuable insights into the type of anemia, including microcytic and macrocytic anemias.

As discussed earlier, normal RBCs have a diameter of 6–8 um, which is comparable to the nucleus of a small lymphocyte and show central pallor corresponding to 1/3rd of the cell diameter **(Fig. 4.16)**.

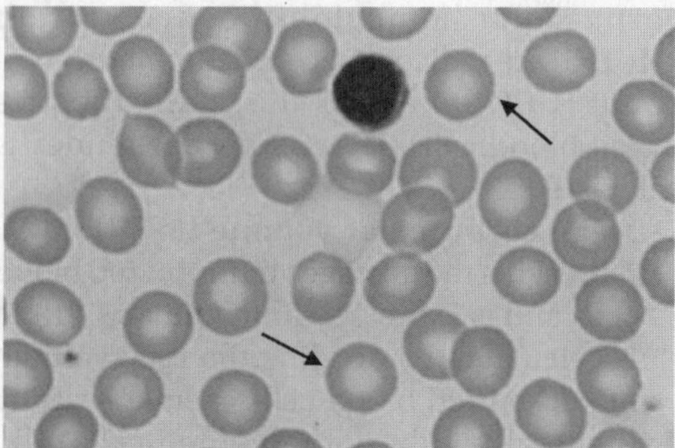

Fig. 4.16: Peripheral blood smear showing normal RBCs. Note the size of the RBC is similar to the size of the nucleus of a small lymphocyte.

(For color version, see Plate 4)

Microcytic anemias are classified into two groups.

1. **Microcytic anemia due to iron deficiency (Table 4.21).**
2. **Microcytic anemia other than iron deficiency (Table 4.21).**

○ Sidroblastic anemia
○ Thalassemia
○ Anemia of chronic disorders.

Iron deficiency anemia is a condition that occurs when there is an insufficient amount of iron available to produce an adequate number of healthy red blood cells. The etiology (causes) of iron deficiency anemia can be categorized into several factors:

○ **Inadequate dietary intake:** A primary cause of iron deficiency anemia is a diet lacking in sufficient iron-rich foods. This can happen due to poor nutrition, limited food availability or dietary choices that do not include enough iron sources such as red meat, poultry, fish, legumes and leafy green vegetables.

○ **Blood loss:** Chronic or acute blood loss can deplete the body's iron stores and lead to iron deficiency anemia. Common causes of blood loss include heavy menstrual periods, gastrointestinal bleeding (from ulcers, gastritis, colon polyps or tumors), trauma,

Table 4.21: Difference between iron deficiency anemia, anemia of chronic disease and thalassemia minor.

Characteristic	Iron deficiency anemia	Anemia of chronic disease	Thalassemia minor
Underlying cause	Inadequate iron intake or absorption	Chronic inflammation or disease	Genetic mutation affecting hemoglobin
Iron status	Low serum iron, ferritin and transferrin saturation	Normal to high serum iron, low transferrin saturation	Normal to high serum iron, normal transferrin saturation
Red blood cell morphology	Microcytic and hypochromic	Normocytic and normochromic	Mild microcytosis
Hemoglobin level	Decreased	Decreased	Normal or slightly decreased
Red blood cell count	Decreased	Normal or slightly decreased	Normal or slightly decreased
Total iron binding capacity	Increased	Normal or decreased	Normal or decreased
Reticulocyte count	Low	Normal or low	Normal or slightly increased

surgery or the use of certain medications that increase the risk of bleeding.

○ **Increased iron requirements:** Some individuals may have increased iron requirements due to growth spurts during childhood, adolescence or pregnancy. In these cases, the body's demand for iron exceeds the available supply, leading to iron deficiency anemia if adequate iron intake is not ensured.

○ **Malabsorption disorders:** Certain medical conditions can impair the absorption of iron from the diet, resulting in iron deficiency anemia. Examples include celiac disease, inflammatory bowel disease (such as Crohn's disease or ulcerative colitis), gastric bypass surgery and certain medications or treatments that affect the absorption of iron.

○ **Chronic diseases:** Chronic diseases, such as kidney disease, cancer or autoimmune disorders can interfere with the body's ability to absorb or utilize iron leading to iron deficiency anemia.

○ **Pregnancy and breastfeeding:** During pregnancy, the body's iron needs increase to support fetal development and the growth of the placenta. If the mother's iron stores are insufficient or her diet lacks adequate iron, iron deficiency anemia can develop. Similarly, breastfeeding mothers may experience iron deficiency if their iron requirements are not met through diet or supplements.

Laboratory Findings in Iron Deficiency Anemia

Blood Picture and Red Cell Indices

The degree of anemia varies. It is usually mild to moderate but occasionally it may be severe due to persistent and severe blood loss. The salient findings in these cases are as under.

○ **Hemoglobin:** The essential feature is a fall in hemoglobin concentration up to a variable degree.

○ **Red blood cells:** Microcytic, hypochromic with poikilocytosis (target cell, pencil cell, tear drop cells) and anisocytosis (RBCs show variation in size, with some being significantly smaller than others) may be seen. Normoblasts (NRBC) are uncommon, RBC count is below normal, dimorphic picture may be present **(Fig. 4.17).**

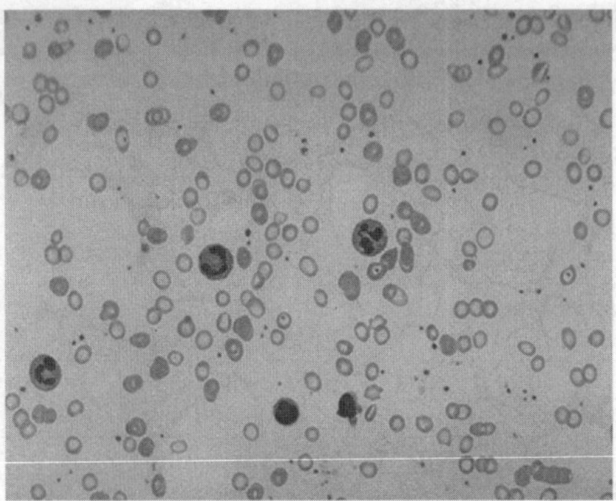

Fig. 4.17: Peripheral blood smear showing microcytes, hypochromic RBCs, and pencil cells.
(For color version, see Plate 4)

○ **The reticulocyte count** is normal or reduced but may be slightly raised (2–5%) in cases after hemorrhage.
○ **Absolute values** The red cell indices reveal a diminished MCV (below 50 fL), diminished MCH (below 15 pg), and diminished MCHC (below 20 g/dL).
○ **Leukocytes** The total and differential white cell counts are usually normal.
○ **Platelets:** Platelet count is usually normal but may be slightly to moderately raised in patients with recent bleeding.

Bone Marrow Findings in Iron Deficiency Anemia

○ **Marrow cellularity:** The marrow cellularity is increased due to **erythroid hyperplasia**.
○ **Erythropoiesis:** There is normoblastic erythropoiesis with predominance of micronormoblasts or polycromatic normoblasts.
Other cells: Myeloid, lymphoid and mega-karyocytic cell are normal in morphology.

Assessment of Iron Stores

Iron can be demonstrated by Prussian blue reaction (Perl Stain) in the bone marrow.

Biochemical Findings in Iron Deficiency Anemia

○ **Decreased hemoglobin (Hb) levels:** In iron deficiency anemia, there is a decrease in hemoglobin levels due to inadequate iron supply for red blood cell production.
○ **Decreased hematocrit (Hct) levels:** Hematocrit levels are decreased in iron deficiency anemia due to a reduced number of red blood cells.
○ **Microcytic and hypochromic red blood cells:** Iron deficiency anemia is often associated with small-sized red blood cells (microcytosis) and decreased red blood cell coloration (hypochromia) due to insufficient iron available for hemoglobin synthesis.
○ **Decreased serum ferritin levels:** There is a decrease in serum ferritin levels, reflecting low iron stores (normal range of serum ferritin is 30–250 ug/dL). This is one of the most reliable indicators of iron deficiency.
○ **Decreased serum iron levels:** Serum iron levels are a measure of the iron bound to transferrin, the iron transport protein (normal range is 40–140 ug/dL).
○ **Increased total iron binding capacity (TIBC):** TIBC represents the total amount of iron that transferrin can bind. In iron deficiency anemia, TIBC levels are increased because the body tries to compensate for low iron levels by producing more transferrin to scavenge any available iron. Normal range for TIBC is 250–450 ug/dL.
○ **Decreased transferrin saturation:** Transferrin saturation refers to the percentage of transferrin that is saturated with iron. In iron deficiency anemia, transferrin saturation is decreased due to inadequate iron supply, reflecting a low percentage of iron-bound transferrin.

Causes of Anemia of Chronic Disease

○ **Chronic inflammatory diseases:** Conditions such as rheumatoid arthritis, systemic lupus erythematosus (SLE), inflammatory bowel disease (Crohn's disease, ulcerative colitis) and chronic infections (such as tuberculosis or HIV) can lead to ACD.

○ **Cancer:** Certain types of cancers, particularly those associated with chronic inflammation can contribute to the development of ACD.

○ **Chronic kidney disease:** Individuals with chronic kidney disease often experience anemia due to impaired production of erythropoietin, a hormone necessary for red blood cell production.

○ **Autoimmune disorders:** Autoimmune conditions like SLE or vasculitis can cause chronic inflammation leading to ACD.

Investigations for Anemia of Chronic Disease

○ **Complete blood count (CBC):** A CBC is performed to measure various parameters, including hemoglobin levels, red blood cell count, hematocrit, mean corpuscular volume (MCV) and red cell distribution width (RDW). A low hemoglobin level and red blood cell parameters consistent with anemia are observed in ACD.

○ **Iron studies:** Iron studies help assess the iron status and provide insights into the underlying cause of anemia. In ACD, iron levels may be normal or even elevated, while the iron transport protein ferritin may be increased due to inflammation.

○ **C-reactive protein (CRP) and erythrocyte sedimentation rate (ESR):** CRP and ESR are markers of inflammation. Elevated levels of these markers can indicate the presence of chronic inflammation, which is often associated with ACD.

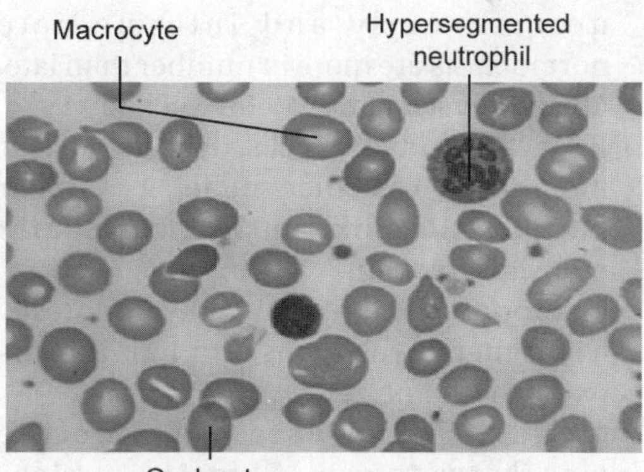

Fig. 4.18: PBS of macrocytic anemia showing macrocytes and a hypersegmented neutrophil.
(For color version, see Plate 4)

Macrocytic Anemia

○ **Macrocytosis:** RBCs appear larger than normal **(Fig. 4.18)**, often with an increased MCV.

○ **Anisocytosis:** RBCs show variation in size, with some being significantly larger than others.

○ **Oval macrocytes:** Oval-shaped RBCs may be present, which are larger than normal RBCs but lack the typical biconcave shape.

○ **Howell-Jolly bodies:** Small, round, basophilic inclusions (DNA remnants) may be seen within RBCs.

○ **Target cells:** RBCs with a central bullseye appearance may be observed.

○ **Hypersegmented neutrophils:** Neutrophils may have more lobes in their nuclei than normal (typically >5 lobes) **(Fig. 4.18)**.

Bone Marrow Findings in Macrocytic Anemia

○ **Cellularity:** Hypercellular

○ **M:E ratio:** Reversed as **erythroid hyperplasia**—1:8

○ **Erythropoiesis:** Erythroid hyperplasia. DNA synthesis is impaired—nuclear replication slowed. Cytoplasm maturation normal—early and intermediate normoblasts are more in number than late.

○ **Megaloblasts:** Early M> Int M> late M.
○ Early M are uniform cells, delicate nuclear membrane, vesicular nuclei, 1–4 linear nucleoli, **sieve like nuclear chromatin** mitosis is frequent.
○ **Myelopoiesis**: Ineffective myelopoiesis. Giant metamyelocytes and band forms pathognomonic.
○ **Megakaryopoiesis**: Ineffective megakaryopoiesis. Complex nuclear hyperlobulation (pseudohyperdiploidy), abnormal nuclear chromatin.
○ Megakaryocytes show fragmentation, forming very few platelets- megathrombocytes.

Biochemical Investigations in Megaloblastic Anemia

○ **Hyperhomocysteinemia:** Both folic acid and vitamin B12 deficiency results in increased homocysteine levels.
○ **Serum LDH levels:** Increased
○ **Serum bilirubin:** Increased: 1–3 mg/dL.
○ Serum folate levels decreased.
○ Serum vitamin B12 levels decreased

THALASSEMIAS

Thalassemias are a group of inherited blood disorders characterized by abnormal production of hemoglobin, the protein responsible for carrying oxygen in red blood cells RBCs. Thalassemias result from mutations or deletions in the genes that control the production of the alpha or beta chains of hemoglobin. The pathogenesis of thalassemias involves impaired production or synthesis of one or more globin chains, leading to a deficiency of functional hemoglobin and subsequent red blood cell abnormalities. Thalassemias can be classified based on which globin chain is affected and the severity of the condition:

Alpha Thalassemia

○ **Alpha thalassemia minor:** In this form, there is a deletion or mutation in one or two of the four alpha globin genes. It typically results in mild or no symptoms.
○ **Hemoglobin H disease:** This form occurs when three out of the four alpha globin genes are affected. It leads to moderate to severe anemia and requires monitoring and management.
○ **Hemoglobin Bart syndrome:** This is the most severe form of alpha thalassemia, occurring when all four alpha globin genes are affected. It leads to a life-threatening condition in newborns, as there is a complete absence of functional hemoglobin.

Beta Thalassemia

○ **Beta thalassemia minor:** Individuals with beta thalassemia minor have a mutation in one of the two beta globin genes, resulting in mild or no symptoms. They are often carriers of the condition.
○ **Beta thalassemia major (Cooley's anemia):** This form occurs when both beta globin genes are affected, leading to a severe deficiency of beta globin chains. It causes severe anemia that requires regular blood transfusions and ongoing medical care.
○ **Beta thalassemia intermedia:** This is a milder form of beta thalassemia, where there is a partial deficiency of beta globin chains. The severity of symptoms varies, and some individuals may not require regular transfusions.

Other less common forms of thalassemia include delta beta thalassemia, gamma delta beta thalassemia, and delta thalassemia. These forms involve mutations in other globin chain genes, leading to abnormalities in the structure and production of hemoglobin.

The clinical manifestations of thalassemias include varying degrees of anemia, jaundice, fatigue, growth and developmental issues (in severe cases), and complications related to iron overload from frequent blood transfusions.

Management of thalassemias involves supportive care, including blood transfusions, iron chelation therapy to manage iron overload and sometimes stem cell transplantation, which can be curative in certain cases.

RETICULOCYTE COUNT

Reticulocyte count is a laboratory test used to evaluate the production of red blood cells (RBCs) in the bone marrow. It measures the percentage of reticulocytes, which are immature RBCs, in the total RBC population. It is useful in assessing bone marrow function and diagnosing various anemias.

Normal Range: The normal range for reticulocyte count is typically expressed as a percentage of the total red blood cell count. The normal range for reticulocytes is approximately 0.5% to 2.5% of the total red blood cells.

Causes of Low Reticulocyte Count

○ **Bone marrow suppression:** Conditions that suppress bone marrow activity can result in a decreased production of reticulocytes. Examples include aplastic anemia, myelodysplastic syndromes and certain medications (e.g., chemotherapy drugs).

○ **Nutritional deficiencies:** Deficiencies in nutrients essential for RBC production, such as iron, vitamin B12 or folate can lead to decreased reticulocyte production.

○ **Chronic diseases:** Certain chronic illnesses such as chronic kidney disease or liver disease can interfere with the production of reticulocytes.

○ **Hypoplastic anemia:** Hypoplastic anemia is characterized by inadequate production of RBCs, including reticulocytes due to bone marrow failure.

○ **Genetic disorders:** Inherited conditions like Diamond-Blackfan anemia and congenital pure red cell aplasia can cause a decreased production of reticulocytes.

Causes of High Reticulocyte Count

○ **Hemolytic anemia:** Hemolytic anemia, where RBCs are destroyed prematurely, leads to an increased demand for new RBC production, resulting in a high reticulocyte count. Causes include autoimmune hemolytic anemia, hereditary spherocytosis and sickle cell disease.

○ **Acute blood loss:** Significant acute blood loss triggers a compensatory increase in RBC production, leading to an elevated reticulocyte count.

○ **Recovery phase:** After a period of bone marrow suppression (e.g., following chemotherapy or treatment for anemia), the reticulocyte count can increase as the bone marrow regains its function and produces more RBCs.

○ **Hemolytic transfusion reaction:** Incompatibility between donor and recipient blood during a blood transfusion can cause hemolysis, leading to an increased reticulocyte count.

○ **Erythropoietin therapy:** Administration of erythropoietin, a hormone that stimulates RBC production, can result in an elevated reticulocyte count.

Reticulocyte Production Index

The reticulocyte count can be further evaluated by calculating the RPI, which takes into account the degree of anemia. The RPI helps assess whether the reticulocyte response is appropriate for the level of anemia.

Measurement: Reticulocyte counts can be determined through manual microscopic examination using special stains such as new methylene blue/brilliant cresyl blue or automated cell counters. Automated analyzers can directly measure the number of reticulocytes using flow cytometry.

Uses

○ Assessing bone marrow function and activity.
○ Evaluating anemias, including iron deficiency anemia, hemolytic anemia and aplastic anemia.
○ Monitoring response to treatment in anemias or erythropoietin therapy.

Method and Procedure

○ **Blood sample collection:** A venous blood sample is collected using standard phlebotomy techniques and anticoagulated with EDTA (ethylenediaminetetraacetic acid).
○ **Reticulocyte staining:** A small amount of the blood sample is mixed with a supravital stain such as new methylene blue or brilliant cresyl blue. This stain precipitates the residual RNA in reticulocytes, making them visible under a microscope.
○ **Blood smear preparation:** A blood smear is made by spreading a thin layer of the stained blood sample on a glass slide.
○ **Microscopic examination:** The stained blood smear is examined under a microscope using an oil immersion lens. Reticulocytes appear bluish in color due to the staining of RNA.
○ **Counting and calculation:** The reticulocytes are manually counted in multiple fields, typically around 500 to 1,000 RBCs and the number of reticulocytes is expressed as a percentage of the total RBCs counted.

Formula: The formula to calculate the reticulocyte count is as follows: Reticulocyte count (%) = (Number of reticulocytes ÷ Total number of RBCs counted) × 100

STAINS IN HEMATOLOGY

Romanowsky stains are a group of hematological stains used in laboratory settings to stain and differentiate various components of blood cells including red blood cells (RBCs), white blood cells (WBCs) and platelets. These stains are commonly used in techniques such as blood smears and bone marrow aspiration smears for the microscopic examination of blood cells.

The most well-known Romanowsky stains are Wright's stain and Giemsa stain. Both stains contain a mixture of dyes that react with different components of cells resulting in distinctive staining patterns. Here is a brief description of these stains:

○ **Wright's stain:** Wright's stain is a combination of eosin (an acidic dye) and methylene blue (a basic dye). It stains different cellular components in various colors:
  ○ Eosin stains the cytoplasm of cells pink to orange.
  ○ Methylene blue stains the nuclei of cells blue-purple.
  ○ The combination of both dyes produces differential staining patterns for RBCs, WBCs and platelets.
○ **Giemsa stain:** Giemsa stain is another Romanowsky stain commonly used in hematological examinations. It contains a mixture of eosin and methylene blue, along with additional components. Giemsa stain produces similar staining patterns to Wright's stain but with slightly different color intensity and clarity. It is particularly useful for staining blood cells to observe cellular details such as nuclear structure and the presence of intracellular parasites (e.g., malaria parasites).

Romanowsky stains, including Wright's stain and Giemsa stain provide excellent contrast and allow for the identification and differentiation of different blood cell types. By using these stains, laboratory technicians and hematologists can analyze blood smears to assess cell morphology, identify abnormal cells and aid in the diagnosis of various blood disorders and infections.

It is important to note that the staining process and specific protocols may vary depending on the laboratory and the purpose of the examination. The use of Romanowsky stains in combination with microscopic examination is a valuable tool in hematology and pathology for evaluating blood cell morphology and assisting in the diagnosis of blood-related disorders.

Leishman Stain

Already discussed.

Cytochemical Stains

Cytochemical stains are the special stains which are used for staining peripheral blood and bone marrow smears which help in classifying and differentiating different types of leukemias.

The advantages are that they are cheap, readily available, time saving and effective in differentiating different types of leukemias easily.

Leukocyte Alkaline Phosphatase

Leukocyte alkaline phosphatase (LAP) stain is used to assess the activity of the enzyme alkaline phosphatase in white blood cells (leukocytes). It provides information about the maturation and function of neutrophil, eosinophils, B lymphocytes, osteoblasts and endothelial cells.

The LAP stain involves a histochemical reaction that identifies the presence and distribution of alkaline phosphatase within neutrophils. The test is typically performed on peripheral blood smears or bone marrow aspirate smears. It works as follows:

○ A thin smear of the sample is prepared on a glass slide and allowed to air dry.
○ The slide is immersed in a solution containing a substrate that reacts with alkaline phosphatase. The substrate produces a colored precipitate at the sites where alkaline phosphatase is present.
○ The stained slide is observed under a microscope. Neutrophils are evaluated based on the intensity and distribution of the colored precipitate within their cytoplasm.

Interpretation

After staining the blood smear with alkaline phosphatase, it is viewed under the microscope and results are interpreted as:

Count 100 neutrophils and score them (0 to +4) based on the intensity of staining. Then the final score is calculated by adding the total scores.

Grading score
○ 0—no stain
○ 1+ is faint staining
○ 2+ is moderate staining
○ 3+ is strong staining with cytoplasmic background
○ 4+ is strong staining without cytoplasmic background.

Normal range: 15–130

The Myeloperoxidase Stain

The myeloperoxidase (MPO) stain is used to detect the presence and distribution of the MPO enzyme in myeloid cells. The MPO enzyme is primarily found in neutrophils, monocytes and some macrophages. The staining procedure utilizes the peroxidase activity of MPO, which catalyzes the oxidation of a substrate in the presence of hydrogen peroxide to produce a colored product. This colored product can be visualized microscopically and indicates the presence of MPO activity. Uses are as follows:

○ **Differentiation of acute myeloid leukemia (AML):** MPO staining is an essential diagnostic tool in distinguishing AML from acute lymphoblastic leukemia (ALL) or other types of leukemia. The presence of MPO activity in blasts (immature cells) is a characteristic feature of AML.

○ **Assessment of myeloid maturation:** MPO staining is used to evaluate the maturation of myeloid cells. It can help determine the stage of differentiation of myeloid cells in bone marrow or peripheral blood smears. The intensity and distribution of MPO staining can provide insights into the lineage and maturity of myeloid cells.

○ **Identification of myeloid cells in tissues:** MPO staining is valuable for identifying myeloid cells in tissue sections. It can be used to assess the presence and distribution of neutrophils, monocytes and macrophages in various tissues, aiding in the diagnosis of infectious, inflammatory or neoplastic conditions.

Interpretation

Interpretation of the MPO stain involves assessing the presence and intensity of MPO activity in cells.

Positive MPO staining: Brown staining or red brown granules in the cytoplasm of cells indicates the presence of MPO activity. This is typically observed in myeloid cells, such as neutrophils, monocytes and macrophages.

Negative MPO staining: Lack of brown staining or absence of the brown precipitate suggests the absence of MPO activity. This is typically seen in lymphoid cells or non-myeloid cells.

Sudan Black B

Sudan black B is a lipophilic dye that selectively stains lipids, particularly neutral lipids and phospholipids. It is commonly used in hematology to assess the presence and distribution of myeloperoxidase-negative granules in myeloid cells. Sudan black B stains these granules, allowing for their visualization under a microscope.

Uses

The Sudan black B stain has several important uses in hematology:

○ **Differentiation of acute myeloid leukemia (AML):** Sudan black B staining is used to help differentiate AML from acute lymphoblastic leukemia (ALL) or other types of leukemia. It aids in identifying myeloblasts with myeloperoxidase-negative granules, a characteristic feature of AML.

○ **Assessment of myeloid maturation:** Sudan black B staining can be utilized to evaluate the maturation and differentiation of myeloid cells in bone marrow or peripheral blood smears. It helps in determining the stage of myeloid cell development based on the presence or absence of granules.

○ **Detection of myeloid leukemia with minimal differentiation:** Sudan black B stain is particularly useful in identifying cases of myeloid leukemia with minimal differentiation, where myeloblasts lack other specific markers of myeloid differentiation.

Interpretation

Interpretation of Sudan black B staining involves evaluating the presence or absence of granules in myeloid cells.

Positive Sudan black B staining: Dark blue or black granules are observed within the cytoplasm of myeloid cells. This indicates the presence of myeloperoxidase-negative granules and suggests myeloid differentiation. It is typically seen in cases of AML or myeloid leukemia with minimal differentiation.

Negative Sudan black B staining: The absence of dark blue or black granules in myeloid cells suggests the absence of myeloperoxidase-negative granules. This may indicate the presence of lymphoid cells or other non-myeloid cells. It is used to distinguish acute myelogenous and monocytic leukemia from acute lymphocytic leukemia.

Periodic Acid-Schiff Stain

The periodic acid-Schiff (PAS) stain is a histochemical technique used in hematology to detect the presence of carbohydrates, particularly glycogen and mucopolysaccharides in cells and tissues.

Purpose

The PAS stain is utilized to identify and characterize specific cells or components within hematological specimens. It can provide valuable information about glycogen storage disorders, certain leukemias, lymphomas and other hematological conditions involving abnormal carbohydrate accumulation or alterations.

Principle

The PAS stain relies on the reaction between periodic acid and the carbohydrates present in the sample. The periodic acid oxidizes the carbohydrates, creating aldehydes. Subsequently, the Schiff reagent is added which reacts with the aldehydes to form a pink to red-purple color, indicating the presence of carbohydrates. Under a microscope, PAS-positive cells or structures will appear pink or red-purple, depending on the staining intensity.

Interpretation

Interpretation of the PAS stain in hematology involves evaluating the presence and intensity of carbohydrate staining within cells or structures.

Positive PAS staining: Pink or red-purple staining indicates the presence of carbohydrates such as glycogen or mucopolysaccharides. PAS-positive cells or structures may be seen in certain leukemias, lymphomas or glycogen storage disorders.

Negative PAS staining: The absence of pink or red-purple staining suggests the absence of detectable carbohydrates within the cells or structures of interest.

ESTERASES

In hematology, esterases are a group of enzymes that hydrolyze ester bonds in various substrates. They play a role in the metabolism and differentiation of cells, particularly in the identification and characterization of specific cell types within hematological specimens. Here's an overview of the role and significance of esterases in hematology:

Specific Esterases

Specific esterases refer to enzymes that exhibit substrate specificity and can be used to differentiate specific cell types within hematological specimens. Some examples include:

○ **Acetylcholinesterase (AChE):** AChE is an enzyme that hydrolyzes acetylcholine, a neurotransmitter. It is particularly useful in the identification of T-cell lymphomas, as AChE staining is positive in T-lymphocytes but negative in B-lymphocytes and myeloid cells.

○ **Butyrylcholinesterase (BChE):** BChE is an enzyme that hydrolyzes butyrylcholine. Its staining can aid in the identification of B-cell lymphomas, as BChE activity is generally detected in B-lymphocytes but not in T-lymphocytes.

Interpretation of Esterase Staining

The staining pattern and intensity can provide information about the differentiation, lineage and maturation stages of hematological cells. Positive esterase staining indicates the presence of esterase activity, while negative staining suggests the absence of esterase activity.

Nonspecific Esterases

Nonspecific esterases (NSEs) are a group of enzymes that hydrolyze ester bonds in various substrates. In hematology, non-specific esterase staining is a histochemical technique used to identify the presence and distribution of esterase activity in cells, particularly myeloid cells.

Purpose

Non-specific esterase staining is employed to differentiate between myeloid and lymphoid cells in hematological samples. It helps in identifying myeloid cells and evaluating their maturation and distribution within tissues. This staining technique can aid in distinguishing between myeloid and lymphoid leukemias, determining the lineage of blasts (immature cells) and assessing the stage of myeloid cell differentiation.

Principle

The non-specific esterase staining procedure utilizes a substrate that reacts with esterases in the cytoplasm of cells. The substrate is typically a naphthol compound that undergoes hydrolysis in the presence of esterase enzymes, producing a colored product. The colored product can be visualized under a microscope and indicates the presence of esterase activity in the cells.

Procedure

The specific procedure for non-specific esterase staining may vary depending on the staining kit or laboratory protocol used. However, it generally involves the following steps:

○ **Preparation of smears or tissue sections:** Prepare thin smears or tissue sections from the hematological sample, such as bone marrow or peripheral blood.

○ **Application of staining solution:** Apply the non-specific esterase staining solution, containing the substrate for esterase activity onto the smears or tissue sections.

○ **Incubation:** Incubate the smears or tissue sections at an appropriate temperature for the recommended duration, typically ranging from several minutes to hours, depending on the staining protocol.

○ **Stop reaction:** After the incubation, rinse the smears or tissue sections to stop the staining reaction.

○ **Counterstaining (optional):** If desired, a counterstain, such as hematoxylin or nuclear fast red, may be applied to provide contrast and aid in the visualization of cellular morphology.

○ **Mounting:** Once staining is complete, mount coverslips over the stained area using an appropriate mounting medium.

Interpretation

The interpretation of non-specific esterase staining involves evaluating the presence and intensity of esterase activity in cells.

Positive non-specific esterase staining: The presence of a colored product, typically red or purple, within the cytoplasm of cells indicates the presence of esterase activity. This is typically observed in myeloid cells, such as monocytes, macrophages, and granulocytes.

Negative non-specific esterase staining: The absence of a colored product suggests the absence of esterase activity. This may indicate the presence of lymphoid cells or other non-myeloid cells.

Perl's Stain

The Perls stain, also known as Perl's Prussian blue stain, is a histochemical staining technique used in hematology to detect the presence of iron deposits, particularly hemosiderin and ferritin, within cells and tissues.

Purpose

The Perls stain is primarily used to identify and characterize iron-containing cells or components within hematological specimens. It aids in the diagnosis and evaluation of iron overload disorders, such as hemochromatosis, as well as iron-deficiency anemia and other conditions involving abnormal iron accumulation or distribution.

Principle

The Perls stain is based on the reaction between potassium ferrocyanide and ferric iron. The reaction produces insoluble Prussian blue pigment, which appears as a blue color. In the presence of iron, the Perls stain will produce a blue reaction product, indicating the presence of iron deposits.

Materials

- 2% potassium ferrocyanide
- 2 N HCl
- 1% aqueous safranin (counterstain)
- Air dried peripheral blood or bone marrow smear.

Method

- Select a sample as a positive control and stain it together with the test sample. Label the slides as control and patient name, registration number (R/N).
- Fix the slides in absolute methanol for 10–20 minutes. Let it dry.
- Prepare the working solution by adding 30 mL potassium ferrocyanide and 30 mL HCl in a Coplin jar (v/v potassium ferrocyanide:HCl = 1:1).
- Submerge the fixed and dried slides into the Coplin jar containing the working solution.
- Leave it at room temperature or incubate in a water bath at 50°C for 20 minutes.
- Wash the slides in running tap water for 3–5 minutes.
- Rinse thoroughly in distilled water, and then counterstain with safranin similar to steps 4–6.
- Dry and cover the slides with cover slips.

Interpretation

The interpretation of the Perls stain involves evaluating the presence and distribution of iron deposits within cells or structures.

Positive Perls staining: The presence of blue staining indicates the presence of iron deposits. This is typically observed as blue granules within cells such as macrophages, hepatocytes, or reticuloendothelial cells.

Negative Perls staining: The absence of blue staining suggests the absence of detectable iron deposits within the cells or structures of interest.

WBC DISORDERS—LEUKEMIAS

Leukemia

- Neoplasms arising from transformation of uncommitted/partially committed hemopoeitic stem cells.
- Classified into acute and chronic.
- Leukemia is classified into two broad groups:

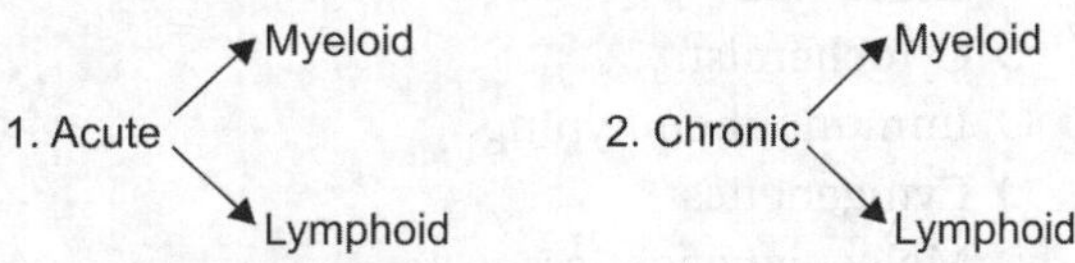

- **Acute leukemia:**
  - ➤ Acute lymphoblastic leukemia (**ALL**)
  - ➤ Acute myeloid leukemia (**AML**)
- **Chronic Leukemia:**
  - ➤ Chronic lymphocytic leukemia (**CLL**)
  - ➤ Chronic myeloid leukemia (**CML**)
- **Subleukemic** leukemia
- **Aleukemic** leukemia

Acute Leukemia

It includes a heterogeneous group of neoplasm that differ with respect to aggressiveness, cell of origin, clinical features and response to therapy. The defect primarily affecting the myeloid stem cell causes acute myeloid leukemia and the defect affecting lymphoid stem cell causes acute lymphoid leukemia.

Table 4.22: Differences between lymphoblast and myeloblast.

Characteristic	Lymphoblast	Myeloblast
Nuclear chromatin	Partially condensed	Dispersed
Nucleoli	0–1, punched out, perinucleolar chromatin condensation	Multiple 2–5, distinct
Cytoplasm	Scant, granules uncommon	Moderate abundant, often with granules, Auer rods
Cytochemistry—myeloperoxidase (MPO) (primary granules)	MPO–	MPO +
SBB (lipid membrane of granules)	SBB–	SBB +
Nonspecific esterase (NSE)	± (Usually T lymphoblast; Resist to sodium fluoride)	(Monoblast + Diffuse, granular; inhibited by sodium fluoride)
Specific (chloroacetate esterase)	–	+

Diagnosis of acute leukemia depends on:
- No. of blasts in the marrow and peripheral blood smear (it should be >20%).
- Morphology of blasts (as shown in **Table 4.22**)
- Cytochemistry
- Immunophenotyping
- Cytogenetics
- Molecular genetics

Acute lymphoblastic leukemia (ALL): ALL is a rapidly progressing leukemia that primarily affects lymphoid cells, which are responsible for the immune response. It is the most common childhood malignancy (about 30% of childhood cancer).

It affects all ages and the highest incidence is between 1–5 years; males are affected more commonly than females.

The patients present with these signs and symptoms.
- Due to BM failure there is decrease in number of RBCs and patients present with pallor, fatigue and lethargy. Decreased WBC function leads to increased chances of infection and fever. Low platelet count lead to purpura and mucosal bleeding.
- Bone pains due to bone erosion. Sternal tenderness is seen due to leukemic involvement of periosteum.
- Extramedullary site involvement by leukemia may be seen as lymphadenopathy and hepatosplenomegaly.
- Due to the CNS involvement patients may present with nausea, vomiting, headache or cranial nerve palsy.
- Testicular involvement may also be seen.

Laboratory findings are as follows:
- **WBC count:** Raised in 60% cases with TLC> 200×10^9 (hyperleukocytosis).
- Subleukemic/aleukemic leukemias.
- Decrease in number of neutrophils.
- Low Hb, decreased platelet counts.
- Approximately 2% patients with aplastic anemia may develop ALL in weeks to months.
- Peripheral smear shows >20% Blasts.
- Bone marrow aspiration shows:
  - Hypercellular marrow with > 20% blasts
  - >20% blasts of all nucleated cells.
  - Decreased erythroid, myeloid series and decreased megakaryocytes.

FAB Classification

- Based on morphology and cytochemistry of blasts into three categories (L1, L2, L3)

Morphology	Classification	Nucleus	Nucleolus	Chromatin	Cytoplasm
	L1 acute lymphoblastic (principally pediatric)	Uniformly round, small	Single, indistinct	Slightly reticulated with pennucleolar clumping	Scant, blue
	L2 lymphoblastic (principally adult)	Irregular	Single to several indistinct	Fine	Moderate, pale
	L3 burkitt-type	Round to oval	Two to five	Course with clear parachromatin	Moderate blue, prominently vacuolated

Fig. 4.19: Morphological, immunophenotypic and cytogenetic features of lymphoblasts.

(For color version, see Plate 5)

Table 4.23: Prognostic markers of ALL.

	Favorable	*Unfavorable*
WBC count	$<10 \times 10^9$/L	$>200 \times 10^9$/L
Age	3–7 years	<1 ; >10
Sex	Female	Male
Ethnicity	White	Black
LN, liver, spleen	–	Massive
Testis	–	+
CNS involvement	–	+
Fab morphology	L1	L2
Ploidy	Hyperploidy	Hypoploidy
Chromosomal abnormality	t(12:21)	t(4:11) , t(1:19), t(9:22)
Time to remission	<14 days	>28 days
Hemoglobin (Hb)	<10 g/dL	Normal
Platelet count	$>100 \times 10^9$/L	<30,000
Immunophenotype	Early Pre B	Pre B ; B/T cell

○ Criteria for acute leukemia was >30% blasts in the peripheral blood smear or bone marrow.

WHO Classification

○ Based on morphological, immunophenotypic and cytogenetic features **(Fig. 4.19)**.
○ Criteria for acute leukemia is >20% blasts in peripheral blood smear or bone marrow.

Prognostic Markers of ALL

Refer **Table 4.23**.

Acute Myeloid Leukemia (AML)

It presents with an uncontrolled proliferation of immature WBCs resulting in an increased number ≥20% myeloblasts in the marrow and peripheral blood.

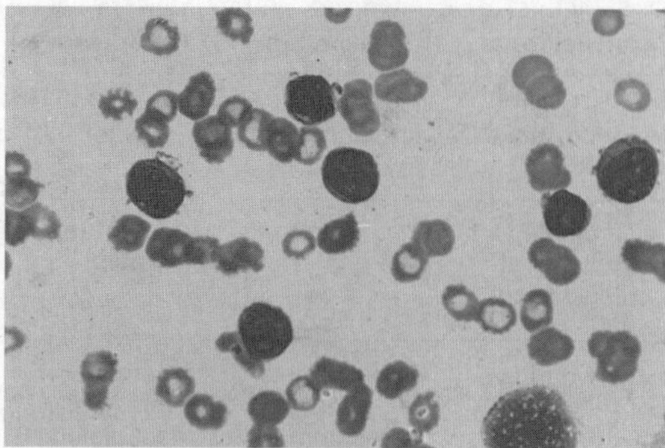

Fig. 4.20: Peripheral blood smear showing blasts.
(For color version, see Plate 5)

Clinical Features of Acute Myeloid Leukemia

- Fever with sweats.
- **DIC:** Acute promyelocytic leukemia
- Organomegaly, adenopathy
- **Skin infiltration:** Violaceous nodular lesions.
- **Gum infiltration:** Monocytic differentiation
- Myeloid sarcoma/chloroma: 2–14%
  - Extramedullary tumor, localized
  - Turns Green in dilute acid because of MPO
  - Involves bone, soft tissues, LN/skin
- CNS involvement

Laboratory Diagnosis of Acute Myeloid Leukemia

- **TLC:** Increased markedly
- **Blast (Fig. 4.20):** Auer rods/Phi bodies (fusiform/spindle shaped)
- Aleukemic rare
- Neutropenia
- Anemia
- Thrombocytopenia
- Bone marrow aspiration shows blasts >20% except acute promyelocytic leukemia
- Cytochemistry, immunophenotyping, cytogenetics
- Investigations for DIC—M3
- Raised uric acid

WHO Classification of Myeloid Neoplasms and Acute Leukemia

Acute myeloid leukemia (AML) and related neoplasms:
- AML with recurrent genetic abnormalities
- AML with t(8;21)(q22q22.1); RUNX1-RUNX1T1
- AML with inv(16)(p13.1q22) or t(16;16)(p13.1;q22); CBFB-MYH11
- APL with PML-RARA
- AML with t(9;11)(p21.3;q23.3); KMT2A-MLLT3
- AML with t(6;9)(p23;q34.1); DEK-NUP214
- AML with inv(3)(q21.3q26.2) or t(3;3)(q21.3;q26.2); GATA2, MECOM
- AML (megakaryoblastic) with t(1;22)(p13.3;q13.1); RBM15-MKL1

Provisional entity: AML with BCR-ABL1
- AML with mutated NPM1
- AML with biallelic mutation of CEBPA

Provisional entity: AML with mutated RUNX1
- AML with myelodysplasia-related changes
- Therapy-related myeloid neoplasms
- AML, not otherwise specified (NOS)
- AML with minimal differentiation
- AML without maturation
- AML with maturation
- Acute myelomonocytic leukemia
- Acute monoblastic and monocytic leukemia
- Pure erythroid leukemia
- Acute megakaryoblastic leukemia
- Acute basophilic leukemia
- Acute panmyelosis with myelofibrosis
- Myeloid sarcoma
- Myeloid proliferations associated with Down syndrome
- Transient abnormal myelopoiesis (TAM) associated with Down syndrome
- Myeloid leukemia associated with Down syndrome

Chronic Lymphoid Leukemia

Accumulation of non-proliferating mature appearing lymphocytes in blood, bone marrow, lymph nodes and spleen. Basic defect is one of cellular accumulation, rather than proliferation. There is a defect in apoptosis due to which majority of cells are long lived with small fraction of proliferating cells. Elderly population is commonly affected.

Clinical Features

- Elderly more than 50 years of age
- **Asymptomatic:** Diagnosed on routine blood examination
- Lymphadenopathy and splenomegaly seen
- Patients present with fatigue and weight loss.
- Pallor due to anemia is common because of replacement of BM with immature cells.
- Bleeding manifestations are rare
- Paraneoplastic syndrome like nephrotic syndrome and pemphigus are common.
- Familial predisposition may be seen.

Laboratory Diagnosis of Chronic lymphoid Leukemia

- Persistent lymphocytosis usually >10 × $10^3/\mu L$
- **Peripheral smear shows** small to medium sized lymphocytes with high nuclear cytoplasmic ratio, clumped chromatin, inconspicuous nucleoli are seen. **Smudge/** basket cell seen.

Criteria for CLL

- Peripheral blood lymphocyte count: >5 × $10^3/\mu L$
- Should have B cell specific Ag: CD 19, 20, 23, 5, 27.
- Monoclonal
- Bone marrow shows >30% lymphocytes.
- **Bone marrow biopsy may show:** Interstitial/nodular/mixed/diffuse pattern of involvement.

Chronic Myeloproliferative Neoplasia

Chronic Myeloproliferative Neoplasia or Disease

- Proliferation with maturation.
- Increase in both mature and immature cells.

MDS/MPD Overlap Syndrome

Feature: Proliferation with dysplasia

- Chronic myelomonocytic leukemia (CMML).
- Juvenile myelomonocytic leukemia (JMML).
- Atypical CML
- Clonal stem cell disorders.
- Aberrant kinase signaling pathway.

Classification of Chronic Myeloproliferative Neoplasia or Disease

1. Chronic myeloid leukemia (CML) t(9, 22) BCR-ABL fusion
2. Polycythemia vera
3. Essential thrombocythemia
4. Chronic idiopathic myelofibrosis
5. Chronic eosinophilic leukemia
6. Chronic neutrophilic leukemia
7. Systemic mastocytosis
8. MPN—unclassifiable

Chronic Myeloid Leukemia

Chronic myeloid leukemia (CML) is a slow-progressing leukemia that affects myeloid cells. It is characterized by the presence of an abnormal chromosome called the Philadelphia chromosome, which results from a genetic mutation.

- It can occur at any age. The average age group is 50–60 years and males are affected more than the females
- Characterized by presence of Philadelphia chromosome/BCR-ABL fusion

○ Involves primarily proliferation of granulocytic cells

○ **Clinical symptoms:** The presence of symptoms associated with CML may prompt further investigation. Common symptoms include fatigue, weight loss, night sweats, abdominal discomfort, and fullness due to an enlarged spleen.

○ **Complete blood count (CBC):** Marked granulocytic leukocytosis (usually > 50,000/µL), particularly increased neutrophils. An increased number of immature white blood cells called myelocytes and metamyelocytes. Prominent peak at neutrophil and myelocyte. Eosinophilia, basophilia, monocytes <3%. Low RBC count (anemia) and/or low platelet count (thrombocytopenia) may be present.

Bone Marrow Findings

Bone Marrow Aspiration

○ Markedly hypercellular
○ Myeloid hyperplasia (M:E ratio >10:1)
○ Myeloblast <5% of all nucleated cells
○ Increased megakaryocytes which may are small with hypolobated nuclei
○ Decreased erythropoiesis

Bone Marrow Biopsy

Increased reticulin fibrosis—bad prognosis.

Special Tests

Neutrophil alkaline phosphatase (NAP): Decreased to zero.

Cytogenetic Study for Philadelphia Chromosome/BCR-ABL

The presence of cells called "Philadelphia chromosome" (Ph chromosome) or the BCR-ABL1 fusion gene is a hallmark of CML. This genetic abnormality occurs due to a reciprocal translocation between chromosomes 9 and 22 [t(9;22)]. It is often detected through genetic testing methods such as fluorescence in situ hybridization (FISH) or polymerase chain reaction (PCR) analysis of blood or bone marrow samples.

The discovery of the Philadelphia chromosome and the development of targeted therapies, such as tyrosine kinase inhibitors (TKIs) that specifically target the BCR-ABL1 protein, have revolutionized the treatment and prognosis of CML. These targeted therapies have significantly improved the outcomes and survival rates for patients with CML.

The essential clinicopathological characteristics of Ph(+) CML in the 2016 WHO classification are defined as follows:

Accelerated phase:

○ **Increased blast count:** The bone marrow or peripheral blood shows 10–19% blasts.

○ **Increased basophils:** Basophils comprise 20% or more of the peripheral blood white cells.

○ **Persistent thrombocytopenia:** Persistent platelet count >1,000 × 10⁹/L that is unresponsive to treatment.

○ **Increasing splenomegaly:** Progressive enlargement of the spleen not controlled by standard therapy.

○ **Additional chromosomal abnormalities:** The presence of new chromosomal abnormalities in addition to the Philadelphia chromosome (BCR-ABL1 fusion gene) may suggest disease progression.

Blast phase (also called blast crisis):

○ **Increased blast count:** The bone marrow or peripheral blood shows 20% or more blasts.

○ **Extramedullary involvement:** The presence of leukemia cells in tissues outside of the bone marrow or blood, such as lymph nodes, liver or central nervous system.

○ **Rapid Progression:** Disease progression characterized by the rapid appearance and accumulation of blasts, often accompanied by worsening symptoms and signs of organ dysfunction.

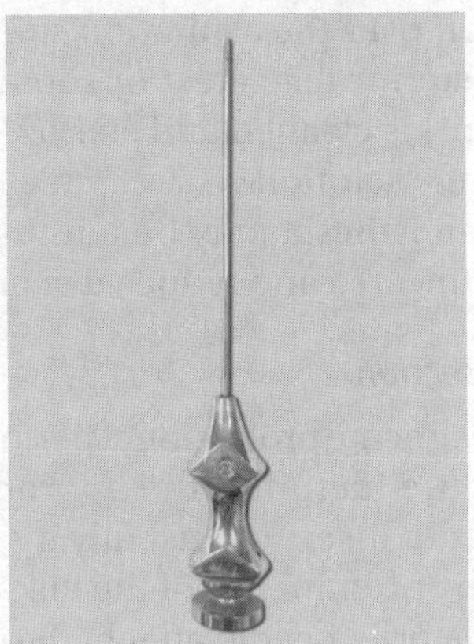

Fig. 4.21: Salah's needle for bone marrow aspiration.

○ **Resistance to therapy:** Failure to achieve a response or loss of response to standard CML treatment, such as tyrosine kinase inhibitors (TKIs).
○ **Additional chromosomal abnormalities:** Acquisition of new chromosomal abnormalities in addition to the Philadelphia chromosome (BCR-ABL1 fusion gene).

BONE MARROW EXAMINATION

Bone marrow examination, includes bone marrow aspiration and biopsy. It is performed to evaluate the cells and structure of the bone marrow. It is commonly used to diagnose and monitor various blood disorders such as leukemia, lymphoma, anemia and other conditions affecting the bone marrow.

Bone Marrow Aspiration

Salah's needle is most commonly used for bone marrow aspiration as shown in **Figure 4.21**.

The common sites for bone marrow aspiration are:
○ The posterior superior iliac spine (hip bone)
○ The anterior superior iliac spine
○ The sternum

○ Tibia in infants.

Bone marrow aspiration is a diagnostic procedure that involves obtaining a small sample of liquid bone marrow for examination. It is commonly performed along with a bone marrow biopsy. Some indications for bone marrow aspiration are:
○ Diagnosis and classification of hematological malignancies (e.g., leukemia, lymphoma, multiple myeloma).
○ Evaluation of unexplained cytopenias (e.g., anemia, leukopenia, thrombocytopenia).
○ Assessment of bone marrow cellularity and architecture.
○ Detection of metastatic cancer involving the bone marrow.
○ Investigation of unexplained fevers or infections.
○ Evaluation of unexplained bone pain or fractures.
○ Monitoring treatment response in hematological malignancies.
○ Assessment of disease progression or remission.
○ Investigation of unexplained splenomegaly.
○ Identification of infiltrative diseases affecting the bone marrow.
○ Workup of unexplained pancytopenia.
○ Evaluation of unexplained hepatomegaly.
○ Identification of genetic or chromosomal abnormalities.
○ Investigation of unexplained organomegaly.
○ Assessment of bone marrow involvement in systemic diseases.

Dry Tap on Bone Marrow Aspiration

A "dry tap" refers to a bone marrow aspiration procedure in which no fluid or only a minimal amount of fluid is obtained despite proper technique. It can be caused by various factors that impede the successful retrieval of bone marrow. Some common causes of dry tap in bone marrow aspiration include:
○ **Fibrosis:** Excessive deposition of fibrous tissue in the bone marrow can make it

difficult to aspirate the liquid component. Fibrosis is often associated with conditions like myelofibrosis, metastatic cancer or certain types of bone marrow disorders.

- **Hypocellular or aplastic bone marrow:** In conditions where the bone marrow is significantly hypocellular or aplastic, the reduced number of hematopoietic cells may result in a dry tap.
- **Marrow adhesions:** Adhesions between the bone and the marrow caused by previous trauma, infections or surgical interventions can make it challenging to aspirate bone marrow.
- **Infiltrative disorders:** In certain conditions, such as lymphoma or metastatic cancer, the bone marrow may be infiltrated by cancer cells, resulting in a reduced volume of liquid marrow available for aspiration.
- **Technical factors:** The dry tap may sometimes occur due to technical issues during the procedure, such as incorrect needle placement or inadequate negative pressure during aspiration.

It is important to note that a dry tap does not necessarily exclude the possibility of a bone marrow disorder or negate the need for further investigation. In cases of suspected bone marrow disorders or unexplained clinical symptoms, additional diagnostic tests, such as a bone marrow biopsy or alternative imaging techniques, may be required to obtain the necessary information for a diagnosis.

Procedure of Bone Marrow Aspiration

The procedure of bone marrow aspiration involves obtaining a sample of liquid bone marrow for examination. Here's a general overview of the bone marrow aspiration procedure:

Preparation

- The patient lies on their side, usually on the examination table, with the hip area exposed.
- The skin over the aspiration site (typically the posterior iliac crest or sometimes the sternum) is cleaned and sterilized with an antiseptic solution.
- Local anesthesia may be administered to numb the area and reduce discomfort.

Needle Insertion

- The healthcare professional performing the procedure identifies the appropriate site for needle insertion, usually by palpating the bony prominence of the iliac crest.
- A thin, sterile needle attached to a syringe is inserted through the skin and into the bone marrow cavity. The needle is typically inserted at an angle to reach the bone marrow space.

Aspiration

- Once the needle is properly positioned within the bone marrow cavity, the healthcare professional applies negative pressure by pulling back on the syringe plunger.
- This negative pressure helps to draw the liquid bone marrow into the syringe.
- The healthcare professional may adjust the needle's position slightly to aspirate from different areas within the bone marrow cavity.

Sample Collection

- Once an adequate amount of bone marrow fluid is obtained, the needle is carefully withdrawn.
- The collected bone marrow sample is then expelled into a container or transferred into appropriate tubes for further processing and examination.

Dressing and Recovery

- The aspiration site is typically covered with a sterile dressing or bandage to protect it.
- Pressure may be applied to the site briefly to promote hemostasis.

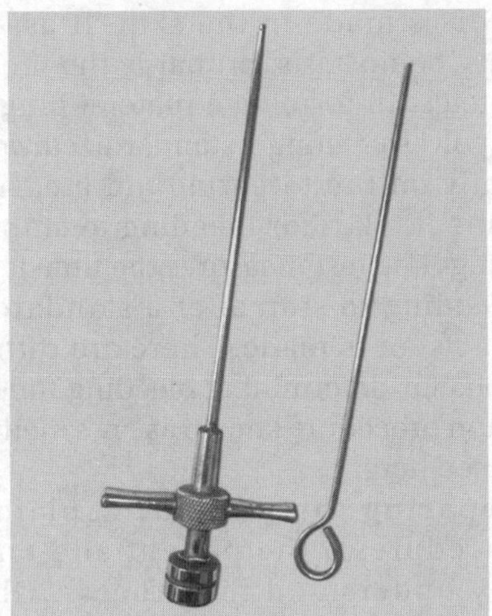

Fig. 4.22: Bone marrow biopsy Jamshidi needle.

○ The patient is usually advised to avoid any strenuous activities involving the aspiration site for a short period following the procedure.

The collected bone marrow sample is sent to a laboratory, where it is processed, stained, and examined under a microscope. The examination helps evaluate the cellular components of the bone marrow, such as hematopoietic stem cells, precursor cells, and supporting cells, assisting in the diagnosis and management of various hematological conditions.

Bone Marrow Biopsy

Bone marrow biopsy is indicated in various clinical scenarios to aid in the diagnosis, staging, and monitoring of various hematological and non-hematological conditions. Jamshidi needle **(Fig. 4.22)** is used for bone marrow biopsy.

Here are some common indications for bone marrow biopsy:

Indications of Bone Marrow Biopsy

○ Evaluation of unexplained anemia.
○ Diagnosis and staging of hematological malignancies (e.g., leukemia, lymphoma, multiple myeloma).
○ Unexplained abnormal blood cell counts (e.g., thrombocytopenia, leukopenia, leukocytosis).
○ Monitoring treatment response in hematological malignancies.
○ Investigation of unexplained fevers or infections.
○ Evaluation of unexplained bone pain or fractures.
○ Identification of infiltrative diseases involving the bone marrow (e.g., amyloidosis, Gaucher disease).
○ Assessment of bone marrow cellularity and architecture.
○ Detection of metastatic cancer involving the bone marrow.
○ Workup of unexplained splenomegaly.
○ Evaluation of unexplained hepatomegaly.
○ Identification of genetic or chromosomal abnormalities.
○ Assessment of bone marrow involvement in systemic diseases.
○ Evaluation of unexplained organomegaly.
○ Workup of unexplained pancytopenia.

Bone Marrow Biopsy

○ **Procedure:** Bone marrow biopsy involves obtaining a small core of bone and the surrounding bone marrow tissue. It is usually performed immediately after the bone marrow aspiration using a slightly larger needle. The biopsy is typically taken from the same site as the aspiration or an alternative site.
○ **Purpose:** The bone marrow biopsy provides a larger tissue sample for the assessment of the bone marrow architecture, including the arrangement and organization of cells, as well as the presence of fibrosis or other abnormalities. It helps evaluate the overall bone marrow health and the presence of

disorders that may affect the bone marrow structure.

○ **Examination:** The collected bone marrow biopsy specimen is processed, embedded in paraffin, and sliced into thin sections. These sections are then stained and examined under a microscope to assess the bone marrow architecture, cellularity, and any abnormalities.

○ Complications are rare but can include bleeding, infection, or damage to surrounding structures.

The results of a bone marrow examination, including both aspiration and biopsy, provide valuable information for diagnosing and monitoring blood disorders. They help guide treatment decisions and provide insights into the underlying causes and progression of various conditions affecting the bone marrow.

HEMOSTASIS

Hemostasis is the physiological process that stops bleeding and maintains blood in a fluid state within the circulatory system. It involves a complex series of events that include platelet activation, formation of a platelet plug, and the coagulation cascade leading to the formation of a fibrin clot. Any defect in the above mechanisms lead to impaired wound healing and bleeding disorders. The various investigations needed to evaluate these patients are:

○ Platelet count and function studies.
○ Bleeding time (BT) and clotting time (CT).
○ Prothrombin time (PT).
○ Activated partial thromboplastin time (aPTT).
○ Thrombin time (TT).
○ D-dimer test.

Bleeding Time

It is a laboratory test that measures the time taken for bleeding to stop after a small incision is made in the skin. It assesses primary hemostasis, primarily the function of platelets in forming a platelet plug. The test involves creating a standardized wound, typically on the forearm, and measuring the time it takes for bleeding to stop. The bleeding time test measures the time it takes for bleeding to stop after a standardized skin incision is made. There are different methods for determining bleeding time, but common procedure known as Ivy's method is discussed here.

○ **Preparing the patient:** Explain the procedure to the patient and ensure they understand the process. Obtain informed consent. It is important to note that certain individuals, such as those with bleeding disorders or taking anticoagulant medications, may not be suitable candidates for this test. Check the patient's medical history and medications before proceeding.

○ **Equipment setup:** Gather the necessary equipment, including a blood pressure cuff, a timer, a sterile lancet or blade, a gauze pad, and a paper template for marking the incision site. Ensure all equipment is sterile and ready for use.

○ **Site preparation:** Typically, the bleeding time test is performed on the volar surface of the forearm. Clean the area with an antiseptic solution and allow it to dry.

○ **Incision site marking:** Place the paper template over the cleaned area and mark the desired length of the incision. The standard length is often 10 millimeters (mm), but it can vary based on the laboratory's protocols.

○ **Incision:** Apply the blood pressure cuff proximally on the patient's upper arm and inflate it to a pressure above systolic pressure, usually around 40 mm Hg. This pressure is meant to occlude blood flow temporarily. Make a clean, shallow incision within the marked area using a sterile lancet or blade. Ensure the incision is perpendicular to the skin surface.

- ○ **Timing and blotting:** Immediately start the timer as the incision is made. Use a gauze pad to gently blot the incision site every 30 seconds until bleeding stops completely. Be careful not to touch the wound directly with your fingers to prevent contamination.
- ○ **Recording the time:** Stop the timer and record the time in seconds once bleeding has ceased entirely. The time recorded represents the bleeding time.
- ○ **Post-procedure care:** Apply an appropriate dressing or bandage to the incision site to protect it from infection and facilitate healing. Instruct the patient on proper care of the wound and any necessary follow-up procedures.

Clotting time: Measures the time it takes for blood to clot in a test tube after the addition of a clotting agent. Clotting time assesses both primary and secondary hemostasis, including the activity of clotting factors involved in the coagulation cascade.

Prothrombin time (PT) is a common laboratory test used to evaluate the extrinsic pathway of the coagulation cascade. It measures the time it takes for blood to clot after the addition of tissue factor and calcium. PT primarily assesses the activity of factors I (fibrinogen), II (prothrombin), V, VII, and X in the coagulation process. It is often used to monitor the effectiveness of oral anticoagulant medications like warfarin and to assess liver function, as many coagulation factors are produced in the liver.

Thrombin time (TT) is a laboratory test that measures the time it takes for fibrinogen in the blood to be converted into fibrin by the enzyme thrombin. It evaluates the final step of the coagulation cascade and assesses the functionality of fibrinogen and thrombin. Thrombin time is primarily used to detect abnormalities in fibrinogen

levels or functionality, such as in cases of dysfibrinogenemia or liver disease.

Activated partial thromboplastin time (aPTT) is a laboratory test that evaluates the intrinsic pathway of the coagulation cascade. It measures the time it takes for blood to clot after the addition of an activator, typically kaolin and phospholipids. aPTT assesses the functionality of various clotting factors, including factors VIII, IX, XI, and XII, as well as other proteins involved in the coagulation process. It is commonly used to diagnose and monitor the treatment of bleeding disorders, such as hemophilia, and to assess the effectiveness of heparin therapy.

D-dimer test is a laboratory test used to measure the levels of D-dimer in the blood. D-dimer is a fibrin degradation product that is produced when a blood clot is broken down by the body's natural fibrinolysis process.

Elevated D-dimer levels suggest increased fibrinolysis, which can be associated with the breakdown of blood clots. The D-dimer test is commonly used in the diagnosis and exclusion of conditions such as deep vein thrombosis (DVT), pulmonary embolism (PE), and disseminated intravascular coagulation (DIC). However, it is important to note that elevated D-dimer levels can also occur in various other clinical situations, including inflammation, trauma, pregnancy, and certain cancers. Therefore, the D-dimer test is often used as a screening tool, and additional diagnostic tests are required to confirm the presence of a blood clot or determine the underlying cause.

Whole Blood Clotting Time

Whole blood clotting time, also known as the Lee-White method or the capillary tube method, is a laboratory test used to assess the time it takes for blood to clot. It measures the overall clotting time of whole blood, including both the intrinsic and extrinsic pathways of coagulation.

Procedure for whole blood clotting time:

○ **Sample collection:** Blood is typically collected from a vein in the patient's arm using a sterile needle and syringe or a vacuum tube system. The blood is collected in a clean, dry tube.

○ **Preparation of capillary tube:** A small, thin capillary tube is filled with the patient's blood. One end of the tube is sealed by melting or using a clay sealant, while the other end remains open.

○ **Timing and observation:** The open end of the capillary tube is held vertically, and the time is started using a stopwatch. The technician or healthcare professional closely observes the tube for the appearance of a visible fibrin clot.

○ **Clot formation:** As the blood clots, a visible fibrin clot starts to form in the capillary tube. The technician continues to observe the tube until a stable clot is present, which is typically indicated by a fixed, non-movable column of blood within the tube.

○ **Recording the time:** The time it takes for the clot to form and stabilize in the capillary tube is recorded as the whole blood clotting time.

It is not commonly being used now a days due to the availability of automated analyzers and more sensitive and specific tests.

The Prothrombin Test

It is a laboratory test used to evaluate the extrinsic pathway of the coagulation cascade and monitor the effectiveness of oral anticoagulant therapy, such as warfarin. It measures the time it takes for blood to clot after the addition of tissue factor and calcium.

Procedure

○ **Sample collection:** Blood is collected from a vein in the patient's arm using a sterile needle and syringe or a vacuum tube system. The blood is collected in a tube containing an anticoagulant, typically citrate.

○ **Preparation of plasma:** The collected blood sample is centrifuged to separate the liquid portion, known as plasma, from the cellular components (red blood cells and platelets). The plasma is used for the prothrombin test.

○ **Addition of reagents:** Tissue factor, also known as thromboplastin, and calcium ions are added to the plasma sample. Tissue factor acts as an activator for the extrinsic pathway of coagulation.

○ **Timing and clot formation:** The stopwatch or automated coagulation analyzer is started as the tissue factor and calcium are added to the plasma sample. The technician or automated system monitors the sample for the formation of a visible clot.

○ **Recording the time:** The time it takes for the clot to form is recorded as the prothrombin time (PT). PT is measured in seconds or in a ratio called the International Normalized Ratio (INR), which standardizes the results across different laboratories and reagents.

Principle

The prothrombin test measures the time it takes for the extrinsic pathway of the coagulation cascade to convert prothrombin (factor II) into thrombin (factor IIa). Thrombin is a key enzyme involved in the conversion of fibrinogen to fibrin, leading to the formation of a blood clot.

The addition of tissue factor to the plasma sample initiates the extrinsic pathway of coagulation, which activates factor VII (proconvertin). Factor VII then activates factor X (Stuart factor) in the presence of calcium ions. The activated factor X leads to the formation of thrombin.

The prothrombin time measures the effectiveness of this extrinsic pathway, and it is commonly used to monitor oral anticoagulant therapy, as these medications interfere with the normal clotting process. The PT results are typically compared to reference ranges or target ranges, and the INR is calculated to ensure appropriate anticoagulant dosage.

The normal range for the International Normalized Ratio (INR) varies depending on the specific clinical situation and the reason for anticoagulant therapy. The INR is a standardized measurement used to monitor and adjust the dosage of oral anticoagulant medications, such as warfarin.

As a general guideline, the target INR range for most individuals on oral anticoagulant therapy is commonly within the range of 2.0 to 3.0. However, the target range may differ based on factors such as the underlying condition being treated, the presence of certain medical conditions, and the individual's overall health status.

Here are some examples of target INR ranges for specific conditions:

○ **Atrial fibrillation:** INR range of 2.0 to 3.0, with a higher range (e.g., 2.5 to 3.5) in certain cases, such as additional risk factors or a history of stroke.

○ **Venous thromboembolism (DVT/PE):** INR range of 2.0 to 3.0, with initial higher intensity therapy (e.g., INR 2.5 to 3.5) in some cases.

○ **Mechanical heart valve:** INR range typically higher, such as 2.5 to 3.5 or even higher depending on the specific type and location of the valve.

Activated Partial Thromboplastin Time (aPTT)

Activated partial thromboplastin time (aPTT) is a laboratory test that measures the intrinsic pathway of the coagulation cascade. It assesses the functionality of various clotting factors and their interactions with platelets.

Principle

The aPTT test measures the time it takes for blood to clot when an activator, usually kaolin or silica, and calcium are added to the plasma sample. The activator triggers the intrinsic pathway of coagulation, leading to the activation of clotting factors, particularly factors XII, XI, IX, VIII, X, and V, as well as fibrinogen and platelets. The time it takes for a fibrin clot to form is recorded as the aPTT.

Procedure

○ **Sample collection:** Blood is collected from a vein in the patient's arm using a sterile needle and syringe or a vacuum tube system. The blood is collected in a tube containing an anticoagulant, typically citrate.

○ **Preparation of plasma:** The collected blood sample is centrifuged to separate the liquid portion, known as plasma, from the cellular components (red blood cells and platelets). The plasma is used for the aPTT test.

○ **Addition of reagents:** The plasma sample is mixed with an activator (kaolin or silica) and calcium ions. These reagents mimic the activation of the intrinsic pathway of coagulation.

○ **Timing and clot formation:** The stopwatch or automated coagulation analyzer is started as the activator and calcium are added to the plasma sample. The technician or automated system monitors the sample for the formation of a visible fibrin clot.

○ **Recording the time:** The time it takes for the clot to form is recorded as the aPTT. The result is typically reported in seconds.

Reference range: The normal range for aPTT is typically between 25 to 35 seconds. It is important to note that the reference range may differ in specific situations, such as when a patient is on anticoagulant therapy or has

Table 4.24: Causes of prolonged aPTT

Causes of prolonged aPTT	Description
Hemophilia A or B	Genetic bleeding disorders characterized by deficiencies in clotting factors VIII (hemophilia A) or IX (hemophilia B)
Von Willebrand disease (VWD)	Inherited bleeding disorder involving deficiency or dysfunction of von Willebrand factor (vWF)
Lupus anticoagulant	Autoimmune disorder associated with abnormal antibodies that interfere with normal blood clotting
Specific factor deficiencies	Deficiencies in clotting factors XI, XII, or prekallikrein
Liver disease	Conditions affecting the liver, such as cirrhosis, hepatitis, or liver failure, leading to impaired clotting factor production
Anticoagulant therapy	Use of anticoagulant medications, such as heparin, warfarin, or direct oral anticoagulants (DOACs)

an underlying bleeding disorder. Therefore, it is essential to interpret the aPTT results in conjunction with the patient's clinical history, medications, and other coagulation tests to ensure accurate assessment and diagnosis. Some of the causes of prolonged aPTT are shown in **Table 4.24**.

Bleeding Disorders

Bleeding disorders are a group of medical conditions characterized by abnormalities in the body's ability to form blood clots, leading to an increased risk of bleeding. These disorders can be inherited or acquired and can affect various aspects of the clotting process, including platelet function, coagulation factor production, or the integrity of blood vessels. Here are some examples of bleeding disorders:

○ **Hemophilia:** Hemophilia is an inherited bleeding disorder caused by deficiencies or defects in specific clotting factors, most commonly factor VIII (hemophilia A) or factor IX (hemophilia B). It results in prolonged bleeding after injury or spontaneous bleeding into joints, muscles or other body tissues.

○ **Von Willebrand disease:** Von Willebrand disease (VWD) is the most common inherited bleeding disorder. It is caused by a deficiency or dysfunction of von Willebrand factor (vWF), a protein that helps platelets adhere to damaged blood vessel walls and carries clotting factor VIII. VWD can lead to mucosal bleeding, easy bruising, and prolonged bleeding after injury or surgery.

○ **Platelet function disorders:** These disorders are characterized by abnormalities in platelet function, leading to impaired platelet aggregation, adhesion, or secretion of clotting factors. Examples include Glanzmann thrombasthenia and Bernard-Soulier syndrome. People with platelet function disorders may experience excessive bleeding or prolonged bleeding from minor injuries or surgeries.

○ **Acquired coagulation factor deficiencies:** Certain medical conditions or medications can lead to acquired deficiencies in clotting factors. For example, liver disease can result in decreased production of multiple clotting factors, while the use of anticoagulant medications (e.g., warfarin) can interfere with the normal functioning of clotting factors.

○ **Disseminated intravascular coagulation (DIC):** DIC is a serious condition that can occur as a result of underlying conditions such as sepsis, trauma, cancer, or complications during pregnancy. It is characterized by widespread activation of the clotting system, leading to both clot formation and excessive bleeding.

○ **Immune thrombocytopenic purpura (ITP):** Also known as idiopathic thrombocytopenic purpura, is an autoimmune disorder characterized by low platelet levels in the blood with bleeding and bruising tendencies. The term "purpura" refers to the characteristic purple-red spots on the skin caused by bleeding under the surface.

○ ITP occurs when the body's immune system mistakenly identifies its platelets as foreign and attacks them, leading to their destruction and removal from circulation. The exact cause of this autoimmune response is not always clear, but it is thought to involve a combination of genetic and environmental factors.

Symptoms of ITP may include:

○ **Petechiae:** Pinpoint-sized, reddish-purple spots on the skin caused by tiny blood vessel bleeds.

○ **Ecchymosis:** Larger, bruise-like patches resulting from bleeding under the skin.

○ Prolonged bleeding from minor cuts or injuries.

○ Nosebleeds or bleeding gums.

○ Menstrual bleeding that is heavier than usual.

○ Blood in urine or stools (in severe cases).

ITP can affect both children and adults. In children, it often follows a viral infection and might resolve on its own without treatment. However, adults may have chronic ITP that requires ongoing management. The difference between acute ITP and chronic ITP is depicted in **Table 4.25**.

Diagnosis of ITP involves a thorough medical history, physical examination, blood tests to assess platelet count and function, and sometimes a bone marrow biopsy to

Table 4.25: Differences between acute ITP and chronic ITP.

Aspect	Acute ITP	Chronic ITP
Duration	Generally resolves within 6 months	Persists for longer than 6 months
Onset	Sudden onset	Insidious or gradual onset
Age group affected	Predominantly affects children, especially after viral infections	Predominantly affects adults, with a peak incidence in middle age
Platelet count	Usually very low (<20,000/mm^3)	Variable platelet count, often above 20,000/mm^3
Spontaneous remission	Common, with many cases resolving spontaneously	Less common, spontaneous remission rates are lower
Treatment response	Typically responds well to initial treatments	More resistant to treatment, may require ongoing management
Underlying conditions	Often follows viral infections or other triggers	Not usually associated with an underlying trigger or infection
Risk of bleeding	Generally higher due to severe thrombocytopenia	Lower risk due to higher platelet counts
Long-term complications	Rarely leads to long-term complications	May lead to chronic bleeding symptoms or require ongoing care
Prognosis	Favorable prognosis in the majority of cases	Variable prognosis, some cases can be persistent or refractory

rule out other possible causes of low platelet levels.

Treatment options for ITP may vary depending on the severity of symptoms and the patient's age. In children with mild symptoms, the condition may resolve spontaneously, and watchful waiting is recommended.

Medications: Corticosteroids, such as prednisone, can help raise platelet counts by suppressing the immune system. Other immunosuppressive drugs may be prescribed if steroids are ineffective or not well-tolerated.

Intravenous immunoglobulin (IVIG): This treatment involves infusing high levels of immunoglobulins to block the immune system's attack on platelets temporarily.

Platelet transfusions: In severe bleeding situations, platelet transfusions might be given to rapidly increase platelet levels.

Splenectomy: If other treatments are unsuccessful, surgical removal of the spleen (splenectomy) may be considered. However, this procedure is not suitable for all cases and is more commonly performed in chronic and refractory cases of ITP.

Newer treatments: In recent years, several novel drugs, such as thrombopoietin receptor agonists, have been approved for the treatment of ITP.

Rare bleeding disorders: There are several other rare bleeding disorders caused by deficiencies or dysfunction of specific clotting factors, such as factor VII deficiency, factor XIII deficiency, or afibrinogenemia.

Disseminated Intravascular Coagulation

Disseminated intravascular coagulation (DIC) is a complex and potentially life-threatening condition characterized by widespread activation of the clotting cascade, leading to the formation of blood clots throughout the body's blood vessels. The excessive clotting can consume clotting factors and platelets, resulting in both clotting and bleeding tendencies. DIC is usually triggered by an underlying condition or event that disrupts the normal balance of coagulation and anticoagulation. Some common causes and triggers of DIC:

- Sepsis
- Trauma
- Obstetric complications such as placental abruption, amniotic fluid embolism, retained fetal material, or severe preeclampsia can trigger DIC during pregnancy or childbirth.
- **Cancer:** Hematologic malignancies, such as acute promyelocytic leukemia, are especially linked to DIC.
- Organ failure such as liver disease (e.g., acute liver failure, cirrhosis), renal failure,

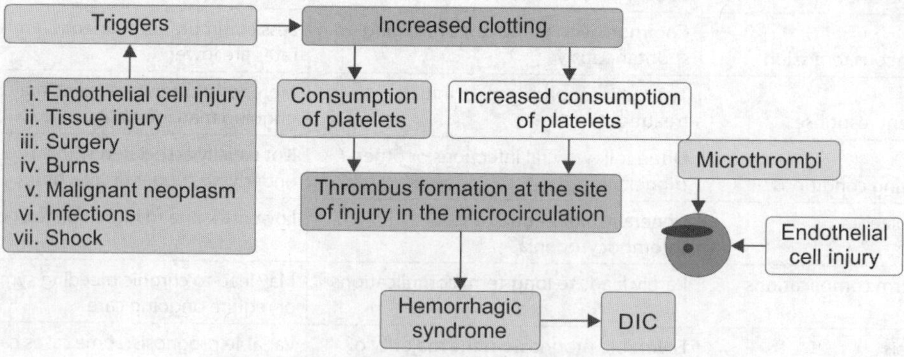

Fig. 4.23: Mechanism of DIC.

or severe respiratory distress syndrome, can trigger DIC.

O **Major vascular disorders:** Conditions like extensive aortic aneurysm, severe vasculitis, or large vessel thrombosis can disrupt blood flow and trigger DIC.

O **Transfusions and incompatible blood products:** Massive blood transfusions or the administration of incompatible blood products can induce DIC due to immune-mediated reactions or other factors.

O **Snake or insect bites:** Certain venomous snake or insect bites can activate the coagulation system, leading to DIC.

The mechanism of disseminated intravascular coagulation (DIC) is shown in **Figure 4.23**.

Laboratory Findings Observed in DIC

O **Platelet count:** Severe thrombocytopenia (platelet count <100,000/mm³) is often observed in advanced stages of DIC.

O **Prothrombin time (PT) and International Normalized Ratio (INR):** PT, is typically prolonged in DIC due to the depletion of clotting factors involved in this pathway. The INR, which is a standardized measurement of PT, may also be elevated.

O **Activated partial thromboplastin time (aPTT):** The aPTT is often prolonged in DIC due to consumption of clotting factors.

O **Fibrinogen level:** Initially, fibrinogen levels may be elevated as a result of acute phase reactants. However, as fibrinogen is consumed in the formation of fibrin clots, the fibrinogen level decreases.

O **D-dimer:** D-dimer levels are elevated in DIC due to the breakdown of cross-linked fibrin by fibrinolysis..

O **Fibrin degradation products (FDPs):** FDPs, which are breakdown products of fibrin, are increased in DIC due to ongoing fibrinolysis. Elevated FDP levels further confirm the presence of ongoing clot formation and breakdown.

O **Peripheral blood smear:** Examination of the peripheral blood smear may reveal the presence of schistocytes (fragmented red blood cells), indicating the presence of microangiopathic hemolysis.

COAGULATION PATHWAYS AND THEIR ABNORMALITIES

The coagulation process, also known as blood clotting, involves a complex series of biochemical reactions that are essential for hemostasis (the prevention and control of bleeding). The coagulation cascade can be divided into two main pathways: the intrinsic pathway and the extrinsic pathway **(Table 4.26)**.

O **Intrinsic pathway:** The intrinsic pathway is initiated by damage to the endothelial lining of blood vessels, exposure of blood to collagen, or contact with certain foreign substances. This pathway occurs within the bloodstream and involves several

Table 4.26: Different pathways of Coagulation cascade

Pathway	Initiation	Key factors
Intrinsic	Activation by contact with negatively charged surfaces	Factors XII (Hageman factor), XI (plasma thromboplastin antecedent), IX (Christmas factor), VIII (antihemophilic factor A), and prekallikrein (Fletcher factor)
Extrinsic	Tissue injury	Tissue factor (factor III) and factor VII (Proconvertin)
Common pathway	Convergence of intrinsic and extrinsic pathways	Factors X (Stuart factor), V (Proaccelerin), II (prothrombin), I (fibrinogen), and XIII (fibrin stabilizing factor)

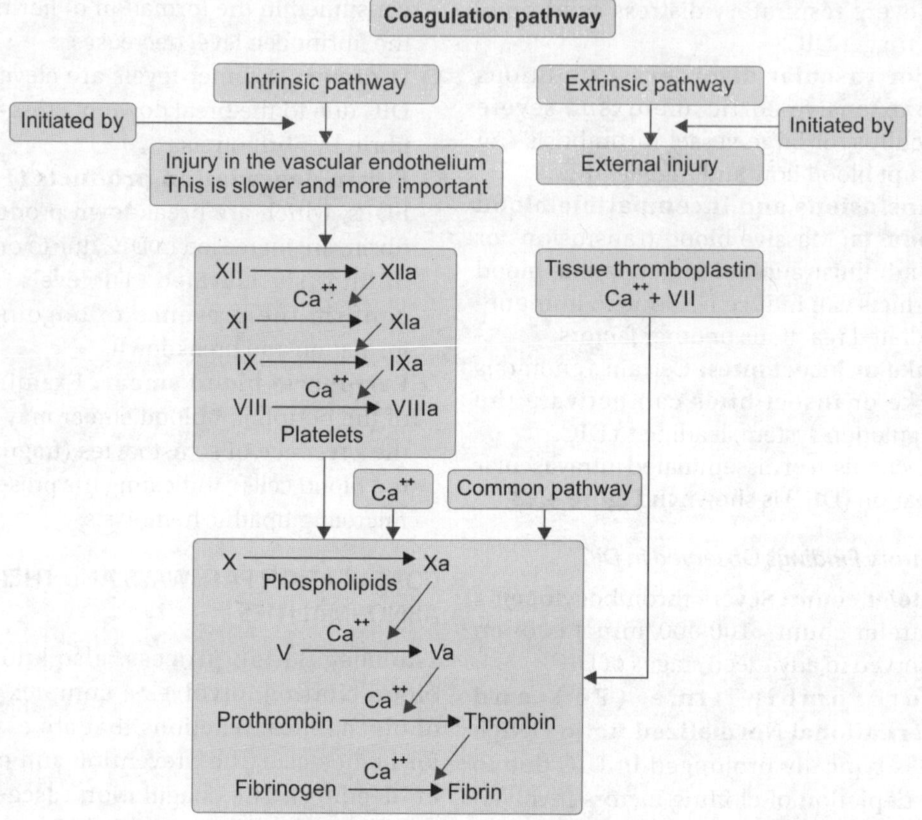

Fig. 4.24: Coagulation pathway.

coagulation factors. Here are the key steps of the intrinsic pathway:

○ **Activation:** In response to vessel injury or contact with foreign substances, factor XII (Hageman factor) is activated.
○ Factor XII activates factor XI, which in turn activates factor IX.
○ Factor IX, in complex with its cofactor factor VIII, is activated by factor XIa. This activated complex, called the intrinsic tenase complex, activates factor X.
○ Factor X then proceeds to activate the common pathway, leading to the formation of a fibrin clot.
○ **Extrinsic pathway:** The extrinsic pathway is triggered by tissue damage and is responsible for the rapid initiation of

clotting. It involves the release of tissue factor (also known as factor III) from damaged tissues into the bloodstream. The steps of the extrinsic pathway are as follows:

○ Tissue factor (factor III) is released from damaged tissues.
○ Tissue factor forms a complex with factor VII, which activates factor VII.
○ Activated factor VII (factor VIIa) then activates factor X.
○ Factor X proceeds to activate the common pathway, leading to clot formation.

The intrinsic and extrinsic pathways converge to activate the common pathway **(Fig. 4.24)**, which involves the activation of factor X and the subsequent generation of

Table 4.27: Coagulation factors.

Coagulation factor	Name	Function
I	Fibrinogen	Converted to fibrin by thrombin, forming the structural framework of blood clots
II	Prothrombin	Converted to thrombin, a key enzyme in the coagulation cascade
III	Tissue factor	Initiates the extrinsic pathway of coagulation
IV	Calcium ions	Essential for the activation of several clotting factors and the formation of a stable fibrin clot
V	Proaccelerin	Serves as a cofactor for the activation of factor X
VII	Proconvertin	Initiates the extrinsic pathway of coagulation, forms a complex with tissue factor to activate factor X
VIII	Antihemophilic factor A	Enhances the activation of factor X by serving as a cofactor for the intrinsic pathway
IX	Christmas factor	Activated by factor XI and participates in the intrinsic pathway of coagulation
X	Stuart factor	Activated by both the intrinsic and extrinsic pathways, plays a crucial role in the common pathway of coagulation
XI	Plasma thromboplastin antecedent	Activated by factor XII and contributes to the intrinsic pathway
XII	Hageman factor	Initiates the intrinsic pathway of coagulation, activates factors XI and prekallikrein

thrombin. Thrombin, in turn, converts fibrinogen into fibrin, forming a stable blood clot.

Factors Involved in Blood Coagulation

Coagulation of blood occurs through a series of reactions due to the activation of a group of substances called clotting factors. There are 13 clotting factors identified and named after the scientists who discovered them or as per the activity as shown in **Table 4.27**. Only factor IX or Christmas factor is named after the patient in whom it was discovered.

AUTOMATION IN HEMATOLOGY

Automation has significantly impacted the field of hematology, revolutionizing laboratory processes and enhancing diagnostic capabilities. Here are some areas where automation has been implemented in hematology:

○ **Complete blood count (CBC):** The CBC is a fundamental test in hematology, providing information about red blood cells, white blood cells, and platelets. Automation has streamlined the process of performing CBCs, reducing the manual labor required and improving accuracy and efficiency. Automated analyzers can quickly and accurately count and classify blood cells, measure cell sizes, and provide information on various parameters such as hemoglobin levels, hematocrit, and differential white blood cell counts.

○ **Hematology analyzers:** Automated hematology analyzers **(Fig. 4.25)** are used to process blood samples and provide comprehensive information about the cellular components of the blood. These analyzers use a combination of technologies such as impedance, flow cytometry, and spectrophotometry to analyze and characterize blood cells. They can handle a high volume of samples, provide rapid results, and often include advanced features like flagging abnormal cells for further investigation.

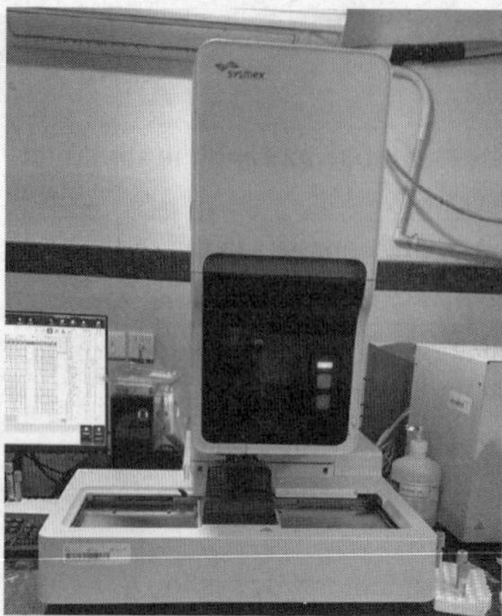

Fig. 4.25: Automated hematology analyzer (6-part).

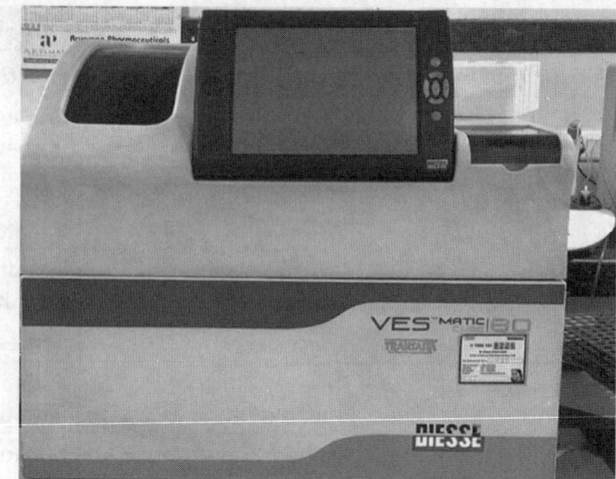

Fig. 4.26: Automated coagulation analyzer.

○ Automated coagulation analyzers **(Fig. 4.26)** are used to perform coagulation tests on blood samples. These analyzers are designed to automate and standardize the coagulation testing process, providing accurate and reliable results in a timely manner. Some common coagulation tests performed on automated analyzers include—prothrombin time (PT), thrombin time (TT), International Normalized Ratio (INR), activated partial thromboplastin time (aPTT), D-dimer and fibrinogen (Factor I).

○ **Slide preparation:** Traditionally, blood smears for microscopic examination were prepared manually by spreading a drop of blood on a glass slide and smearing it. However, automated slide preparation systems are now available that can perform this process with consistent quality and speed. These systems improve standardization and reduce the variability introduced by manual preparation.

○ **Morphological analysis:** Manual examination of blood smears under a microscope is a crucial aspect of hematology diagnosis. While automation cannot replace the expertise of a skilled hematologist, it can aid in the analysis by digitizing the slides and providing computer-assisted image analysis. Automated image recognition algorithms can identify and classify blood cells, flagging abnormal cells for further scrutiny by the hematologist. This can improve efficiency and accuracy, especially in high-volume laboratories.

○ **Data management:** Automation has also greatly improved data management in hematology laboratories. Laboratory information systems (LIS) are now commonly used to automate sample tracking, result reporting, and integration with other laboratory systems. This allows for faster turnaround times, improved accuracy, and seamless integration with electronic health records (EHR) systems.

Overall, automation in hematology has transformed laboratory processes, reducing human error, increasing throughput, and enhancing diagnostic capabilities. It has enabled faster and more accurate analysis of blood samples, leading to improved patient care and outcomes.

BLOOD BANKING

Blood Grouping

Blood grouping refers to the classification of blood into different types based on the presence or absence of certain antigens on the surface of red blood cells. At least 100 blood grouping antigens have been defined and the important blood group systems are ABO, Rh, MNS P, Lutheran, Kell, Lewis, Duffy, Kidd, Diego, Li, Yt Xg, Dombrock, and Colton. The two most common blood grouping systems are the ABO system and the Rh system.

ABO System of Blood Grouping

The ABO blood group system is the most well-known and widely used blood grouping system. It classifies human blood into four major types based on the presence or absence of two antigens, A and B, on the surface of red blood cells:

- **Blood Type A:** Individuals with blood type A have the A antigen on their red blood cells. Their plasma contains antibodies against the B antigen, called anti-B antibodies.
- **Blood Type B:** Individuals with blood type B have the B antigen on their red blood cells. Their plasma contains antibodies against the A antigen, called anti-A antibodies.
- **Blood Type AB:** Individuals with blood type AB have both the A and B antigens on their red blood cells. They do not naturally produce antibodies against either A or B antigens.
- **Blood Type O:** Individuals with blood type O do not have either the A or B antigens on their red blood cells. However, they have both anti-A and anti-B antibodies in their plasma, which can react against the corresponding antigens in other blood types.
- The ABO blood type is determined by inheriting genes from parents. The ABO alleles responsible for the A, B, and O blood types are denoted as IA, IB, and i, respectively. The possible genotypes and resulting blood types are as follows:
  - Blood type A: IAIA or IAi
  - Blood type B: IBIB or IBi
  - Blood type AB: IAIB
  - Blood type O: ii

- The ABO blood group system is important in blood transfusions to ensure compatibility. Generally, individuals with blood type A can receive blood from donors with blood types A or O, individuals with blood type B can receive blood from donors with blood types B or O, individuals with blood type AB can receive blood from donors with any blood type (A, B, AB, or O), and individuals with blood type O can only receive blood from donors with blood type O.
- The ABO system also plays a role in determining compatibility for organ transplantation and can influence certain medical conditions and disease susceptibility.

Rh System of Blood Grouping

- The Rh system is a blood group system named after the Rhesus monkey, in which the factor was first discovered.
- It is one of the most important blood group systems in humans, along with the ABO system.
- The Rh system determines the presence or absence of the Rh antigen on the surface of red blood cells.
- If the Rh antigen is present, an individual is said to be Rh positive (Rh+).
- If the Rh antigen is absent, the individual is Rh negative (Rh–).
- The most important Rh antigen is called RhD, and it is what determines whether someone is Rh+ or Rh–
- The Rh system is particularly significant in situations where blood transfusions or pregnancies are involved.
- In blood transfusions, Rh compatibility is crucial to prevent the recipient's immune system from attacking the transfused red blood cells.
- Rh incompatibility can also cause complications during pregnancy if an Rh-mother carries an Rh+ fetus, as the mother's

immune system may produce antibodies against the Rh antigen, potentially affecting future pregnancies.

Bombay Blood Group

○ The Bombay blood group is also known as the Bombay phenotype.
○ It is a rare blood group type that was first discovered in Bombay (now Mumbai), India.
○ Individuals with the Bombay blood group do not express the ABO antigens on their red blood cells and are typed as "O" since they lack the A and B antigens.
○ These individuals have additional antibodies that target the A and B antigens, which are naturally absent in their blood.
○ It is considered to be extremely rare, with an estimated frequency of 1 in every 250,000 individuals in the general population
○ Symbol Oh is used for this blood group. These individuals cannot form basic H antigen. It results in RBCs with no H, A, or B antigen (patient types as O) that is why Bombay blood group people have abs against A, B, H antigen.
○ These individuals require blood from other rare Bombay blood group donors or from individuals who are genetically HH or Hh and do not produce the A or B antigens.

There are several less common blood group systems in addition to the well-known ABO and Rh systems. These blood group systems are characterized by different antigens present on the surface of red blood cells:

○ **Kell blood group system:** The Kell system is one of the most clinically significant blood group systems after ABO and Rh. It includes antigens such as K, k, Kp(a), and Kp(b). Kell antibodies can cause severe reactions during transfusions and can also lead to hemolytic disease of the newborn.
○ **Duffy blood group system:** The Duffy system consists of antigens that determine the susceptibility to malaria infection. The antigens include Fya and Fyb. People lacking the Duffy antigens [Fy(a-b-)] are generally resistant to certain strains of malaria.
○ **Kidd blood group system:** The Kidd system comprises the Jka and Jkb antigens. Antibodies against these antigens can cause transfusion reactions. The Kidd antigens can also play a role in the rejection of transplanted kidneys.
○ **MNS blood group system:** The MNS system includes a variety of antigens, such as M, N, S, and s. Antibodies against these antigens can cause transfusion reactions and hemolytic disease of the newborn.
○ **Diego blood group system:** The Diego system includes antigens such as Di(a) and Di(b). Antibodies against these antigens can cause transfusion reactions and hemolytic disease of the newborn.
○ **Lutheran blood group system:** The Lutheran system includes antigens Lu(a) and Lu(b). Antibodies against these antigens can cause transfusion reactions and hemolytic disease of the newborn.
○ **P blood group system:** The P system includes antigens P1, P, and Pk. Antibodies against these antigens can cause transfusion reactions and are associated with paroxysmal cold hemoglobinuria.

There are several methods used to determine blood groups, including:

○ **Forward typing (cell typing):** This method involves mixing the donor's blood sample with specific antibodies that are known to react with certain blood group antigens. The blood group can be determined by observing the agglutination (clumping) of red blood cells. For example, if clumping occurs when anti-A antibodies are added to the blood sample, it indicates the presence of A antigen, and the blood type is classified as A.

○ **Reverse typing (serum typing):** In this method, the donor's serum (liquid portion of the blood) is mixed with red blood cells of known blood types. If agglutination occurs, it indicates the presence of antibodies against the corresponding antigens in the donor's serum. This helps determine the blood group by identifying the antibodies present.

○ **Slide method:** This method involves placing a drop of blood on a microscope slide and adding specific reagents (known as antisera) containing antibodies against A, B, and Rh antigens. The appearance of agglutination or lack thereof helps determine the blood type.

○ **Gel method:** This is a more advanced technique that uses a gel matrix containing specific antibodies. The donor's blood sample is mixed with the gel, and the antigens in the blood react with the corresponding antibodies in the gel. Agglutination or lack thereof helps determine the blood group **(Figs. 4.27 to 4.29)**.

○ **Tube method:** The tube method involves a series of test tubes, each containing different reagents (known antibodies) that react with the specific antigens on the red blood cells. In this method the RBCs and antibodies mixture is centrifuged, and the result is easily interpreted by visual examination. If the RBC sediment is undisturbed after centrifugation for a few minutes and gently shaking the test tube, it is considered complete agglutination. On the other hand, uniform distribution suspension of the RBCs indicates non-agglutination. In the event of a lack of any obvious agglutination, the RBC suspension is dropped on a glass slide, and the degree of agglutination is observed under a microscope. The interpretation of these results varies on individual interpretation and lacks a unified standard. In addition,

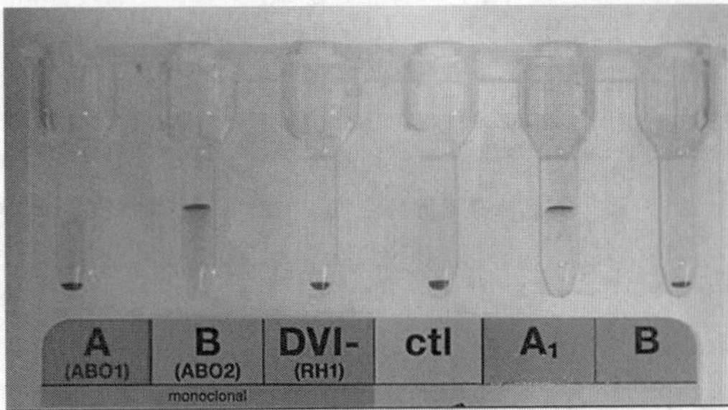

Fig. 4.27: Blood group B –ve by forward cell typing method.

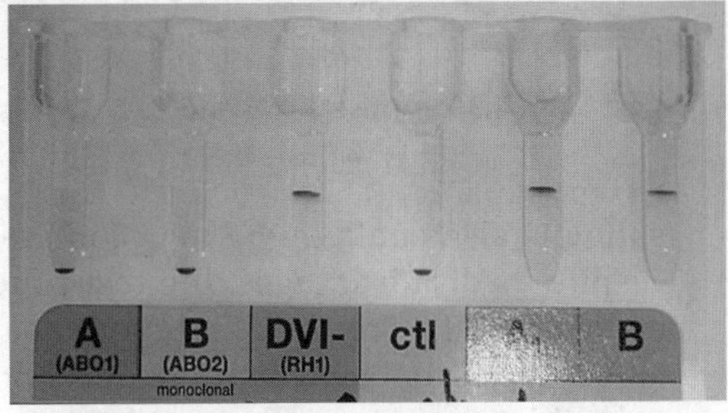

Fig. 4.28: Blood group O +ve by forward cell typing method.

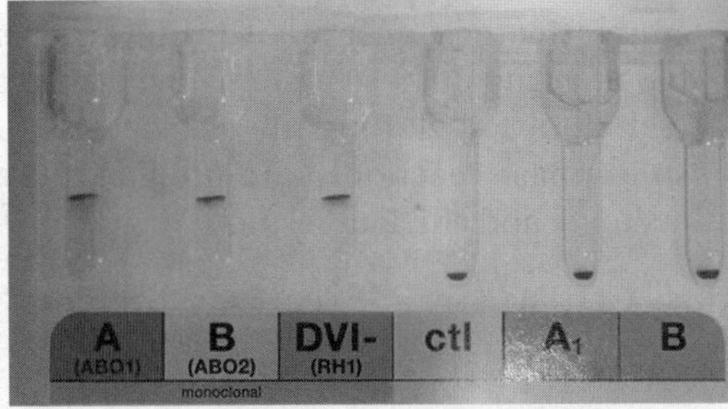

Fig. 4.29: Blood group AB +ve by forward cell typing method.

(For color version, see Plate 5)

this method cannot be used to accurately determine the blood group in infants (reverse typing), leukemia patients with weak antigens, and patients with low antibody titers, etc. It is imperative to clean test tubes, be precise with the centrifugation time and speed, and observe the results under ambient conditions to assure the accuracy of this testing. Tube

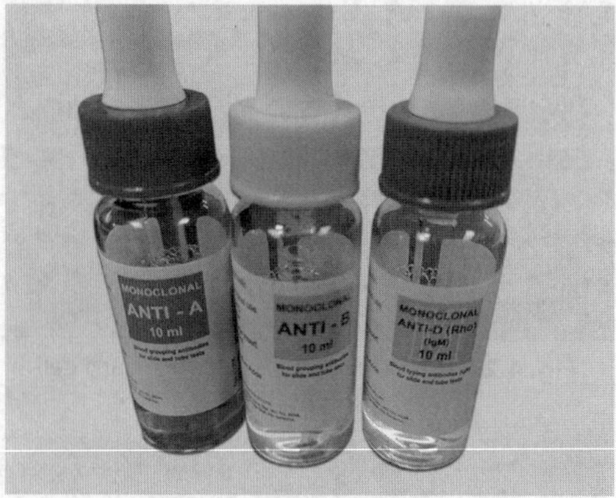

Fig. 4.30: Antisera A, B and D.

(For color version, see Plate 5)

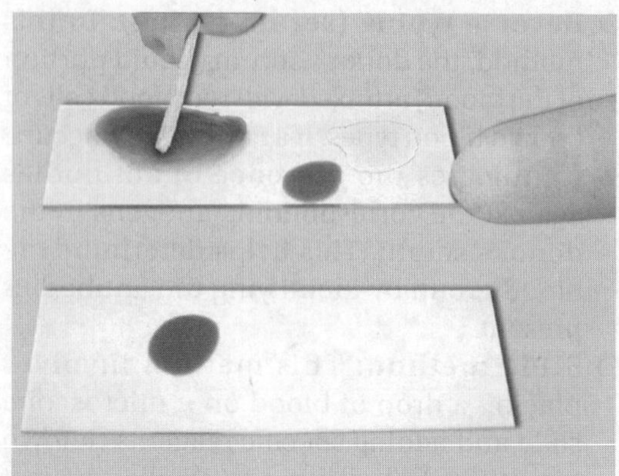

Fig. 4.31: Method of mixing of antisera and blood sample.

(For color version, see Plate 5)

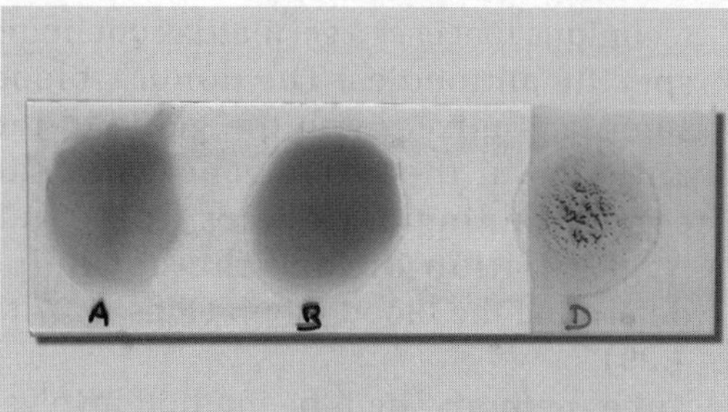

Fig. 4.32: Depicting O +ve blood group.

(For color version, see Plate 6)

testing is also challenging to automate. Despite its disadvantages, the test-tube method is still a prevalent technique that has been used for blood type identification and validation.

○ **Automated methods:** Modern laboratories often use automated systems that employ sophisticated equipment to determine blood groups. These systems use various techniques, including the gel method or solid-phase reactions, and provide more accurate and efficient results.

Slide Method

Procedure

○ **Preparation of the slide:** Clean the glass slide thoroughly to ensure it is free of contaminants. Label the slide with the donor's identification information.

○ **Adding blood sample:** Using a sterile lancet or needle, puncture the donor's fingertip to obtain a small drop of blood and carefully place the drop in the center of the slide. The blood sample collected in EDTA vial can also be used.

○ **Addition of reagents:** Add a drop of anti-A serum to one side of the blood drop and a drop of anti-B serum to the other side. For Rh typing, a drop of anti-Rh(D) serum is added separately **(Fig. 4.30)**.

○ Antisera stored at 4–6°C to preserve their potency

○ **Mixing:** Using a separate applicator stick for each reagent, gently mix the blood drop with the corresponding antisera. Ensure that the blood and antisera are thoroughly mixed but avoid spreading the mixture beyond the designated areas **(Fig. 4.31)**.

○ **Observing agglutination:** After mixing, observe the slide under a microscope or with the naked eye. Look for the presence or absence of agglutination (clumping) of red blood cells.

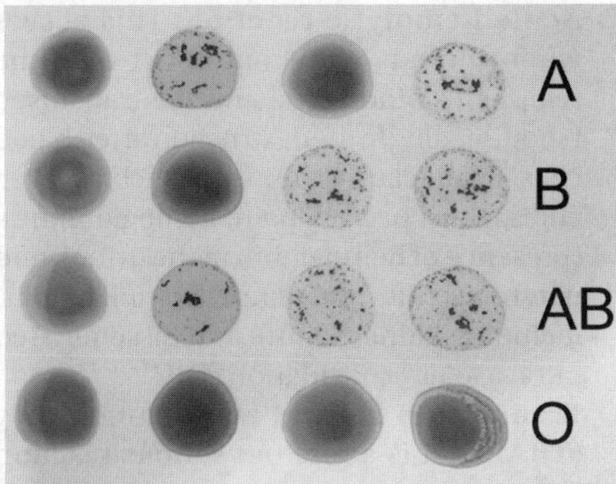

Fig. 4.33: Blood grouping based on agglutination.
(For color version, see Plate 6)

If agglutination occurs:
- Agglutination with anti-A serum indicates the presence of A antigen, and the blood type is classified as A.
- Agglutination with anti-B serum indicates the presence of B antigen, and the blood type is classified as B.
- Agglutination with anti-Rh(D) serum indicates the presence of the Rh(D) antigen, and the blood type is classified as Rh-positive (Rh+).
- If no agglutination occurs:
  - No agglutination with anti-A and anti-B sera indicates blood type O **(Fig. 4.32)**.
  - No agglutination with anti-Rh(D) serum indicates Rh-negative (Rh-) blood type.

Record the results within two minutes.

Based on the presence or absence of agglutination, record the donor's blood type as shown in **Figure 4.33**.

Advantage:
- Quick and easy technique that can be used in blood donation camps and in emergency
- Used for emergency ABO typing (in outdoor camps where centrifuge is not available)

Disadvantage:
- Less sensitive
- Not reliable for weakly reactive antigens in forward typing and antibodies in reverse typing.
- Drying of reaction mixture can cause aggregation mistaken for agglutination—false positive.

Crossmatch

Crossmatching is a critical process performed in blood banks to ensure compatibility between donor blood and recipient blood before transfusion. It involves testing the recipient's serum or plasma against the donor's red blood cells to identify any potential incompatibilities. There are two main methods of crossmatching used in blood banks:

Major Crossmatch

In the major crossmatch, the recipient's serum or plasma is tested against the donor's red blood cells. This test is designed to detect any preformed antibodies present in the recipient's blood that could react with the donor's red blood cells.

The process involves combining the recipient's serum or plasma with the donor's red blood cells and observing for any visible agglutination (clumping) or hemolysis (rupture of red blood cells).

If agglutination or hemolysis occurs, it indicates an incompatible match, and the blood should not be transfused to the recipient.

Minor Crossmatch

The minor crossmatch is performed to detect any antibodies present on the surface of the recipient's red blood cells that could react with the donor's plasma or serum. In this test, the recipient's red blood cells are mixed with the donor's serum or plasma.

Again, any visible agglutination or hemolysis indicates an incompatible match, and the blood should not be transfused.

It is important to note that crossmatching procedures may vary between blood banks, and additional techniques may be used to ensure compatibility. These methods can include computerized crossmatching, which involves the use of software algorithms to predict compatibility based on previous antibody screening results. This technique is often used as a rapid screening method but may still require confirmation with a major crossmatch.

In certain situations, such as emergencies or when time is limited, an abbreviated crossmatch may be performed. The abbreviated crossmatch involves testing the recipient's serum or plasma against a limited panel of donor red blood cells that are representative of the most common antigens. If no agglutination or hemolysis occurs, the blood is considered compatible for transfusion.

The crossmatching process is crucial for ensuring safe and compatible blood transfusions, and the specific method used may depend on the resources, policies, and preferences of the individual blood bank.

Blood transfusions are generally considered safe, but like any medical procedure, they carry a risk of adverse reactions. Adverse reactions to blood transfusions can be classified into two main categories: immediate reactions and delayed reactions. Here are some examples of adverse reactions that can occur during or after a blood transfusion:

Immediate Reactions

○ **Allergic reactions:** These can range from mild to severe and may include symptoms such as hives, itching, flushing, or wheezing. In severe cases, it can lead to anaphylaxis, a life-threatening allergic reaction.
○ **Febrile non-hemolytic reaction:** This is characterized by fever during or after the transfusion without evidence of hemolysis (breakdown of red blood cells).

○ **Acute hemolytic reaction:** This occurs when there is a mismatch between the recipient's blood type and the transfused blood, leading to the destruction of red blood cells. It can cause symptoms such as fever, chills, chest or back pain, hemoglobinuria (presence of hemoglobin in the urine), and potentially life-threatening complications, including kidney failure and disseminated intravascular coagulation (DIC).
○ **Transfusion-related acute lung injury (TRALI):** It is a rare but serious reaction characterized by acute respiratory distress shortly after a transfusion. It is thought to be caused by antibodies in the donor blood that react with cells in the recipient's lungs.
○ **Circulatory overload:** Excessive volume or rapid transfusion can lead to fluid overload, causing symptoms like shortness of breath, cough, and elevated blood pressure.

Delayed Reactions

○ **Delayed hemolytic reaction:** It occurs when antibodies in the recipient's blood gradually destroy the transfused red blood cells. Symptoms may include a drop in hemoglobin levels, jaundice, and mild to moderate anemia.
○ **Iron overload:** Multiple blood transfusions can lead to excessive accumulation of iron in the body, which can cause organ damage over time.
○ **Infections:** Although strict screening and testing of donated blood help minimize the risk, there is still a small chance of transmitting infectious agents such as bacteria, viruses [including human immunodeficiency virus (HIV), hepatitis B and C], or other pathogens.

Precautions to be Taken During Blood Transfusion

During a blood transfusion, several precautions should be taken to ensure the safety and well-being of the recipient. Here are some important precautions to be followed:

- **Proper patient identification:** Verify the patient's identity using at least two unique identifiers (e.g., name, date of birth) before initiating the transfusion. Match the patient's identification with the blood product and the transfusion order to prevent any errors.
- **Blood compatibility:** Ensure compatibility between the blood product and the recipient's blood type. ABO and Rh typing should be accurately performed and matched with the blood product to avoid transfusion reactions.
- **Visual inspection:** Carefully inspect the blood bag and label before starting the transfusion. Check for any signs of leakage, discoloration, or abnormalities in the blood product. The label should match the patient's identification and the transfusion order.
- **Proper blood storage:** Blood products must be stored and transported under appropriate conditions to maintain their integrity. Verify that the blood product has been stored properly and is within the specified temperature range before use.
- **Infusion equipment:** Use dedicated, sterile infusion sets and blood administration sets specifically designed for blood transfusions. Avoid using the same infusion set for multiple blood products or patients to prevent cross-contamination.
- **Infusion rate:** Follow the prescribed infusion rate for the specific blood product and monitor the recipient closely during the initial stages of the transfusion. Start with a slower rate (usually 2 mL/minute) for the first 15 minutes and then increase if there are no adverse reactions.
- **Monitoring:** Observe the patient closely throughout the transfusion for any signs of adverse reactions, including fever, chills, shortness of breath, rash, or changes in vital signs. Regularly check vital signs (temperature, blood pressure, heart rate) and assess the patient's overall condition.
- **Documentation:** Document the transfusion process accurately, including the patient's identification, blood product details, vital signs before, during, and after the transfusion, and any adverse reactions or interventions.
- **Response to reactions:** If any adverse reactions occur, promptly stop the transfusion, maintain intravenous access, and initiate appropriate management according to the specific reaction type. Notify the healthcare team immediately for further guidance.
- **Post-transfusion monitoring:** Monitor the patient for a period after the transfusion to ensure there are no delayed reactions or complications. Document any post-transfusion instructions or observations.

Complications

ABO Incompatibility

- ABO incompatibility occurs when the mother's blood type is different from the fetus's blood type. The ABO blood types include A, B, AB, and O. In general, if a mother is type O, she can safely carry a fetus of any blood type without ABO incompatibility concerns. However, if the mother is type A, B, or AB, and the fetus has a different blood type, ABO incompatibility issues can arise.
- The most significant ABO incompatibility occurs when an Rh-negative mother carries an Rh-positive fetus. In this case, the mother's immune system may produce antibodies against the Rh antigen present in the fetus's blood. This can occur during pregnancy or delivery and may also affect subsequent pregnancies if the mother is sensitized to the Rh antigen.

Rh Incompatibility

- ❍ Rh incompatibility specifically refers to a mismatch between the Rh blood types of a mother and her fetus or between a blood donor and recipient. An Rh-positive individual has the Rh antigen, while an Rh-negative individual lacks it. If an Rh-negative mother, is exposed to Rh-positive blood (such as during pregnancy or blood transfusion), she may develop antibodies against the Rh antigen. This can occur if the fetus is Rh-positive and the mother is sensitized to the Rh antigen during pregnancy or delivery.

- ❍ In subsequent pregnancies with an Rh-positive fetus, the antibodies produced by the mother's immune system can cross the placenta and attack the fetal red blood cells, causing hemolytic disease of the newborn (HDN) or erythroblastosis fetalis. HDN can lead to severe anemia, jaundice, and other complications in the newborn.

- ❍ To prevent Rh incompatibility, Rh-negative mothers receive an injection of Rh immunoglobulin (RhIg) called RhoGAM during pregnancy and after delivery. RhIg prevents the mother's immune system from producing antibodies against the Rh antigen, reducing the risk of sensitization and subsequent complications.

- ❍ In cases of severe Rh incompatibility during pregnancy, close monitoring, fetal blood sampling, and intrauterine transfusions may be necessary to manage fetal anemia and prevent complications.

Erythroblastosis Fetalis

- ❍ Erythroblastosis fetalis, also known as hemolytic disease of the newborn (HDN), is a condition that occurs when there is a significant incompatibility between the blood types of a pregnant woman and her fetus, specifically regarding the Rh antigen.

- ❍ Erythroblastosis fetalis develops when an Rh-negative mother is sensitized to the Rh antigen during pregnancy or delivery. If the fetus is Rh-positive (inheriting the Rh antigen from the father), the mother's immune system may produce antibodies against the Rh antigen. These antibodies can cross the placenta and attack the red blood cells of the Rh-positive fetus.

- ❍ The severity of erythroblastosis fetalis can vary, depending on factors such as the level of Rh antibody production and the degree of fetal red blood cell destruction. The condition can lead to the following complications in the fetus or newborn:

  - ○ **Anemia:** The destruction of fetal red blood cells can result in a shortage of red blood cells, leading to anemia. Severe anemia can negatively impact fetal development and oxygen delivery.

  - ○ **Jaundice:** The breakdown of red blood cells releases a substance called bilirubin, which can accumulate and cause yellowing of the skin and eyes (jaundice) in the newborn.

  - ○ **Enlarged liver and spleen:** Due to the increased destruction of red blood cells, the liver and spleen may become enlarged.

  - ○ **Hydrops fetalis:** In severe cases, extensive red blood cell destruction and anemia can lead to the accumulation of fluid in various body tissues, a condition known as hydrops fetalis. This can be life-threatening for the fetus.

- ❍ To prevent or manage erythroblastosis fetalis, healthcare providers closely monitor Rh-negative mothers during pregnancy. If the mother has been sensitized to the Rh antigen, interventions may include:

  - ○ **Administration of Rh immunoglobulin (RhIg) during pregnancy and after delivery:** RhIg is given to Rh-negative mothers to prevent them from producing antibodies against the Rh antigen. This helps prevent sensitization and subsequent complications in future pregnancies.

- ○ **Monitoring fetal well-being:** Regular ultrasound examinations and blood tests may be performed to assess the severity of anemia and other potential complications.
- ○ **Intrauterine transfusions:** In severe cases, where fetal anemia is life-threatening, blood transfusions may be performed directly into the fetus's bloodstream while still in the womb.
- ○ **Phototherapy or exchange transfusions:** After birth, if the newborn develops jaundice, phototherapy (exposure to special lights) or exchange transfusions may be performed to treat or prevent complications related to high bilirubin levels.
- ❍ Erythroblastosis fetalis is now relatively rare due to the widespread use of RhIg and improved monitoring and treatment approaches. Regular prenatal care and appropriate medical interventions help manage the condition effectively and reduce potential risks to the fetus or newborn.

These precautions are essential for ensuring the safety and effectiveness of blood transfusions. Healthcare providers should follow established protocols and guidelines specific to their clinical setting to minimize the risks associated with transfusions.

Anticoagulants in Blood Bank

In blood banks, anticoagulants are added to whole blood or blood components to prevent clotting and preserve the viability of the blood cells during storage. The choice of anticoagulant depends on the intended use and duration of storage. Here are some commonly used anticoagulants in blood storage:

- ○ **Citrate phosphate dextrose (CPD):** CPD is an anticoagulant solution used for the collection and storage of whole blood. It contains trisodium citrate, sodium phosphate, and dextrose. CPD helps prevent clotting by binding calcium ions required for coagulation. It is commonly used when the blood will be processed into various components, such as packed red blood cells, platelets, and plasma.
- ○ **Citrate phosphate dextrose adenine (CPDA-1):** CPDA-1 is a modified version of CPD that contains an additional adenine component. Adenine helps maintain ATP levels in red blood cells, providing energy for cell viability during storage. CPDA-1 is typically used for the collection and storage of whole blood when an extended storage duration is required, such as for red blood cell units intended for transfusion.
- ○ **Citrate phosphate double dextrose (CP2D):** CP2D is another anticoagulant solution used for the collection and storage of whole blood. It is similar to CPD but with a higher concentration of dextrose. CP2D is commonly used in countries where the availability of refrigeration during blood storage is limited.
- ○ **Heparin:** Heparin is an anticoagulant that works by inhibiting the coagulation cascade. It is used for specific purposes in blood banking, such as in the collection of blood for specialized tests or in the preparation of platelet concentrates. Heparin is not commonly used for long-term storage of whole blood or blood components due to its potential adverse effects on cell viability.

It is important to note that different anticoagulants have specific storage requirements, and the appropriate anticoagulant is selected based on the intended use of the blood product and the duration of storage. The use of anticoagulants in blood storage help to maintain the quality and functionality of blood components, ensuring their safety and effectiveness when used for transfusion or other medical purposes.

MULTIPLE CHOICE QUESTIONS

1. **Which blood component is responsible for carrying oxygen to body tissues?**
   a. Red blood cells (erythrocytes)
   b. White blood cells (leukocytes)
   c. Platelets
   d. Plasma

2. **Which type of blood cells are involved in the body's immune response?**
   a. Red blood cells (erythrocytes)
   b. Neutrophils
   c. Platelets
   d. Plasma

3. **Which blood component plays a crucial role in blood clotting?**
   a. Red blood cells (erythrocytes)
   b. Neutrophils
   c. Platelets
   d. Plasma

4. **Which of the following is NOT a constituent of plasma?**
   a. Water
   b. Proteins
   c. Platelets
   d. Nutrients

5. **Which blood component is responsible for defending the body against pathogens?**
   a. Red blood cells (erythrocytes)
   b. Neutrophils
   c. Platelets
   d. Plasma

6. **Which type of blood cells are involved in transporting carbon dioxide in the bloodstream?**
   a. Red blood cells (erythrocytes)
   b. Neutrophils
   c. Eosinophils
   d. Platelets

7. **What is the primary function of red blood cells?**
   a. Initiating the immune response
   b. Transporting oxygen to body tissues
   c. Forming blood clots
   d. Regulating blood pressure

8. **Which component of red blood cells is responsible for carrying oxygen?**
   a. Hemoglobin
   b. Nucleus
   c. Cytoplasm
   d. Plasma membrane

9. **Red blood cells are produced in which organ?**
   a. Liver
   b. Kidneys
   c. Spleen
   d. Bone marrow

10. **What is the typical lifespan of a red blood cell in the human body?**
    a. 1 day
    b. 7 days
    c. 30 days
    d. 120 days

11. **What is the shape of mature red blood cells in humans?**
    a. Spherical
    b. Cuboidal
    c. Discoid or biconcave
    d. Irregular or amoeboid

12. **What is the approximate percentage of red blood cells in total blood volume?**
    a. 20%
    b. 40%
    c. 60%
    d. 80%

Answers:

1. a	2. b	3. c	4. c
5. b	6. a	7. b	8. a
9. d	10. d	11. c	12. b

13. **Which hormone stimulates the production of red blood cells?**
    a. Insulin
    b. Estrogen
    c. Testosterone
    d. Erythropoietin

14. **Which of the following is NOT a function of white blood cells?**
    a. Carrying oxygen to body tissues
    b. Defending against pathogens
    c. Initiating immune responses
    d. Removing dead cells and debris

15. **Which type of white blood cell is primarily responsible for phagocytosis?**
    a. Neutrophils
    b. Lymphocytes
    c. Monocytes
    d. Eosinophils

16. **Which type of white blood cell is involved in allergic reactions and parasitic infections?**
    a. Neutrophils
    b. Lymphocytes
    c. Monocytes
    d. Eosinophils

17. **Which type of white blood cell produces antibodies?**
    a. Neutrophils
    b. Lymphocytes
    c. Monocytes
    d. Basophils

18. **Which white blood cell is the largest in size?**
    a. Neutrophils
    b. Lymphocytes
    c. Monocytes
    d. Eosinophils

19. **Which white blood cells are involved in antigen presentation?**
    a. Neutrophils
    b. Lymphocytes
    c. Monocytes
    d. Basophils

20. **Which type of white blood cell is responsible for coordinating immune responses?**
    a. Neutrophils
    b. Lymphocytes
    c. Monocytes
    d. Basophils

21. **Which of the following types of white blood cells is the most numerous in a typical WBC differential cell count?**
    a. Neutrophils
    b. Lymphocytes
    c. Monocytes
    d. Eosinophils

22. **Which type of WBCs are characterized by their multilobed nucleus and granular cytoplasm?**
    a. Neutrophils
    b. Lymphocytes
    c. Monocytes
    d. Eosinophils

23. **Which white blood cells play a crucial role in the immune response, including the production of antibodies?**
    a. Neutrophils
    b. Lymphocytes
    c. Monocytes
    d. Eosinophils

24. **Which white blood cells are involved in phagocytosis and the defense against bacterial infections?**
    a. Neutrophils
    b. Lymphocytes
    c. Monocytes
    d. Eosinophils

25. **Which white blood cells have a bilobed nucleus and are involved in the release of histamine during allergic reactions?**
    a. Neutrophils
    b. Lymphocytes
    c. Monocytes
    d. Basophils

Answers:	13. d	14. a	15. a	16. d
	17. b	18. c	19. b	20. b
	21. a	22. a	23. b	24. a
	25. d			

26. **Which type of white blood cells are characterized by their kidney-shaped or horseshoe-shaped nucleus and are involved in the phagocytosis of pathogens and debris?**
    a. Neutrophils
    b. Lymphocytes
    c. Monocytes
    d. Eosinophils

27. **During fetal life, hematopoiesis commences in the bone marrow by:**
    a. 2nd to 3rd month
    b. 4th to 5th month
    c. 6th to 7th month
    d. 7th to 8th month

28. **Bone marrow trephine biopsy has advantage over aspiration since:**
    a. The former method is less time-consuming
    b. Romanowsky stains can be done in the former
    c. Architectural pattern of marrow is better in the former
    d. Cell morphology is better appreciated in the former

29. **Erythroid cells continue to proliferate up to the stage of:**
    a. Reticulocytes
    b. Late normoblasts
    c. Intermediate normoblasts
    d. Early normoblasts

30. **Weight of hemoglobin in RBC is:**
    a. 50%
    b. 70%
    c. 90%
    d. 99%

31. **Red cell membrane defects include the following, *except*:**
    a. Spherocytosis
    b. Ovalocytosis
    c. Leptocytosis
    d. Echinocytosis

32. **The following factors determine the release of oxygen from hemoglobin in tissue capillaries, *except*:**
    a. Nature of globin chains in Hb
    b. Bicarbonate ions in blood
    c. pH of blood
    d. Concentration of 2,3-BPG

33. **Absorption of iron is enhanced by the following, *except*:**
    a. Ascorbic acid
    b. Citric acid
    c. Tannates
    d. Sugars

34. **In iron deficiency anemia, TIBC is:**
    a. Low
    b. Normal
    c. High
    d. Borderline

35. **Pappenheimer bodies are found in:**
    a. Sideroblasts
    b. Siderocytes
    c. Late normoblasts
    d. Intermediate normoblasts

36. **In anemia of chronic disorders, serum ferritin is:**
    a. Normal
    b. Low
    c. Increased
    d. Absent

37. **Folate circulates in plasma as:**
    a. Methyl tetrahydrofolate
    b. Polyglutamate
    c. Monoglutamate
    d. Diglutamate

38. **Measurement of formiminoglutamic acid (FIGLU) for folate deficiency is done in:**
    a. Whole blood
    b. Serum
    c. Plasma
    d. Urine

Answers:

26. c	27. a	28. c	29. b
30. d	31. c	32. b	33. c
34. c	35. b	36. c	37. a
38. d			

39. **Pernicious anemia causes pathologic changes in the anatomic region of stomach as under, *except*:**
    a. Antrum b. Body
    c. Body-fundic area d. Fundus

40. **In warm antibody autoimmune hemolytic anemia antibody is commonly:**
    a. IgA b. IgG
    c. IgM d. Ig D

41. **Which of the following is NOT a function of white blood cells?**
    a. Phagocytosis
    b. Antibody production
    c. Oxygen transport
    d. Immune response activation

42. **Which white blood cell is involved in the production of antibodies to fight against infections?**
    a. Neutrophils b. Lymphocytes
    c. Basophils d. Monocytes

43. **Which type of white blood cell releases histamine and other chemicals during an allergic reaction?**
    a. Neutrophils b. Lymphocytes
    c. Eosinophils d. Basophils

44. **Which white blood cell plays a crucial role in coordinating the immune response and killing infected cells?**
    a. Neutrophils b. Lymphocytes
    c. Eosinophils d. Monocytes

45. **Which type of white blood cell is the most abundant in the human body?**
    a. Neutrophils
    b. Lymphocytes
    c. Eosinophils
    d. Monocytes

46. **Which white blood cell is involved in wound healing and tissue repair?**
    a. Neutrophils
    b. Lymphocytes
    c. Eosinophils
    d. Monocytes

47. **What is the term used to describe the percentage of each type of white blood cell in a differential count?**
    a. Hemoglobin count
    b. Erythrocyte sedimentation rate
    c. White blood cell differential
    d. Platelet count

48. **Which type of white blood cell is most commonly increased during bacterial infections?**
    a. Neutrophils b. Lymphocytes
    c. Eosinophils d. Monocytes

49. **Which type of white blood cell is primarily responsible for combating parasitic infections and allergic reactions?**
    a. Neutrophils b. Lymphocytes
    c. Eosinophils d. Monocytes

50. **Which white blood cell is elevated in response to viral infections and plays a critical role in immune response coordination?**
    a. Neutrophils b. Lymphocytes
    c. Eosinophils d. Basophils

51. **A high percentage of neutrophils in a differential count may indicate which of the following conditions?**
    a. Allergic reaction
    b. Viral infection
    c. Bacterial infection
    d. Autoimmune disease

Answers:	39. a	40. b	41. c	42. b
	43. d	44. b	45. a	46. d
	47. c	48. a	49. c	50. b
	51. c			

52. **Which white blood cell type is associated with phagocytosis and engulfing foreign particles?**
    a. Neutrophils
    b. Lymphocytes
    c. Eosinophils
    d. Monocytes

53. **Which type of white blood cell is responsible for presenting antigens to other immune cells and activating the immune response?**
    a. Neutrophils
    b. Lymphocytes
    c. Eosinophils
    d. Monocytes

54. **Which type of white blood cell is most commonly increased during bacterial infections?**
    a. Neutrophils
    b. Lymphocytes
    c. Eosinophils
    d. Monocytes

55. **What does ESR measure?**
    a. Red blood cell count
    b. White blood cell count
    c. Rate of sedimentation of red blood cells
    d. Hemoglobin concentration

56. **Which method is commonly used to estimate ESR?**
    a. Hemocytometer counting
    b. Flow cytometry
    c. Automated blood cell counters
    d. Westergren method

57. **What is the unit of measurement for ESR?**
    a. mm Hg
    b. mm/hr (millimeters per hour)
    c. mL/min (milliliters per minute)
    d. g/dL (grams per deciliter)

58. **PCV estimation is a measure of:**
    a. Red blood cell count
    b. White blood cell count
    c. Plasma volume in the blood
    d. Volume occupied by red blood cells in a given volume of blood

59. **What is the PCV value that represents the normal range in adult males?**
    a. 20–30%
    b. 30–40%
    c. 40–50%
    d. 50–60%

60. **Which method is commonly used to estimate PCV?**
    a. Hemocytometer counting
    b. Flow cytometry
    c. Automated blood cell counters
    d. Microhematocrit centrifugation

61. **PCV is also known as:**
    a. Erythrocyte sedimentation rate
    b. Hemoglobin concentration
    c. Red blood cell count
    d. Hematocrit

62. **Which type of tissue is blood ?**
    a. Epithelial tissue
    b. Muscle tissue
    c. Nervous tissue
    d. Connective tissue

63. **What is the difference between plasma and serum?**
    a. Plasma contains more water
    b. Plasma contains iron
    c. Plasma does not contain fibrinogen
    d. Plasma contain fibrinogen

64. **New methylene blue reagent is used for staining of which blood cells?**
    a. Platelets.
    b. Reticulocytes
    c. WBC's
    d. Heinz bodies

Answers:

52. a	53. b	54. a	55. c
56. d	57. b	58. d	59. c
60. d	61. d	62. d	63. d
64. b			

65. **What is the ratio of dilution of blood when Turk's fluid is used for counting WBC manually?**
    a. 1:20
    b. 1:50
    c. 1:100
    d. 1:200

66. **All of the following are functions of blood, *except*:**
    a. Buffer system
    b. Oxygen transport
    c. Nutrient absorption
    d. Hormone production

67. **What is the primary purpose of performing a manual count of WBCs?**
    a. To assess red blood cell count
    b. To determine platelet count
    c. To evaluate the immune response
    d. To measure hemoglobin levels

68. **Which type of microscope is commonly used for manual counting of WBCs?**
    a. Compound microscope
    b. Electron microscope
    c. Fluorescence microscope
    d. Scanning electron microscope

69. **What is the preferred staining method for manual counting of WBCs?**
    a. Hematoxylin and eosin (H&E) stain
    b. Wright stain
    c. Gram stain
    d. Periodic acid-Schiff (PAS) stain

70. **How is the WBC count reported in a manual count?**
    a. Per cubic millimeter (mm³) of blood
    b. Per microliter (µL) of blood
    c. Per deciliter (dL) of blood
    d. As a percentage of total blood volume

71. **What is the normal range for the total WBC count in adults?**
    a. 4,500–11,000 cells/mm³
    b. 7,000–18,000 cells/mm³
    c. 12,000–20,000 cells/mm³
    d. 20,000–30,000 cells/mm³

72. **Which factor is critical for ensuring accurate manual counting of WBCs?**
    a. Proper calibration of the microscope
    b. Use of automated cell counters
    c. High-powered magnification
    d. Rapid staining techniques

73. **What does an automated CBC measure?**
    a. Red blood cell count, white blood cell count, and platelet count
    b. Hemoglobin, hematocrit, and mean corpuscular volume (MCV)
    c. Red blood cell indices, white blood cell differential, and platelet indices
    d. All of the above

74. **The CBC provides information about:**
    a. The overall health of the blood
    b. The presence of infection or inflammation
    c. The oxygen-carrying capacity of the blood
    d. All of the above

75. **Which of the following is not typically included in an automated CBC?**
    a. Red blood cell distribution width (RDW)
    b. Mean corpuscular hemoglobin (MCH)
    c. Mean platelet volume (MPV)
    d. Serum electrolyte levels

Answers: 65. a   66. d   67. c   68. a
          69. b   70. a   71. a   72. a
          73. d   74. d   75. d

76. What is the primary technology used in automated CBC analyzers?
a. Flow cytometry
b. Microscopic examination
c. Spectrophotometry
d. Polymerase chain reaction (PCR)

77. The term "differential" in a CBC refers to:
a. The percentage breakdown of different types of white blood cells
b. The variation in red blood cell size
c. The presence of abnormal cells in the blood
d. The ratio of platelets to red blood cells

78. Which parameter of the CBC is used to assess the oxygen-carrying capacity of the blood?
a. Hemoglobin
b. Hematocrit
c. Mean corpuscular volume (MCV)
d. Red blood cell distribution width (RDW)

79. Why is an automated CBC preferred over a manual blood count?
a. It provides more accurate and consistent results
b. It requires less time and labor
c. It can analyze a larger number of samples quickly
d. All of the above

80. Red blood cell indices are calculated using measurements from a complete blood count (CBC) and provide information about:
a. Hemoglobin levels
b. Red blood cell size and volume
c. Oxygen-carrying capacity of the blood
d. All of the above

81. Which of the following red cell indices measures the average size of red blood cells?
a. Mean corpuscular hemoglobin (MCH)
b. Mean corpuscular volume (MCV)
c. Mean corpuscular hemoglobin concentration (MCHC)
d. Red blood cell distribution width (RDW)

82. The mean corpuscular volume (MCV) is expressed in which unit?
a. Picograms (pg)
b. Micrometers (μm)
c. Femtoliters (fL)
d. Milliliters (mL)

83. The mean corpuscular hemoglobin concentration (MCHC) represents:
a. The amount of hemoglobin in each red blood cell
b. The average size of red blood cells
c. The concentration of red blood cells in a given volume of blood
d. The variation in red blood cell size

84. Which red cell index can be helpful in distinguishing between different types of anemia?
a. MCV
b. MCH
c. MCHC
d. RDW

85. A high RDW (red blood cell distribution width) indicates:
a. Variation in red blood cell size
b. Low hemoglobin levels
c. Presence of abnormal cells
d. Decreased red blood cell count

Answers: 76. a   77. a   78. a   79. d
80. d   81. b   82. c   83. a
84. d   85. a

86. **Red cell indices are useful in diagnosing and classifying different types of anemias based on:**
    a. Hemoglobin levels only
    b. Red blood cell count only
    c. Red blood cell size and hemoglobin content
    d. White blood cell count and platelet count

87. **A blood donor diagnosed with HbsAg positive should be differed for how long?**
    a. For 3 months
    b. For 6 months
    c. For 1 year
    d. Permanently

88. **What is the name of this tube in picture?**

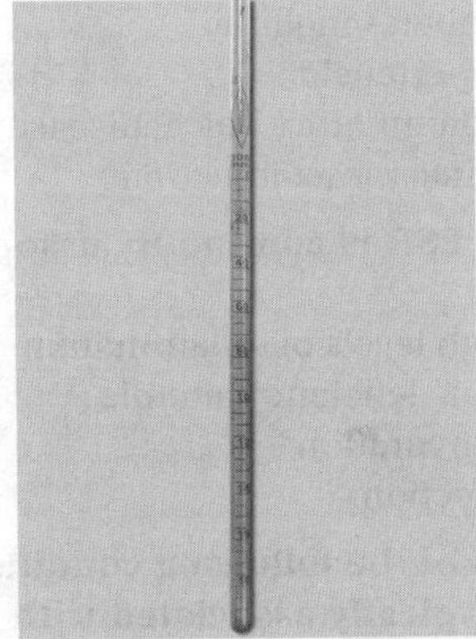

    a. Westergren's pipette
    b. ESR pipette
    c. WBC pipette
    d. Wintrobe's tube

89. **What is the usage of tube shown in the above question?**
    a. Measuring RBC count
    b. Measuring WBC count
    c. Measuring hematocrit
    d. Measuring reticulocyte count

90. **PCV, also known as hematocrit, refers to:**
    a. The percentage of red blood cells in the total blood volume
    b. The number of platelets in the blood
    c. The level of hemoglobin in the blood
    d. The size of red blood cells

91. **The normal range of PCV in adult males is typically:**
    a. 30–40%
    b. 40–50%
    c. 50–60%
    d. 60–70%

92. **ESR is a laboratory test that measures:**
    a. The speed at which red blood cells settle in a tube of blood
    b. The number of white blood cells in the blood
    c. The amount of hemoglobin in the blood
    d. The concentration of platelets in the blood

93. **ESR is commonly used as an indicator of:**
    a. Inflammation or infection
    b. Anemia
    c. Blood clotting disorders
    d. Liver function

94. **The normal range of ESR in adult females is typically:**
    a. 0–10 mm/hr
    b. 10–20mm/hr
    c. 20–30 mm/hr
    d. 30–40mm/hr

95. **Factors that can increase ESR include:**
    a. Inflammation or infection
    b. Anemia
    c. Pregnancy
    d. All of the above

Answers:

86. c	87. d	88. d	89. c
90. a	91. b	92. a	93. a
94. b	95. d		

96. Factors that can decrease ESR include:
a. Anemia
b. Hyperalbuminemia
c. Polycythemia
d. None of the above

97. Erythroblastosis fetalis occurs due to:
a. ABO incompatibility
b. RH incompatibility
c. Hemophilia
d. Leukemia

98. An elevated ESR is commonly associated with:
a. Decreased inflammation
b. Iron deficiency anemia
c. Infection or inflammation
d. Dehydration

99. Which of the following conditions is NOT typically associated with a raised ESR?
a. Rheumatoid arthritis
b. Bacterial infection
c. Anemia
d. Hypothyroidism

100. The ESR is a nonspecific marker and may be increased in various diseases due to:
a. Increased red blood cell count
b. Increased white blood cell count
c. Decreased platelet count
d. Inflammation or tissue injury

101. A significantly raised ESR in an elderly individual may raise suspicion for:
a. Iron deficiency anemia
b. Polycythemia vera
c. Temporal arteritis
d. Thalassemia

102. Factors that can affect ESR levels include:
a. Age and gender
b. Pregnancy
c. Medications
d. All of the above

103. The ESR is measured by:
a. Counting the number of red blood cells
b. Determining the rate at which red blood cells settle in a tube
c. Assessing the shape and size of red blood cells
d. Measuring the hemoglobin level in red blood cells

104. An elevated ESR is useful in diagnosing and monitoring the progress of:
a. Diabetes mellitus
b. Hypertension
c. Inflammatory bowel disease
d. Urinary tract infection

105. A low ESR is commonly associated with:
a. High levels of inflammation
b. Iron-deficiency anemia
c. Dehydration
d. Infection

106. Which of the following conditions is NOT typically associated with a low ESR?
a. Polycythemia vera
b. Sickle cell anemia
c. Hypothyroidism
d. Thalassemia

Answers:	96. c	97. a	98. c	99. d
	100. d	101. c	102. d	103. b
	104. c	105. c	106. d	

107. The ESR is a nonspecific marker and may be decreased in certain conditions such as:
a. Severe infection
b. Chronic liver disease
c. Acute inflammatory conditions
d. Autoimmune disorders

108. A significantly low ESR may raise suspicion for:
a. Hypovolemia
b. Iron overload (hemochromatosis)
c. Systemic lupus erythematosus (SLE)
d. Chronic kidney disease

109. A low ESR is useful in diagnosing and monitoring the progress of:
a. Acute bacterial infection
b. Hyperthyroidism
c. Rheumatoid arthritis
d. Anemia

110. The most commonly used technique for estimating PCV is:
a. Microhematocrit centrifugation
b. Optical absorbance measurement
c. Coulter counter analysis
d. Impedance-based cell counting

111. Microhematocrit centrifugation involves:
a. Spinning a capillary tube of blood in a centrifuge
b. Measuring the light absorption of the blood sample
c. Utilizing electrical impedance for cell counting
d. Analyzing the blood cells using flow cytometry

112. The principle behind microhematocrit centrifugation is:
a. Separation of blood components based on their density
b. Direct measurement of red blood cell size
c. Estimation of hemoglobin concentration in the blood
d. Calculation of the mean corpuscular volume (MCV)

113. Optical absorbance measurement for PCV estimation involves:
a. Shining light through a diluted blood sample and measuring the transmitted light
b. Counting the number of red blood cells in a given volume
c. Measuring the electrical resistance of the blood sample
d. Utilizing a laser to determine red blood cell size and volume

114. Coulter counter analysis for PCV estimation relies on:
a. Measurement of light scattering by red blood cells
b. Detection of electrical impedance changes caused by blood cells
c. Separation of blood components using a magnetic field
d. Calculation of mean corpuscular hemoglobin concentration (MCHC)

Answers: 107. d   108. a   109. b   110. a
         111. a   112. a   113. a   114. b

115. Impedance-based cell counting for PCV estimation involves:
a. Passing blood cells through a small orifice and measuring changes in electrical impedance
b. Measuring the absorbance of light by the blood sample
c. Utilizing flow cytometry for cell analysis
d. Direct microscopic examination of the blood cells

116. Microcytic hypochromic anemia is characterized by:
a. Small red blood cells with reduced hemoglobin content
b. Large red blood cells with increased hemoglobin content
c. Normal-sized red blood cells with reduced hemoglobin content
d. Abnormally shaped red blood cells with varied hemoglobin content

117. The most common cause of microcytic hypochromic anemia worldwide is:
a. Iron deficiency
b. Vitamin B12 deficiency
c. Folate deficiency
d. Chronic kidney disease

118. Iron deficiency anemia is commonly caused by:
a. Inadequate dietary intake of iron
b. Chronic blood loss
c. Impaired iron absorption
d. All of the above

119. Anemia of chronic disease can present as microcytic hypochromic anemia and is associated with:
a. Inflammatory conditions
b. Infections
c. Autoimmune diseases
d. All of the above

120. Thalassemia, an inherited disorder, can cause microcytic hypochromic anemia due to:
a. Defects in globin chain synthesis
b. Defective iron absorption
c. Impaired heme production
d. Abnormal red blood cell membrane structure

121. Lead poisoning can lead to microcytic hypochromic anemia by:
a. Inhibiting heme synthesis
b. Causing iron overload
c. Disrupting red blood cell membrane integrity
d. Reducing red blood cell production

122. Macrocytic anemia is characterized by:
a. Large red blood cells
b. Small red blood cells
c. Normal-sized red blood cells
d. Abnormally shaped red blood cells

123. The most common cause of macrocytic anemia is:
a. Iron deficiency
b. Vitamin B12 deficiency
c. Folate deficiency
d. Chronic kidney disease

124. Vitamin B12 deficiency can lead to macrocytic anemia due to:
a. Impaired DNA synthesis in red blood cells
b. Increased red blood cell destruction
c. Defective iron absorption
d. Autoimmune destruction of red blood cells

Answers:	115. a	116. a	117. a	118. d
	119. d	120. a	121. a	122. a
	123. b	124. a		

125. **Folate deficiency can cause macrocytic anemia by:**
    a. Impairing DNA synthesis in red blood cells
    b. Disrupting red blood cell membrane integrity
    c. Causing iron overload
    d. Increasing red blood cell destruction

126. **Alcoholism can contribute to macrocytic anemia through:**
    a. Vitamin B12 deficiency
    b. Folate deficiency
    c. Impaired iron absorption
    d. Autoimmune destruction of red blood cells

127. **Pernicious anemia is a type of macrocytic anemia caused by:**
    a. Inherited genetic mutations affecting red blood cell production
    b. Impaired absorption of vitamin B12
    c. Autoimmune destruction of intrinsic factor
    d. Defective iron utilization in red blood cells

128. **Thalassemia is a genetic disorder that affects:**
    a. Red blood cell production
    b. White blood cell production
    c. Platelet production
    d. Plasma production

129. **Thalassemia is characterized by:**
    a. Abnormally shaped red blood cells
    b. Defective hemoglobin production
    c. Reduced red blood cell count
    d. All of the above

130. **The two main types of thalassemia are:**
    a. Alpha and beta thalassemia
    b. Delta and gamma thalassemia
    c. Epsilon and zeta thalassemia
    d. A and B thalassemia

131. **In alpha thalassemia, there is a deficiency in:**
    a. Alpha globin chains
    b. Beta globin chains
    c. Gamma globin chains
    d. Delta globin chains

132. **In beta thalassemia, there is a deficiency in:**
    a. Alpha globin chains
    b. Beta globin chains
    c. Gamma globin chains
    d. Delta globin chains

133. **Severe forms of thalassemia can result in:**
    a. Cooley's anemia
    b. Sickle cell anemia
    c. Hemolytic anemia
    d. Iron-deficiency anemia

134. **The diagnosis of alpha thalassemia is confirmed by:**
    a. Complete blood count (CBC)
    b. Hemoglobin electrophoresis
    c. Bone marrow biopsy
    d. Genetic testing

135. **Anemia of chronic diseases is characterized by:**
    a. Decreased red blood cell production
    b. Increased red blood cell destruction
    c. Impaired iron absorption
    d. All of the above

Answers: 125. a   126. a   127. b   128. a
129. d   130. d   131. a   132. b
133. a   134. d   135. d

136. Anemia of chronic diseases is commonly seen in patients with:
a. Inflammatory conditions
b. Infections
c. Autoimmune diseases
d. All of the above

137. The primary cause of anemia of chronic diseases is:
a. Iron deficiency
b. Vitamin B12 deficiency
c. Impaired erythropoietin production
d. Chronic inflammation

138. In anemia of chronic diseases, the levels of circulating iron are:
a. Increased   b. Decreased
c. Normal   d. Variable

139. Anemia of chronic diseases is typically characterized by:
a. Fragmented red blood cells
b. Microcytic hypochromic red blood cells
c. Macrocytic red blood cells
d. Abnormally shaped red blood cells

140. Treatment of anemia of chronic diseases primarily focuses on:
a. Iron supplementation
b. Erythropoietin therapy
c. Treating the underlying cause
d. Blood transfusion

141. Chronic kidney disease is a common cause of anemia of chronic diseases due to:
a. Impaired iron absorption
b. Decreased production of erythropoietin
c. Increased red blood cell destruction
d. Autoimmune destruction of red blood cells

142. Sickle cell anemia is a genetic disorder characterized by:
a. Abnormal shape of red blood cells
b. Decreased red blood cell production
c. Impaired iron absorption
d. Chronic inflammation

143. Sickle cell anemia is caused by a mutation in the:
a. Alpha globin chains
b. Beta globin chains
c. Gamma globin chains
d. Delta globin chains

144. In sickle cell anemia, the abnormal hemoglobin causes red blood cells to:
a. Become fragile and easily destroyed
b. Decrease in size and volume
c. Lose their ability to carry oxygen
d. Increase in size and volume

145. Hemolytic anemia is characterized by:
a. Increased destruction of red blood cells
b. Decreased red blood cell production
c. Impaired iron absorption
d. Chronic inflammation

146. Common causes of hemolytic anemia include:
a. Autoimmune disorders
b. Infections
c. Inherited conditions
d. All of the above

147. The direct Coombs test is used to diagnose:
a. Sickle cell anemia
b. Iron-deficiency anemia
c. Hemolytic anemia
d. Thalassemia

Answers: 136. d   137. d   138. a   139. b
140. c   141. b   142. a   143. b
144. a   145. a   146. d   147. c

148. **Treatment options for sickle cell anemia and hemolytic anemia may include:**
a. Blood transfusions
b. Medications to manage symptoms
c. Bone marrow transplantation
d. All of the above

149. **Hereditary spherocytosis is characterized by:**
a. Abnormal shape of red blood cells
b. Decreased production of red blood cells
c. Impaired iron absorption
d. Autoimmune destruction of red blood cells

150. **The primary abnormality in hereditary spherocytosis is related to:**
a. Defects in the red blood cell membrane proteins
b. Abnormal hemoglobin production
c. Impaired DNA synthesis in red blood cells
d. Autoantibodies against red blood cells

151. **G6PD deficiency is an inherited condition affecting:**
a. Red blood cell membrane structure
b. Hemoglobin synthesis
c. Red blood cell enzyme function
d. Iron absorption

152. **G6PD deficiency can lead to hemolysis due to:**
a. Increased oxidative stress on red blood cells
b. Impaired iron utilization in red blood cells

c. Autoimmune destruction of red blood cells
d. Defective hemoglobin production

153. **Triggers for hemolysis in individuals with G6PD deficiency can include:**
a. Certain medications
b. Infections
c. Fava beans (broad beans)
d. All of the above

154. **The diagnostic test for G6PD deficiency is:**
a. Complete blood count (CBC)
b. Hemoglobin electrophoresis
c. Direct Coombs test
d. G6PD enzyme assay

155. **Leukemia is a type of cancer that affects:**
a. Bone marrow and blood cells
b. Lymph nodes and lymphocytes
c. Liver and kidney cells
d. Lung tissue and bronchial cells

156. **The two main types of leukemia are:**
a. Acute and chronic leukemia
b. Lymphocytic and myeloid leukemia
c. Hodgkin and non-Hodgkin leukemia
d. Primary and secondary leukemia

157. **Acute leukemia is characterized by:**
a. Rapid progression of the disease
b. Slow and indolent course of the disease
c. Prevalence in older adults
d. Involvement of lymph nodes

158. **Chronic leukemia is characterized by:**
a. Slow progression of the disease
b. Rapid and aggressive course of the disease
c. Prevalence in younger individuals
d. Involvement of solid organs

Answers: 148. d 149. a 150. a 151. c
152. a 153. d 154. d 155. a
156. a 157. a 158. a

159. The hallmark feature of leukemia is:
a. Abnormal proliferation of white blood cells
b. Reduced production of red blood cells
c. Enlarged lymph nodes
d. Decreased platelet count

160. The diagnostic test commonly used to confirm leukemia is:
a. Complete blood count (CBC)
b. Bone marrow biopsy and aspiration
c. Lymph node biopsy
d. Chest X-ray

161. The treatment for leukemia may include:
a. Chemotherapy
b. Radiation therapy
c. Stem cell transplantation
d. All of the above

162. Acute myeloid leukemia is a type of cancer that affects:
a. Red blood cells
b. White blood cells
c. Platelets
d. Bone marrow cells

163. AML is characterized by the proliferation of:
a. Immature myeloid cells
b. Lymphocytes
c. Plasma cells
d. Megakaryocytes

164. The most common age group affected by AML is:
a. Children
b. Adolescents
c. Young adults
d. Older adults

165. AML is diagnosed by:
a. Complete blood count (CBC)
b. Bone marrow biopsy and aspiration
c. Lymph node biopsy
d. Chest X-ray

166. The symptoms of AML can include:
a. Fatigue and weakness
b. Easy bruising and bleeding
c. Fever and infections
d. All of the above

167. The treatment for AML may include:
a. Chemotherapy
b. Radiation therapy
c. Stem cell transplantation
d. All of the above

168. The presence of specific genetic mutations can influence the prognosis and treatment approach in AML. One such mutation is:
a. FLT3 mutation
b. BRCA1 mutation
c. EGFR mutation
d. HER2 mutation

169. Acute lymphoblastic leukemia (ALL) is a type of cancer that affects:
a. Red blood cells
b. White blood cells
c. Platelets
d. Bone marro cells with erythrocytes

170. ALL is characterized by the proliferation of:
a. Immature lymphoid cells
b. Myeloid cells
c. Plasma cells
d. Megakaryocytes

171. The most common age group affected by ALL is:
a. Children
b. Adolescents
c. Young adults
d. Older adults

Answers:

159. a	160. b	161. d	162. d
163. a	164. d	165. b	166. d
167. d	168. a	169. b	170. a
171. a			

172. **ALL is diagnosed by:**
    a. Complete blood count (CBC)
    b. Bone marrow biopsy and aspiration
    c. Lymph node biopsy
    d. Chest X-ray

173. **The symptoms of ALL can include:**
    a. Fatigue and weakness
    b. Easy bruising and bleeding
    c. Fever and infections
    d. All of the above

174. **The treatment for ALL may include:**
    a. Chemotherapy
    b. Radiation therapy
    c. Stem cell transplantation
    d. All of the above

175. **The presence of specific genetic mutations can influence the prognosis and treatment approach in ALL. One such mutation is:**
    a. BCR-ABL fusion gene
    b. BRCA1 mutation
    c. EGFR mutation
    d. HER2 mutation

176. **CML is characterized by the proliferation of abnormal cells in the:**
    a. Red blood cell lineage
    b. White blood cell lineage
    c. Platelet lineage
    d. Lymphocyte lineage

177. **The genetic abnormality associated with CML is:**
    a. Philadelphia chromosome
    b. HER2 mutation
    c. TP53 mutation
    d. JAK2 mutation

178. **The chronic phase of CML is characterized by:**
    a. Mild symptoms and slow disease progression
    b. Rapid disease progression and severe symptoms
    c. Asymptomatic phase with normal blood counts
    d. Increased production of normal blood cells

179. **The diagnostic test used to confirm CML is:**
    a. Complete blood count (CBC)
    b. Bone marrow biopsy and aspiration
    c. Lymph node biopsy
    d. Chest X-ray

180. **The treatment of CML often involves targeted therapy with:**
    a. Tyrosine kinase inhibitors (TKIs)
    b. Chemotherapy
    c. Radiation therapy
    d. Stem cell transplantation

181. **CLL is characterized by the proliferation of abnormal cells in the:**
    a. Red blood cell lineage
    b. White blood cell lineage
    c. Platelet lineage
    d. Lymphocyte lineage

182. **The most common leukemia in adults is:**
    a. Acute lymphoblastic leukemia (ALL)
    b. Acute myeloid leukemia (AML)
    c. Chronic lymphocytic leukemia (CLL)
    d. Chronic myeloid leukemia (CML)

Answers:	172. **b**	173. **d**	174. **d**	175. **a**
	176. **b**	177. **a**	178. **a**	179. **b**
	180. **a**	181. **d**	182. **c**	

183. **The hallmark feature of CLL is the presence of:**
a. Abnormal lymphocytes called "smudge cells"
b. Blast cells in the bone marrow
c. Reed-Sternberg cells
d. Hypersegmented neutrophils

184. **The treatment approach for CLL depends on the stage and risk factors but may include:**
a. Watchful waiting
b. Chemotherapy
c. Immunotherapy
d. All of the above

185. **The characteristic translocation in chronic myeloid leukemia (CML) involves the reciprocal exchange of genetic material between chromosomes:**
a. Chromosome 9 and chromosome 22
b. Chromosome 13 and chromosome 14
c. Chromosome 11 and chromosome 22
d. Chromosome 4 and chromosome 7

186. **The French-American-British (FAB) classification system is used to classify:**
a. Acute lymphoblastic leukemia (ALL)
b. Acute myeloid leukemia (AML)
c. Chronic lymphocytic leukemia (CLL)
d. Chronic myeloid leukemia (CML)

187. **AML is characterized by the proliferation of abnormal cells in the:**
a. Red blood cell lineage
b. White blood cell lineage
c. Platelet lineage
d. Lymphocyte lineage

188. **The genetic abnormality associated with AML is:**
a. Philadelphia chromosome
b. BCR-ABL fusion gene
c. FLT3 mutation
d. JAK2 mutation

189. **The diagnostic test used to confirm AML is:**
a. Complete blood count (CBC)
b. Bone marrow biopsy and aspiration
c. Lymph node biopsy
d. Chest X-ray

190. **The World Health Organization (WHO) classification system for AML incorporates:**
a. Cytogenetic and molecular genetic information
b. Patient's age and sex
c. Symptoms and physical examination findings
d. Blood cell counts

191. **The characteristic feature of AML blasts on peripheral blood smear is:**
a. Presence of Auer rods
b. Hypersegmented neutrophils
c. Smudge cells
d. Reed-Sternberg cells

192. **Secondary AML can arise as a result of:**
a. Previous chemotherapy or radiation therapy
b. Inherited genetic mutations
c. Exposure to certain chemicals or toxins
d. All of the above

Answers:

183. a	184. d	185. a	186. b
187. b	188. c	189. b	190. a
191. a	192. d		

193. **ALL is characterized by the proliferation of abnormal cells in the:**
    a. Red blood cell lineage
    b. White blood cell lineage
    c. Platelet lineage
    d. Megakaryocytic lineage

194. **The most common age group affected by ALL is:**
    a. Children
    b. Adolescents
    c. Young adults
    d. Older adults

195. **The genetic abnormality associated with a significant proportion of ALL cases is:**
    a. Philadelphia chromosome
    b. BCR-ABL fusion gene
    c. FLT3 mutation
    d. TEL-AML1 fusion gene

196. **The diagnostic test used to confirm ALL is:**
    a. Complete blood count (CBC)
    b. Bone marrow biopsy and aspiration
    c. Lymph node biopsy
    d. Chest X-ray

197. **The treatment for ALL often involves induction chemotherapy followed by:**
    a. Maintenance chemotherapy
    b. Radiation therapy
    c. Stem cell transplantation
    d. Immunotherapy

198. **The World Health Organization (WHO) classification system for ALL incorporates:**
    a. Cytogenetic and molecular genetic information
    b. Patient's age and sex
    c. Symptoms and physical examination findings
    d. Blood cell counts

199. **The risk stratification in ALL is based on factors such as:**
    a. Age and white blood cell count
    b. Hemoglobin level and platelet count
    c. Cytogenetic abnormalities
    d. All of the above

200. **The genetic abnormality associated with CML is:**
    a. HER2 mutation
    b. BCR-ABL fusion gene
    c. FLT3 mutation
    d. JAK2 mutation

201. **The World Health Organization (WHO) classification system for CML incorporates:**
    a. Cytogenetic and molecular genetic information
    b. Patient's age and sex
    c. Symptoms and physical examination findings
    d. Blood cell counts

202. **The risk stratification in CML is based on factors such as:**
    a. Age and white blood cell count
    b. Hemoglobin level and platelet count
    c. Cytogenetic abnormalities
    d. All of the above

203. **The accelerated phase of CML is characterized by:**
    a. Increased blast cells in the blood or bone marrow
    b. Progressive increase in symptoms
    c. Resistance to tyrosine kinase inhibitors
    d. All of the above

Answers:	193. b	194. a	195. c	196. b
	197. c	198. a	199. d	200. b
	201. a	202. d	203. d	

204. The blast crisis phase of CML resembles:
a. Acute myeloid leukemia (AML)
b. Acute lymphoblastic leukemia (ALL)
c. Chronic lymphocytic leukemia (CLL)
d. Multiple myeloma

205. The initial treatment choice for most patients with CML is:
a. Tyrosine kinase inhibitors (TKIs)
b. Chemotherapy
c. Stem cell transplantation
d. Radiation therapy

206. The tyrosine kinase inhibitor commonly used as first-line therapy in CML is:
a. Imatinib
b. Dasatinib
c. Nilotinib
d. Bosutinib

207. Monitoring response to treatment in CML is done through:
a. Regular blood tests and bone marrow biopsies
b. Imaging studies
c. Genetic testing
d. Physical examination findings

208. Thrombocytopenia is defined as a decrease in platelet count below:
a. 150,000/mm³   b. 300,000/mm³
c. 200,000/mm³   d. 250,000/mm³

209. The most common cause of acquired thrombocytopenia is:
a. Idiopathic thrombocytopenic purpura (ITP)
b. Thrombotic thrombocytopenic purpura (TTP)
c. Hemolytic uremic syndrome (HUS)
d. Drug-induced thrombocytopenia

210. Idiopathic thrombocytopenic purpura (ITP) is characterized by:
a. Autoimmune destruction of platelets
b. Increased platelet production
c. Platelet aggregation defects
d. Abnormal platelet adhesion

211. Von Willebrand disease is characterized by a deficiency or dysfunction of:
a. Factor VIII
b. Factor IX
c. Factor XI
d. von Willebrand factor

212. Bernard-Soulier syndrome is characterized by:
a. Deficiency of platelet factor 3
b. Deficiency of von Willebrand factor
c. Deficiency of glycoprotein Ib-IX-V complex
d. Deficiency of factor V

213. Glanzmann's thrombasthenia is characterized by:
a. Deficiency of platelet factor 3
b. Deficiency of von Willebrand factor
c. Deficiency of glycoprotein Ib-IX-V complex
d. Deficiency of glycoprotein IIb/IIIa complex

214. Immune thrombocytopenic purpura (ITP) primarily affects which age group?
a. Children
b. Adolescents
c. Young adults
d. Older adults

Answers: 204. a   205. a   206. a   207. a
208. a   209. a   210. a   211. d
212. c   213. d   214. a

215. Hemophilia A is characterized by a deficiency of:
a. Factor VIII
b. Factor IX
c. Factor XI
d. Factor XIII

216. Thrombotic thrombocytopenic purpura (TTP) is characterized by:
a. Microangiopathic hemolytic anemia and thrombocytopenia
b. Abnormal platelet aggregation
c. Deficiency of von Willebrand factor
d. Factor V Leiden mutation

217. Heparin-induced thrombocytopenia (HIT) is caused by:
a. An immune reaction to heparin
b. Direct toxicity of heparin on platelets
c. Platelet aggregation defects
d. von Willebrand factor deficiency

218. Essential thrombocythemia is characterized by:
a. Excessive production of platelets
b. Destruction of platelets by autoantibodies
c. Deficiency of von Willebrand factor
d. Impaired platelet adhesion

219. Platelet function disorders can be caused by defects in:
a. Platelet adhesion
b. Platelet aggregation
c. Platelet secretion
d. All of the above

220. The most common inherited bleeding disorder is:
a. Hemophilia A
b. von Willebrand disease
c. Bernard-Soulier syndrome
d. Glanzmann's thrombasthenia

221. May-Hegglin anomaly is characterized by:
a. Giant platelets and thrombocytopenia
b. Increased platelet production
c. Platelet aggregation defects
d. Abnormal platelet adhesion

222. The diagnostic test used to evaluate platelet function is:
a. Bleeding time
b. Platelet count
c. Coagulation profile
d. Bone marrow biopsy

223. Immune thrombocytopenic purpura (ITP) is primarily treated with:
a. Corticosteroids
b. Platelet transfusion
c. Anticoagulants
d. Immune globulin therapy

224. A normal platelet count ranges from:
a. 150,000 to 450,000/mm^3
b. 100,000 to 300,000/mm^3
c. 200,000 to 500,000/mm^3
d. 50,000 to 150,000/mm^3

225. Thrombocytopathy refers to:
a. Platelet disorder
b. Abnormal platelet count
c. Decreased platelet production
d. Increased platelet destruction

226. Platelet aggregation is primarily mediated by:
a. von Willebrand factor
b. Fibrinogen
c. Platelet factor 3
d. Thromboxane A2

Answers:

215. a	216. a	217. a	218. a
219. d	220. b	221. a	222. a
223. a	224. a	225. a	226. a

227. Platelet storage pool deficiency is characterized by defects in:
a. Platelet adhesion
b. Platelet aggregation
c. Platelet secretion
d. Platelet production

228. Blood typing involves the determination of:
a. ABO group
b. Rh factor
c. Both ABO group and Rh factor
d. HLA typing

229. The most common blood type in the ABO system is:
a. A
b. B
c. AB
d. O

230. The Rh factor refers to the presence or absence of the:
a. A antigen
b. B antigen
c. D antigen
d. O antigen

231. The universal blood donor type is:
a. A
b. B
c. AB
d. O

232. The universal blood recipient type is:
a. A
b. B
c. AB
d. O

233. A unit of whole blood typically contains approximately:
a. 200 mL
b. 400 mL
c. 500 mL
d. 700 mL

234. Packed red blood cells (PRBCs) are primarily used to:
a. Increase oxygen-carrying capacity
b. Increase platelet count
c. Provide coagulation factors
d. Increase white blood cell count

235. Fresh frozen plasma (FFP) is rich in:
a. Red blood cells
b. Platelets
c. Plasma proteins
d. Coagulation factors

236. Cryoprecipitate is used to treat deficiencies in:
a. Red blood cells
b. Platelets
c. Plasma proteins
d. Coagulation factors

237. The process of separating blood components using a centrifuge is called:
a. Apheresis
b. Filtration
c. Irradiation
d. Fractionation

238. The term "crossmatching" refers to:
a. Compatibility testing between donor and recipient
b. Blood typing and grouping
c. Collection of blood samples
d. Platelet count estimation

239. Indirect Coombs' test is used to detect:
a. ABO incompatibility
b. Rh incompatibility
c. Hemolytic disease of the newborn
d. Platelet dysfunction

240. The purpose of leukoreduction in blood products is to:
a. Decrease the risk of febrile transfusion reactions
b. Increase platelet count
c. Enhance clotting capabilities
d. Improve oxygen-carrying capacity

Answers:
227. c	228. c	229. d	230. c
231. d	232. c	233. c	234. a
235. d	236. d	237. a	238. a
239. c	240. a		

241. Irradiation of blood products is necessary for patients at risk of:
a. Graft-versus-host disease (GVHD)
b. Hemolytic disease of the newborn
c. Thrombocytopenia
d. Coagulopathy

242. Platelet apheresis is a procedure to collect:
a. Whole blood
b. Red blood cells
c. Platelets
d. Plasma

243. The maximum shelf life of packed red blood cells (PRBCs) is typically:
a. 7 days   b. 14 days
c. 21 days   d. 30 days

244. Blood products should be stored at:
a. Room temperature
b. Refrigerated temperature
c. Frozen temperature
d. Varies depending on the product

245. The term "autologous donation" refers to:
a. Donating blood for oneself
b. Donating blood for a family member
c. Donating blood for a friend
d. Donating blood for a stranger

246. The term "directed donation" refers to:
a. Donating blood for oneself
b. Donating blood for a family member
c. Donating blood for a friend
d. Donating blood for a stranger

247. Blood products are typically transfused via:
a. Intravenous (IV) infusion
b. Intramuscular (IM) injection
c. Subcutaneous injection
d. Oral administration

248. The term "apheresis" refers to:
a. Donating blood for oneself
b. Donating blood for a family member
c. Collection of specific blood components
d. Blood typing and grouping

249. The term "apheresis platelets" refers to:
a. Whole blood collected for transfusion
b. Red blood cells collected for transfusion
c. Platelets collected for transfusion
d. Plasma collected for transfusion

250. The term "platelet refractoriness" refers to:
a. Reduced platelet count in the blood
b. Inability of platelets to aggregate
c. Failure to respond to platelet transfusions
d. Excessive platelet activation

251. The term "transfusion-related acute lung injury (TRALI)" refers to:
a. A transfusion reaction resulting in fever and chills
b. A transfusion reaction causing severe allergic reactions
c. A transfusion reaction causing acute kidney injury
d. A transfusion reaction causing acute respiratory distress

252. The term "hemolytic transfusion reaction" refers to:
a. A transfusion reaction resulting in fever and chills
b. A transfusion reaction causing severe allergic reactions
c. A transfusion reaction causing acute kidney injury
d. A transfusion reaction causing destruction of red blood cells

---

Answers: 241. a   242. c   243. c   244. b
         245. a   246. b   247. a   248. c
         249. c   250. c   251. d   252. d

253. **The term "febrile non-hemolytic transfusion reaction" refers to:**
    a. A transfusion reaction resulting in fever and chills
    b. A transfusion reaction causing severe allergic reactions
    c. A transfusion reaction causing acute kidney injury
    d. A transfusion reaction causing destruction of red blood cells

254. **The term "transfusion-associated circulatory overload (TACO)" refers to:**
    a. A transfusion reaction resulting in fever and chills
    b. A transfusion reaction causing severe allergic reactions
    c. A transfusion reaction causing acute kidney injury
    d. A transfusion reaction causing fluid overload

255. **The term "transfusion-related immunomodulation (TRIM)" refers to:**
    a. A transfusion reaction resulting in fever and chills
    b. A transfusion reaction causing severe allergic reactions
    c. A transfusion reaction causing acute kidney injury
    d. A transfusion reaction causing immunological effects

256. **The term "plateletpheresis" refers to:**
    a. Collection of platelets from whole blood
    b. Collection of platelets from packed red blood cells
    c. Collection of platelets from fresh frozen plasma
    d. Collection of platelets from cryoprecipitate

257. **The term "rare donor registry" refers to a database of individuals who have:**
    a. Rare blood types
    b. High platelet counts
    c. Hemophilia
    d. Anemia

258. **The term "liquid plasma" refers to:**
    a. Plasma stored at room temperature
    b. Plasma stored under refrigeration
    c. Plasma stored frozen
    d. Plasma mixed with an anticoagulant

259. **The term "reagent red blood cells" refers to:**
    a. Donor red blood cells
    b. Patient red blood cells
    c. Universal donor red blood cells
    d. Reagent used for blood typing

260. **The term "extended phenotype" refers to the testing of:**
    a. ABO and Rh antigens
    b. Donor-recipient compatibility
    c. HLA typing
    d. Blood product sterility

261. **The term "antibody screen" refers to testing for:**
    a. Antibodies in donor blood
    b. Antibodies in patient blood
    c. Compatibility of blood types
    d. Hemoglobin levels

262. **The term "pretransfusion testing" refers to:**
    a. Testing for bloodborne pathogens in donor blood
    b. Testing for bloodborne pathogens in patient blood
    c. Compatibility testing between donor and recipient
    d. ABO and Rh typing

Answers:

253. a	254. d	255. d	256. c
257. a	258. a	259. d	260. c
261. b	262. c		

263. **The term "apheresis red blood cells" refers to:**
   a. Whole blood collected for transfusion
   b. Red blood cells collected for transfusion
   c. Platelets collected for transfusion
   d. Plasma collected for transfusion

264. **The term "hemovigilance" refers to the surveillance and reporting of:**
   a. Blood-borne pathogens
   b. Transfusion reactions and adverse events
   c. Donor eligibility criteria
   d. Blood product availability

265. **The term "autologous directed donation" refers to:**
   a. Donating blood for oneself
   b. Donating blood for a family member
   c. Donating blood for a friend
   d. Donating blood for a stranger

266. **The term "universal leukodepletion" refers to the removal of:**
   a. Red blood cells from blood products
   b. Platelets from blood products
   c. White blood cells from blood products
   d. Plasma from blood products

267. **The term "compatibility testing" refers to testing for:**
   a. Antibodies in donor blood
   b. Antibodies in patient blood
   c. Compatibility of blood types
   d. Hemoglobin levels

268. **The term "hyperhemolysis" refers to:**
   a. Increased red blood cell production
   b. Increased destruction of red blood cells

   c. Increased production of platelets
   d. Increased clotting factors

269. **The term "autologous stem cell transplant" refers to the transplantation of:**
   a. Donor stem cells
   b. Patient's own stem cells
   c. Universal donor stem cells
   d. Blood product components

270. **The term "HLA typing" refers to testing for:**
   a. ABO and Rh antigens
   b. Donor-recipient compatibility
   c. HLA antigens on white blood cells
   d. Blood product sterility

271. **The term "delayed hemolytic transfusion reaction" refers to:**
   a. A transfusion reaction resulting in fever and chills
   b. A transfusion reaction causing severe allergic reactions
   c. A transfusion reaction causing destruction of red blood cells
   d. A transfusion reaction causing acute respiratory distress

272. **The term "microbial testing" refers to testing for:**
   a. Antibodies in donor blood
   b. Antibodies in patient blood
   c. Blood-borne pathogens in donor blood
   d. Blood-borne pathogens in patient blood

273. **The term "thawed plasma" refers to:**
   a. Plasma stored at room temperature
   b. Plasma stored under refrigeration
   c. Plasma stored frozen and then thawed
   d. Plasma mixed with an anticoagulant

Answers: 263. b   264. b   265. b   266. c
        267. c   268. b   269. b   270. c
        271. c   272. c   273. c

274. Which blood grouping method involves the use of gel cards?
- a. Slide method
- b. Tube method
- c. Gel method
- d. Centrifugation method

275. The gel method of blood grouping is based on:
- a. Agglutination reactions
- b. Hemolysis reactions
- c. Precipitation reactions
- d. Coagulation reactions

276. The gel method of blood grouping is commonly used for:
- a. ABO typing
- b. Rh typing
- c. Antibody screening
- d. Cross-matching

277. In the gel method, if agglutination occurs, it is visualized as:
- a. Clumps in the gel column
- b. Precipitate at the bottom of the tube
- c. Cloudiness in the gel column
- d. No visible change in the gel column

278. The slide method of blood grouping involves mixing the patient's blood with:
- a. Anti-A and anti-B sera
- b. Anti-D serum
- c. Anti-Rh serum
- d. Anti-Kell serum

279. In the slide method, agglutination is observed under a:
- a. Microscope
- b. Centrifuge
- c. Incubator
- d. UV light

280. The slide method is commonly used for:
- a. ABO typing
- b. Rh typing
- c. Antibody screening
- d. Direct Coombs test

281. In the slide method, which of the following indicates a positive reaction?
- a. Clear separation of cells and serum
- b. Clumps of cells visible
- c. No visible change
- d. Hemolysis of red blood cells

282. The slide method is less sensitive than the gel method in detecting:
- a. ABO incompatibilities
- b. Rh incompatibilities
- c. Antibodies in the serum
- d. Hemolytic reactions

283. Which method allows for simultaneous testing of multiple blood samples?
- a. Slide method
- b. Tube method
- c. Gel method
- d. Centrifugation method

284. Which of the following is not a type of white blood cell?
- a. Neutrophil
- b. Eosinophil
- c. Thrombocyte
- d. Lymphocyte

285. Which of the following is the most abundant leukocyte in the peripheral blood?
- a. Neutrophil
- b. Eosinophil
- c. Basophil
- d. Monocyte

Answers:
274. c	275. a	276. c	277. a
278. a	279. a	280. c	281. b
282. c	283. c	284. c	285. a

286. **Which laboratory test is used to evaluate the oxygen-carrying capacity of red blood cells?**
    a. Hematocrit
    b. Hemoglobin
    c. Platelet count
    d. Prothrombin time

287. **Which type of anemia is characterized by a deficiency of iron in the body?**
    a. Aplastic anemia
    b. Hemolytic anemia
    c. Iron-deficiency anemia
    d. Sickle cell anemia

288. **Which of the following is the correct sequence of red cell development in the bone marrow?**
    a. Myeloblast → Promyelocyte → Myelocyte → Metamyelocyte → Band form
    b. Proerythroblast → Normoblast → Reticulocyte → Erythrocyte
    c. Megakaryoblast → Megakaryocyte → Platelet
    d. Lymphoblast → Prolymphocyte → Lymphocyte

289. **Which of the following is an abnormal increase in the number of circulating red blood cells?**
    a. Leukopenia
    b. Thrombocytopenia
    c. Polycythemia
    d. Hemophilia

290. **Which laboratory test is used to evaluate the intrinsic and common coagulation pathways?**
    a. Prothrombin time (PT)
    b. Activated partial thromboplastin time (aPTT)
    c. Fibrinogen level
    d. D-dimer test

291. **Which of the following conditions is characterized by the presence of abnormal sickle-shaped red blood cells?**
    a. Hemophilia A
    b. Von Willebrand disease
    c. Sickle cell disease
    d. Hemochromatosis

292. **Which anticoagulant is commonly used for collecting blood samples for coagulation studies?**
    a. Sodium citrate
    b. Ethylenediaminetetraacetic acid (EDTA)
    c. Heparin
    d. Sodium fluoride

293. **Which of the following is a disorder characterized by a decreased number of platelets in the blood?**
    a. Leukocytosis
    b. Neutropenia
    c. Thrombocytopenia
    d. Lymphocytosis

294. **Which of the following cells are responsible for phagocytosis in the immune system?**
    a. Neutrophils   b. Eosinophils
    c. Basophils   d. Monocytes

295. **Which of the following is a commonly used stain for peripheral blood smear examination?**
    a. H&E stain
    b. Giemsa stain
    c. Prussian blue stain
    d. Periodic acid-Schiff (PAS) stain

Answers: 286. b   287. c   288. b   289. c
290. b   291. c   292. a   293. c
294. a   295. b

296. **Which of the following is a red blood cell disorder characterized by a crescent or sickle shape of the cells?**
    a. Hemophilia
    b. Thalassemia
    c. Sickle cell anemia
    d. Polycythemia vera

297. **Which laboratory test is used to assess the average lifespan of red blood cells?**
    a. Erythrocyte sedimentation rate (ESR)
    b. Red blood cell count
    c. Reticulocyte count
    d. Hemoglobin electrophoresis

298. **Which of the following is the main function of platelets in the blood?**
    a. Oxygen transport
    b. Clot formation
    c. Immune response
    d. Iron storage

299. **Which of the following is the correct order of the clotting factors in the coagulation cascade?**
    a. VII → X → II → I
    b. XII → X → VIII → II
    c. VIII → IX → X → XI
    d. V → XII → XI → X

300. **Which of the following blood group systems is based on the presence or absence of the Rh factor?**
    a. ABO system
    b. Lewis system
    c. Kell system
    d. Rh system

301. **Which of the following is a hereditary bleeding disorder characterized by a deficiency of clotting factor VIII?**
    a. Hemophilia A
    b. Hemophilia B
    c. Von Willebrand disease
    d. Factor V Leiden deficiency

302. **Which of the following laboratory tests is used to evaluate the extrinsic and common coagulation pathways?**
    a. Prothrombin time (PT)
    b. Activated partial thromboplastin time (aPTT)
    c. Thrombin time
    d. Bleeding time

303. **Which of the following is the correct term for an increase in the number of white blood cells?**
    a. Leukopenia
    b. Leukocytosis
    c. Lymphopenia
    d. Thrombocytosis

304. **Which of the following is a cell fragment involved in blood clotting?**
    a. Neutrophil
    b. Erythrocyte
    c. Monocyte
    d. Platelet

305. **Which of the following is the correct term for a decrease in the number of red blood cells or hemoglobin in the blood?**
    a. Erythrocytosis
    b. Anemia
    c. Leukemia
    d. Hemolysis

Answers: 296. c   297. c   298. b   299. a
300. d   301. a   302. a   303. b
304. d   305. b

306. Which of the following is the correct order of cell maturation in the megakaryocyte-platelet lineage?
a. Megakaryoblast → Promegakaryocyte → Megakaryocyte → Platelet
b. Proerythroblast → Normoblast → Reticulocyte → Erythrocyte
c. Myeloblast → Promyelocyte → Myelocyte → Metamyelocyte → Band form
d. Lymphoblast → Prolymphocyte → Lymphocyte

307. Which laboratory test measures the volume of red blood cells in a given volume of whole blood?
a. Hematocrit
b. Hemoglobin
c. Platelet count
d. Erythrocyte sedimentation rate (ESR)

308. Which of the following is an inherited disorder characterized by an abnormal hemoglobin molecule?
a. Aplastic anemia
b. Thalassemia
c. Sickle cell anemia
d. Idiopathic thrombocytopenic purpura (ITP)

309. Which of the following cells are responsible for producing antibodies in response to foreign antigens?
a. Neutrophils
b. Eosinophils
c. Basophils
d. Lymphocytes

310. Which laboratory test is used to detect the presence of abnormal hemoglobin variants?
a. Red blood cell count
b. Hemoglobin electrophoresis
c. Reticulocyte count
d. Erythrocyte sedimentation rate (ESR)

311. Which of the following is a primary function of the lymphatic system?
a. Production of red blood cells
b. Oxygen transport
c. Immune response
d. Clot formation

312. Which of the following is a genetic disorder characterized by a decreased production of clotting factor IX?
a. Hemophilia A
b. Hemophilia B
c. Von Willebrand disease
d. Factor V Leiden deficiency

313. Which of the following cells are responsible for initiating the clotting process in response to tissue injury?
a. Neutrophils
b. Eosinophils
c. Basophils
d. Platelets

314. Which of the following is a red blood cell disorder characterized by a decreased production of hemoglobin?
a. Hemophilia
b. Thalassemia
c. Sickle cell trait
d. Polycythemia vera

Answers: 306. a   307. a   308. c   309. d
310. b   311. c   312. b   313. d
314. b

315. **Which laboratory test measures the time it takes for blood to clot after adding a thromboplastin reagent?**
    a. Prothrombin time (PT)
    b. Activated partial thromboplastin time (aPTT)
    c. Thrombin time
    d. Bleeding time

316. **Which of the following is the correct term for an abnormal decrease in the number of white blood cells?**
    a. Leukopenia
    b. Leukocytosis
    c. Lymphopenia
    d. Thrombocytopenia

317. **Which of the following is the most common inherited bleeding disorder?**
    a. Hemophilia A
    b. Hemophilia B
    c. Von Willebrand disease
    d. Factor V Leiden deficiency

318. **Which laboratory test is used to assess platelet function and evaluate primary hemostasis?**
    a. Prothrombin time (PT)
    b. Activated partial thromboplastin time (aPTT)
    c. Bleeding time
    d. D-dimer test

319. **Which of the following is the correct term for an abnormal increase in the number of platelets in the blood?**
    a. Thrombocytopenia
    b. Thrombocytosis
    c. Polycythemia
    d. Hemophilia

320. **Which of the following is a condition characterized by a deficiency of all types of blood cells?**
    a. Aplastic anemia
    b. Hemolytic anemia
    c. Iron-deficiency anemia
    d. Sickle cell anemia

321. **Which laboratory test measures the time it takes for a blood clot to dissolve?**
    a. Prothrombin time (PT)
    b. Activated partial thromboplastin time (aPTT)
    c. Thrombin time
    d. D-dimer test

322. **Which of the following is an abnormal decrease in the number of circulating red blood cells?**
    a. Leukopenia
    b. Thrombocytopenia
    c. Anemia
    d. Hemophilia

323. **Which of the following is the correct term for a decrease in the number of platelets in the blood?**
    a. Leukocytosis
    b. Neutropenia
    c. Thrombocytopenia
    d. Lymphocytosis

324. **Which laboratory test measures the ability of platelets to aggregate and form clumps?**
    a. Prothrombin time (PT)
    b. Activated partial thromboplastin time (aPTT)
    c. Platelet count
    d. Platelet aggregation test

Answers: 315. a   316. a   317. c   318. c
319. b   320. a   321. a   322. c
323. c   324. d

325. Which of the following cells are responsible for the release of histamine during allergic reactions?
a. Neutrophils
b. Eosinophils
c. Basophils
d. Monocytes

326. Which laboratory test is used to evaluate the intrinsic coagulation pathway and monitor heparin therapy?
a. Prothrombin time (PT)
b. Activated partial thromboplastin time (aPTT)
c. Thrombin time
d. Fibrinogen level

327. Which of the following is an acquired autoimmune disorder characterized by the destruction of platelets?
a. Aplastic anemia
b. Idiopathic thrombocytopenic purpura (ITP)
c. Iron-deficiency anemia
d. Sickle cell anemia

328. Which of the following is a red blood cell disorder characterized by an abnormal increase in the number of red blood cells?
a. Leukocytosis
b. Polycythemia
c. Anemia
d. Hemophilia

329. Which laboratory test measures the time it takes for a blood clot to form after adding calcium and a clotting reagent?
a. Prothrombin time (PT)
b. Activated partial thromboplastin time (aPTT)
c. Thrombin time
d. D-dimer test

330. Which of the following is a blood clotting disorder characterized by a deficiency of clotting factor IX?
a. Hemophilia A
b. Hemophilia B
c. Von Willebrand disease
d. Factor V Leiden deficiency

331. Which of the following cells are responsible for transporting oxygen to tissues?
a. Neutrophils
b. Eosinophils
c. Basophils
d. Erythrocytes

332. Which laboratory test is used to evaluate the extrinsic coagulation pathway and monitor warfarin therapy?
a. Prothrombin time (PT)
b. Activated partial thromboplastin time (aPTT)
c. Thrombin time
d. Fibrinogen level

333. Which of the following cells are responsible for antibody-mediated immunity?
a. Neutrophils
b. Eosinophils
c. B lymphocytes
d. T lymphocytes

334. Which laboratory test measures the rate at which red blood cells settle in a vertical tube over a given period?
a. Hematocrit
b. Hemoglobin
c. Erythrocyte sedimentation rate (ESR)
d. Reticulocyte count

Answers: 325. c 326. b 327. b 328. b
329. a 330. b 331. d 332. c
333. c 334. c

335. Which of the following is a hereditary bleeding disorder characterized by a deficiency of von Willebrand factor?
a. Hemophilia A
b. Hemophilia B
c. Von Willebrand disease
d. Factor V Leiden deficiency

336. Which of the following is an inherited disorder characterized by excessive iron absorption and deposition in various organs?
a. Aplastic anemia
b. Hemochromatosis
c. Iron-deficiency anemia
d. Sickle cell anemia

337. Which laboratory test is used to evaluate the overall clotting function of the blood?
a. Prothrombin time (PT)
b. Activated partial thromboplastin time (aPTT)
c. Thrombin time
d. Bleeding time

338. Which of the following is an acquired bleeding disorder characterized by the presence of an autoantibody against platelet glycoproteins?
a. Aplastic anemia
b. Idiopathic thrombocytopenic purpura (ITP)
c. Hemolytic anemia
d. Sickle cell anemia

339. Which laboratory test is used to evaluate the concentration of fibrinogen in the blood?
a. Prothrombin time (PT)
b. Activated partial thromboplastin time (aPTT)
c. Fibrinogen level
d. D-dimer test

340. Which of the following is a red blood cell disorder characterized by a defect in hemoglobin synthesis?
a. Hemophilia
b. Thalassemia
c. Sickle cell anemia
d. Polycythemia vera

341. Which laboratory test measures the time it takes for blood to clot and form a fibrin clot?
a. Prothrombin time (PT)
b. Activated partial thromboplastin time (aPTT)
c. Thrombin time
d. D-dimer test

342. Which of the following cells are responsible for releasing heparin to prevent blood clotting?
a. Neutrophils
b. Eosinophils
c. Basophils
d. Monocytes

343. Which of the following is a hereditary bleeding disorder characterized by a deficiency of clotting factor XIII?
a. Hemophilia A
b. Hemophilia B
c. Von Willebrand disease
d. Factor XIII deficiency

344. Which laboratory test measures the concentration of red blood cells in a given volume of whole blood?
a. Hematocrit
b. Hemoglobin
c. Platelet count
d. Reticulocyte count

Answers: 335. c | 336. b | 337. a | 338. b
339. c | 340. b | 341. c | 342. c
343. d | 344. a

345. Which of the following is a red blood cell disorder characterized by an abnormal increase in the number of red blood cells?
a. Leukocytosis
b. Polycythemia
c. Anemia
d. Hemophilia

346. Which laboratory test is used to evaluate the activation of the final step in the coagulation cascade?
a. Prothrombin time (PT)
b. Activated partial thromboplastin time (aPTT)
c. Thrombin time
d. D-dimer test

347. Which laboratory test is used to detect the presence of fibrin degradation products in the blood?
a. Prothrombin time (PT)
b. Activated partial thromboplastin time (aPTT)
c. Thrombin time
d. D-dimer test

348. Which of the following is a red blood cell disorder characterized by an abnormal decrease in the number of red blood cells?
a. Leukocytosis
b. Polycythemia
c. Anemia
d. Hemophilia

349. Which laboratory test measures the time it takes for blood to clot after adding calcium and a thromboplastin reagent?
a. Prothrombin time (PT)
b. Activated partial thromboplastin time (aPTT)
c. Thrombin time
d. D-dimer test

350. Which of the following cells are responsible for the phagocytosis of foreign particles and cellular debris?
a. Neutrophils
b. Eosinophils
c. Basophils
d. Monocytes

351. Which laboratory test measures the concentration of hemoglobin in a given volume of whole blood?
a. Hematocrit
b. Hemoglobin
c. Platelet count
d. Erythrocyte sedimentation rate (ESR)

352. Which of the following is a red blood cell disorder characterized by an abnormal increase in the number of red blood cells?
a. Leukocytosis
b. Polycythemia
c. Anemia
d. Hemophilia

353. Which laboratory test is used to evaluate the activation of the final step in the coagulation cascade?
a. Prothrombin time (PT)
b. Activated partial thromboplastin time (aPTT)
c. Thrombin time
d. D-dimer test

354. Which of the following cells are responsible for the production of antibodies?
a. Neutrophils
b. Eosinophils
c. Basophils
d. B lymphocytes

Answers: 345. **b**   346. **c**   347. **d**   348. **c**
349. **a**   350. **a**   351. **b**   352. **b**
353. **c**   354. **d**

355. Which of the following is a red blood cell disorder characterized by a defect in hemoglobin synthesis?
a. Hemophilia
b. Thalassemia
c. Sickle cell anemia
d. Polycythemia vera

356. Which of the following is a red blood cell disorder characterized by abnormal hemoglobin synthesis?
a. Hemophilia
b. Thalassemia
c. Sickle cell anemia
d. Polycythemia vera

Answers: 355. b   356. b

SECTION

Histopathology and Cytology

Section Outline

5

CHAPTER

Histopathology

INTRODUCTION TO HISTOPATHOLOGY

Histopathology is a branch of pathology associated with the microscopic study of diseases in tissue section. It acts as an important link between anatomy and pathology for the correct diagnosis of diseases.

There are a series of steps that a tissue undergoes before a pathologist examines it under a microscope to reach a particular diagnosis.

Steps of Histological Techniques

Specimen brought to the histopathological laboratory is first logged, identified by a histotechnician and then subjected to specimen preparation and further sent for tissue processing.

Steps of histopathology techniques are shown in **Flowchart 5.1**.

Flowchart 5.1: Steps of histopathology techniques.

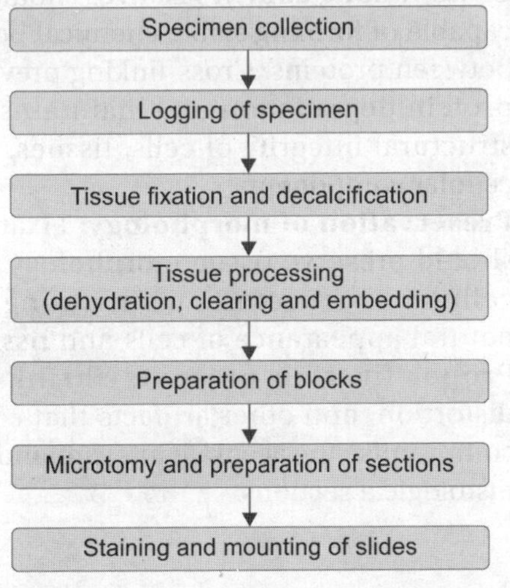

Responsibilities of a Technician

In the histopathology laboratory, the technician is responsible for:
- Preservation of specimen.
- Labeling, logging and identification of the specimen.
- Preparing the specimen to facilitate its grossing and microscopy.
- Maintenance of records.

To fulfill these aims the following points need to be considered.
- On receiving the specimen in the laboratory, the technician must check the labelling of the specimen. Name, age, Hospital Registration No. and the nature of the tissue to be examined should be mentioned on the label. The requisition form accompanying the specimen should also be checked.
- Checking the fixative of the specimen. The technician should ensure that the fixative is around fifteen to twenty times the volume of the specimen for proper fixation of the specimen.
- The biopsy/specimen received should be entered in the register and given a unique pathology number. The allotted number should be written over the specimen container and requisition form. This number will act as the identification number of the specimen in the histopathological laboratory.
- Large specimen received should be informed to the pathologist so that specimen is given further cuts for adequate fixation of the specimen.

○ After preparation of slides, blocks should be preserved properly with their histopathology number as they have to be preserved lifelong.

○ Slides should also be stored properly after the reporting by a pathologist is complete.

○ Discarding of the specimen should be done after checking with pathologist.

FIXATION

In histopathology, fixation is crucial in preparing tissue samples for microscopic examination. The principle of fixation is to preserve the tissue structure and cellular components in a stable and unaltered state, preventing decay, autolysis, and putrefaction. Fixation also allows for the retention of antigenicity, which is essential for immunohistochemical staining and other molecular techniques.

The primary objectives of fixation in histopathology are:

○ **Preservation of tissue morphology:** Fixation helps maintain the tissue sample's architecture and cellular details as close to their natural state as possible. It prevents distortion and shrinkage, ensuring that the cells and structures are accurately represented in the subsequent histological sections.

○ **Prevention of autolysis and putrefaction:** Immediately after tissue removal from the body, enzymatic and bacterial degradation processes start to occur, leading to tissue deterioration. Fixation halts these processes by inactivating endogenous enzymes and denaturing proteins, thus preventing the breakdown of cellular components.

○ **Inactivation of infectious agents:** Fixatives such as formalin have antimicrobial properties and can kill or inactivate infectious microorganisms in the tissue, reducing the risk of handling and processing infectious samples.

○ **Cross-linking of proteins:** Fixatives form chemical bonds between proteins, primarily by creating covalent cross-links. This stabilizes the tissue structure and cellular proteins, preventing their degradation and maintaining their antigenicity.

Properties of Fixatives

○ **Stability:** Fixatives should be chemically stable and not undergo degradation or decomposition over time. Stability ensures the consistent performance of the fixative and helps maintain its effectiveness during storage.

○ **Compatibility:** Fixatives should be compatible with various tissue types and capable of effectively preserving the cellular components of different tissues. Compatibility ensures that the fixative can penetrate the tissue and cross-link proteins without causing significant damage or altering the tissue's characteristics.

○ **Penetration:** Fixatives should have good penetration properties, allowing them to diffuse into the tissue quickly and evenly. Adequate penetration ensures that the fixative reaches all areas of the tissue, ensuring uniform fixation and preservation of cellular structures.

○ **Cross-linking ability:** Fixatives should be capable of forming stable chemical bonds between proteins. Cross-linking prevents protein degradation and maintains the structural integrity of cells, tissues, and cellular components.

○ **Preservation of morphology:** Fixatives should preserve tissue morphology and cellular architecture, maintaining the natural appearance of cells and tissues. Proper fixation prevents shrinkage, distortion, and other artifacts that could compromise the accurate interpretation of histological sections.

○ **Retention of antigenicity:** Fixatives should retain the antigenicity of tissues, allowing for subsequent immunohistochemical staining and molecular analysis. Preserving antigenicity enables the detection of specific markers and the identification of cellular components and pathological processes.

○ **Safety:** Fixatives should be safe to handle and not pose significant health risks to laboratory personnel. Proper precautions should be taken during the handling, storage, and disposal of fixatives to ensure the safety of individuals and the environment.

○ **Compatibility with downstream processing:** Fixatives should be compatible with subsequent processing steps, including tissue processing, embedding, sectioning, and staining. They should not interfere with the quality of histological sections or the performance of staining methods.

○ **Archival properties:** Fixatives should allow for long-term preservation of tissue samples without significant degradation. This quality is essential for archival purposes, retrospective studies, and the long-term storage of specimens.

○ **Availability and cost-effectiveness:** Fixatives should be readily available and cost-effective, as histopathology laboratories typically process a large number of samples. Availability and affordability ensure that the fixative can be obtained and used without compromising the quality of fixation.

○ **Amount of fixative:** The general rule of thumb is to use at least 20 times the volume of fixative as compared to the volume of the tissue specimen. This ratio ensures sufficient coverage and penetration of the fixative throughout the tissue.

○ **Tissue size:** Larger tissue specimen may require more fixative to adequately cover and penetrate the entire sample. Sections are made in large specimen such that slices of 1.5 cm are made for easy penetration of fixative.

○ **Container size:** The size of the container holding the fixative should be large enough to accommodate the tissue specimen without overcrowding. Sufficient space allows for proper immersion and even distribution of the fixative.

Factors Affecting Fixation

○ **Penetration ability:** The fixative's ability to penetrate tissues is crucial for uniform and effective fixation. Fixatives with good penetration properties can efficiently diffuse through the tissue, reaching all cellular layers and ensuring consistent preservation.

○ **Chemical composition:** The composition of the fixative solution plays a significant role in fixation. Different fixatives have varying chemical properties that determine their ability to cross-link proteins, stabilize cellular structures, and inhibit autolysis. The choice of fixative should be based on the specific requirements of the tissue and the desired diagnostic or research objectives.

○ **pH:** The pH of the fixative solution affects the rate and extent of fixation. Optimal pH conditions are necessary for effective protein cross-linking and preservation of tissue morphology. Deviations from the appropriate pH range can lead to incomplete fixation, tissue damage, or alteration of cellular structures.

○ **Osmolarity:** The osmolarity of the fixative solution refers to its concentration of solute particles. Fixatives with osmolarity similar to that of the tissue cytoplasm can minimize tissue shrinkage and maintain cellular integrity during fixation. Proper osmolarity helps preserve tissue morphology and prevent artifacts.

○ **Fixation time:** The duration of tissue immersion in the fixative solution influences fixation quality. Longer fixation times allow for more extensive cross-linking of proteins and preservation of cellular structures. However, over-fixation can lead to tissue hardening and potential loss of antigenicity. The optimal fixation time varies depending on the fixative, tissue type, and desired diagnostic outcomes.

○ **Temperature:** The temperature at which fixation occurs affects the rate of fixation, fixative penetration, and preservation of cellular components. Lower temperatures can slow down fixation processes and enzymatic activity, preserving tissue integrity. However, excessively low temperatures can hinder fixative penetration. Higher temperatures can accelerate fixation but may result in tissue shrinkage and artifact formation.

Types of Fixation

There are several types of fixation techniques used, depending on the specific requirements of the tissue and the desired diagnostic or research objectives.

Some commonly used types of fixation are:

○ **Chemical fixation:** Chemical fixation involves immersing tissue samples in a fixative solution containing various chemicals. The most commonly used chemical fixative is formalin (10% neutral buffered formalin), which contains formaldehyde. Other chemical fixatives include paraformaldehyde, glutaraldehyde, and alcohol-based fixatives. Chemical fixation cross-links proteins and stabilizes cellular structures to preserve tissue morphology.

○ **Cold fixation:** Cold fixation involves fixing tissues at lower temperatures, usually around 4°C (refrigeration). Lower temperatures slow down enzymatic activity and reduce autolysis, allowing for extended fixation times and better preservation of tissue integrity. Cold fixation is commonly used for delicate tissues, such as biopsies or surgical specimens.

○ **Heat fixation:** Heat fixation involves using heat to fix tissue samples onto glass slides. This technique is often used for cytological preparations, such as smears or fine needle aspirates. Heat fixation promotes adhesion of cells to the slide and helps preserve cellular morphology. Examples of heat fixation methods include flame fixation (passing the slide through a flame) or heating slides on a hot plate.

○ **Microwave-assisted fixation:** Microwave-assisted fixation combines the use of a fixative solution with microwave energy to accelerate fixation. The heat generated by the microwave helps enhance the penetration and reaction of the fixative with the tissue, reducing fixation time compared to traditional methods. Microwave-assisted fixation is commonly used for rapid fixation in certain protocols.

○ **Freeze fixation:** Freeze fixation involves rapidly freezing tissue samples using cryogens, such as liquid nitrogen or freezing sprays. Freezing halts cellular activity and preserves cellular structures in a near-native state. This technique is often used for preserving certain antigens or delicate structures, such as lipids or enzyme activities, that may be altered by chemical fixation.

○ **In vivo fixation:** In vivo fixation involves the fixation of tissues while they are still inside the living organism. It is commonly used for research purposes to study specific cellular processes or to preserve tissues for specialized analyzes. In vivo fixation can be achieved by perfusing fixative solutions directly into the blood vessels or organs of an anesthetized animal.

Types of chemical fixatives are depicted in **Flowchart 5.2**.

Flowchart 5.2: Types of chemical fixatives.

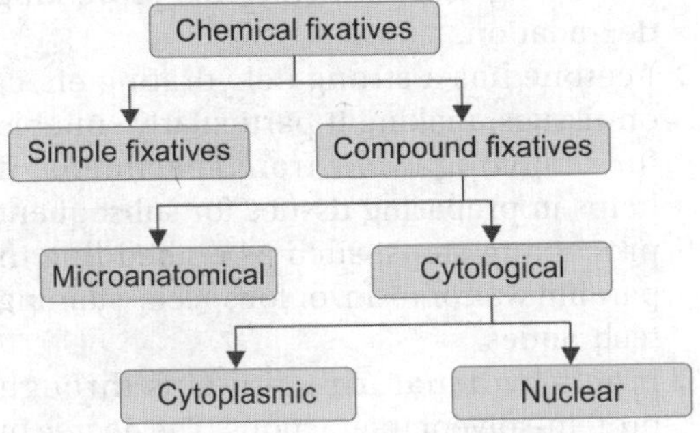

Simple Fixatives

Formaldehyde

It is a simple fixative commonly used in histopathology and other biological sciences. It is a colorless gas with a pungent odor and is highly reactive. In the laboratory, formaldehyde is typically used in the form of a 37–40% aqueous solution called formalin. Here are some key points about formaldehyde as a fixative:

- **Fixative properties:** Formaldehyde acts as a cross-linking fixative, forming covalent bonds between proteins and stabilizing cellular structures. It preserves tissue morphology and prevents degradation by inhibiting autolysis and enzymatic activity.
- **Fixation mechanism:** Formaldehyde reacts with primary amino groups of proteins, mainly forming methylene bridges ($-CH_2-$) between adjacent protein molecules. This cross-linking leads to the stabilization of cellular proteins and prevents their degradation.
- **Cross-linking effects:** The extent of cross-linking and tissue preservation can be influenced by factors such as fixation time, temperature, and formaldehyde concentration. Overfixation with formaldehyde may lead to tissue hardening and masking of certain antigens, while underfixation can result in poor preservation and tissue damage.
- **Formalin preparation:** Formalin is prepared by dissolving formaldehyde gas in water, typically in a buffered solution to maintain a slightly acidic pH. The most commonly used formulation is 10% neutral buffered formalin (NBF), which has a pH of around 7.
- On standing for a long period formalin oxidizes to formic acid which is neutralized by phosphates or calcium carbonate, else it leads to brown colored artifact formation in tissues. For removal of this pigment picric acid or saturated alcoholic sodium hydroxide is used.
  Commercially available formalin becomes cloudy on standing due to formation of a precipitate of paraformaldehyde which can be filtered.
- **Safety considerations:** Formaldehyde is a hazardous substance and is classified as a carcinogen by some regulatory agencies. Proper precautions should be taken when handling formaldehyde, including working in a well-ventilated area, using appropriate personal protective equipment, and following proper waste disposal protocols.

Limitations

- While formaldehyde is widely used and provides good preservation for routine histopathological examination, it may not be suitable for certain specialized applications or preserving specific antigens. In such cases, alternative fixatives or modifications to the fixation protocols may be necessary.

Alcohol (Ethyl Alcohol)

It is commonly used as a fixative in histopathology and other biological sciences. Ethanol acts as a coagulating fixative, denaturing proteins and causing their precipitation. It leads to forming a protein coagulum that helps preserve tissue structure and prevent degradation.

○ It provides good preservation of cellular structures, including nuclei, cytoplasm, and extracellular components. It allows for subsequent processing, embedding in paraffin wax, sectioning, and staining for microscopic examination.

○ Ethanol has a dehydrating effect on tissues, which helps in removing water and preparing tissues for subsequent steps in the processing, such as embedding in paraffin wax. The dehydration property of ethanol makes it an essential component in the tissue processing workflow.

○ It acts by denaturing proteins through protein-alcohol interactions and cross-linking. The degree of protein denaturation and fixation can be influenced by factors such as the concentration of ethanol, fixation time, and temperature.

○ Ethanol is commonly used in different concentrations for fixation, such as 70%, 95%, or absolute (100%) ethanol. The choice of concentration depends on the specific requirements of the tissue type and downstream processing techniques.

○ Ethanol is a flammable substance, and proper precautions should be taken when handling it, including working in a well-ventilated area and following proper storage and handling guidelines. Additionally, ethanol can cause tissue hardening and shrinkage if overexposed, so careful control of fixation time is important.

○ While ethanol fixation is widely used, it may not provide the same level of tissue preservation as other fixatives, such as formalin. Ethanol fixation is particularly suitable for certain applications, such as preserving enzyme activity, lipid-rich tissues, or specific antigens.

Acetone

Acetone is a volatile organic compound that can be used as a fixative in histopathology and other biological sciences.

○ It acts as a coagulating fixative, similar to ethanol, by denaturing proteins and causing their precipitation. It helps in preserving tissue structure and preventing degradation.

○ Acetone has a strong dehydrating effect on tissues, making it particularly suitable for removing water from specimens. It helps in preparing tissues for subsequent processing steps, such as embedding in paraffin wax or resin, or for special staining techniques.

○ It acts by denaturing proteins through protein-solvent interactions. The degree of fixation can be influenced by factors such as the concentration of acetone, fixation time, and temperature.

○ Acetone fixation is particularly useful for preserving lipids and for certain immunohistochemical staining protocols. It is commonly used for lipid staining techniques, such as Sudan stains, where preservation of lipid content is critical.

Limitations

While acetone fixation can be effective for certain applications, it may not provide the same level of tissue preservation as formalin or other fixatives. It may cause tissue shrinkage and can result in some loss of antigenicity, requiring optimization of staining protocols for immunohistochemistry.

Mercuric Chloride

Mercuric chloride ($HgCl_2$) is a chemical compound historically used as a fixative in histopathology and other biological applications. However, its use as a fixative has declined due to safety concerns associated with its toxicity.

It acts as a cross-linking fixative, similar to formaldehyde, by forming covalent bonds with proteins and stabilizing cellular structures. It helps preserve tissue morphology and prevent degradation.

The thickness of the tissue to be fixed in mercuric chloride should be around 4 mm; if it is more, the tissue gets hardened at the periphery while the central part is soft and under-fixed.

Tissues fixed in it contain black pigment which are the precipitates of mercury that can be removed by treating with 0.5% iodide solution in 70% ethanol for 5–10 minutes.

Picric Acid

Picric acid, also known as 2,4,6-trinitrophenol (TNP), is a chemical compound that has been historically used as a fixative in histopathology. However, its use as a fixative has significantly declined due to safety concerns and the availability of safer alternatives.

It acts as a coagulating fixative, similar to other fixatives like formaldehyde and ethanol. It denatures proteins and causes their precipitation, preserving tissue structure.

Picric acid fixation provides good preservation of cellular structures, including nuclei, cytoplasm, and extracellular components.

Osmium Tetroxide

Osmium tetroxide (OsO4) is a chemical compound used as a fixative in histopathology and electron microscopy. It is primarily used for preserving ultrastructural details in biological samples. Osmium tetroxide is a heavy metal stain that imparts a dark brown or black color to biological samples. This staining property helps highlight cellular structures and provides contrast for electron microscopy imaging. Osmium tetroxide is a heavy metal stain that imparts a dark brown or black color to biological samples. This staining property helps highlight cellular structures and provides contrast for electron microscopy imaging.

Compound Fixatives

Compound fixatives are made by combining multiple chemicals or compounds to achieve specific fixation properties. These fixatives are often formulated to address tissue preservation needs or enhance specific staining techniques.

They are further divided into:
- Microanatomical fixatives
- Cytological fixatives

Microanatomical Fixatives

Microanatomical fixatives, or special or specific fixatives, are a category of fixatives used to preserve specific microanatomical structures or components within tissues. These fixatives are often tailored to preserve delicate structures, cellular components, or molecular targets of interest.

1. **10% formol saline solution:** A 10% formol saline solution, also known as 10% formalin saline solution, is a commonly used fixative solution in histology and pathology. It is a mixture of formaldehyde (typically in the form of formalin) and physiological saline (0.9% sodium chloride solution). It is mostly used for fixation of tissue from the central nervous system and postmortem tissue. It has a slow action and requires 24 hours or long for the fixation of tissue.

2. **Neutral buffered formalin:** Neutral buffered formalin (NBF) is a commonly used fixative in histopathology and clinical laboratories. It is a formaldehyde solution in a buffered aqueous solution, usually phosphate buffer, to maintain a neutral pH. It is widely available in most laboratories and medical facilities. It is a standard fixative used in routine histopathology, and laboratory staff are usually familiar with its handling and processing protocols.

3. **Formal sublimate (Zenker's fluid):** Formal sublimate, also known as Zenker's fixative or Zenker's fluid, is a chemical

fixative commonly used in histopathology to preserve tissue specimens. It is a specialized fixative that combines the properties of formaldehyde and mercuric chloride.

Composition: Formal sublimate is typically composed of the following ingredients:

○ *Formaldehyde (37–40% aqueous solution):* Provides cross-linking and preservation of tissue proteins.

○ *Mercuric chloride:* Enhances the fixation properties and aids in preserving cellular structures.

○ *Potassium dichromate:* Acts as an oxidizing agent and further contributes to the fixation process.

○ *Glacial acetic acid:* Helps to stabilize and acidify the fixative.

Formal sublimate is particularly effective in preserving glycogen and connective tissue fibers. It is commonly used in special staining techniques to demonstrate these specific components.

Tissues fixed with formal sublimate can be processed for routine histological techniques such as paraffin embedding, sectioning, and staining. However, it is important to note that mercuric chloride can interfere with some histochemical staining methods, requiring proper removal or neutralization of mercuric residues before staining.

4. **Bouin's fluid:** Bouin's fluid is a fixative commonly used in histopathology to preserve tissue specimen. French pathologist Pol Bouin developed it in the early 20th century. Bouin's fluid is particularly useful for preserving delicate structures and antigens, making it suitable for certain histological staining techniques.

Composition:

○ Saturated aqueous picric acid—75 mL

○ Formalin—25 mL

○ Glacial acetic acid—5 mL

It penetrates rapidly and provides little shrinkage. It acts as an excellent fixative for intestinal and testicular biopsies as it gives very good nuclear details.

Bouin's fluid is particularly effective in preserving glycogen, mucins, and certain enzyme activities. It is commonly used for special staining techniques that require the demonstration of these specific components.

It is commonly used for the fixation of small tissue specimens, such as biopsies or small surgical specimens. Larger tissue samples may require longer fixation times or alternative fixatives to ensure proper penetration and fixation.

5. **Helly's fluid:** Helly's fluid, also known as Helly's solution, is a fixative used in histopathology for the preservation of tissue specimens. It is named after the German histologist August Helly. Helly's fluid is a modified formulation of Bouin's fluid, which is another commonly used fixative.

Composition: Helly's fluid typically consists of the following ingredients:

○ *Picric acid:* Acts as a fixative and helps preserve tissue structures.

○ *Formaldehyde (37–40% aqueous solution):* Cross-links and preserves tissue proteins.

○ *Glacial acetic acid:* Acidifies the fixative solution.

Helly's fluid is particularly useful for preserving delicate structures, such as glycogen, mucins, and certain enzyme activities. It is often used for special staining techniques that require the demonstration of these specific components.

Cytological Fixatives

Nuclear Fixatives

Nuclear fixatives are a type of fixative that specifically target and preserve nuclear components within cells. They are designed to provide optimal preservation of nuclear morphology and structures, which is essential for many histological and cytological studies. Here are some common nuclear fixatives:

○ **Carnoy's fixative:** Carnoy's fixative is a mixture of ethanol, chloroform, and glacial acetic acid. It is a rapid-acting fixative that effectively preserves nuclear and cytoplasmic components. Carnoy's fixative is commonly used in cytology for preserving nuclear morphology in fine-needle aspiration (FNA) specimens.

○ **Methanol:** Methanol is a simple alcohol fixative that is frequently used for preserving nuclear antigens and DNA/RNA in cytology and immunocytochemistry. It provides excellent preservation of nuclear structures and is commonly used in Papanicolaou (Pap) staining and fluorescence in situ hybridization (FISH) techniques.

○ **Ethanol:** Ethanol is another commonly used fixative for preserving nuclear components. It acts by denaturing proteins and preserving DNA/RNA structures. Ethanol fixation is commonly used in cytology and molecular biology applications.

○ **Formaldehyde-free fixatives:** There are formaldehyde-free fixatives available that are specifically designed to preserve nuclear antigens while avoiding the cross-linking effects of formaldehyde. These fixatives, such as PAXgene, RCL2, and CytoLyt, are used in molecular pathology and molecular diagnostics for preserving nuclear material for subsequent nucleic acid analysis.

Cytoplasmic Fixatives

Cytoplasmic fixatives are specialized fixatives used to preserve the cytoplasmic components of cells while minimizing changes to the cellular morphology and structure. These fixatives are particularly important in cytology and cytochemistry, where the focus is on studying the cytoplasmic contents and organelles of cells , e.g., Helly's fluid.

Histochemical Fixatives

Histochemical fixatives are a category of fixatives specifically designed for preserving tissue structures and components while retaining the biochemical and enzymatic activities within the tissue. These fixatives are used in histochemical techniques, which involve the visualization and localization of specific molecules, enzymes, or chemical reactions within tissues. Here are a few examples of histochemical fixatives:

○ **Formaldehyde-based fixatives:** Formaldehyde-based fixatives, such as formalin or paraformaldehyde, are the most commonly used in histology and histochemistry. They effectively preserve tissue morphology and cellular structures while retaining many enzyme activities and molecular antigens. Formaldehyde-based fixatives are versatile and widely compatible with various histochemical staining techniques.

○ **Acetone:** Acetone is a widely used fixative in histochemistry, particularly for preserving antigens and enzymatic activities. It is commonly used in immunohistochemistry and enzyme histochemistry techniques. Acetone fixation effectively preserves tissue antigenicity and facilitates the penetration of antibodies or enzyme substrates into the tissue.

○ **Methanol:** Methanol is another common fixative used in histochemistry, especially for preserving enzymes and antigens. It is often used with acetone for sequential fixation and permeabilization steps in immunohistochemistry protocols. Methanol fixation is rapid and efficient, providing good preservation of antigenicity.

○ **Carnoy's fixative:** It is commonly used in histochemistry for preserving enzyme activities, particularly for enzyme histochemistry studies involving specific enzymes or metabolic pathways.

○ **Zenker's fixative** is particularly useful for preserving glycogen and connective tissue fibers in tissues.

Vapor Fixatives

Vapor fixatives, also known as gas fixatives or fumigation fixatives, act by exposure to vapors or gases rather than direct immersion of the specimen in a liquid fixative solution. These fixatives are particularly useful for preserving delicate or difficult-to-fix specimens or preserving the integrity of volatile or easily damaged substances. Here are some examples of vapor fixatives:

○ **Osmium tetroxide:** Osmium tetroxide is a commonly used vapor fixative in electron microscopy. It is typically used as a post-fixative by exposing the specimen to its vapors, penetrating and reacting with the tissue to preserve ultrastructural details. Osmium tetroxide is highly volatile and toxic, requiring caution during handling.

○ **Formaldehyde vapor:** Formaldehyde can be used as a vapor fixative by exposing the specimen to formaldehyde gas. This method is often used for preserving large specimens, such as whole organs or surgical specimens, or preserving the integrity of volatile substances, such as certain neurotransmitters or chemicals. Formaldehyde gas is typically generated by heating paraformaldehyde or formalin solution.

○ **Glutaraldehyde vapor:** Glutaraldehyde can also be a vapor fixative in certain applications. It is commonly used in electron microscopy, where glutaraldehyde vapors are employed to fix specimens before further processing and embedding.

Secondary Fixatives

Secondary fixatives, also known as post-fixatives, are additional fixatives used after the initial fixation step to enhance the preservation of specific components or structures in the tissue specimen. These fixatives are applied following the primary fixation with a primary fixative, such as formalin or alcohol. Secondary fixatives can help improve the quality of histological preparations and facilitate the detection of specific targets. Here are a few examples of secondary fixatives:

○ **Osmium tetroxide:** Osmium tetroxide is a commonly used secondary fixative, particularly in electron microscopy. It is applied after primary fixation to enhance the preservation of lipids and membrane structures, providing improved ultrastructural details.

○ **Potassium permanganate:** Potassium permanganate is used as a secondary fixative in certain staining techniques, such as the periodic acid-Schiff (PAS) stain. It oxidises and fixes carbohydrates, enhancing their staining properties and visibility.

○ **Iodine:** Iodine is often used as a secondary fixative in iodine-based stains, such as Lugol's iodine solution in Schiller's test for cervical cytology. It enhances the fixation and visualization of glycogen in cells.

○ **Ruthenium red:** Ruthenium red is a secondary fixative used in electron microscopy to preserve and enhance the visualization of extracellular matrices, such as basement membranes and collagen fibers.

Points to Remember

When working with fixation and fixatives in histopathology, several important points must be remembered. Here are some key considerations:

○ **Timely fixation:** Fixation should be performed as soon as possible after specimen collection to prevent tissue degradation and preserve cellular

Table 5.1: Common fixatives used in histopathology.

Tissue	Fixative of choice	Time for fixation
Routine biopsies	Formalin	10–12 hours
GIT biopsy Liver biopsy	Neutral buffered formalin	5–12 hours
Testicular biopsy	Bouin's fixative	4–6 hours
Bone marrow biopsy	Bouin's fixative in running	4–6 hours
Spleen	Zenker's fluid	1–6 hours
Lymph node	B5	12–18 hours

morphology. Delayed fixation can lead to artefacts and compromised results.

○ **Proper specimen handling:** Specimen should be handled carefully to avoid damage or distortion before fixation. Gentle handling, appropriate labelling, and proper container selection are essential.

○ **Adequate fixative volume:** Sufficient volume of fixative should be used to ensure complete coverage and penetration of the specimen. The general rule is to use at least 10 times the volume of the specimen.

○ **Fixative concentration:** It is crucial to follow the recommended concentration of the fixative to achieve optimal results. Under- or over-concentration of fixatives may lead to inadequate fixation or tissue damage.

○ **Fixation time:** Fixation duration should be optimized based on the type of tissue, specimen size, and fixative used. Insufficient fixation can result in poor preservation, while excessive fixation may lead to overfixation and tissue artifacts.

○ **Fixative compatibility:** Consider the compatibility of the fixative with subsequent processing steps and staining techniques. Some fixatives may interfere with specific stains or molecular analysis methods, requiring appropriate rinsing and neutralization steps.

○ **Safety precautions:** Many fixatives, such as formaldehyde and osmium tetroxide, can be toxic, corrosive, or irritating. Proper safety measures should be followed, including using appropriate personal protective equipment (PPE), working in well-ventilated areas, and following local regulations for disposal.

○ **Quality control:** Regularly monitor and maintain the quality of fixatives, such as checking pH, stability, and expiration dates. Poor-quality fixatives can compromise fixation results.

○ **Documentation:** Accurate and detailed documentation of fixation protocols, including the fixative used, concentration, fixation time, and any special considerations, is essential for consistent and reproducible results and for quality assurance.

○ **Consult established protocols:** It is important to follow established protocols, guidelines, and literature recommendations for specific fixatives and fixation techniques. Different tissues and applications may require different fixatives and optimized protocols.

Common fixatives are shown in **Table 5.1**.

DECALCIFICATION

Decalcification is a process used in histopathology to remove mineralized deposits, mainly calcium, from tissue specimens that contain bone or calcified structures. The purpose of decalcification is to soften the tissue, making it easier to cut into thin sections for histological examination.

Preparation of Tissue for Decalcification

Preparing tissue for decalcification involves several important steps to ensure effective and successful removal of mineralized deposits. Here is a general outline of the tissue preparation process for decalcification:

O **Fixation:** Begin by properly fixing the tissue specimen using an appropriate fixative. Common fixatives include formalin, buffered formalin, or alcohol.

O **Trimming and sectioning:** Trim the tissue specimen to a suitable size that allows adequate penetration of the decalcifying solution.

O **Sample labeling:** Properly label the tissue specimen with relevant information, including patient identification, specimen type, and any other necessary details. Accurate labeling is essential for tracking and identification during the decalcification and subsequent histological processes.

O **Penetration enhancement:** Enhance the penetration of the decalcifying solution into the tissue specimen by creating perforations or small incisions in the dense areas, such as bone or calcified tissues. This helps to facilitate the decalcification process.

O **Selection of decalcifying solution:** Choose an appropriate decalcifying solution based on the type of tissue, desired decalcification rate, and compatibility with subsequent histological procedures. Commonly used decalcifying solutions include formic acid, hydrochloric acid, EDTA, citric acid, or a combination of these agents.

O **Decalcification container and volume:** Place the tissue specimen in a suitable container that allows sufficient immersion in the decalcifying solution. The volume of the decalcifying solution should be adequate to cover the tissue specimen completely, ensuring efficient decalcification.

O **Decalcification duration:** The duration of decalcification varies depending on the type of tissue, size, and density of the mineralized deposits, as well as the decalcifying solution used. It is important to follow established protocols and guidelines to determine the appropriate decalcification time. Regularly monitor the progress of decalcification by taking small tissue samples for testing.

O **Agitation or shaking:** Agitate or gently shake the decalcification container at regular intervals to enhance the contact between the tissue specimen and the decalcifying solution. This promotes efficient decalcification by facilitating the exchange of the decalcifying solution and promoting better penetration.

O **Monitoring decalcification progress:** Regularly assess the progress of decalcification by testing small tissue samples with a calcium-specific stain, such as Alizarin red. The stain will indicate the presence of residual calcium deposits in the tissue. Adjust the decalcification time accordingly until the desired level of decalcification is achieved.

O **Rinse and tissue processing:** Once the tissue is adequately decalcified, thoroughly rinse the tissue specimen in running water or a neutralizing solution to remove any traces of the decalcifying agent. The tissue is then dehydrated, cleared, and processed for embedding, sectioning, and subsequent histological staining.

Methods of Decalcification

There are several methods of decalcification available for removing mineralized deposits from tissue specimens. The choice of method depends on factors such as the type of tissue, the extent of calcification, the desired speed of decalcification, and the compatibility with subsequent histological processing. Here are some common methods of decalcification:

Acid-based Decalcification

Acid-based decalcification methods use acids to dissolve mineralized deposits. Common acids used include hydrochloric acid, nitric acid, formic acid, and acetic acid. Acid decalcification is effective for most calcified tissues but may lead to tissue damage if not properly controlled. It is the most common method used for decalcification.

In decalcification, the choice between strong and weak acid solutions depends on the extent and composition of the mineralized deposits, the nature of the tissue, and the desired speed of decalcification. Here's a comparison of strong and weak acid solutions for decalcification:

Strong Acid Solutions

○ **Hydrochloric acid (HCl):** Strong hydrochloric acid solutions, typically ranging from 5% to 10% concentration, are commonly used for decalcification. Hydrochloric acid is effective in dissolving calcium salts and is particularly useful for routine decalcification of most calcified tissues.

○ **Nitric acid (HNO$_3$):** Nitric acid is a strong acid commonly used for decalcification, especially when dealing with harder or more resistant calcifications. Nitric acid solutions are generally used at concentrations ranging from 5% to 15%. However, it is important to note that nitric acid is more aggressive and can cause greater tissue damage compared to hydrochloric acid.

Weak Acid Solutions

○ **Formic acid (HCOOH):** Formic acid is a weak acid often used in decalcification, especially for delicate tissues. It is generally used at concentrations ranging from 5% to 10%. Formic acid has a milder decalcifying effect compared to strong acids, which reduces the risk of tissue damage but may require longer decalcification times.

○ **Acetic acid (CH$_3$COOH):** Acetic acid, also a weak acid, is occasionally used for decalcification. It is typically used at concentrations ranging from 5% to 10%. Acetic acid has a gentler action on tissue, making it suitable for delicate samples. However, decalcification with acetic acid may take longer compared to strong acid solutions.

Choosing the appropriate acid solution depends on factors such as the type of tissue, the extent and density of the mineralized deposits, the desired speed of decalcification, and the preservation of tissue morphology. Strong acids like hydrochloric acid and nitric acid are generally more effective in rapidly dissolving calcium salts, but they can cause more tissue damage. Weak acids like formic acid and acetic acid are milder and better suited for delicate tissues, but they may require longer decalcification times.

Chelating Agent-based Decalcification

Chelating agents are compounds that bind to metal ions, including calcium, to form soluble complexes. Ethylenediaminetetraacetic acid (EDTA) and ethylene glycol-bis-(β-aminoethyl ether)-N,N,N',N'-tetraacetic acid (EGTA) are commonly used chelating agents for decalcification. Chelating agents are milder than acids and are suitable for delicate tissues.

Combination Decalcification

Some decalcification methods combine acid-based and chelating agent-based approaches to enhance decalcification efficiency. For example, a common combination is using formic acid followed by an EDTA solution.

Enzymatic Decalcification

Enzymatic decalcification involves the use of enzymes, such as trypsin or collagenase, to break down the collagen matrix surrounding calcium deposits. This method is useful for decalcifying dense calcified tissues, such as bone.

Physical Decalcification

Physical methods involve the use of mechanical forces to break down or remove mineralized deposits. Grinding, shaving, or using ultrasonic vibrations can be employed to mechanically disrupt the calcified tissues.

Microwave-assisted Decalcification

Microwave-assisted decalcification utilizes microwave energy to accelerate the decalcification process. This method reduces the time required for decalcification while maintaining tissue morphology.

Ion Exchange Resins

Ion exchange resins can be used for decalcification by exchanging calcium ions with other ions, such as hydrogen ions. Commonly used resins include strong cation exchange resins, such as sulfonated polystyrene-based resins. These resins contain negatively charged functional groups that attract and bind calcium ions. This method is often used for smaller tissue samples or when preserving delicate structures is a priority.

The choice of decalcification method should be based on factors such as the nature of the tissue, the desired speed of decalcification, preservation of tissue morphology, and compatibility with downstream processing techniques, including staining and immunohistochemistry.

Surface Decalcification

Surface decalcification is a technique used to selectively remove calcium deposits from the surface of a tissue specimen while preserving the underlying structure. It is commonly employed when the calcification is limited to the outer layers of the tissue and deeper decalcification is not required. Surface of paraffin blocks are immersed in 5% HCl for an hour. In this method, around 30 microns from top is decalcified. The blocks are then thoroughly washed before they are subjected for cutting.

Endpoint Decalcification

Endpoint decalcification refers to the process of decalcifying a tissue specimen until a specific endpoint or desired level of decalcification is reached. The endpoint is determined based on the absence of visible calcium deposits and the ability to section the tissue easily.

Methods for Determining Endpoint Decalcification

- **Visual inspection:** One of the simplest ways to determine the endpoint is through visual inspection. As the decalcification progresses, the tissue should appear softer and more pliable. Check for the absence of visible calcium deposits or a translucent appearance in the previously calcified areas.
- **Palpation:** Gently palpate the tissue specimen throughout the decalcification process. Initially, the tissue will feel hard and rigid due to the presence of calcium deposits. As decalcification progresses, the tissue should become softer and more flexible. The absence of firmness or resistance can indicate the endpoint.
- **Microscopic evaluation:** Take small tissue samples at regular intervals during the decalcification process. Process these samples, embed them in paraffin, and prepare thin sections. Stain the sections with a calcium-specific stain, such as

Alizarin red. Evaluate the stained sections under a microscope to determine the presence or absence of residual calcium deposits. The endpoint is reached when no visible calcium deposits are observed.

○ **X-ray examination:** X-ray imaging can be used to visualize the presence or absence of calcium deposits in the tissue. Take X-ray images of the tissue specimen at various stages of the decalcification process. Compare the images to determine when the calcium deposits are no longer visible, indicating the endpoint of decalcification.

○ **Mechanical testing:** In some cases, mechanical testing can be employed to determine the endpoint. This involves subjecting the tissue specimen to gentle pressure or bending and observing its response. If the tissue is pliable and easily deforms without resistance, it suggests the absence of calcium deposits.

○ **Chemical method:** Ammonium hydroxide can be used as a chemical method to determine the endpoint of decalcification. The basic principle behind this method is the reaction between ammonium hydroxide and residual calcium ions in the tissue specimen. As decalcification progresses, the concentration of calcium ions decreases, resulting in a weaker reaction with ammonium hydroxide.
The reaction between ammonium hydroxide and residual calcium ions may result in the release of carbon dioxide gas, leading to effervescence. Initially, the reaction may be vigorous due to the presence of a higher concentration of calcium ions. As decalcification progresses and the concentration of calcium ions decreases, the effervescence reaction will gradually decrease in intensity. Observe the tissue samples over time and note the point at which the effervescence becomes minimal or ceases completely.

○ **Endpoint determination:** The endpoint of decalcification is typically reached when the tissue samples show little to no effervescence in the ammonium hydroxide solution. This indicates that the majority of the calcium ions have been removed, and the tissue is adequately decalcified.

TISSUE PROCESSING

Tissue processing is a series of steps performed after fixation and decalcification (if required) to prepare tissue samples for microscopic examination. The goal of tissue processing is to embed the tissue in a solid medium, typically paraffin wax, which allows for thin sectioning and subsequent staining. Here are the general steps involved in tissue processing:

○ **Dehydration:** The tissue specimen is dehydrated by gradually replacing water with alcohol. This is typically done through a series of alcohol solutions of increasing concentration (e.g., 70%, 80%, 95%, and 100% ethanol). Dehydration removes water from the tissue, making it compatible with the subsequent steps of tissue processing.

○ **Clearing:** After dehydration, the tissue is cleared by placing it in a clearing agent, such as xylene or other organic solvents. Clearing agents remove the alcohol from the tissue and render it transparent, allowing for better infiltration of the embedding medium.

○ **Infiltration:** Infiltration involves impregnating the tissue with a suitable embedding medium, commonly paraffin wax. The tissue is placed in melted paraffin wax, which infiltrates the tissue, replacing the clearing agent. This step ensures that the tissue is adequately supported for sectioning and prevents distortion.

○ **Embedding:** The infiltrated tissue is placed in a mold with fresh molten paraffin wax and allowed to solidify. The mold is typically a small cassette or a specialized embedding mold. The tissue becomes embedded in the solidified wax block, providing structural support for sectioning.

○ **Trimming:** Once the wax has solidified, the excess wax around the tissue block is trimmed using a microtome or a specialized trimming instrument. Trimming ensures that the tissue is exposed for sectioning and removes any unnecessary wax.

○ **Sectioning:** The embedded tissue block is cut into thin sections, typically ranging from 3 to 5 micrometers in thickness. Microtomes or other sectioning instruments are used to obtain consistent and precise sections. The sections are collected on glass slides or other appropriate surfaces.

○ **Mounting:** The sections are mounted onto glass slides by spreading a thin layer of adhesive, such as a mounting medium or adhesive tape, on the slide. The sectioned tissue is carefully transferred onto the slide, ensuring proper orientation and arrangement.

○ **Drying:** The mounted sections are allowed to dry completely. This step is essential to remove any residual moisture and ensure proper adhesion of the tissue sections to the slide.

After tissue processing, the slides with mounted sections are ready for further staining, such as hematoxylin and eosin (HandE) staining or immunohistochemical staining, which facilitate the visualization and characterization of different tissue components under a microscope.

Dehydration

Dehydration is a crucial step in tissue preparation that removes water from the tissue samples, allowing for effective impregnation with an embedding medium such as paraffin wax. Dehydration is typically performed after tissue fixation and prior to embedding.

Histological dehydration is achieved by immersing the fixed tissue specimens in a series of alcohol solutions of increasing concentrations. Commonly used dehydrating agents include ethanol or isopropanol. The alcohol solutions gradually replace water in the tissue, dehydrating it and preparing it for embedding.

Dehydration is typically performed in a series of alcohol solutions, starting from lower concentrations and gradually increasing the alcohol concentration. For example, a typical dehydration protocol may include a series of ethanol solutions, such as 70%, 80%, 95%, and 100% ethanol. Each step allows for a gradual removal of water from the tissue while minimizing tissue shrinkage and distortion.

The duration of dehydration can vary depending on the tissue type and size. It is important to ensure sufficient time for each step to allow thorough dehydration. The tissue samples are usually left in each alcohol solution for a specific period, typically ranging from several minutes to a few hours.

During the process, it is essential to monitor the tissue's appearance to assess the progress of dehydration. Tissues are translucent when adequately dehydrated, indicating the removal of water and successful penetration of the alcohol. Overdehydration should be avoided as it can lead to tissue shrinkage and artifact formation.

Dehydrating Agents

Common dehydrating agents include:

○ **Ethanol:** Ethanol (ethyl alcohol) is widely used as a dehydrating agent in histopathology. It is available in different concentrations, such as 70%, 80%, 95%, and 100% ethanol. These solutions are used in a graded series to gradually remove water from the tissue samples.

○ **Isopropanol:** Isopropanol (isopropyl alcohol) is another commonly used dehydrating agent. It functions similarly to ethanol and is available in various concentrations. Isopropanol is often used as an alternative to ethanol or in combination with ethanol in dehydration protocols.

○ **Methanol:** Methanol (methyl alcohol) is occasionally used as a dehydrating agent in certain histological techniques. It has a higher affinity for water than ethanol and is sometimes preferred for specific applications.

○ **Acetone:** Acetone is a rapid dehydrating agent commonly used in frozen sectioning and certain special staining techniques. It has a high volatility and quickly removes water from tissues. Acetone is particularly useful when rapid processing is required.

○ **Tert-butyl alcohol (TBA):** Tert-butyl alcohol is used as a dehydrating agent in some specialized applications. It has a relatively low toxicity and is often used in combination with other dehydrating agents or as a substitute for ethanol or acetone.

○ **Dioxane:** Dioxane, also known as 1,4-dioxane or diethylene dioxide, is a clear, colorless liquid organic compound. It is used as a dehydrating as well as clearing agent in histopathology and tissue processing.

Advantages: Dioxane has a relatively low boiling point, which facilitates the removal of water from tissues without excessively high temperatures. It is also considered a gentle dehydrating agent that can preserve tissue morphology and antigenicity, making it suitable for immunohistochemical studies.

Disadvantages: It is a toxic substance and is expensive than alcohol.

Clearing

Clearing is a crucial step in histopathology and tissue processing that follows dehydration.

After removing water from tissue samples, clearing agents are used to replace the dehydrating agent and render the tissue transparent or translucent. Clearing enhances tissue visibility, allowing for improved penetration of the embedding medium and subsequent microscopic examination.

Various clearing agents can be used in histopathology, depending on the desired level of transparency, compatibility with subsequent processing steps, and the specific application. Commonly used clearing agents include xylene, toluene, benzene, limonene, and other organic solvents. Xylene is one of the most commonly used clearing agents due to its effectiveness and widespread availability.

The duration of tissue clearing can vary depending on the clearing agent used and the specific tissue type. Tissue samples are typically immersed in the clearing agent for a sufficient amount of time to allow complete penetration and removal of the dehydrating agent. The duration can range from a few minutes to several hours, depending on the tissue's size and composition.

During the clearing step, it is essential to handle the tissue samples gently to avoid damage or distortion. Excessive agitation or rough handling can lead to tissue disruption or detachment from the supporting substrates.

It is crucial to ensure compatibility between the clearing agent and the subsequent embedding medium (e.g., paraffin wax). The clearing agent should be compatible with the embedding medium to ensure optimal infiltration and preservation of tissue morphology.

After clearing, the tissue samples are ready for embedding in an appropriate medium (e.g., paraffin wax) for sectioning and further histological processing, including staining and microscopic examination.

Clearing Agents

Clearing agents are substances used in histopathology and tissue processing to render the tissue transparent or translucent after the dehydration step. Several clearing agents are commonly used in histopathology, including:

○ **Xylene:** Xylene is one of the most widely used and effective clearing agents in histopathology. It is a colorless, aromatic hydrocarbon that has good clearing properties and high compatibility with various embedding media. Xylene is volatile and easily evaporates, making it suitable for subsequent steps in tissue processing.

○ **Toluene:** Toluene is another commonly used clearing agent that shares similar properties with xylene. It is also an aromatic hydrocarbon and can effectively clear tissues. Toluene is often used as an alternative to xylene, especially in laboratories where xylene may be restricted or when a less toxic alternative is desired.

○ **Benzene:** Benzene is an aromatic hydrocarbon with clearing properties. However, its use as a clearing agent has significantly declined due to safety concerns associated with its carcinogenic properties. It is now less commonly used in histopathology laboratories.

○ **Limonene:** Limonene is a natural, citrus-derived clearing agent that is considered a safer alternative to xylene and benzene. It is an effective clearing agent and has low toxicity, making it suitable for routine tissue processing.

○ **Citrus-based clearing agents:** Various citrus-based clearing agents are available, which are derived from citrus fruits. These agents are often used as safer alternatives to traditional hydrocarbon-based clearing agents, such as xylene or toluene. They offer good clearing properties and are generally considered less hazardous.

Impregnation/Infiltration

Impregnation, also known as infiltration, is a crucial step in histopathology and tissue processing that follows dehydration and clearing. It involves the impregnation of tissue samples with a suitable embedding medium to provide structural support and facilitate sectioning. The embedding medium fills the intercellular spaces and surrounds the tissue components, preserving their morphology and allowing for thin sectioning for microscopic examination.

The embedding medium used for impregnation can vary depending on the specific application and subsequent processing steps. The most commonly used embedding medium in histopathology is paraffin wax. Paraffin wax is heated until it becomes molten and then infiltrates the dehydrated and cleared tissue. Other embedding media, such as plastic resins (e.g., methyl methacrylate), are used for specialized techniques and applications.

Impregnation techniques: There are different techniques for impregnating tissue samples with embedding media. The most widely used technique is the routine paraffin wax embedding, where tissue samples are immersed in molten paraffin wax. Vacuum impregnation is also employed to enhance penetration of the embedding medium into the tissue.

Embedding Medium

Paraffin Wax

Paraffin wax is the most commonly used embedding medium in histopathology for the impregnation of tissue samples. It provides structural support to the tissue and facilitates thin sectioning for microscopic examination. Here are some key points about paraffin wax for embedding:

Composition: Paraffin wax is a mixture of long-chain hydrocarbons derived from petroleum or other sources. It is a solid at room temperature and has a melting point typically ranging from 50 to 65°C (122 to 149°F).

Paraffin wax has several properties that make it suitable for tissue embedding. It is translucent and allows light to pass through, enabling the visualization of tissue structures under a microscope. It is also chemically inert, providing stability to the embedded tissue during subsequent processing steps.

Paraffin wax is melted at an appropriate temperature, typically around 56 to 60°C (132 to 140°F), to create a molten liquid. Tissue samples that have undergone dehydration and clearing are immersed in the molten paraffin wax to impregnate them. After impregnation, the molten paraffin wax is allowed to cool and solidify, forming a solid block that contains the embedded tissue.

It is compatible with a wide range of histological stains, allowing for various staining techniques and protocols to be used for microscopic examination. It allows for proper penetration and adherence of the staining solutions, leading to accurate visualization of cellular and tissue structures.

Volume of the wax should be around 25–50 times the volume of tissue. The tissue is subjected to 3 changes of wax. The temperature of the wax bath should be 2–3°C above the melting point of wax.

Plastic Resins

Plastic resins, such as methyl methacrylate (MMA) or epoxy resins, are used as embedding media in specialized histopathology techniques. These resins offer excellent tissue preservation, durability, and resistance to chemical and physical stresses. Plastic embedding is often employed in studies requiring thick sections or for special staining techniques.

Glycerol

Glycerol is a clear, viscous liquid that can be used as an embedding medium for frozen sections. It is commonly used in research and clinical laboratories for immediate processing of fresh tissue samples. Glycerol embedding allows for rapid sectioning and is suitable for immunofluorescence studies.

Gelatin

Gelatin can be used as an embedding medium for embedding small specimens, such as biopsy samples or small animal tissues. It offers easy sectioning and can be dissolved away after sectioning, leaving the tissue sections on the slide. Gelatin embedding is often employed in special techniques like enzyme histochemistry or immunohistochemistry.

Agar

Agar, a polysaccharide derived from seaweed, is sometimes used as an embedding medium for larger specimens. It provides stability and support during sectioning and allows for subsequent staining and analysis. Agar embedding is commonly used in research settings or when preserving the overall structure of the tissue is crucial.

Celloidin

Celloidin is a nitrocellulose-based embedding medium that provides excellent preservation of tissue morphology. It is commonly used in neurohistology for embedding brain tissue. Celloidin embedding allows for the sectioning of thick sections and is compatible with various staining techniques.

Embedding

Embedding is a crucial step in histopathology that involves the infiltration and embedding of tissue specimens into a solid medium to facilitate sectioning and microscopic examination.

Paraffin wax is the most widely used embedding medium in histopathology.

The impregnated specimens are placed in melted paraffin wax, which infiltrates the tissue and fills the intercellular spaces. The wax provides support and stability to the tissue during sectioning and ensures that the tissue sections adhere to microscope slides.

Embedding molds: Embedding molds, typically made of metal or plastic, are used to hold the tissue specimens during the embedding process. The molds have various sizes and shapes to accommodate different tissue sizes and orientations.

○ **Metal Embedding molds:** Metal embedding molds are typically made of stainless steel or aluminum. They are durable and can withstand high temperatures during the embedding process. These molds are available in various sizes and shapes, such as rectangular, round, or square. Leuckhart's L molds are most commonly used. They are two 'L' shaped metal pieces mostly made of brass, which rest on a flat metal or glass plate.

○ **Plastic embedding molds:** Plastic embedding molds are made of disposable plastic materials, such as polyethylene or polypropylene. They are convenient to use and eliminate the need for cleaning and sterilization. Plastic molds are available in different sizes and shapes, including cassettes, rectangular molds, or embedding rings.

○ **Tissue cassettes:** Tissue cassettes are commonly used in automated tissue processing systems. They are usually made of plastic, such as polypropylene, and have a square or rectangular shape. Tissue cassettes have a mesh or biopsy pad at the bottom to hold the tissue sample securely.

○ **Embedding rings:** Embedding rings, also known as biopsy rings or embedding capsules, are small circular molds made of metal or plastic. They have an open top and a closed bottom. Tissue samples are placed inside the ring, and the liquid embedding medium is poured over the sample to form a solid block.

The molds are filled with the melted paraffin wax containing the impregnated tissue specimens. Place the specimen in the embedding mold with careful attention to its orientation. Ensure that the specimen is aligned according to the desired orientation, such as longitudinal, transverse, or specific anatomical landmarks.

Once the specimens are placed in the embedding molds, the molds are transferred to a cooling plate or a cold water bath. The rapid cooling solidifies the paraffin wax, embedding the tissue specimens within it. The solidified wax block, also known as the tissue block, can be easily handled and stored. Proper labeling of the embedding blocks is essential to ensure accurate identification and tracking of tissue samples throughout the subsequent processing steps. Information such as patient identifiers, specimen type, and processing dates should be recorded on the blocks.

Automated Tissue Processor

A tissue processor is a vital piece of equipment used in histopathology laboratories for automating and standardizing the tissue processing workflow. It plays a crucial role in the dehydration, clearing, impregnation, and paraffin wax embedding of tissue samples.

It offers programmable automation, allowing users to set specific processing protocols and parameters for different types of tissues or samples. The processor can automatically move tissue samples through various processing steps, controlling the duration of each step, the reagent exchange, and temperature control. Tissue processors have multiple containers or chambers for holding the different processing reagents, including dehydration agents (alcohols), clearing agents (such as xylene or alternatives), and embedding media (e.g., molten paraffin wax). These reagents are sequentially introduced to the tissue samples, ensuring proper dehydration, clearing, and impregnation. They have temperature-controlled chambers or baths for maintaining optimal temperatures during processing steps.

There are two types of tissue processor devices available:

1. Tissue transfer (Histokinette)
2. Fluid transfer

Time required for tissue processing:

Automated Processing Schedule

1.	80% alcohol (holding point)	1 hour
2.	95% alcohol	2 hours
3.	95% alcohol	1 hour
4.	100% alcohol	1 hour
5.	100% alcohol	1 hour
6.	100% alcohol	1 hour
7.	Xylene	1 hour
8.	Xylene	1 hour
9.	Xylene	1 hour
10.	Paraffin wax	2 hours
11.	Paraffin wax	2 hours
12.	Paraffin wax	2 hours

SECTION CUTTING

Section cutting is a critical step in histopathology that involves the process of cutting thin sections from embedded tissue blocks for microscopic examination. The quality and technique of section cutting play a significant role in obtaining well-preserved tissue sections with optimal thickness. Here are some key points to consider regarding section cutting:

○ **Microtome selection:** Microtome is a specialized instrument designed for cutting thin sections of tissue. Microtomes can be manual or automated and are equipped with a cutting blade and controls for adjusting the section thickness.

○ **Block trimming:** Before section cutting, trim the tissue block to expose the area of interest and achieve the desired orientation. Trimming helps ensure that the tissue sections will include the target tissue and relevant structures.

○ **Block orientation:** Ensure that the tissue block is properly oriented in the microtome. Align the block according to the desired orientation established during embedding. Use the markings made on the block to guide correct alignment.

○ **Blade selection:** Choose an appropriate cutting blade for sectioning. The blade should be sharp, clean, and properly aligned in the microtome. Commonly used blades include disposable steel blades, glass knives, or diamond knives, depending on the specific requirements of the tissue and staining technique.

○ **Section thickness:** Adjust the microtome controls to achieve the desired section thickness. The typical range for tissue sections is around 3–5 micrometers, although this can vary depending on the tissue type and staining method. Proper section thickness ensures clear visualization of cellular details without compromising tissue integrity.

○ **Section collection:** Collect the cut sections as they are produced. Use a brush, water bath, or other appropriate methods to transfer the sections to microscope slides or water baths for further processing and staining.

○ **Quality control:** Inspect the sections under a microscope to ensure they meet the desired quality standards. Look for artifacts, folds, wrinkles, or other anomalies that may affect the interpretation of the tissue. Make adjustments to the cutting technique or blade as needed.

○ **Section handling:** Handle the sections with care to avoid damage or contamination. Use fine-pointed forceps or other suitable tools to lift and transfer the sections without causing folds or tears.

○ **Section mounting:** Once the sections are collected, mount them onto microscope slides using appropriate mounting media, such as adhesive or water baths. Ensure proper alignment and avoid air bubbles or wrinkles during mounting.

Equipment Required for Section Cutting

To perform section cutting in histopathology, the following equipment is typically required:

○ **Microtome:** A microtome is a precision instrument used to cut thin tissue sections. It consists of a base, a knife holder, and a mechanism to control the thickness of the sections. Microtomes can be manual or motorised, depending on the specific model.

○ **Microtome knife:** Microtome knives, also known as microtome blades, are used for cutting the tissue sections. Different types of knives, such as disposable steel blades, glass knives, or diamond knives, may be used based on the application and the desired section quality.

○ **Slide holder:** A slide holder or slide tray is used to hold glass slides during section cutting. It provides a stable platform for collecting the sections as they are cut.

○ **Water bath or warm water tray:** A water bath or warm water tray collects the sections as they are cut. The water helps to float the sections onto the surface, making retrieving and transferring them to glass slides easier. The temperature of the water bath is set 5 degree below the melting point of paraffin wax.

○ **Hot plate:** It is used for drying sections. The temperature of the hot plate is set 5 degrees above the melting point of the wax.

○ **Brushes or fine-pointed needles:** Brushes or fine-pointed needles separate and collect the sections from the water bath.

These tools help handle delicate sections without causing damage.

○ **Glass slides:** Glass slides are the surfaces on which the tissue sections are mounted for further processing and examination. The slides should be clean and free from dust or debris.

○ Section adhesive

○ **Diamond marker pencil:** Used for writing the identification number over the slides.

○ **Slide racks or slide boxes:** Slide racks or slide boxes are used to store the glass slides with the mounted tissue sections. They provide a safe and organized way to store the slides until they are ready for staining or analysis.

○ **Safety equipment:** Safety equipment such as gloves and protective eyewear should be worn during section cutting to ensure personal safety and prevent contamination of the sections.

Microtome

A microtome is a specialized instrument used in histopathology and other biological disciplines for cutting thin sections of tissue samples for microscopic examination. It allows for precise and controlled sectioning of embedded tissues into thin slices of uniform thickness. Here are some key features and components of a microtome:

○ **Blade holder:** The microtome features a blade holder that holds the cutting blade securely in place. The blade can be a disposable steel blade, a glass knife, or a diamond knife, depending on the specific requirements of the tissue and staining technique.

○ **Sample holder:** The sample holder, also known as the specimen chuck or object holder, securely holds the tissue block during sectioning. It ensures stability and proper orientation of the tissue for accurate cutting.

○ **Feed mechanism:** Microtomes have a feed mechanism that allows for controlled movement of the sample holder and the tissue block during sectioning. This mechanism can be manual, semi-automatic, or fully automated, depending on the type of microtome.

○ **Thickness adjustment:** Microtomes have a mechanism for adjusting the thickness of the sections. This can be done by adjusting the position of the knife or by controlling the movement of the sample holder.

○ **Knife angle adjustment:** Some microtomes allow for the adjustment of the angle at which the cutting blade contacts the tissue. This feature is particularly useful for achieving optimal section quality and reducing artifacts.

○ **Waste tray:** Microtomes often include a waste tray or blade guard that collects the cut sections and waste materials to keep the work area clean and prevent contamination.

○ **Coarse and fine adjustment knobs:** Microtomes are equipped with knobs for coarse and fine adjustments. These knobs allow for precise movement of the sample holder and enable the user to control the cutting process.

Types of Microtome

Several types of microtomes are used in histopathology and other biological research fields, each with advantages and applications. The common types of microtomes include:

○ **Rotary microtome:** Rotary microtomes **(Fig. 5.1)** are histopathology laboratories' most widely used microtomes. They employ a rotating mechanism to cut thin sections of embedded tissues. The tissue block is attached to a sample holder, and as the handle is rotated, the sample is brought into contact with the cutting blade, resulting in sectioning. Rotary microtomes

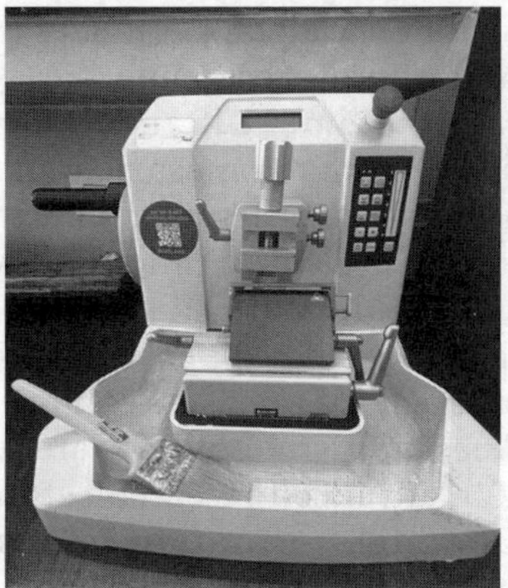

Fig. 5.1: Rotary microtome.

are versatile, easy to use, and suitable for routine sectioning of various tissue types.

○ **Sliding microtome:** Sliding microtomes operate on a sliding principle, where the sample holder and the knife move horizontally along a track. The tissue block is fixed on the sample holder, and sections are cut as the knife moves across the block. Sliding microtomes are particularly useful for large or hard tissue samples requiring greater cutting force.

○ **Cryostat microtome:** Cryostat microtomes are specialized for cutting frozen tissue sections. They are used when rapid freezing of tissues is necessary for preservation. Cryostat microtomes have a freezing chamber that maintains the tissue at low temperatures, allowing for precise sectioning of frozen tissue samples. They are commonly used for rapid diagnosis or research applications requiring immediate fresh tissue freezing.

○ **Vibrating microtome:** Vibrating microtomes utilize high-frequency vibrations to cut tissue sections. The sample is typically fixed to a vibrating platform, and the blade oscillates, resulting in precise and consistent sectioning. Vibrating microtomes are particularly useful for delicate or soft tissues prone to distortion during sectioning.

O **Ultramicrotome:** Ultramicrotomes are specialized microtomes used for cutting ultra-thin sections (less than 1 micrometer) required for electron microscopy. They utilize an ultrathin diamond or glass knife and are equipped with precision mechanisms to precisely control section thickness. Ultramicrotomes are typically used in advanced research settings that require high-resolution imaging and analysis.

Microtome Knives

Microtome knives, also known as microtome blades, are essential components of microtomes used for cutting thin sections of tissue samples in histopathology and other biological research fields. Different types of microtome knives are available, and the choice depends on the specific application, tissue type, and desired section quality.

Some commonly used microtome knives are:

O **Disposable steel blades:** Disposable steel blades are the most commonly used microtome knives. They are made of high-quality stainless steel and come in different shapes and sizes, such as low-profile, high-profile, and slotted blades. Disposable steel blades are suitable for routine sectioning of paraffin-embedded tissues and provide good section quality at an affordable cost. They are easy to use and widely available.

O **Glass knives:** Glass knives are made of thin glass rods that are shaped and honed to create a cutting edge. They are commonly used for cutting thin sections of hard or delicate tissues, such as bone or certain plant tissues. Glass knives provide excellent section quality due to their sharpness and smooth cutting action. They are particularly useful for specialized applications that

require precise sectionings, such as neuroanatomy or specific tissue types with delicate structures.

O **Diamond knives:** Diamond knives are the highest precision microtome knives available. They have a cutting edge coated with synthetic diamond particles, which makes them extremely sharp and durable. Diamond knives are commonly used for ultrathin sectioning in electron microscopy and other advanced research applications. They allow for precise and consistent sectioning of tissues with minimal distortion or artefacts. However, diamond knives are expensive and require careful handling and maintenance.

O **Tungsten carbide knives:** Tungsten carbide knives are known for their durability and long blade life. Bonding tungsten carbide particles make them into a stainless-steel blade. Tungsten carbide knives are suitable for cutting hard tissues, frozen sections, or materials like plastic or resin-embedded samples. They maintain their sharpness for longer and are more resistant to wear than disposable steel blades.

O **Sapphire knives:** Sapphire knives are made of synthetic sapphire, an extremely hard and durable material. They are used for specialized applications that require high precision and longevity, such as serial sectioning or cutting hard materials. Sapphire knives offer excellent cutting performance, minimal wear, and high section quality. However, they are expensive and require careful handling and maintenance.

Sharpening of Microtome Knife

Honing and stropping are additional techniques for sharpening microtome knives, particularly those with razor or wedge-cutting edges. Here's a brief explanation of honing and stropping:

○ **Honing:** Honing is a process that involves using a honing stone or sharpening stone to refine and realign the cutting edge of a microtome knife. Honing helps remove small burrs or irregularities that may have formed during sectioning or sharpening. It is usually performed after initial sharpening to achieve a finer, smoother cutting edge.

To hone a microtome knife, follow these steps:
○ Select a honing stone with fine grit.
○ Apply a few drops of lubricating or honing oil to the stone's surface.
○ Hold the microtome knife at the appropriate angle and gently glide it back and forth across the honing stone, maintaining consistent pressure and the same angle throughout.
○ Repeat the honing process several times, checking the cutting edge for smoothness and sharpness.
○ After honing, carefully clean the knife and remove any residue before using it for sectioning.

○ **Stropping:** Stropping is a technique used to refine further and polish the cutting edge of a microtome knife, enhancing its sharpness and smoothness. It involves stroking the knife blade against a strop, typically a leather or fabric strip coated with a polishing compound.

To strop a microtome knife, follow these steps:
○ Attach the strop securely to a flat surface, ensuring it is taut and stable.
○ Apply a small amount of polishing compound or stropping paste to the surface of the strop.
○ Hold the microtome knife at the appropriate angle and gently slide it back and forth across the strop, maintaining consistent pressure and the same angle throughout.
○ Repeat the stropping process several times, alternating the direction of the strokes to ensure even polishing of the cutting edge.
○ After stropping, carefully clean the knife to remove any residue before using it for sectioning.

Section Adhesives

Section adhesive, also known as mounting medium or mounting adhesive, is a substance used in histopathology to adhere tissue sections to glass slides. It helps to secure the tissue sections in place, prevent their detachment during subsequent processing steps, and maintain the structural integrity of the sections for microscopic examination. Some of the commonly used adhesives are—Albumin, gelatin, Poly-L-lysine, starch, cellulose, resin.

Paraffin Section Cutting

Paraffin section cutting is a critical step in histopathology that involves obtaining thin, uniform sections of tissue for microscopic examination. Here is an overview of the process of paraffin section cutting:
○ **Preparation:** Ensure that the paraffin blocks containing the embedded tissue are ready for sectioning. The blocks should be properly labeled, oriented, and securely attached to the microtome chuck.
○ **Microtome Setup:** Set up the microtome according to the manufacturer's instructions. This involves adjusting the cutting thickness, setting the speed, and positioning the knife holder.
○ **Knife selection:** Choose an appropriate microtome knife based on the tissue type, section thickness required, and the cutting edge's condition. Ensure that the knife is securely mounted in the knife holder.
○ **Block trimming:** Trim the paraffin block to expose the tissue surface of interest.

Use a sharp razor blade or a block trimmer to remove excess paraffin and achieve a flat surface for sectioning. The section thickness adjusters are set at 15 microns to trim away any surplus wax and to expose a suitable area of tissue for sectioning.

○ **Wetting the knife:** Wet the cutting edge of the microtome knife with distilled water or a suitable wetting agent. This helps prevent the sections from sticking to the knife during cutting.

○ **Sectioning:** Lower the knife holder to make contact with the block surface. Use the microtome handle to advance the block against the knife, allowing the knife to cut thin sections of tissue. Maintain a steady and smooth motion to obtain consistent section thickness. For routine purpose, the section thickness is set at 4–6 microns.

○ **Water bath:** As the sections are cut, they will float onto the surface of a water bath or warm water tray so as to remove the creases in the sections. The temperature of water bath is set 5° below the melting point of wax. Gently separate and collect the sections using a brush or a fine-pointed needle.

○ **Mounting:** Transfer the sections from the water bath onto glass slides. The glass slides are smeared with egg albumin which acts as the adhesive for the sections. Arrange them in the desired orientation and ensure they are free from folds or wrinkles. Press gently to flatten the sections on the slide.

○ **Drying:** Allow the slides with sections to dry on a slide warmer or in incubator. The temperature is set 5° above the melting point of wax. This helps the sections adhere to the slides and facilitates subsequent staining procedures.

○ **Storing:** Once the sections are completely dry, store the slides in slide racks or slide boxes for further processing or staining.

STAINING

Staining is a fundamental technique used in histopathology to enhance the visualization of tissue structures, cells, and cellular components under a microscope. It involves applying specific dyes or chemicals to tissue sections to impart color or produce contrast, allowing for better identification and examination of the tissue's microscopic details.

Types of Staining

○ Routine or routine histology staining refers to standard techniques used in histopathology laboratories to visualize and study tissue sections under a microscope. These stains provide general information about the cellular and tissue components, allowing for the identification of different cell types and structures. For example, HandE staining, Giemsa stain, etc.

○ **Special stains:** Special stains are diverse staining techniques used to highlight specific cellular components or structures. Examples include periodic acid-Schiff (PAS) staining for carbohydrates, Masson's trichrome staining for collagen and connective tissue, and silver stains for reticular fibers or microorganisms.

○ **Vital staining:** Vital staining selectively stains living cells or tissues without causing significant harm or damage. It involves using dyes or stains specifically taken up by living cells and can provide information about their structure, function, or viability. Vital staining is often used in biological and medical research to observe and analyze living cells and tissues in their natural state. For example, Trypan blue, Propidium iodide, etc.

○ **Supravital staining:** Supravital staining is a technique used to stain cells or tissues while they are still alive or shortly after they have been removed from the body.

Unlike vital staining, which stains living cells, supravital staining involves staining cells isolated or treated outside their normal physiological conditions. For example, Neutral red or Janus green.

○ **Metachromatic staining:** Metachromatic staining is a special technique used in histology and histopathology to stain certain components of cells or tissues exhibiting metachromasia selectively. Metachromasia refers to the phenomenon where certain structures or substances within cells or tissues appear differently colored than the staining dye. Metachromatic staining is commonly used to identify and characterize mucins, mast cell granules, and amyloid deposits, which display metachromasia. These substances change color during staining, appearing different from the dye used.

Toluidine Blue is the most widely used metachromatic stain, a basic dye that stains acidic components. Toluidine Blue selectively stains substances rich in sulfated or carboxylated acidic polysaccharides, such as mucins and mast cell granules, when applied to a tissue section. These substances appear purple or blue, contrasting the surrounding tissue. Other metachromatic stains include Alcian Blue, which stains acidic polysaccharides, and Congo Red, which stains amyloid deposits. These stains can help identify and differentiate pathological conditions, such as abnormal mucins or amyloidosis.

Classification of Stains

Based on Application

Stains can be classified based on their applications in various fields of study. Here are some common classifications of stains based on their applications:

○ **Histological stains:** These stains are specifically designed to visualize and study tissues in histology and histopathology. Examples include Hematoxylin and Eosin (HandE), Masson's Trichrome, and Periodic Acid-Schiff (PAS) stains.

○ **Cytochemical stains:** These stains study specific cellular components or functions. They can help identify and visualize cellular structures, organelles, or specific cellular activities. Examples include stains for mitochondria (MitoTracker dyes), nuclei (Hoechst or DAPI), and cytoskeletal elements (Phalloidin).

○ **Microbiological stains:** These stains are used to study microorganisms, such as bacteria, fungi, and parasites. Examples include Gram stain for bacterial cell wall visualization, Acid-fast stain for mycobacteria, and Giemsa stain for malaria parasites.

○ **Immunohistochemical stains:** Involve using specific antibodies to detect and visualize specific proteins or antigens within tissues. Immunohistochemical stains are commonly used for diagnostic purposes and to study protein expression patterns in normal and diseased tissues.

○ **Cytogenetic stains:** These are used in cytogenetics to study chromosomes and genetic material. Examples include Giemsa stain for banding patterns (G-banding) and fluorescence in situ hybridization (FISH) stains for specific DNA sequences.

○ **Fluorescent stains:** These stains emit fluorescence when exposed to specific wavelengths of light. They are widely used in fluorescence microscopy to study cellular structures, protein localization, and intracellular processes. Examples include fluorescent dyes like DAPI, FITC, and Rhodamine.

○ **Vital stains:** These stains are used to study living cells or tissues without causing significant harm or damage. They can selectively stain specific structures or identify viable cells. Examples include trypan blue for cell viability assessment and dyes like calcein AM or fluorescein diacetate for live cell imaging.

○ **Special stains:** These stains are used for specific purposes or to visualize specific substances. Examples include silver stains for reticulin fibers, Alcian Blue for acidic mucins, and Congo Red for amyloid deposits.

Based on Tissue Affinities

Stains can also be classified based on their affinities for specific tissue components. Here are some common classifications of stains based on tissue affinities:

○ **Nuclear stains:** These stains have a strong affinity for nuclear material, including DNA and RNA. They selectively stain cell nuclei and aid in visualizing nuclear morphology and chromatin patterns. Examples include Hematoxylin, DAPI, and Hoechst stains.

○ **Cytoplasmic stains:** These stains selectively stain the cytoplasm of cells, highlighting the presence and distribution of various cytoplasmic components. Examples include Eosin, eosin Y, and certain eosinophilic dyes.

○ **Connective tissue stains:** These stains have an affinity for connective tissue components, such as collagen and elastic fibers. They help in visualizing the structural organization of connective tissues and detecting pathological changes. Examples include Masson's Trichrome, Van Gieson, and Elastic Van Gieson stains.

○ **Epithelial stains:** These stains are specific to epithelial tissues and help differentiate various types of epithelial cells. They can also highlight pathological changes in epithelial tissues. Examples include Cytokeratin stains for differentiating epithelial cells and PAS stains for detecting mucin in epithelial cells.

○ **Nerve stains:** These stains selectively stain nervous tissue components, such as neurons, axons, and myelin sheaths. They aid in studying neural morphology and identifying pathological changes in nerve tissues. Examples include Luxol Fast Blue for myelin, Bielschowsky stain for neurons, and S100 protein immunostains for neural cells.

○ **Vascular stains:** These stains target blood vessels and highlight their morphology and distribution. They can help in the study of vascular structures and the detecting of abnormalities in blood vessels. Examples include Hematoxylin and Eosin (HandE) stains, Verhoeff's stain for elastic fibers in blood vessels, and CD31 immunostains for endothelial cells.

○ **Specialised stains:** These target specific tissue components or structures, such as amyloid deposits, reticulin fibers, or specific cell types. Examples include Congo Red stain for amyloid, Reticulin stain for reticulin fibers, and immunostains for specific cell markers (e.g., CD3 for T cells, CD20 for B cells).

Based on Source

Stains can also be classified based on their source or origin. Here are some common classifications of stains based on their source:

○ **Natural stains:** These are derived from natural sources, such as plants, minerals, or biological materials. Examples include Hematoxylin (derived from the logwood tree) and safranin (derived from saffron).

○ **Synthetic stains:** These stains are chemically synthesized in the laboratory. They are designed to have specific affinities for certain tissue components or structures. Examples include Eosin Y and Fast Green.

○ **Biological stains:** These are derived from biological sources, such as bacteria or fungi. They may be produced by the organisms themselves or extracted from them.

Examples include Gram stain (derived from bacteria) and lactophenol cotton blue (derived from fungi).

○ **Fluorescent stains:** These stains are specifically designed to emit fluorescence when exposed to specific wavelengths of light. They are often synthetic dyes that are conjugated with fluorescent molecules. Examples include fluorescent dyes like fluorescein, rhodamine, and Alexa Fluor dyes.

○ **Nucleic acid stains:** These stains target nucleic acids, such as DNA or RNA. They are used for nucleic acid visualization, DNA sequencing, and gel electrophoresis applications. Examples include ethidium bromide, SYBR Green, and propidium iodide.

Methods of Staining

Direct staining and indirect staining are two different approaches used in staining techniques.

○ **Direct staining:** A single stain or dye is applied directly to the specimen or tissue section. The stain directly binds to the target component or structure, leading to its visualization. This method is relatively simple and quick, not requiring additional steps or reagents. Examples of direct staining include basic stains like Crystal Violet, Safranin, and Methylene Blue. Direct staining is commonly used in simple techniques to visualize the overall morphology and basic cellular structures.

○ **Indirect staining:** In this process, the action of dye is intensified by adding mordant, which acts as a link or bridge between tissue and dye.

MORDANT—A substance or solution is used to enhance or fix the staining process. It helps to intensify the color of the stain, improve its adherence to the specimen, and increase its resistance to fading or washing out. Mordants form insoluble complexes with the stain, which are more tightly bound to the target tissue.

Commonly used mordants include:

○ **Iodine:** Iodine is commonly used as a mordant in Gram staining. It forms a complex with the crystal violet stain, helping to fix it to the peptidoglycan layer of Gram-positive bacteria.

○ **Tannic acid:** Tannic acid is used as a mordant in some histological staining techniques. It helps to intensify the staining of certain tissue components, such as collagen fiber.

○ **Alum:** Alum (aluminum potassium sulfate) is a commonly used mordant in various staining techniques. It forms insoluble complexes with stains like hematoxylin, enhancing their color and binding to tissue structures.

○ **Schiffs reagent:** Schiff's reagent is a mordant used in Periodic Acid-Schiff (PAS) staining. It reacts with the oxidized carbohydrates generated by periodic acid, forming a pink or magenta color.

Bluing

Bluing is a step in certain staining techniques, particularly in hematoxylin-based staining methods, such as Hematoxylin and Eosin (HandE) staining. The purpose of the bluing step is to enhance the contrast and appearance of stained nuclei.

After staining with a hematoxylin solution, which imparts a blue-purple color to the nuclei, excessive stain needs to be removed and the nuclei need to be properly differentiated from the surrounding cytoplasm. This is achieved through the bluing step.

Bluing agents, also known as differentiation agents or "bluing reagents," are used to counteract the natural red color that develops in nuclei when exposed to air. These agents convert the red color to a more desirable blue color, thus improving the visibility of the nuclei.

Commonly used bluing agents include:

○ **Scott's tap water substitute:** Scott's tap water substitute is a commonly used bluing reagent. It is a mildly alkaline solution that helps to neutralize the acidic hematoxylin and enhance the blue color of the nuclei.

○ **Ammonium hydroxide:** In dilute form, ammonium hydroxide is sometimes used as a bluing agent. It helps to neutralize the acid in the stained sections and enhance the blue color of the nuclei.

Hematoxylin and Eosin Stain

Hematoxylin is a natural dye commonly used in histopathology for staining cell nuclei. It is derived from the heartwood of certain trees, such as logwood trees (Haematoxylum campechianum). Hematoxylin is a basic or cationic dye, which carries a positive charge when dissolved in water or other aqueous solutions.

When used in staining, hematoxylin selectively binds to acidic structures in tissues, particularly DNA and RNA in cell nuclei. It forms complexes with these acidic components, resulting in a blue to purple color. Hematoxylin staining provides contrast and allows for the visualization of nuclei, essential for evaluating tissue morphology and identifying cellular features.

Different formulations of hematoxylin stains are available, such as Harris hematoxylin, Mayer's hematoxylin, Gill's hematoxylin, and Ehrlich's hematoxylin. These formulations may vary in composition and staining characteristics, but their basic principle remains the same.

Hematoxylin staining is typically performed as part of the Hematoxylin and Eosin (HandE) staining method, a routine staining technique used in histopathology. After staining with hematoxylin, the excess stain is usually differentiated and blued to enhance the contrast and visibility of nuclei.

Hematein can be extracted from hematoxylin by a process called oxidation. Hematein is the oxidized form of hematoxylin and is responsible for the staining properties of hematoxylin.

The oxidation of hematoxylin refers to a chemical process that occurs during the preparation of hematoxylin staining solutions. Hematoxylin, the natural dye derived from the heartwood of certain trees, is initially in a reduced form, referred to as hematein. Hematein is not readily soluble in water and does not have the desired staining properties. To convert hematein into a soluble and effective staining dye, it needs to be oxidized.

The oxidation of hematein to hematoxylin is typically achieved by exposing the hematein solution to an oxidizing agent. Common oxidizing agents used in this process include sodium iodate, periodic acid, or other oxidizing agents that can convert the reduced form of hematein into its oxidized form, hematoxylin.

The oxidation process allows the hematoxylin to exhibit enhanced staining properties, including a stronger affinity for target structures such as cell nuclei. The oxidized form of hematoxylin is soluble in water—or alcohol-based solutions, making it more suitable for staining tissue sections.

The commercially available hematoxylin staining solutions are prepared and contain the oxidized form of hematoxylin ready for use.

After extraction of hematein from hematoxylin it is linked to a mordant that can either be an aluminum salt or iron or tungsten. Depending on the mordant, hematoxylins are further grouped.

Alum hematoxylin utilizes aluminum salts, commonly aluminum sulfate or ammonium aluminum sulfate (alum), as a mordant Mayer's hematoxylin, Harris hematoxylin, and Ehrlich's hematoxylin.

Iron hematoxylin—Ferric chloride or ferrous sulphate is the mordant. Weigert's hematoxylin.

Tungsten Hematoxylin—Mallory's phosphotungstic acid hematoxylin.

Staining Approaches

Progressive and regressive staining are two different approaches to staining in histopathology. Here's an explanation of each:

1. **Progressive staining:** In progressive staining, the tissue sections are exposed to a staining solution for a specific period until the desired staining intensity is achieved. The staining time is determined based on the desired level of contrast and intensity required to visualize the target structures. With progressive staining, the stain accumulates in the target structures over time, resulting in a darker colouration. Excess stain is then washed off, and the sections are typically counterstained with a contrasting dye to enhance the visualization of other tissue components. Progressive staining is commonly used when a strong and uniform intensity is desired throughout the tissue section.

2. **Regressive staining:** The tissue sections are first overstained with a relatively concentrated staining solution in regressive staining. The excess stain is then removed by subjecting the sections to a differentiation or decolorising solution for a specific duration. The differentiation solution selectively removes the excess stain, leaving a reduced and controlled staining intensity behind. The differentiation time is carefully monitored to achieve the desired level of color reduction. Regressive staining is often employed when a selective and controlled intensity is desired, allowing for better visualization of specific tissue structures while minimising background

staining. After differentiation, the sections may be counterstained if necessary.

The choice between progressive and regressive staining depends on the specific staining requirements and the tissue's characteristics. Progressive staining is suitable for uniform staining and when a strong intensity is desired. Regressive staining is useful for achieving selective and controlled staining intensity, allowing for better contrast and differentiation of specific tissue structures.

Procedure of H and E Staining

HandE staining, short for Hematoxylin and Eosin staining, is a widely used staining technique in histology. It provides valuable information about tissues' overall structure and morphology under a microscope. HandE staining involves a sequential application of two dyes: hematoxylin and eosin. Harris hematoxylin is used for routine HandE staining.

Here's a step-by-step overview of the HandE staining process:

○ **Deparaffinisation:** The paraffin-embedded tissue sections are deparaffinized to remove the wax. This is typically done by immersing the slides in xylene or a xylene substitute and gradually transferring them through descending ethanol concentrations.

○ **Hydration:** The deparaffinized sections are rehydrated by immersing them in a series of descending concentrations of ethanol. This process helps to remove any remaining xylene and prepare the tissue for staining.

○ **Hematoxylin staining:** The tissue sections are immersed in a hematoxylin solution, Hematoxylin has an affinity for acidic components in the cell, such as nucleic acids. It stains the nuclei of cells blue-purple. The sections are usually left in the hematoxylin solution for 15 minutes for proper staining.

○ **Differentiation:** After the hematoxylin staining, the excess stain is removed by differentiating the sections in an acidic alcohol solution, typically called acid alcohol or differentiation solution. This step selectively removes excess hematoxylin from the tissue while retaining the blue-purple color in the nuclei.

○ **Bluing:** The sections are then "blued" by rinsing them in water or a bluing solution, which stabilizes and intensifies the blue color of the nuclei. This step is crucial for achieving optimal staining quality.

○ **Eosin staining:** The sections are next immersed in an eosin solution. Eosin is an acidic dye that stains cytoplasm, extracellular matrix, and other acidic structures in shades of pink or red. Eosin staining contrasts the blue nuclei and allows visualization of cellular details and tissue architecture.

○ **Dehydration:** To remove excess water from the tissue sections, they are dehydrated by transferring them through ascending ethanol concentrations.

○ **Clearing:** Finally, the sections are cleared by immersing them in xylene or a xylene substitute to remove any remaining water and prepare them for mounting with a coverslip.

After the staining process, the HandE-stained slides can be observed under a light microscope. Nuclei will appear blue-purple, while cytoplasm and extracellular structures will appear pink or red, providing information about cell types, tissue organization, and abnormalities, if present.

Coverslipping and Mounting

Coverslips are thin, transparent pieces of glass or plastic placed over the tissue section on a slide after mounting. The coverslip protects the tissue and holds it in place for microscopic examination. Coverslips are 22 mm or 24 mm wide, but the length varies to suit the size of the section.

Mounting Medium

A mounting medium is a substance used to secure a coverslip onto a tissue section mounted on a glass slide. The mounting medium acts as an adhesive, providing a clear, protective layer between the coverslip and the tissue, and helps to minimise air bubbles and preserve the sample for microscopic examination. The choice of mounting medium depends on the staining technique, the sample type, and the final slide's desired characteristics.

Here are a few common types of mounting media used in histology:

○ **Aqueous-based mounting media:** These mounting media are water-based and suitable for tissue sections stained with aqueous or water-soluble dyes. Examples include glycerine jelly, aqueous mountants like glycerol or glycerol-gelatin, and commercial mounting media such as Aqua-Poly/Mount.

○ **Organic-based mounting media** are organic solvents or resins typically used with tissue sections stained with organic dyes or chromogens. Examples include DPX (dibutylphthalate Polystyrene Xylene), Permount, Entellan, and Canada balsam. Due to their potentially toxic nature, these mounting media are often xylene-based and require careful handling in a well-ventilated area.

○ **Fluorescent mounting media:** When working with fluorescently labelled samples, specialized mounting media preserve the fluorescent signal and minimise fading. Fluoromount or Vectashield are examples of mounting media specifically designed for preserving fluorescence.

Characteristics of Good Mounting Medium

A good mounting medium should possess several characteristics to ensure optimal preservation and visualization of the tissue section. Here are some important characteristics to consider when selecting a mounting medium:

○ **Transparency:** The mounting medium should be transparent to visualize the tissue section and any stained components. A transparent medium ensures that the microscopic details of the sample are easily observable.

○ **Refractive index:** The refractive index of the mounting medium should closely match that of the coverslip and the microscope objective lens, i.e., between 1.53 and 1.54. A close match in the refractive index helps to minimise light refraction and improve the quality of the image. This reduces the distortion and loss of resolution that can occur due to refractive index mismatches.

○ **Compatibility with staining methods:** The mounting medium should be compatible with the staining method used for the tissue section. It should not interfere with the staining process or alter the color or intensity of the stain. Ensure that the mounting medium does not cause fading or degradation of the staining over time.

○ **Long-term stability:** A good mounting medium should provide the mounted tissue section long-term stability. It should protect the sample from degradation, fading, or discoloration. The mounting medium should be resistant to environmental factors, such as light, moisture, and temperature changes, to maintain the integrity of the slide.

○ **Adhesive properties:** The mounting medium should have sufficient adhesive properties to hold the coverslip securely. It should create a strong bond between the coverslip and the glass slide to prevent detachment or movement during handling and microscopic examination. Adequate adhesion helps to avoid air bubbles and provides stability to the sample.

○ **Compatibility with microscopy techniques:** The mounting medium should suit the microscopy technique. For example, if fluorescent microscopy is performed, the mounting medium should preserve the fluorescence signal and minimise fading or photobleaching.

○ **Easy application and drying:** A good mounting medium should be easy to apply onto the tissue section and allow quick and uniform drying. It should spread evenly without forming bubbles or streaks. Fast drying minimises the risk of contaminants settling on the slide and ensures timely examination.

SPECIAL STAINS

Special stains, also known as histochemical stains, are a group of staining techniques used in histology to highlight specific tissue components, structures, or substances that are not readily visualized with routine HandE staining. These stains provide additional information about the composition, distribution, and function of various cellular and extracellular components in tissues.

Stains for Carbohydrates

Staining techniques for carbohydrates are commonly used in histology to identify and visualize specific carbohydrate-rich structures within tissues. Here are two commonly used stains for carbohydrates:

1. **Periodic acid-Schiff (PAS) stain:** PAS staining is widely used to detect and highlight carbohydrates, such as glycogen, glycoproteins, and mucins. Carbohydrates appear as magenta or pink under the microscope, PAS staining is useful for

identifying glycogen in tissues, basement membranes, and mucus-producing cells. It can also reveal glycoproteins in different tissues.

2. **Alcian Blue stain:** Alcian Blue is another technique commonly used to detect acidic carbohydrates, such as mucins and glycosaminoglycans (GAGs). Acidic mucins and GAGs stain blue with Alcian Blue, allowing their identification and localization within the tissue.

3. **Mucicarmine:** Mucicarmine stain is a specialized staining technique used to identify and highlight acidic mucopolysaccharides and mucins, which are specific types of carbohydrates, in histological sections. This stain is particularly useful for identifying mucin-producing cells and evaluating mucin-rich tissues, such as those found in certain tumors or gastrointestinal tract samples. Under the microscope, the mucicarmine-stained mucins and mucopolysaccharides will appear red or pink.

Connective Tissue Stains

Connective tissue stains help identify and differentiate components such as collagen fibers, elastic fibers, and ground substances. Here are some stains specifically used for connective tissue:

○ **Masson's trichrome stain:** Masson's trichrome stain is widely used to differentiate collagen fibers (blue/green), muscle fibers (red), and cell nuclei (dark brown/black). This stain is commonly used to assess fibrosis and to visualize connective tissue in various organs.

○ **Van Gieson's stain:** Van Gieson's stain differentiates collagen (red) from other tissue components (yellow/orange). It highlights collagen fibers in connective tissue and helps assess collagen distribution and organization.

○ **Verhoeff's stain:** Verhoeff's stain is specifically for elastic fibers. It stains black or dark brown elastic fibers and is useful for visualizing elastic fibers in tissues such as blood vessels, skin, and ligaments.

○ **Movat's pentachrome stain:** Movat's pentachrome stain is a combination of stains that allows for the differentiation of various tissue components in connective tissue. It includes stains for collagen (blue), nuclei (black), elastic fibers (black), fibrin (pink/red), and ground substance (yellow).

○ **Orcein stain:** Orcein stain is another stain used specifically for elastic fibers. It stains elastic fibers a reddish-brown color and can be used to assess elastic fiber integrity and distribution in tissues.

○ **Mallory's PTAH stain:** Mallory's phosphotungstic acid-hematoxylin (PTAH) stain primarily highlights reticular fibers in connective tissue. With this stain, reticular fibers appear blue or purple and can be observed in tissues such as lymph nodes, liver, and spleen.

Stains for Amyloid

Amyloid refers to an abnormal accumulation of protein fibrils that can occur in various tissues and organs in certain diseases, such as amyloidosis. Staining techniques specific for amyloid can aid in its identification and visualization in histological samples.

○ **Congo Red stain:** Congo Red is a classic stain for amyloid.

○ **Thioflavin T stain:** Thioflavin T is another commonly used fluorescent dye for amyloid staining. It provides sensitive and specific detection of amyloid deposits and is particularly useful when fluorescent microscopy is available.

Stains for Pigments and Minerals

○ **Fontana-Masson stain:** Fontana-Masson stain is a silver impregnation technique used to identify and visualize melanin, a brown-black pigment found in melanocytes.

Melanin-containing cells or structures will appear black or dark brown.

It is commonly used in dermatopathology to detect and assess melanin pigment in skin samples.

- **Prussian blue stain:** Prussian blue stain is used to detect and localize iron in tissues. Iron can be present in various forms, such as hemosiderin, ferritin, or iron deposits. Iron-containing structures will appear as blue or blue-green.

  It is commonly used to evaluate iron accumulation in tissues, such as in cases of hemochromatosis or hemosiderosis.

- **Von Kossa stain:** Von Kossa stain identifies and visualizes calcium deposits in tissues. Calcium deposits will appear black or brown.

  It is commonly used to detect and evaluate calcium deposition in tissues, such as calcified blood vessels or pathological mineralization.

- **Alizarin Red S:** It is used to identify calcium. The calcium deposits turn orange-red.

- **Rubeanic acid:** This stain is used for the depiction of copper pigment. The copper pigment appears greenish-black, and the nuclei appear pale red.

Stains for Lipids

- **Oil Red O stain:** Oil Red O is a lipophilic dye that specifically stains neutral lipids, such as triglycerides and cholesterol esters. Lipid-rich areas, such as fat droplets or lipid-filled cells, appear red under the microscope.

  It is commonly used to visualize and quantify lipid droplets in adipose tissue, liver samples (to detect steatosis), and other lipid-rich tissues.

- **Sudan Black B stain:** Sudan Black B is a lipophilic dye that stains lipids, including neutral and phospholipids.

  Lipid-rich structures, such as lipocytes or myelin sheaths, will be stained black or dark blue-black.

  Sudan Black B stain is commonly used to visualize lipids in various tissues, including nervous tissue, adipose tissue, and myelin-rich areas.

- **Sudan III or Sudan IV stain:** Sudan III and Sudan IV are lipophilic dyes that stain neutral lipids, particularly triglycerides.

  Lipid-rich structures or lipid droplets appear red-orange or dark red.

  Sudan III or Sudan IV stains are commonly used to visualize lipids in tissues, such as adipose tissue or lipid-containing cells.

Stains for Microorganisms

- **Gram stain:** The Gram stain is a differential staining technique that distinguishes between gram-positive and gram-negative bacteria based on their cell wall composition differences. The gram stain is widely used to differentiate bacteria into gram-positive (purple) and gram-negative (pink) categories.

- **Ziehl-Nelson's (Acid-fast) stain:** The acid-fast stain is used to identify acid-fast bacteria, including the *Mycobacterium tuberculosis* species, which have a waxy cell wall. Acid-fast staining is primarily used to detect acid-fast bacteria that appear red/magenta colored under the microscope, particularly in diagnosing tuberculosis.

- **Fite-wade stain:** It is used for the identification of Lepra bacilli which appear red under the microscope.

- **Shikata's orcein stain:** It is used to identify Hepatitis B surface antigen, which appear brown to black in color.

- **Lendrum's phloxine tartrazine method:** It is used for the identification of viral bodies which appear bright red under the microscope.

○ **Schleifstein's method:** It is used for the identification of Negri bodies of humans and canines. On staining, negri bodies appear deep magenta, cytoplasm, bluish violet and erythrocytes copper red.

○ **Giemsa stain:** Giemsa stain is a versatile stain used to identify various microorganisms, including bacteria, parasites, and blood-borne pathogens. Giemsa stain is commonly used to diagnose malaria, Chlamydia, and other bacterial and parasitic infections.

○ **Periodic acid-Schiff (PAS) stain:** While primarily used for carbohydrates, the PAS stain can also highlight certain fungal cell walls. Fungal organisms, such as Candida or Pneumocystis, can be identified with the PAS method's characteristic magenta or pink staining.

Silver Stains

These stains are particularly useful for highlighting various components, including nerve fibers, reticular fibers, microorganisms, and specific proteins.

○ **Golgi-Cox stain:** The Golgi-Cox stain visualizes neurons' morphology and processes. This stain impregnates a small number of neurons with silver chromate, allowing for the visualization of the entire neuron, including dendrites, cell bodies, and axons.

○ **Gomori silver impregnation:** The Gomori silver impregnation method is used to visualize reticular fibers, which form the supporting framework of various tissues. This stain is commonly used in liver, spleen, and lymph node samples to highlight the delicate reticular network. Reticular fibers appear black or brown with this stain.

○ **Warthin-Starry stain:** The Warthin-Starry stain detects and visualizes certain

bacteria, particularly spirochetes and *Helicobacter pylori*. It uses silver nitrate to impregnate the microorganisms, which subsequently appear black or dark brown against a background of surrounding tissue. This stain is commonly used to diagnose conditions such as syphilis or infections caused by *Helicobacter pylori*.

○ **Bielschowsky silver stain:** The Bielschowsky silver stain visualizes neurofibrillary tangles and senile plaques, characteristic pathological features of Alzheimer's disease. This stain selectively impregnates the abnormal structures, allowing their visualization under the microscope. Neurofibrillary tangles and senile plaques appear black or brown with this stain.

Nucleic Acid Stains

Nucleic acid stains are commonly used in laboratory techniques to visualize and detect DNA and RNA within cells and tissues. These stains bind specifically to nucleic acids, allowing for their identification and localization.

DAPI (4′,6-diamidino-2-phenylindole): DAPI is a fluorescent stain that binds to DNA. It emits blue fluorescence when excited with ultraviolet (UV) light. DAPI is commonly used in fluorescence microscopy to visualize nuclear DNA in fixed cells and tissues.

○ **Propidium iodide (PI):** Propidium iodide is a fluorescent dye that binds to DNA. It is impermeable to live cells but can enter cells with compromised cell membranes, such as dead or apoptotic cells. PI emits red fluorescence when excited with appropriate wavelengths. It is frequently used in flow cytometry and fluorescence microscopy to distinguish between live and dead cells.

○ **Ethidium bromide (EtBr):** Ethidium bromide is a fluorescent dye that intercalates into DNA, causing it to fluoresce. It emits orange-red fluorescence when excited with UV light. Ethidium bromide was commonly used for DNA visualization but is now less favored due to safety concerns. However, it is still used in some laboratories with proper safety precautions.

○ **SYBR Green:** SYBR Green is a family of fluorescent dyes that bind to double-stranded DNA. When bound to DNA, it exhibits green fluorescence. SYBR Green is commonly used in techniques like real-time PCR (polymerase chain reaction) or gel electrophoresis to detect and quantify DNA.

○ **Acridine Orange:** Acridine Orange is a fluorescent dye that can bind to both DNA and RNA. It emits green fluorescence when bound to DNA and red fluorescence when bound to RNA. Acridine Orange is often used in fluorescence microscopy to differentiate between DNA and RNA in cells and tissues.

AUTOMATION IN HISTOPATHOLOGY

Automation plays a crucial role in modern histopathology laboratories, streamlining processes, improving efficiency, and enhancing accuracy in diagnostic procedures. Here are some key areas where automation is commonly employed in histopathology:

○ **Tissue processing:** Automated tissue processors process tissue samples, including fixation, dehydration, clearing, and infiltration with paraffin wax. These instruments help standardize processing times and improve the quality of tissue sections.

○ **Embedding:** Automated embedding systems automate the placement of processed tissue samples into molds and facilitate embedding in paraffin wax. This eliminates the manual handling of samples and ensures consistent orientation and positioning.

○ **Microtomy:** Automated microtomes are used to section the paraffin-embedded tissue blocks into thin slices (usually around 4–6 micrometers thick). These instruments offer precision, speed, and consistency, reducing technician fatigue and improving section quality.

○ **Staining:** Automated staining systems automate the staining process, reducing the labor-intensive and time-consuming nature of manual staining. These systems can handle multiple slides simultaneously, precisely controlling staining times and reagent volumes to ensure consistent and reproducible results.

○ **Immunohistochemistry (IHC):** Automated IHC platforms perform the entire IHC process, including antigen retrieval, primary antibody incubation, secondary antibody application, and detection steps. These systems increase accuracy, minimise technician variability, and improve turnaround times.

○ **Slide scanning:** Slide scanners digitize glass slides, creating high-resolution digital images of entire tissue sections. Automated scanning enables efficient storage, retrieval, and remote slide access, facilitating consultation, research, and collaboration.

○ **Image analysis:** Automated image analysis software assists in quantifying and interpreting histopathological images. These tools can identify and measure various features, such as cell counts, nuclear characteristics, and staining intensity, aiding in diagnostic and research applications.

○ **Laboratory information systems (LIS):** LIS platforms automate the management of patient information, specimen tracking, workflow management, and result reporting. These systems enhance communication, reduce errors, and improve overall laboratory efficiency.

The integration of automation in histopathology helps laboratories increase productivity, reduce turnaround times, enhance accuracy, and improve standardization. It enables pathologists and laboratory staff to focus on more complex tasks, data interpretation, and diagnostic decision-making, ultimately benefiting patient care.

IMMUNOHISTOCHEMISTRY

Immunohistochemistry (IHC) is a laboratory technique to detect and visualize specific proteins or antigens within tissue sections. It combines principles of immunology and histology to identify the presence, location, and abundance of target proteins in tissues. The IHC process involves several steps:

- **Tissue preparation:** Tissue sections are prepared by embedding in paraffin wax, frozen sectioning, or cytological preparations such as cell smears or cytospins. The choice of preparation depends on the type of tissue and the study's specific objectives.
- **Antigen retrieval:** For formalin-fixed paraffin-embedded (FFPE) tissues, antigen retrieval is typically required to expose target antigens masked by fixation. Common methods for antigen retrieval include heat-induced epitope retrieval (HIER) using heat or pressure or enzyme digestion for enzyme-labile antigens.
- **Blocking:** Non-specific binding sites on tissue sections are blocked using blocking agents such as serum or protein-based solutions. Blocking reduces background staining caused by non-specific antibody binding.
- **Primary antibody incubation:** Tissue sections are incubated with a primary antibody that specifically binds to the target antigen. The primary antibody can be polyclonal or monoclonal, raised against the target protein or specific epitopes of interest.
- **Washing:** After incubation with the primary antibody, the tissue sections are washed to remove unbound antibodies and reduce background staining.
- **Secondary antibody incubation:** Tissue sections are incubated with a secondary antibody conjugated to a detection molecule, such as an enzyme (e.g., horseradish peroxidase) or a fluorophore (e.g., fluorescein isothiocyanate). The secondary antibody binds to the primary antibody, amplifying the signal and allowing visualization of the target antigen.
- **Signal detection:** For enzyme-based detection, a chromogenic substrate reacts with the enzyme, producing a visible colored precipitate at the site of the target antigen. The fluorophore-conjugated secondary antibody emits fluorescence when excited with specific wavelengths for fluorescence-based detection.
- **Counterstaining and mounting:** Tissue sections may be counterstained with dyes such as hematoxylin to visualize cellular morphology. Finally, the slides are mounted with a coverslip using an appropriate mounting medium.
- **Microscopic examination:** The stained tissue sections are observed under a microscope, and the presence, localization, and intensity of staining for the target protein are assessed.

Immunohistochemistry is widely used in research, clinical diagnostics, and pathology to study protein expression patterns, identify tumor markers, classify diseases, and guide treatment decisions. It provides valuable insights into cellular and tissue-level protein

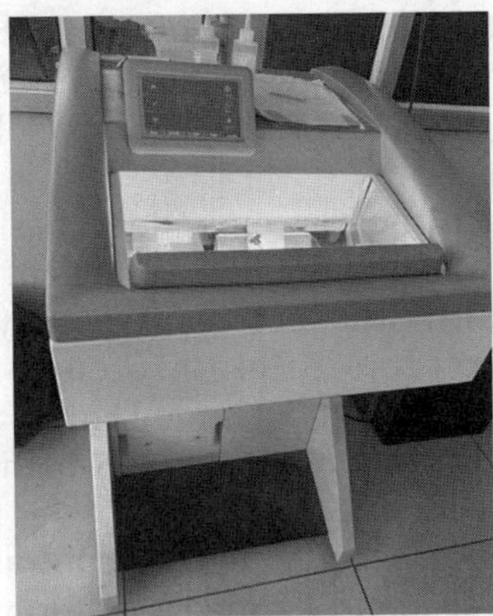

Fig. 5.2: Cryostat.

localization, allowing for the correlation of protein expression with pathological conditions and clinical outcomes.

Frozen Section

Frozen section processing is a technique used in histopathology to prepare and evaluate tissue samples rapidly during surgery. It provides real-time information about the tissue's nature, such as tumors, inflammation, infection, or other abnormalities. This technique is particularly valuable during surgical procedures when immediate diagnosis is crucial for determining the course of action. The **Figure 5.2** depicts the cryostat.

The process of frozen section preparation involves the following steps:

○ **Tissue excision:** A small piece of tissue is removed from the patient during surgery using a scalpel or other surgical instruments. The tissue is selected based on the surgeon's judgment and the specific diagnostic question.

○ **Tissue orientation:** The excised tissue is carefully oriented to ensure proper sectioning and accurate interpretation of the results. Orientation is particularly important when the tissue has distinct anatomical features or when the location of a lesion is critical for diagnosis.

○ **Freezing:** The tissue is rapidly frozen using a cryostat, a specialized freezing device. Depending on the laboratory protocols, the cryostat cools the tissue to a very low temperature, typically around –20 to –30°C or even lower.

○ **Sectioning:** Once the tissue is frozen, it is cut into thin sections using a microtome within the cryostat. The microtome produces slices that are usually between 5 to 10 micrometers thick. These sections are mounted onto glass slides or other suitable substrates for further processing.

○ **Staining:** The frozen tissue sections are stained using various dyes or specific antibodies to enhance the visibility of different cell types or structures. Common stains used in frozen section processing include hematoxylin and eosin (HandE), which contrast cell nuclei and cytoplasm, and special stains that highlight specific cellular components or pathologies.

○ **Examination:** The stained slides are examined under a microscope by a pathologist. They evaluate the tissue morphology and rapidly diagnose based on the observed features. The pathologist communicates the diagnosis to the surgeon, who can make informed decisions during the ongoing surgery.

It is important to note that frozen section processing has limitations compared to traditional formalin-fixed, paraffin-embedded tissue processing. Frozen sections are typically lower quality, and artefacts can be introduced during the freezing and sectioning steps. Therefore, frozen section diagnosis is preliminary and may require confirmation with permanent tissue sections processed using formalin fixation and paraffin embedding techniques.

Frozen section processing plays a vital role in surgical pathology despite its limitations. It provides rapid intraoperative information, allowing surgeons to make immediate decisions regarding the surgical approach and patient management.

Electron Microscopy

Electron microscopy (EM) is a specialized technique used in histopathology to examine tissue samples at a high resolution, allowing for detailed visualization of cellular structures and ultrastructural abnormalities. The processing of tissue samples for electron microscopy involves several steps, which are outlined below:

○ **Fixation:** The tissue sample is first fixed to preserve its cellular structure and prevent degradation. Unlike traditional histopathology, where formalin fixation is commonly used, electron microscopy requires specialized fixatives that preserve ultrastructural details. Common fixatives for EM include glutaraldehyde and paraformaldehyde.

○ **Postfixation:** After the initial fixation, the tissue sample may undergo additional postfixation steps to stabilize further and enhance the cellular structures. This may involve secondary fixation with osmium tetroxide or other chemical agents.

○ **Dehydration:** The fixed tissue is dehydrated through a series of alcohol solutions with increasing concentrations. This process removes water from the tissue while preserving the cellular structures.

○ **Infiltration and embedding:** The dehydrated tissue is then infiltrated with a resin, such as epoxy resin or acrylic resin, which provides structural support and allows for thin sectioning. The tissue is placed in a mixture of resin and a solvent, which gradually replaces the alcohol in the tissue. Finally, the tissue is embedded in a resin block and cured to form a solid tissue block.

○ **Sectioning:** The embedded tissue block is trimmed to the desired area of interest, and ultrathin sections (typically 40–100 nanometers thick) are cut using an ultramicrotome. Diamond knives are often used for sectioning to achieve high-quality, thin sections.

○ **Staining:** To enhance the contrast of the tissue sections, staining is performed using heavy metals, such as uranyl acetate and lead citrate. These stains selectively bind to cellular components, allowing for better visualization of the ultrastructural details.

○ **Mounting:** The stained sections are mounted onto copper grids or other suitable substrates. These grids allow the sections to be easily handled and transferred for examination under the electron microscope.

○ **Examination:** The prepared grids with tissue sections are placed in an electron microscope, which uses a beam of electrons to image the sample. The electron beam interacts with the tissue, generating detected and converted signals into an image. This imaging process enables the visualization of cellular structures at high magnification and resolution.

Electron microscopy in histopathology provides valuable insights into the ultrastructure of cells and tissues, allowing for the identification of ultrastructural abnormalities and the investigation of various pathological conditions. It is particularly useful for studying diseases affecting subcellular structures, such as mitochondrial disorders, renal pathology, muscle diseases, and certain tumors.

MULTIPLE CHOICE QUESTIONS

1. **Histopathology is the study of:**
   a. Tissue
   b. Diseased tissue
   c. Morphology of cells
   d. Blood cells

2. **Which of the following is NOT the responsibility of histotechnician?**
   a. Logging of specimen
   b. Record maintenance
   c. Microscopy of slides
   d. Checking the fixative of the specimen

3. **Which of the following is the correct stage of tissue processing?**
   a. Fixation-Embedding-Clearing-Dehydration-Infiltration
   b. Dehydration-Fixation-Clearing-Infiltration-Embedding
   c. Fixation-Dehydration-Clearing-Infiltration-Embedding
   d. Clearing-Fixation-Dehydration-Infiltration-Embedding

4. **Which of the following statement is NOT true regarding fixatives?**
   a. Fixatives should be chemically stable and not undergo degradation or decomposition over time
   b. Fixatives should be compatible with various tissue types and capable of effectively preserving the cellular components of different tissues

   c. Fixatives should have good penetration properties, allowing them to diffuse into the tissue quickly and evenly
   d. Fixatives should not retain the antigenicity of tissues.

5. **Which of the following statements are correct about fixation?**
   a. Preservation of tissue morphology
   b. Prevention of autolysis and putrefaction
   c. Inactivation of infectious agents
   d. All of the above

6. **What is the primary purpose of fixation in histopathology?**
   a. Preservation of tissue structure and morphology
   b. Enhancement of antigen detection
   c. Staining of cellular components
   d. Removal of cellular debris

7. **Which of the following fixatives is commonly used for routine histopathological processing?**
   a. Glutaraldehyde
   b. Osmium tetroxide
   c. Ethanol
   d. Formalin

8. **Which fixative is preferred for electron microscopy studies?**
   a. Formalin
   b. Acetone
   c. Glutaraldehyde
   d. Ethanol

Answers: 1. b   2. c   3. c   4. d
             5. d   6. a   7. d   8. c

9. **Which statement regarding fixation is true?**
   a. Fixation prevents all changes in tissue structure and composition
   b. Overfixation can lead to excessive tissue hardening
   c. Fixation can reverse autolysis and decomposition processes
   d. Fixation does not affect antigenicity

10. **What is the purpose of antigen retrieval in immunohistochemistry?**
    a. To enhance antigen binding to antibodies
    b. To remove non-specific antibodies
    c. To remove excess fixative
    d. To enhance tissue staining

11. **Which property of a fixative is crucial for preserving tissue morphology and cellular structures?**
    a. Antigen retrieval capability
    b. Dehydration ability
    c. Cross-linking ability
    d. High pH level

12. **Which property of a fixative is important for minimizing autolysis and preserving cellular antigens?**
    a. Penetration ability
    b. Rapid fixation speed
    c. Antibacterial properties
    d. Neutral pH level

13. **Which property of a fixative is desirable for preventing tissue shrinkage and hardening?**
    a. High osmolality
    b. Low viscosity
    c. Low osmolality
    d. High viscosity

14. **Which property of a fixative is advantageous for easy handling and storage?**
    a. Compatibility with other reagents
    b. Low cost
    c. Long shelf life
    d. Compatibility with different tissue types

15. **Which property of a fixative is important for maintaining the stability of proteins and enzymes?**
    a. Antimicrobial properties
    b. Neutral pH level
    c. High reactivity
    d. Low reactivity

16. **Which fixative is commonly used for preserving lipid-rich tissues?**
    a. Formalin
    b. Glutaraldehyde
    c. Ethanol
    d. OsO4 (Osmium tetroxide)

17. **Which fixative is used for preserving cytoskeletal components, such as microtubules and intermediate filaments?**
    a. Formalin
    b. Glutaraldehyde
    c. Ethanol
    d. Carnoy's solution

18. **Which fixative is commonly used for rapid frozen section analysis during surgery?**
    a. Formalin
    b. Glutaraldehyde
    c. Ethanol
    d. Liquid nitrogen

Answers: 9. b   10. a   11. c   12. b
            13. c   14. c   15. b   16. d
            17. b   18. d

19. **What should be the ratio between the volume of tissue and the fixative?**
    a. 1:5
    b. 1:10
    c. 1:20
    d. 1:100

20. **What is the usual concentration of the commercial formaldehyde available?**
    a. 17% to 30%
    b. 7% to 10%
    c. 37% to 40%
    d. 45% to 50%

21. **Yellow color of Bouin's fluid is due to the presence of:**
    a. Picric acid
    b. Formalin
    c. Mercury
    d. Chloroform

22. **Zenker's fluid is best for fixation of which tissue biopsy:**
    a. Gastrointestinal biopsy
    b. Spleen
    c. Testicular biopsy
    d. Liver biopsy

23. **What is the purpose of decalcification in histopathology?**
    a. Removal of excess fixative
    b. Preservation of tissue morphology
    c. Removal of calcium deposits from tissues
    d. Enhancement of antigen detection

24. **Which of the following is a commonly used decalcifying agent in histopathology?**
    a. Formalin
    b. Ethanol
    c. Acetic acid
    d. Ethylenediaminetetraacetic acid (EDTA)

25. **Which type of tissue often requires decalcification before histopathological processing?**
    a. Skin
    b. Muscle
    c. Lung
    d. Bone

26. **Which method of decalcification involves the use of acid as the decalcifying agent?**
    a. Chemical decalcification
    b. Physical decalcification
    c. Enzymatic decalcification
    d. Ion exchange decalcification

27. **Which factor affects the duration of decalcification?**
    a. Tissue fixation time
    b. Tissue thickness
    c. Decalcifying agent concentration
    d. Room temperature

28. **Common fixatives for electron microscopy include glutaraldehyde and paraformaldehyde.**
    a. True
    b. False

29. **Which acids are commonly used for acid decalcification?**
    a. Hydrochloric acid (HCl) and acetic acid
    b. Nitric acid and formic acid
    c. Sulfuric acid and phosphoric acid
    d. Hydrochloric acid (HCl) and formic acid

Answers:	19. c	20. c	21. a	22. b
	23. c	24. d	25. d	26. a
	27. c	28. a	29. a	

30. **Which factor affects the duration of acid decalcification?**
    a. Tissue thickness
    b. Acid concentration
    c. Temperature
    d. pH of the solution

31. **What should be monitored during acid decalcification to ensure optimal results?**
    a. pH of the solution
    b. Temperature of the solution
    c. Appearance of the tissue
    d. Odor of the solution

32. **What is the recommended method for neutralizing the acid after decalcification?**
    a. Rinsing with distilled water
    b. Rinsing with alcohol
    c. Immersion in alkaline solution
    d. Immersion in acidic solution

33. **What is the purpose of endpoint decalcification in histopathology?**
    a. Preservation of tissue morphology
    b. Removal of calcium deposits from tissues
    c. Enhancement of antigen detection
    d. Removal of excess fixative

34. **Which method is commonly used for endpoint decalcification?**
    a. Chemical decalcification
    b. Physical decalcification
    c. Enzymatic decalcification
    d. Chelation decalcification

35. **What is the criterion used to determine the endpoint in endpoint decalcification?**
    a. Color change of the decalcifying solution

    b. pH of the decalcifying solution
    c. Time duration of the decalcification process
    d. Hardness of the tissue sample

36. **Which indicator is often used to monitor the progress of endpoint decalcification?**
    a. Methyl red
    b. Bromothymol blue
    c. Alizarin red
    d. Toluidine blue

37. **When is endpoint decalcification typically employed in histopathological processing?**
    a. Before tissue fixation
    b. After tissue fixation
    c. Simultaneously with tissue fixation
    d. Before staining

38. **Which method of decalcification involves the use of chemical agents to remove calcium deposits from tissues?**
    a. Acid decalcification
    b. Physical decalcification
    c. Enzymatic decalcification
    d. Chelation decalcification

39. **Which of the following is an example of physical decalcification?**
    a. Immersion in decalcifying solution
    b. Grinding or milling the tissue
    c. Digestion with enzymes
    d. Treatment with chelating agents

40. **What is the advantage of enzymatic decalcification over other methods?**
    a. Rapid decalcification process
    b. Preservation of tissue morphology
    c. Minimal impact on antigenicity
    d. Ability to remove all types of calcification

Answers:

30. b	31. a	32. a	33. b
34. a	35. a	36. c	37. b
38. a	39. b	40. c	

41. **Which method of decalcification involves the use of chelating agents that bind to calcium ions?**
    a. Acid decalcification
    b. Physical decalcification
    c. Enzymatic decalcification
    d. Chelation decalcification

42. **What is the primary disadvantage of physical decalcification?**
    a. Longer decalcification time
    b. Loss of tissue morphology
    c. Destruction of cellular antigens
    d. Difficulty in removing all calcium deposits

43. **What is the primary purpose of surface decalcification in histopathology?**
    a. Removal of calcium deposits from tissue surfaces
    b. Preservation of tissue morphology
    c. Enhancement of antigen detection
    d. Removal of excess fixative

44. **Which method is commonly used for surface decalcification?**
    a. Acid decalcification
    b. Physical decalcification
    c. Enzymatic decalcification
    d. Chelation decalcification

45. **Which tissues or samples are suitable for surface decalcification?**
    a. Bone sections
    b. Teeth
    c. Calcified plaques
    d. All of the above

46. **What is the typical duration for surface decalcification?**
    a. Several hours
    b. Overnight
    c. Several days
    d. Weeks

47. **What is the recommended method for neutralizing the decalcifying agent after surface decalcification?**
    a. Rinsing with distilled water
    b. Rinsing with alcohol
    c. Immersion in alkaline solution
    d. Immersion in acidic solution

48. **What is the purpose of dehydration in histopathology?**
    a. Removal of excess fixative
    b. Preservation of tissue morphology
    c. Enhancement of antigen detection
    d. Removal of water from tissues

49. **Which common solvent is commonly used for dehydration in histopathology?**
    a. Xylene
    b. Ethanol
    c. Acetone
    d. Chloroform

50. **Which property of the solvent affects the dehydration process?**
    a. Viscosity
    b. Boiling point
    c. pH
    d. Refractive index

51. **What is the typical sequence of increasing concentration of alcohol used in dehydration?**
    a. 70%–80%–90%–100%
    b. 100%–90%–80%–70%
    c. 80%–90%–100%
    d. 100%–80%–70%

52. **What is the purpose of dehydration in relation to the subsequent steps in histopathology?**
    a. To enhance tissue staining
    b. To remove remaining cellular debris
    c. To allow for infiltration of embedding medium
    d. To prevent tissue shrinkage

Answers:

41. d	42. b	43. a	44. b
45. d	46. a	47. a	48. d
49. b	50. a	51. a	52. c

53. **Which dehydration agent is commonly used as an intermediate step between water and the final clearing agent?**
    a. Xylene
    b. Ethanol
    c. Acetone
    d. Chloroform

54. **Which dehydration agent is preferred for delicate tissues or tissues with lipids?**
    a. Xylene
    b. Ethanol
    c. Acetone
    d. Chloroform

55. **Which dehydration agent is commonly used in immunohistochemistry for antigen retrieval?**
    a. Xylene
    b. Ethanol
    c. Acetone
    d. Chloroform

56. **Which factor should be considered when selecting a dehydration agent?**
    a. Cost of the agent
    b. Compatibility with the subsequent steps
    c. Speed of dehydration
    d. Availability of the agent

57. **What is the purpose of clearing in histopathology?**
    a. Removal of excess fixative
    b. Preservation of tissue morphology
    c. Enhancement of antigen detection
    d. Removal of dehydrating agents and rendering tissues transparent

58. **Which common clearing agent is commonly used in histopathology?**
    a. Xylene
    b. Ethanol
    c. Acetone
    d. Chloroform

59. **Which property of the clearing agent is important for rendering tissues transparent?**
    a. High refractive index
    b. Low viscosity
    c. High boiling point
    d. Low volatility

60. **What is the typical sequence of clearing agents used in histopathology?**
    a. Xylene–Ethanol–Acetone
    b. Acetone–Xylene–Ethanol
    c. Ethanol–Xylene–Acetone
    d. Ethanol–Acetone–Xylene

61. **What is the purpose of clearing in relation to the subsequent steps in histopathology?**
    a. To enhance tissue staining
    b. To remove remaining cellular debris
    c. To allow for infiltration of embedding medium
    d. To prevent tissue shrinkage

62. **Which clearing agent is known for its high refractive index and ability to render tissues transparent?**
    a. Xylene
    b. Ethanol
    c. Acetone
    d. Chloroform

63. **Which clearing agent is commonly used for delicate tissues or tissues with lipids?**
    a. Xylene
    b. Ethanol
    c. Acetone
    d. Chloroform

64. **Which clearing agent is commonly used for immunohistochemistry staining?**
    a. Xylene
    b. Ethanol
    c. Acetone
    d. Chloroform

Answers:

53. a	54. c	55. c	56. b
57. d	58. a	59. a	60. d
61. c	62. a	63. c	64. a

65. Which factor should be considered when selecting a clearing agent?
a. Cost of the agent
b. Compatibility with subsequent steps
c. Speed of clearing
d. Availability of the agent

66. What is the purpose of impregnation in histopathology?
a. Removal of excess fixative
b. Preservation of tissue morphology
c. Enhancement of antigen detection
d. Replacement of clearing agents with an infiltrating medium

67. Which common impregnating medium is commonly used in histopathology?
a. Paraffin wax   b. Acetone
c. Ethanol   d. Xylene

68. Which property of the impregnating medium is important for its penetration into the tissue?
a. High refractive index
b. Low viscosity
c. High boiling point
d. Low volatility

69. What is the typical sequence of impregnation steps used in histopathology?
a. Impregnation–Embedding–Sectioning
b. Embedding–Impregnation–Sectioning
c. Sectioning–Impregnation–Embedding
d. Embedding–Sectioning–Impregnation

70. What is the purpose of impregnation in relation to the subsequent steps in histopathology?
a. To enhance tissue staining
b. To remove remaining cellular debris
c. To provide structural support for sectioning
d. To prevent tissue shrinkage

71. Which property of the embedding medium is important for its solidification and stability?
a. High refractive index
b. Low viscosity
c. High boiling point
d. High melting point

72. Which of the following is a commonly used embedding medium in histopathology?
a. Paraffin wax   b. Acetone
c. Ethanol   d. Xylene

73. Which property of the embedding medium is important for sectioning thin and consistent tissue sections?
a. High refractive index
b. Low viscosity
c. High boiling point
d. High melting point

74. What is the primary advantage of using paraffin wax as an embedding medium?
a. It provides excellent tissue support and sectioning quality
b. It allows for easy removal of excess fixative
c. It enhances antigen detection in immunohistochemistry
d. It prevents tissue shrinkage during sectioning

Answers: 65. **b**   66. **d**   67. **a**   68. **b**
            69. **a**   70. **c**   71. **d**   72. **a**
            73. **b**   74. **a**

75. Which factor should be considered when selecting an embedding medium?
a. Cost of the medium
b. Compatibility with subsequent steps
c. Availability of the medium
d. Viscosity of the medium

76. What is the primary purpose of using paraffin wax in histopathology?
a. Preservation of tissue morphology
b. Enhancement of antigen detection
c. Removal of excess fixative
d. Facilitation of tissue sectioning

77. What is the typical melting point range of paraffin wax used in histopathology?
a. 10–20°C
b. 40–50°C
c. 55–65°C
d. 90–100°C

78. How is paraffin wax typically melted and maintained in a liquid state during embedding?
a. Heating on a hot plate
b. Use of a water bath
c. Use of a microwave oven
d. Use of an open flame

79. What is the purpose of embedding molds in histopathology?
a. Preservation of tissue morphology
b. Enhancement of antigen detection
c. Shaping and holding the embedding medium
d. Removal of excess fixative

80. Which material is commonly used for embedding molds in histopathology?
a. Plastic
b. Glass
c. Metal
d. Silicone

81. What is the advantage of using disposable plastic embedding molds?
a. The are cost-effective and reduce contamination risks
b. They provide better heat conductivity for uniform cooling
c. They are reusable and more durable than other materials
d. They are resistant to embedding medium infiltration

82. How are tissue samples placed in embedding molds during the embedding process?
a. Upside down
b. Random orientation
c. Specific orientation
d. Placed in a separate cassette

83. Which factor should be considered when selecting embedding molds?
a. Cost of the molds
b. Compatibility with the embedding medium
c. Availability of the molds
d. Heat resistance of the molds

84. Why is the orientation of tissue important during the embedding process in histopathology?
a. To ensure even distribution of staining agents
b. To maintain consistency in tissue sectioning
c. To prevent tissue shrinkage during sectioning
d. To enhance antigen detection

Answers:

75. b	76. d	77. c	78. b
79. c	80. a	81. a	82. c
83. b	84. b		

85. **Which orientation is commonly used for embedding tissues with a specific anatomical structure?**
    a. Random orientation
    b. Longitudinal orientation
    c. Cross-sectional orientation
    d. Upside-down orientation

86. **In which situation is random orientation of tissue preferred during embedding?**
    a. When specific tissue structures need to be preserved
    b. When tissue orientation is not crucial for analysis
    c. When precise sectioning along a particular plane is required
    d. When tissue is too large to fit in the embedding mold

87. **What is the recommended orientation for embedding a tube-like tissue specimen, such as a blood vessel or a gastrointestinal tract section?**
    a. Random orientation
    b. Longitudinal orientation
    c. Cross-sectional orientation
    d. Upside-down orientation

88. **Why is cross-sectional orientation preferred for tube-like tissue specimens during embedding?**
    a. It allows for better visualization of tissue layers and structures
    b. It ensures consistent sectioning along the long axis of the tissue
    c. It helps in preserving the three-dimensional shape of the tissue
    d. It reduces tissue compression during embedding

89. **What is the recommended orientation for embedding a skin biopsy specimen?**
    a. Random orientation
    b. Longitudinal orientation
    c. Cross-sectional orientation
    d. Upside-down orientation

90. **Why is cross-sectional orientation not commonly used for skin biopsy specimens during embedding?**
    a. It can disrupt the natural alignment of skin layers
    b. It hinders the visualization of epidermal and dermal structures
    c. It results in inconsistent sectioning of the tissue
    d. It leads to tissue distortion during embedding

91. **What can be done to ensure proper orientation of tube and skin biopsy specimens during embedding?**
    a. Using embedding molds with specific orientations
    b. Marking the tissue with ink or dyes before embedding
    c. Embedding tissues within a supporting medium
    d. Using specialized embedding cassettes

92. **What is the primary purpose of automated tissue processors in histopathology?**
    a. Preservation of tissue morphology
    b. Enhancement of antigen detection
    c. Removal of excess fixative
    d. Streamlining and standardization of tissue processing steps

Answers: 85. c   86. b   87. c   88. a
          89. b   90. b   91. b   92. d

93. **Which component of an automated tissue processor is responsible for fluid circulation and exchange?**
    a. Vacuum system
    b. Reagent containers
    c. Agitation mechanism
    d. Temperature control unit

94. **How does an automated tissue processor facilitate consistent and reproducible tissue processing?**
    a. By maintaining optimal temperature and timing parameters
    b. By allowing manual adjustments for each processing step
    c. By reducing the use of reagents and optimizing cost-effectiveness
    d. By eliminating the need for fixation and dehydration steps

95. **What is the advantage of using an automated tissue processor over manual processing methods?**
    a. Increased flexibility and customization of processing protocols
    b. Decreased processing time and improved turnaround time
    c. Lower overall cost and reduced instrument maintenance
    d. Enhanced quality of tissue sections and staining results

96. **How are reagents typically delivered and exchanged in an automated tissue processor?**
    a. Through manual pipetting by the operator
    b. Through pre-filled disposable cartridges or cassettes
    c. Through a separate reagent mixing and dispensing system
    d. Through a direct connection to reagent storage containers

97. **The tissue processing unit is also known as:**
    a. Histotech
    b. Histokinette
    c. Histoform
    d. Microtome

98. **What are the qualities of a good clearing agent?**
    a. Can dissolve lipids
    b. Is able to impede wax penetration
    c. Both a and b
    d. None

99. **What is the purpose of section cutting in histopathology?**
    a. Removal of excess fixative
    b. Preservation of tissue morphology
    c. Enhancement of antigen detection
    d. Preparation of thin tissue sections for microscopic examination

100. **Which instrument is commonly used for section cutting in histopathology?**
    a. Microtome
    b. Centrifuge
    c. Incubator
    d. Autoclave

101. **Which type of microtome is commonly used for routine section cutting in histopathology?**
    a. Rotary microtome
    b. Vibrating microtome
    c. Cryostat microtome
    d. Ultramicrotome

102. **What is the ideal thickness range for routine tissue sections in histopathology?**
    a. 3–5 micrometers
    b. 10–20 micrometers
    c. 50–100 micrometers
    d. 200–500 micrometers

Answers:

93. c	94. a	95. b	96. b
97. b	98. c	99. d	100. a
101. a	102. a		

103. **What should be considered when selecting the cutting speed during sectioning?**
    a. Tissue fixation time
    b. Tissue thickness
    c. Tissue type and consistency
    d. Room temperature

104. **What is the principle of operation for a rotary microtome?**
    a. Tissue sections are cut using a vibrating blade
    b. Tissue sections are cut using a diamond knife
    c. Tissue sections are cut using a rotating knife edge
    d. Tissue sections are cut using a freezing mechanism

105. **Which component of a microtome allows for adjustment of section thickness?**
    a. Knife holder
    b. Specimen clamp
    c. Feed mechanism
    d. Elevation mechanism

106. **How is sectioning accuracy maintained during microtome operation?**
    a. Regular calibration of the microtome
    b. Selection of cutting speed
    c. Operator's experience and skill
    d. Application of anti-static solutions

107. **Which type of microtome is specifically designed for cutting frozen tissue sections?**
    a. Rotary microtome
    b. Vibrating microtome
    c. Cryostat microtome
    d. Ultramicrotome

108. **Which type of microtome is used for sectioning hard and difficult-to-cut specimens, such as bone or teeth?**
    a. Rotary microtome
    b. Vibrating microtome
    c. Cryostat microtome
    d. Ultramicrotome

109. **Which type of microtome is used for cutting ultra-thin sections for electron microscopy?**
    a. Rotary microtome
    b. Vibrating microtome
    c. Cryostat microtome
    d. Ultramicrotome

110. **Which type of microtome is commonly used for sectioning soft and delicate specimens, such as brain or liver?**
    a. Rotary microtome
    b. Vibrating microtome
    c. Cryostat microtome
    d. Ultramicrotome

111. **What is the primary purpose of microtome blades in histopathology?**
    a. Preservation of tissue morphology
    b. Enhancement of antigen detection
    c. Removal of excess fixative
    d. Cutting of thin tissue sections during sectioning

112. **Which type of microtome blade is commonly used for routine section cutting in histopathology?**
    a. Disposable blades
    b. Cryostat blades
    c. Glass knives
    d. Tungsten carbide blades

Answers: 103. c   104. c   105. c   106. a
107. c   108. a   109. d   110. b
111. d   112. a

113. What is the advantage of using disposable microtome blades?
a. Superior cutting quality and precision
b. Cost-effectiveness and ease of replacement
c. Longevity and durability
d. Compatibility with all types of microtomes

114. Which microtome blade type is commonly used for cutting hard and difficult-to-cut specimens, such as bone or teeth?
a. Disposable blades
b. Diamond blades
c. Glass knives
d. Tungsten carbide blades

115. How often should microtome blades be replaced to ensure optimal cutting performance?
a. After every use
b. After every 10 uses
c. After every 50 uses
d. After every 100 uses

116. What is the purpose of honing microtome blades?
a. Preservation of tissue morphology
b. Enhancement of antigen detection
c. Removal of excess fixative
d. Restoration of blade sharpness and cutting efficiency

117. What does honing involve in the context of microtome blades?
a. Cleaning the blade with solvents
b. Grinding the blade to a finer edge
c. Adjusting the blade angle for optimal cutting
d. Replacing the blade with a new one

118. How does honing affect the cutting performance of microtome blades?
a. It increases the lifespan of the blade.
b. It improves the sectioning quality and precision
c. It reduces the risk of tissue artifacts during cutting
d. It enhances the compatibility of the blade with various microtomes

119. Which tool is commonly used for honing microtome blades?
a. Diamond knife
b. Glass knife
c. Honing stone or strop
d. Tissue adhesive

120. What is the purpose of stropping microtome blades?
a. Preservation of tissue morphology
b. Enhancement of antigen detection
c. Removal of excess fixative
d. Polishing the blade edge and enhancing cutting performance

121. What does stropping involve in the context of microtome blades?
a. Cleaning the blade with solvents
b. Grinding the blade to a finer edge
c. Aligning the blade angle for optimal cutting
d. Polishing the blade edge with a strop or leather

122. How does stropping affect the cutting performance of microtome blades?
a. It increases the lifespan of the blade
b. It improves the sectioning quality and precision
c. It reduces the risk of tissue artefacts during cutting
d. It enhances the compatibility of the blade with various microtomes

Answers: 113. b 114. b 115. c 116. d
117. b 118. b 119. c 120. d
121. d 122. b

123. **What material is commonly used for stropping microtome blades?**
    a. Diamond
    b. Glass
    c. Metal
    d. Leather or fabric strop

124. **How often should microtome blades be stropped to maintain optimal cutting efficiency?**
    a. After every use
    b. After every ten uses
    c. After every 50 uses
    d. After every 100 uses

125. **What is the primary purpose of a water bath in histopathology?**
    a. Preservation of tissue morphology
    b. Enhancement of antigen detection
    c. Removal of excess fixative
    d. Temperature-controlled incubation and specimen processing

126. **How does a water bath facilitate temperature control during histopathological procedures?**
    a. It uses hot air to heat the specimens
    b. It circulates cold water to cool the specimens
    c. It maintains a constant temperature using heated water
    d. It monitors and adjusts humidity levels during processing

127. **Which histopathological procedure commonly utilizes a water bath?**
    a. Tissue embedding
    b. Section cutting
    c. Immunohistochemistry staining
    d. Tissue fixation

128. **Which equipment is commonly used for temperature control during section cutting in histopathology?**
    a. Hot plate
    b. Water bath
    c. Centrifuge
    d. Incubator

129. **How does a hot plate facilitate temperature control during section cutting?**
    a. It circulates hot water to maintain a constant temperature
    b. It provides a heated surface for warming the sections
    c. It generates hot air for drying the sections
    d. It cools the sections quickly after cutting

130. **What is the primary advantage of using a hot plate in section cutting?**
    a. Precise temperature control for optimal cutting conditions
    b. Prevention of tissue loss during cutting
    c. Reduction of tissue compression during sectioning
    d. Enhanced tissue morphology preservation

131. **Which equipment is commonly used for keeping water at a specific temperature during section cutting?**
    a. Hot plate
    b. Water bath
    c. Centrifuge
    d. Incubator

Answers: 123. d   124. b   125. d   126. c
127. a   128. b   129. b   130. a
131. b

132. How does a water bath facilitate section cutting?
a. It provides a heated surface for warming the sections
b. It cools the sections quickly after cutting
c. It ensures the sections remain hydrated during cutting
d. It generates hot air for drying the sections

133. Temperature of water bath is maintained at:
a. 5° below the melting point of paraffin wax
b. 5° above the melting point of paraffin wax
c. 10° below the melting point of paraffin wax
d. 10° below the melting point of paraffin wax

134. Temperature of hot plate is maintained at:
a. 5° below the melting point of paraffin wax
b. 5° above the melting point of paraffin wax
c. 10° below the melting point of paraffin wax
d. 10° below the melting point of paraffin wax

135. What is the purpose of using section adhesives in histopathology?
a. Preservation of tissue morphology
b. Enhancement of antigen detection
c. Removal of excess fixative
d. Attachment of tissue sections to slides for staining

136. Which type of section adhesive is commonly used in histopathology?
a. Glue
b. Tape
c. Albumin
d. Charged slides

137. How does a section adhesive facilitate the attachment of tissue sections to slides?
a. It helps in preventing tissue detachment during staining procedures
b. It enhances tissue morphology preservation during sectioning
c. It reduces tissue compression during embedding
d. It improves antigen accessibility for immunohistochemistry

138. What is the advantage of using a charged slide as a section adhesive?
a. It provides a strong and permanent attachment of tissue sections
b. It enhances the quality of staining results
c. It allows for easy removal of excess fixative
d. It improves sectioning quality and precision

139. How should section adhesives be applied to slides for optimal results?
a. Apply a thin and even layer across the slide surface
b. Apply the adhesive only to the edges of the slide
c. Apply a thick layer to ensure strong tissue attachment
d. Apply the adhesive after sectioning is complete

Answers: 132. c   133. a   134. b   135. d
136. c   137. a   138. b   139. a

140. **What is the purpose of staining in histopathology?**
a. Preservation of tissue morphology
b. Enhancement of antigen detection
c. Removal of excess fixative
d. Visualization and differentiation of tissue components

141. **Which type of staining is commonly used to visualize the nuclei of cells?**
a. Hematoxylin staining
b. Eosin staining
c. Masson's trichrome staining
d. Periodic acid-Schiff (PAS) staining

142. **What is the purpose of counterstaining in histopathological staining?**
a. To increase the intensity of the primary stain
b. To differentiate specific tissue components
c. To remove excess fixative from the tissue
d. To provide contrast and enhance the visualization of the primary stain

143. **Which staining technique is commonly used for highlighting collagen fibers in tissue sections?**
a. Hematoxylin and eosin (H&E) staining
b. Periodic acid-Schiff (PAS) staining
c. Masson's trichrome staining
d. Giemsa staining

144. **How can the staining intensity be controlled during the staining process?**
a. By adjusting the staining time
b. By increasing the temperature of the staining solution
c. By diluting the staining reagents
d. By changing the pH of the staining solution

145. **Which staining technique is commonly used to differentiate acidophilic and basophilic cellular components?**
a. Hematoxylin and eosin (H&E) staining
b. Giemsa staining
c. Silver staining
d. Alcian blue staining

146. **Which staining technique is commonly used to detect carbohydrates and glycogen in tissues?**
a. Hematoxylin and eosin (H&E) staining
b. Periodic acid-Schiff (PAS) staining
c. Masson's trichrome staining
d. Giemsa staining

147. **Which staining technique is commonly used to identify microorganisms, such as bacteria or parasites, in tissue sections?**
a. Hematoxylin and eosin (H&E) staining
b. Giemsa staining
c. Immunohistochemical staining
d. Alcian blue staining

Answers: 140. d 141. a 142. d 143. c
144. a 145. a 146. b 147. b

148. **What is the purpose of vital staining in histopathology?**
    a. Preservation of tissue morphology
    b. Enhancement of antigen detection
    c. Visualization of living cells or tissues
    d. Removal of excess fixative

149. **How does vital staining differ from routine histological staining techniques?**
    a. Vital staining requires fixation of the tissue
    b. Vital staining uses non-toxic stains that do not damage living cells
    c. Vital staining involves multiple steps and longer staining times
    d. Vital staining is used only for specific cellular components

150. **What is the purpose of supravital staining in histopathology?**
    a. Preservation of tissue morphology
    b. Enhancement of antigen detection
    c. Visualization of intracellular components in living cells
    d. Removal of excess fixative

151. **Which of the following is the example of vital stain?**
    a. Toluidine blue
    b. Propidium Iodide
    c. Trypan blue
    d. All of the above

152. **Which of the following is the example of supravital stain?**
    a. Brilliant cresyl blue
    b. New methylene blue
    c. Crystal violet
    d. All of the above

153. **What is the underlying principle of metachromatic staining?**
    a. Differential uptake of stains by various cellular components
    b. Utilization of fluorescence microscopy for visualization
    c. Conversion of dyes into different colors by cellular components
    d. Binding of dyes to specific antigens

154. **Which type of cellular components often exhibit metachromasia in metachromatic staining?**
    a. Nuclei
    b. Cytoplasm
    c. Cell membranes
    d. Connective tissue elements, such as mucopolysaccharides

155. **Which dye is commonly used for metachromatic staining?**
    a. Hematoxylin   b. Eosin
    c. Alcian blue   d. Giemsa

156. **How does metachromatic staining appear under the microscope?**
    a. Components of interest appear in the same color as the dye
    b. Components of interest appear in a contrasting color to the dye
    c. Components of interest appear as fluorescent signals
    d. Components of interest appear colorless

157. **All of these are nucleic acid stains, *except:***
    a. Ethidium bromide
    b. SYBR green
    c. Propidium iodide
    d. Safranin

Answers: 148. c   149. b   150. c   151. d
152. d   153. a   154. d   155. c
156. b   157. d

158. Stains can also be classified based on the chemical nature of the dye. Which type of stain involves the use of synthetic dyes that contain chromophores?
  a. Basic stains
  b. Acidic stains
  c. Metachromatic stains
  d. Differential stains

159. Stains can be classified based on their application in specific staining techniques. Which type of stain is commonly used in immunohistochemistry to detect specific antigens?
  a. Basic stains
  b. Acidic stains
  c. Metachromatic stains
  d. Immunostains

160. Which type of stain is commonly used to visualize cell nuclei?
  a. Hematoxylin stain
  b. Eosin stain
  c. Acidic stain
  d. Basic stain

161. What is the primary purpose of nuclear staining in histopathology?
  a. To enhance the visualization of cytoplasmic structures
  b. To differentiate specific cell types
  c. To highlight the presence of nucleoli
  d. To assess the proliferation rate of cells

162. Which stain is commonly used as a nuclear counterstain in hematoxylin and eosin (H&E) staining?
  a. Hematoxylin stain
  b. Eosin stain
  c. Acidic stain
  d. Basic stain

163. Which type of stain is commonly used to visualize cytoplasmic components?
  a. Hematoxylin stain
  b. Eosin stain
  c. Acidic stain
  d. Basic stain

164. How do nuclear and cytoplasmic stains differ in terms of color?
  a. Nuclear stains are typically blue, while cytoplasmic stains are pink/red
  b. Nuclear stains are typically pink/red, while cytoplasmic stains are blue
  c. Both nuclear and cytoplasmic stains are typically blue
  d. Both nuclear and cytoplasmic stains are typically pink/red

165. What is the primary difference between forward staining and reverse staining?
  a. The order in which different stains are applied to the specimen
  b. The specific cellular components targeted by the stains
  c. The use of different types of dyes in each staining technique
  d. The staining method used (e.g., immersion staining versus contact staining)

166. In forward staining, which stain is typically applied first to the specimen?
  a. Basic stain
  b. Acidic stain
  c. Metachromatic stain
  d. Immunostain

Answers: 158. a   159. d   160. a   161. c
162. a   163. b   164. a   165. a
166. a

167. In reverse staining, which stain is typically applied first to the specimen?
a. Basic stain
b. Acidic stain
c. Metachromatic stain
d. Immunostain

168. What is the purpose of using a mordant in staining?
a. To enhance the staining intensity of the dye
b. To remove excess fixative from the specimen
c. To preserve tissue morphology during staining
d. To prevent fading of the stain over time

169. What is the role of a mordant in the Gram staining technique?
a. It acts as a counterstain to differentiate gram-positive and gram-negative bacteria
b. It enhances the penetration of the primary stain into the bacterial cell wall
c. It fixes the dye onto the bacterial cells, making the stain more permanent
d. It neutralizes the effect of the decolorizing agent in the staining process

170. The commonly used mordant in the Gomori's trichrome staining for connective tissue fibers is:
a. Lugol's iodine
b. Ferric chloride
c. Copper sulfate
d. Sodium thiosulfate

171. How does a mordant work in the staining process?
a. It forms a complex with the dye, increasing its affinity to the target
b. It acts as a solvent, dissolving excess stain from the tissue
c. It fixes the dye onto the tissue, preventing its leaching during subsequent steps
d. It enhances the contrast between different tissue components

172. What is the consequence of inadequate mordanting in staining?
a. Reduced staining intensity and poor visualization of the target
b. Excessive staining intensity, leading to tissue artifacts
c. Loss of tissue morphology and cellular details
d. Ineffective removal of excess fixative, affecting subsequent steps of staining

173. Which mordant is commonly used in the Gram staining technique?
a. Iodine
b. Ferric chloride
c. Copper sulfate
d. Sodium thiosulfate

174. Which mordant is commonly used in the Schmorl's stain for demonstrating hemosiderin deposits?
a. Iodine
b. Ferric chloride
c. Copper sulfate
d. Sodium thiosulfate

Answers: 167. b	**168. a**	**169. c**	**170. c**
171. a	**172. a**	**173. a**	**174. b**

175. **Which mordant is commonly used in the Mallory's trichrome stain for collagen fibers?**
   a. Iodine
   b. Ferric chloride
   c. Copper sulfate
   d. Sodium thiosulfate

176. **Which mordant is commonly used in the periodic acid-Schiff (PAS) staining technique?**
   a. Iodine
   b. Ferric chloride
   c. Copper sulfate
   d. Sodium thiosulfate

177. **What is the purpose of bluing in staining?**
   a. To enhance the staining intensity of the dye
   b. To remove excess fixative from the specimen
   c. To change the soluble reddish-purple hematoxylin into an insoluble blue components
   d. To preserve tissue morphology during staining

178. **Which commonly used reagent is used for bluing in hematoxylin staining?**
   a. Ammonia water
   b. Hydrochloric acid
   c. Sodium hydroxide
   d. Ethanol

179. **How does bluing affect the staining of nuclei in histopathology?**
   a. It intensifies the nuclear staining
   b. It reduces the nuclear staining
   c. It changes the color of the nuclear stain
   d. It has no effect on the nuclear staining

180. **What is the consequence of inadequate bluing in staining?**
   a. Overly intense staining, leading to tissue artifacts
   b. Insufficient contrast and poor visualization of the target
   c. Loss of tissue morphology and cellular details
   d. Ineffective removal of excess fixative, affecting subsequent steps of staining

181. **What is the recommended bluing time during staining procedures?**
   a. 1–2 minutes
   b. 5–10 minutes
   c. 15–30 minutes
   d. 60–90 minutes

182. **Which of the following statement is false regarding hematoxylin?**
   a. Hematoxylin is a synthetic dye
   b. It is derived from heartwood of Haematoxylum campechianum
   c. Hematoxylin selectively binds to acidic structures in tissues, particularly DNA and RNA in cell nuclei
   d. Hematein can be extracted from hematoxylin by a process called oxidation

183. **Hematoxylin is commonly used in histopathology as a staining agent. What is the purpose of oxidizing hematoxylin?**
   a. To enhance its stability and shelf life
   b. To increase its solubility in staining solutions
   c. To convert it into its active form for staining
   d. To remove impurities and contaminants

Answers: 175. b   176. d   177. c   178. a
179. a   180. b   181. b   182. a
183. c

184. What is the common oxidizing agent used to convert hematoxylin into its active form?
a. Hydrogen peroxide
b. Potassium permanganate
c. Sodium hydroxide
d. Acetic acid

185. What is the color of oxidized hematoxylin?
a. Red   b. Blue
c. Purple   d. Colorless

186. How does oxidation affect the staining properties of hematoxylin?
a. Oxidation increases the affinity of hematoxylin for specific tissue components
b. Oxidation reduces the affinity of hematoxylin for specific tissue components
c. Oxidation changes the color of the stained tissue
d. Oxidation has no significant effect on the staining properties

187. Which factor can be adjusted to control the oxidation process of hematoxylin?
a. Concentration of the oxidizing agent
b. Temperature of the oxidation reaction
c. Duration of the oxidation process
d. All of the above

188. Hematoxylin staining in histopathology can be achieved using different types of hematoxylin solutions. Which type of hematoxylin is commonly used in routine histological staining?
a. Harris hematoxylin
b. Mayer's hematoxylin
c. Ehrlich's hematoxylin
d. Weigert's hematoxylin

189. Which type of hematoxylin is often used for staining nuclear details and counterstaining in H&E staining?
a. Harris hematoxylin
b. Mayer's hematoxylin
c. Ehrlich's hematoxylin
d. Weigert's hematoxylin

190. Which type of hematoxylin is commonly used for staining connective tissue fibers, such as collagen?
a. Harris hematoxylin
b. Mayer's hematoxylin
c. Ehrlich's hematoxylin
d. Weigert's hematoxylin

191. Which type of hematoxylin is used in specific staining techniques for demonstrating elastic fibers?
a. Harris hematoxylin
b. Mayer's hematoxylin
c. Ehrlich's hematoxylin
d. Weigert's hematoxylin

192. Which factor can be adjusted to control the staining intensity and differentiation of hematoxylin staining?
a. Staining time
b. pH of the staining solution
c. Concentration of the hematoxylin solution
d. All of the above

Answers:	184. a	185. b	186. a	187. d
	188. b	189. a	190. d	191. d
	192. d			

193. Hematoxylin and eosin (H&E) stain is a widely used staining technique in histopathology. Which component of the tissue does hematoxylin primarily stain?
   a. Nuclei
   b. Cytoplasm
   c. Collagen fibers
   d. Red blood cells

194. Eosin is the counterstain used in H&E staining. Which component of the tissue does eosin primarily stain?
   a. Nuclei
   b. Cytoplasm
   c. Collagen fibers
   d. Red blood cells

195. What is the color of nuclei after staining with hematoxylin in H&E staining?
   a. Blue
   b. Red
   c. Pink
   d. Purple

196. What is the color of cytoplasm after staining with eosin in H&E staining?
   a. Blue
   b. Red
   c. Pink
   d. Purple

197. How does the combination of hematoxylin and eosin staining aid in histopathological analysis?
   a. It provides information about the presence of microorganisms
   b. It helps differentiate between various cell types
   c. It enhances the visibility of collagen fibers
   d. It allows for the detection of specific antigens

198. How does the staining intensity of hematoxylin affect tissue visualization?
   a. Darker staining intensity enhances tissue visibility
   b. Lighter staining intensity enhances tissue visibility
   c. Staining intensity does not significantly affect tissue visibility
   d. Staining intensity affects the color of the tissue components

199. Which factor influences the staining affinity and intensity of hematoxylin?
   a. pH of the staining solution
   b. Staining time
   c. Temperature of the staining solution
   d. All of the above

200. All of these are alum hematoxylin, *except:*
   a. Harris hematoxylin
   b. Mayer hematoxylin
   c. Heidenhain's hematoxylin
   d. Cole's hematoxylin

201. Sodium iodate is used as an oxidizing agent in which hematoxylin?
   a. Harris hematoxylin
   b. Mayer hematoxylin
   c. Delafield's hematoxylin
   d. Cole's hematoxylin

202. All of the following act as mordants for hematoxylin, *except:*
   a. Copper
   b. Potash alum
   c. Iron
   d. Iodine

Answers: 193. a   194. b   195. a   196. c
         197. b   198. a   199. d   200. c
         201. b   202. d

203. **What is the first step in the H&E staining procedure?**
a. Deparaffinization of the tissue sections
b. Fixation of the tissue sections
c. Washing the tissue sections with water
d. Application of eosin stain

204. **Which stain is applied after the hematoxylin stain in the H&E staining procedure?**
a. Eosin stain
b. Acid fuchsin stain
c. Fast green stain
d. Safranin stain

205. **After applying the hematoxylin stain, what is the next step in the H&E staining procedure?**
a. Differentiation
b. Bluing
c. Dehydration
d. Counterstaining with eosin

206. **What is the purpose of bluing in the H&E staining procedure?**
a. To enhance the nuclear staining with hematoxylin
b. To remove excess eosin stain from the tissue sections
c. To increase the contrast between different tissue components
d. To dehydrate the tissue sections

207. **What is the final step in the H&E staining procedure?**
a. Mounting the stained sections with a coverslip
b. Washing the stained sections with water

c. Applying a clearing agent to remove excess stain
d. Performing a dehydration step

208. **Which stain is commonly used for the visualization of carbohydrates in histopathology?**
a. Periodic acid-Schiff (PAS) stain
b. Hematoxylin stain
c. Eosin stain
d. Giemsa stain

209. **What is the underlying principle of the Periodic acid-Schiff (PAS) stain?**
a. Selective binding of the stain to carbohydrates
b. Utilization of fluorescence microscopy for visualization
c. Conversion of the stain into a different color by carbohydrates
d. Generation of contrast through differential solubility of carbohydrates

210. **How do carbohydrates appear after staining with the Periodic acid-Schiff (PAS) stain?**
a. Blue
b. Red
c. Purple
d. Pink

211. **What is the purpose of diastase digestion in the Periodic acid-Schiff (PAS) stain?**
a. To enhance the visualization of carbohydrates
b. To remove excess stain from the tissue
c. To block the staining of carbohydrates
d. To facilitate the binding of the stain to carbohydrates

Answers: **203.** a **204.** a **205.** b **206.** a
207. a **208.** a **209.** a **210.** d
211. c

212. **Besides the Periodic acid-Schiff (PAS) stain, which stain is commonly used to visualize glycogen specifically?**
   a. Alcian blue
   b. Alizarin red
   c. Masson's trichrome
   d. Periodic acid-thiosemicarbazide-silver proteinate (PATAg)

213. **Alcian blue staining is commonly used for the visualization of which type of tissue component?**
   a. Nuclei
   b. Cytoplasm
   c. Glycosaminoglycans (GAGs)
   d. Collagen fibers

214. **What is the underlying principle of Alcian blue staining?**
   a. Selective binding of the stain to nuclei
   b. Utilization of fluorescence microscopy for visualization
   c. Binding of the stain to GAGs through electrostatic interactions
   d. Conversion of the stain into a different color by GAGs

215. **How do GAGs appear after staining with Alcian blue?**
   a. Blue
   b. Red
   c. Purple
   d. Pink

216. **Which pH is commonly used for the staining solution in Alcian blue staining?**
   a. Acidic pH
   b. Neutral pH
   c. Alkaline pH
   d. It varies depending on the target tissue component

217. **Besides Alcian blue, which stain is commonly used in combination to distinguish neutral mucins from acid mucins?**
   a. Hematoxylin
   b. Eosin
   c. Periodic acid-Schiff (PAS)
   d. Masson's trichrome

218. **Mucicarmine staining is commonly used to visualize which type of tissue component?**
   a. Nuclei
   b. Cytoplasm
   c. Mucin
   d. Collagen fibers

219. **What is the underlying principle of mucicarmine staining?**
   a. Selective binding of the stain to nuclei
   b. Utilization of fluorescence microscopy for visualization
   c. Binding of the stain to mucin through chelation
   d. Conversion of the stain into a different color by mucin

220. **How does mucin appear after staining with mucicarmine?**
   a. Blue
   b. Red
   c. Purple
   d. Pink

221. **Which component of the mucicarmine staining solution is responsible for staining mucin?**
   a. Carmine
   b. Hematoxylin
   c. Periodic acid
   d. Sodium metabisulfite

Answers: 212. d   213. c   214. c   215. a
216. a   217. c   218. c   219. c
220. b   221. a

222. Besides mucicarmine which stain is commonly used to demonstrate mucin?
a. Periodic acid-Schiff (PAS)
b. Alcian blue
c. Both of the above
d. None of the above

223. Van Gieson staining is commonly used to visualize which type of tissue component?
a. Nuclei
b. Cytoplasm
c. Collagen fibers
d. Glycogen

224. What is the underlying principle of Van Gieson staining?
a. Selective binding of the stain to nuclei
b. Utilization of fluorescence microscopy for visualization
c. Binding of the stain to collagen fibers
d. Conversion of the stain into a different color by specific tissue components

225. How do collagen fibers appear after staining with Van Gieson?
a. Blue
b. Red
c. Purple
d. Pink

226. Which components are used in the Van Gieson staining solution?
a. Acid fuchsin and picric acid
b. Hematoxylin and eosin
c. Alcian blue and periodic acid
d. Methylene blue and safranin

227. Besides collagen fibers, which tissue component is also stained by Van Gieson?
a. Nuclei
b. Cytoplasm
c. Elastic fibers
d. Glycogen

228. Which hematoxylin is used in Van Gieson staining?
a. Harris hematoxylin
b. Mayer's hematoxylin
c. Cole's hematoxylin
d. Weigert's hematoxylin

229. Which stain is commonly used to visualize collagen fibers in connective tissue?
a. Masson's trichrome stain
b. Periodic acid-Schiff (PAS) stain
c. Alizarin red stain
d. Toluidine blue stain

230. Masson's trichrome stain is a widely used staining technique for connective tissue. What are the colors of collagen fibers and muscle fibers, respectively, in Masson's trichrome stain?
a. Collagen fibers: Blue; Muscle fibers: Red
b. Collagen fibers: Red; Muscle fibers: Blue
c. Collagen fibers: Purple; Muscle fibers: Green
d. Collagen fibers: Green; Muscle fibers: Purple

231. Which stain is commonly used to visualize elastic fibers in connective tissue?
a. Van Gieson stain
b. Verhoeff's stain
c. Alcian blue stain
d. Wright-Giemsa stain

Answers: 222. c   223. c   224. c   225. b
226. a   227. c   228. d   229. a
230. a   231. b

232. What is the underlying principle of Verhoeff's stain for elastic fibers?
a. Selective binding of the stain to elastic fibers
b. Utilization of fluorescence microscopy for visualization
c. Oxidation of elastic fibers for enhanced visibility
d. Conversion of the stain into a different color by elastic fibers

233. Which stain is commonly used to visualize reticular fibers in connective tissue?
a. Periodic acid-Schiff (PAS) stain
b. Gomori's silver stain
c. Congo red stain
d. Alcian blue stain

234. Which stain is commonly used to visualize amyloid deposits in histopathology?
a. Congo red stain
b. Hematoxylin stain
c. Eosin stain
d. Masson's trichrome stain

235. What is the characteristic color change observed in amyloid deposits after staining with Congo red under polarized light?
a. Red
b. Blue
c. Green
d. Apple-green

236. What is the underlying principle of Congo red staining for amyloid?
a. Selective binding of the stain to amyloid deposits
b. Utilization of fluorescence microscopy for visualization
c. Conversion of the stain into a different color by amyloid
d. Oxidation of amyloid for enhanced visibility

237. After staining with Congo red, how do amyloid deposits appear when viewed under polarized light?
a. They appear yellow-orange in color
b. They exhibit apple-green birefringence
c. They appear pink in color
d. They exhibit blue-purple birefringence

238. Besides Congo red staining, which stain is commonly used to confirm the presence of amyloid by immunohistochemistry?
a. Periodic acid-Schiff (PAS) stain
b. Thioflavin T stain
c. Hematoxylin and eosin (H&E) stain
d. Masson's trichrome stain

239. Which stain is commonly used to visualize hemosiderin deposits in histopathology?
a Prussian blue stain
b. Oil red O stain
c. Periodic acid-Schiff (PAS) stain
d. Masson's trichrome stain

240. What is the characteristic color observed in hemosiderin deposits after staining with Prussian blue?
a. Blue
b. Red
c. Green
d. Yellow

241. Which stain is commonly used to detect lipid droplets or fat deposits?
a. Prussian blue stain
b. Oil red O stain
c. Periodic acid-Schiff (PAS) stain
d. Masson's trichrome stain

Answers: 232. **a**   233. **b**   234. **a**   235. **d**
236. **a**   237. **b**   238. **b**   239. **a**
240. **a**   241. **b**

242. What is the characteristic color observed in lipid droplets or fat deposits after staining with oil red O?
a. Blue
b. Red
c. Green
d. Yellow

243. Which stain is commonly used to identify calcium deposits or calcifications?
a. Von Kossa stain
b. Oil red O stain
c. Periodic acid-Schiff (PAS) stain
d. Masson's trichrome stain

244. Silver stains are commonly used to visualize which type of tissue component?
a. Nuclei
b. Cytoplasm
c. Connective tissue fibers
d. Lipid droplets

245. What is the underlying principle of silver stains?
a. Selective binding of the stain to nuclei
b. Utilization of fluorescence micros-copy for visualization
c. Reduction of silver ions by target tissue components
d. Oxidation of target tissue compo-nents for enhanced visibility

246. Which stain is commonly used to visualize reticular fibers in connective tissue?
a. Gomori's silver stain
b. Periodic acid-Schiff (PAS) stain
c. Congo red stain
d. Alcian blue stain

247. What is the characteristic color of reticular fibers after staining with Gomori's silver stain?
a. Blue
b. Red
c. Purple
d. Black or brown

248. Which stain is commonly used to visualize neurofibrillary tangles in the brain?
a. Bielschowsky stain
b. Verhoeff's stain
c. Alizarin red stain
d. Masson's trichrome stain

249. Which stain is commonly used to visualize bacterial cells in histopathology?
a. Gram stain
b. Periodic acid-Schiff (PAS) stain
c. Acid-fast stain
d. Hematoxylin and eosin (H&E) stain

250. Gram stain is a differential staining technique that helps classify bacteria into which two major groups?
a. Gram-positive and gram-negative
b. Acid-fast and non-acid-fast
c. Aerobic and anaerobic
d. Spore-forming and non-spore-forming

251. Acid-fast stain is commonly used to visualize which type of microorganisms?
a. Fungi
b. Viruses
c. Protozoa
d. Mycobacteria

Answers: 242. b   243. a   244. c   245. c
246. a   247. d   248. a   249. a
250. a   251. d

252. **What is the characteristic color of acid-fast microorganisms after staining with acid-fast stains such as Ziehl-Neelsen or Kinyoun stain?**
     a. Blue
     b. Red
     c. Green
     d. Pink or red

253. **Which stain is commonly used to visualize fungi, such as Candida or Aspergillus?**
     a. Gomori's methenamine silver (GMS) stain
     b. Gram stain
     c. Periodic acid-Schiff (PAS) stain
     d. Acid-fast stain

254. **Which stain is commonly used to visualize DNA and RNA in histopathology?**
     a. Hematoxylin stain
     b. Eosin stain
     c. Acridine orange stain
     d. Masson's trichrome stain

255. **Acridine orange is a fluorescent stain commonly used to visualize nucleic acids. What color does DNA appear under fluorescent microscopy when stained with acridine orange?**
     a. Red
     b. Green
     c. Blue
     d. Yellow

256. **Which stain is commonly used to detect apoptotic cells, which often exhibit fragmented DNA?**
     a. Toluidine blue stain
     b. TUNEL (Terminal deoxynucleotidyl transferase dUTP nick end labeling) stain
     c. Congo red stain
     d. Alizarin red stain

257. **What is the principle of the TUNEL (Terminal deoxynucleotidyl transferase dUTP nick end labeling) assay?**
     a. Selective binding of the stain to apoptotic cells
     b. Utilization of fluorescence microscopy for visualization of fragmented DNA
     c. Conversion of the stain into a different color by fragmented DNA
     d. Oxidation of fragmented DNA for enhanced visibility

258. **Which stain is commonly used to visualize nucleoli within the nuclei of cells?**
     a. Hematoxylin stain
     b. Eosin stain
     c. Silver stain
     d. Giemsa stain

259. **Which stain is commonly used to visualize melanin pigment in histopathology?**
     a. Masson's trichrome stain
     b. Fontana-Masson stain
     c. Congo red stain
     d. Periodic acid-Schiff (PAS) stain

260. **What is the underlying principle of the Fontana-Masson stain?**
     a. Selective binding of the stain to melanin pigment
     b. Utilization of fluorescence microscopy for visualization
     c. Conversion of the stain into a different color by melanin pigment
     d. Oxidation of melanin pigment for enhanced visibility

Answers: 252. d 253. a 254. c 255. b
          256. b 257. b 258. d 259. b
          260. a

261. Which color does melanin pigment appear after staining with the Fontana-Masson stain?
a. Black
b. Red
c. Green
d. Blue

262. Which stain is commonly used to visualize copper deposits, such as in Wilson's disease?
a. Rubeanic acid stain (Rhodanine stain)
b. Oil red O stain
c. Periodic acid-Schiff (PAS) stain
d. Masson's trichrome stain

263. What is the characteristic color of copper deposits after staining with the Rubeanic acid (Rhodanine) stain?
a. Blue
b. Red
c. Brown
d. Yellow

264. Which stain is commonly used to visualize melanin pigment in histopathology?
a. Masson's trichrome stain
b. Fontana-Masson stain
c. Congo red stain
d. Shikata's Orcein stain

265. What is the purpose of mounting slides in histopathology?
a. To protect the tissue sections from damage
b. To enhance the visibility of the stained tissue sections
c. To provide a permanent record of the specimen
d. All of the above

266. Which mounting medium is commonly used for permanent mounting of histopathology slides?
a. Water
b. Glycerol
c. Xylene
d. Canada balsam

267. Which mounting medium is suitable for both brightfield and fluorescence microscopy?
a. Glycerol jelly
b. Permount
c. Entellan
d. Polyvinyl alcohol (PVA)

268. How should the coverslip be placed on the slide during mounting?
a. With slight pressure to evenly distribute the mounting medium
b. With a gentle touch to prevent air bubbles
c. With a twisting motion to secure it in place
d. It depends on the type of mounting medium used

269. What is the recommended drying time for mounted slides before examination?
a. 5 minutes
b. 30 minutes
c. 24 hours
d. It varies depending on the mounting medium used

270. Which mounting medium is commonly used for immunofluorescence microscopy?
a. Glycerol jelly
b. Permount
c. Entellan
d. Polyvinyl alcohol (PVA)

Answers:
261. a 262. a 263. c 264. b
265. d 266. d 267. b 268. b
269. d 270. b

271. **Which mounting medium is suitable for preserving fluorescence and preventing photobleaching?**
   a. Water
   b. Glycerol
   c. Xylene
   d. Anti-fading mounting medium

272. **Which mounting medium provides a refractive index similar to glass, allowing for clear microscopic visualization?**
   a. Glycerol jelly
   b. Permount
   c. Entellan
   d. Polyvinyl alcohol (PVA)

273. **Which mounting medium is commonly used for temporary mounting of slides?**
   a. Water
   b. Glycerol
   c. Xylene
   d. Mounting oil

274. **The refractive index of a mounting medium affects which aspect of microscopic visualization?**
   a. Contrast
   b. Resolution
   c. Magnification
   d. Depth of field

275. **Which mounting medium has a refractive index closest to that of glass coverslips?**
   a. Glycerol jelly
   b. Permount
   c. Xylene
   d. Polyvinyl alcohol (PVA)

276. **A higher refractive index of the mounting medium helps reduce which phenomenon?**
   a. Chromatic aberration
   b. Spherical aberration
   c. Photobleaching
   d. Background noise

277. **Which of the following mounting media has a lower refractive index?**
   a. Glycerol jelly
   b. Permount
   c. Xylene
   d. Polyvinyl alcohol (PVA)

278. **How does the refractive index of the mounting medium affect the quality of microscopic images?**
   a. Higher refractive index improves image resolution
   b. Lower refractive index improves image contrast
   c. Similar refractive index to the sample reduces artifacts
   d. Refractive index does not significantly affect image quality

279. **Frozen sections are commonly used for which of the following purposes?**
   a. Rapid diagnosis during surgery
   b. Long-term preservation of tissue samples
   c. Staining of fixed tissue sections
   d. Electron microscopy analysis

280. **What is the main advantage of frozen sections over paraffin sections?**
   a. Preservation of cellular morphology
   b. Better staining of intracellular components
   c. Enhanced visualization of extracellular matrix
   d. Higher resolution for electron microscopy

Answers: 271. **d**   272. **c**   273. **a**   274. **a**
       275. **b**   276. **b**   277. **c**   278. **c**
       279. **a**   280. **a**

281. What is the temperature range of cryostat?
a. 2°C to 10°C
b. –80°C to –70°C
c. –20°C to –30°C
d. 4°C to 10°C

282. How are frozen sections typically prepared for microscopic examination?
a. Sectioning with a microtome and mounting on glass slides
b. Embedding in paraffin wax and sectioning with a microtome
c. Freezing with liquid nitrogen and examination without sectioning
d. Staining without sectioning, directly on the frozen tissue block

283. What is the primary staining technique used for visualizing frozen sections?
a. Hematoxylin and eosin (H&E) stain
b. Gram stain
c. Periodic acid-Schiff (PAS) stain
d. Oil red O stain

284. What is a cryostat commonly used for in histopathology?
a. Sectioning frozen tissue samples
b. Fixing tissue samples
c. Dehydrating tissue samples
d. Embedding tissue samples in paraffin wax

285. What is the working principle of a cryostat?
a. It uses a cryogenic chamber to freeze tissue samples
b. It uses heat to thaw frozen tissue samples
c. It uses a microtome to section frozen tissue samples
d. It uses chemicals to preserve tissue samples

286. Which of the following components is found in a cryostat?
a. Freezing stage
b. Cryogenic gas supply
c. Microtome blade
d. All of the above

287. How is temperature controlled in a cryostat?
a. By using liquid nitrogen or other cryogenic gases
b. By using an electrical heating element
c. By using a water bath
d. By using a cooling fan

288. What is the purpose of the cryostat chamber in the instrument?
a. To hold the tissue samples during sectioning
b. To freeze the tissue samples to a specific temperature
c. To regulate the temperature of the microtome blade
d. To store the cryogenic gases used for cooling

289. Automation in histopathology refers to the use of technology to automate which aspect of the laboratory workflow?
a. Tissue fixation
b. Section cutting
c. Staining
d. All of the above

Answers:	281. c	282. a	283. a	284. a
	285. c	286. d	287. a	288. a
	289. d			

290. **Which of the following is an example of an automated slide stainer used in histopathology?**
   a. Cryostat
   b. Microtome
   c. Immunohistochemistry (IHC) stainer
   d. Embedding station

291. **What is the primary advantage of automated slide staining systems?**
   a. Faster processing time
   b. Greater accuracy and consistency
   c. Reduced risk of human error
   d. All of the above

292. **Automation in histopathology has contributed to improved laboratory efficiency by:**
   a. Reducing manual labor and hands-on time
   b. Increasing the number of required personnel
   c. Slowing down the workflow due to technical issues
   d. Eliminating the need for quality control and validation

293. **What is the primary purpose of immunohistochemistry in histopathology?**
   a. To visualize cellular structures under a microscope
   b. To detect and localize specific antigens in tissue samples
   c. To stain nuclei for better contrast
   d. To identify infectious organisms in tissues

294. **What is the detection system used in immunohistochemistry to visualize the antigen-antibody complex?**
   a. Enzyme-linked immunosorbent assay (ELISA)
   b. Fluorescence microscopy
   c. Chromogenic substrates
   d. Radioactive isotopes

295. **Which stain is commonly used as a counterstain in immunohistochemistry to provide contrast to the target antigen?**
   a. Hematoxylin
   b. Eosin
   c. DAB (3,3'-Diaminobenzidine)
   d. Alcian blue

296. **What is the purpose of blocking in immunohistochemistry?**
   a. To prevent nonspecific binding of antibodies
   b. To enhance the binding of primary antibodies to antigens
   c. To increase the sensitivity of the staining reaction
   d. To deactivate enzymes used in the detection system

297. **What type of beam is used in electron microscopy?**
   a. X-ray beam
   b. Ultraviolet beam
   c. Proton beam
   d. Electron beam

298. **Which component in electron microscopy is responsible for focusing the electron beam onto the specimen?**
   a. Objective lens
   b. Condenser lens
   c. Stigmator
   d. Electromagnetic coil

Answers:	290. c	291. d	292. a	293. b
	294. c	295. a	296. a	297. d
	298. a			

299. **What is the purpose of the electron-sensitive photographic film or detector in electron microscopy?**
a. To capture and record the image formed by the electron beam
b. To generate a visible light image of the specimen
c. To enhance the contrast of the image
d. To control the intensity of the electron beam

300. **Which staining method is commonly used in electron microscopy to enhance the contrast of the specimen?**
a. Hematoxylin and eosin (H&E) stain
b. Immunohistochemistry (IHC)
c. Negative staining
d. Fluorescent staining

Answers: 299. a   **300. c**

6 Cytology

INTRODUCTION TO CYTOLOGY

Cytology, or cytopathology, is the branch of science that studies cells shed from body fluids or tissues. The cells can be collected by scraping, brushing or through interventions. Interpretation of cells shed from epithelial surfaces or tissues is an important diagnostic tool for detecting various diseases, and it was introduced by George N Papanicolaou in 1928. Cytology is divided into two types:

1. Exfoliative cytology
2. Intervention cytology

Exfoliative cytology deals with studying cells shed from the body naturally or scrapped manually. Some examples of exfoliative cytology are listed in **Table 6.1**.

Intervention cytology is the type of cytology in which the sample (cells/fluid, etc.) is collected with the help of some intervention procedures. One of the most common procedures used for intervention cytology is FNAC (fine needle aspiration cytology).

Uses of Diagnostic Cytology

- To differentiate between benign and malignant lesions.
- For screening or diagnosis of premalignant lesions.
- For the diagnosis of malignant lesions.
- For diagnosis of infectious or inflammatory diseases.
- Follow up of the malignant lesions.
- Monitoring the response to therapy.
- In addition to diagnostic, it also have therapeutic applications.

Advantages of Diagnostic Cytology

- It is a minimally invasive and relatively simple diagnostic procedure.
- It is cost-effective.
- There are fewer chances of discomfort or complications.
- Early delivery of diagnostic reports.
- OPD procedures that usually do not require anesthesia.

Table 6.1: Examples of exfoliative cytology.

S. No.	Organs	Procedure for collection of cells
1.	Gynecological samples	Pap smear
2.	Gastrointestinal tract samples	Brushing off the cells from epithelial lining during endoscopy or ascitic fluid
3.	Skin or mucus membrane	Scrapping off the cells
4.	Respiratory tract samples	Collection of fluid from respiratory tract
5.	Genital tract samples	Urine collection
6.	Breast	Nipple discharge/aspirated fluid

- Early screening of premalignant or malignant lesions is possible.
- The procedure can be repeated if adequate material is not obtained.

Disadvantages of Diagnostic Cytology

- Grading of tumor is not possible
- The margins and extent of the tumor cannot be evaluated
- Biopsy of the tissue is required to reach the definitive diagnosis

FINE NEEDLE ASPIRATION CYTOLOGY

It is a cytological procedure by which cells/tissue or fluid can be aspirated from the pathological lesion with the help of the needle under negative pressure. This procedure is done in the swellings or lesions that are apparent or easily palpable. For the deep-seated lesions, it is guided with other imaging techniques, such as ultrasonography (USG) and computed tomography (CT).

Requirements

- **Franzen handle:** used for the aspiration of a sample **(Fig. 6.1)**

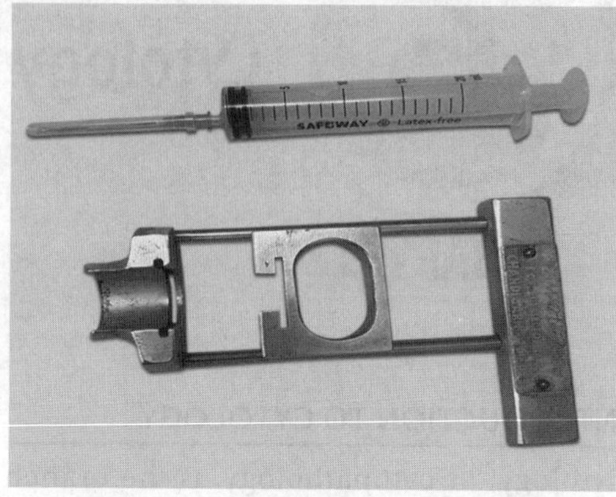

Fig. 6.1: Franzen handle and a syringe with a needle.

- 22–27 gauge needle
- Syringes (20, 10 and 5 mL)
- Gloves
- Gauze/Cotton
- Clean, grease-free, dry slides

Procedure of FNAC

To obtain an adequate specimen, it is important to follow each step appropriately:

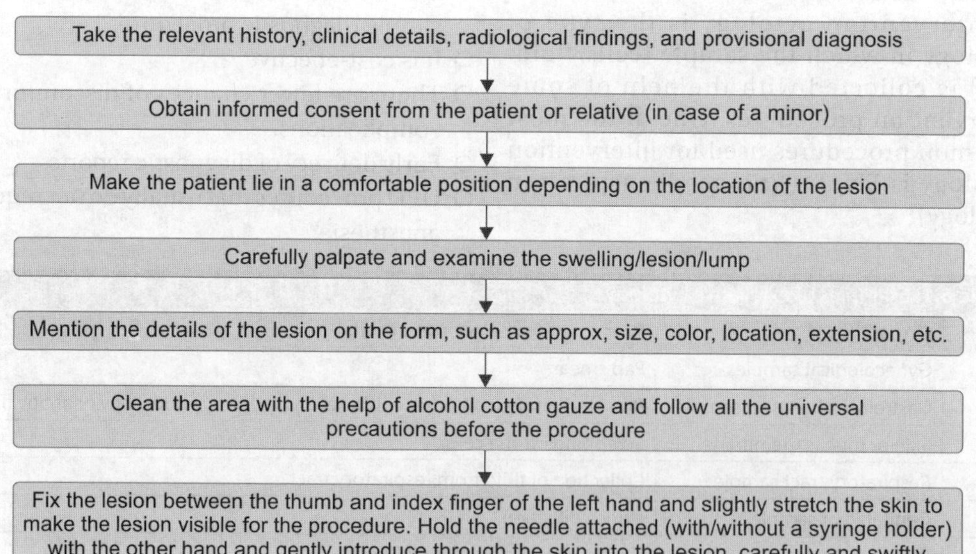

Contd...

Contd...

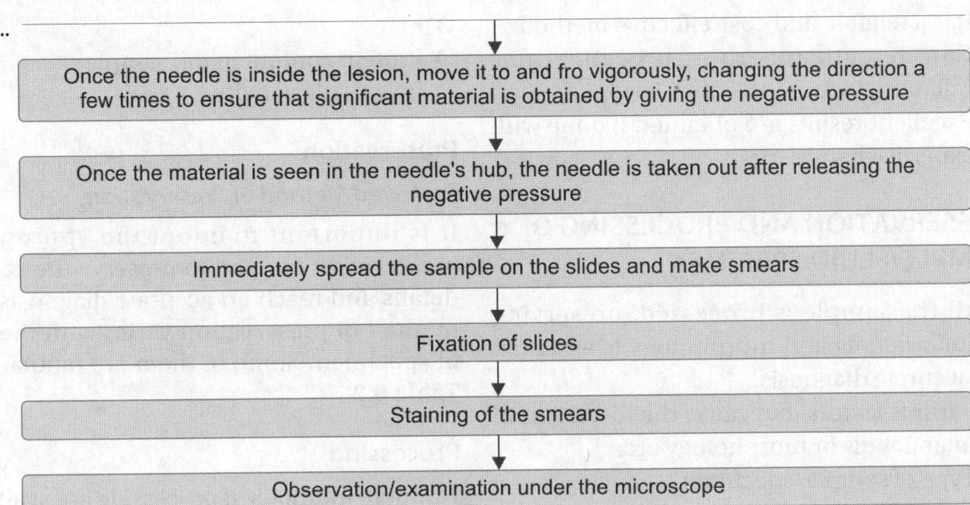

If, during aspiration, any cork of tissue is obtained, then it is to be fixed in formalin and processed like any other tissue sample in the histopathology section.

Techniques of Aspiration

Aspiration or Suction Method

❍ In this method, a needle attached to the Franzen handle is inserted into the lesion or mass or area of interest, and negative pressure is applied. Once the needle is in the lesion, multiple fast jabbing movements are done to obtain the maximum material. While removing the needle from the lesion, negative pressure is released to prevent the aspiration of the material in the syringe. The needle is detached from the syringe, and smears are made.

Non-aspiration Method

❍ In this method, a needle is passed into the lesion without any syringe or handle. After passing the needle into the lesion, multiple fast jabbing movements are given in different directions to obtain the material. Once the material is visible in the needle's hub, it is taken out to make the smears. This method is also known as fine needle capillary method or non-suction method. Admixture with blood is less with this technique and is useful in thyroid aspiration. The advantage of this method is that there is less hemorrhage; thus, it is more suitable in areas with high vascularity, like the thyroid.

Adequacy of FNAC Reporting

Reporting of the smears depends upon the adequacy of the specimen.

Following are the fundamental requirements for accurate reporting and diagnosis of FNAC smears.

❍ The sample should be representative of the lesion under investigation.
❍ The sample should be adequate.
❍ The sample should be properly smeared.
❍ The sample should be properly processed.
❍ Sufficient data, including clinical details and investigations, should be accompanied.

Advantages

❍ It is a simple procedure that can be done in OPD without any need for anesthesia.

- It is a reliable and cost-effective method.
- Can detect cancerous, precancerous, inflammatory or infectious lesions.
- Excellent results are obtained if done with expertise hands.

PRESERVATION AND PROCESSING OF SAMPLE/FLUID SPECIMEN

Until the sample is processed, preserving cellular details and morphology is essential for accurate diagnosis.

Various factors that cause the distortion of cellular details or morphology are:
- Type of sample/specimen
- Type of fixative used
- The duration between sample collection and processing

- pH
- Protein content in the sample
- Enzymatic activity

Preservation

Preferred Method of Preservation

It is important to adopt the appropriate preservation method to preserve the cellular details and reach an accurate diagnosis. The method of preservation varies with the type of specimen. Some of them are tabulated in **Table 6.2**.

Processing

Different methods of processing are available.

Some of the methods of processing with their advantages and disadvantages are tabulated in **Table 6.3**.

Table 6.2: Different types of specimen with their preferred mode of preservation.

Type of specimen	Example	Mode of preservation	Duration of preservation	Mechanism of action
Specimen with high mucus content	Sputum, bronchial aspirates, mucocele fluid	Refrigeration	12–24 hours	Refrigeration slows down the bacterial growth thereby preventing cell damage
Specimen with high protein content	Pleural, peritoneal or pericardial fluids	Refrigeration	24–48 hours	Refrigeration slows down the bacterial growth
Specimen with low mucus or protein content	Urine or CSF	Refrigeration	1–2 hours	Refrigeration slows down the bacterial growth
Specimen with low pH	Gastric material	Should be collected on ice	Few minutes	

Table 6.3: Advantages and limitations of different processing methods.

S. No.	Method	Advantages	Limitations
1.	Centrifugation (**Fig. 6.2**)	Simple to use	Risk of contamination to the user during processing
2.	Cytospin	• Easy to use • Minimal cell loss	Air drying artefacts
3.	Slow sedimentation technique	Cell distortion is minimum	
4.	Membrane filtration	Simple to use	Sample should be fresh as prefixed sample coagulates protein and clog the filter pores

Fluid/specimen rich in proteins or bloody aspirates, or thin/serous fluids need to be processed especially to ensure an accurate diagnosis. Some of the methods are tabulated in **Table 6.4**.

STAINING OF CYTOLOGICAL SAMPLES

Preparation of Smear

There are two methods of preparation of a smear:

1. **Direct smear:** As soon as the sample appears in the hub of the needle in FNAC, detach the needle from the syringe, draw the air in the syringe, reattach the needle and slowly express the material in the center of the pre-labeled slides. Put the other slide on the 1st slide and pull the slides apart by gently pressing to obtain the smears.
2. **Indirect smear:** If the material obtained is diluted with the blood or fluid or when a large sample is aspirated, the smears are made after processing the sample.

   Methods like centrifugation, cytospin, filtration, etc., are used in the case of body fluids to make smears.

Fixation and Staining

The method of fixation used depends upon the stain being used for staining the smears.

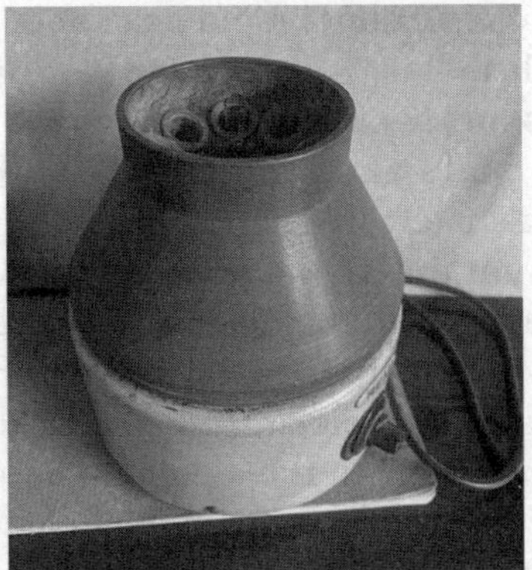

Fig. 6.2: Centrifuge.

Properties of Ideal Cytologic Fixatives

○ It should not excessively shrink or swell cells.
○ It should not distort or dissolve cellular components.
○ It should preserve nuclear details and enhance staining.
○ It should kill microbes.

Type of Fixation

○ **Rapid staining or Diff-Quik staining:** It is useful to check the adequacy of the sample. The smears are stained rapidly, and if the sample is found to be inadequate, the procedure can be repeated simultaneously, thereby preventing unnecessary delay in the diagnosis.

Table 6.4: Different techniques of processing of body fluids.

S. No.	Type of specimen/fluid	Can result in	Technique used	Mechanism of action
1.	Proteinaceous fluid	Can cause excessive background staining, therefore causing hindrance in cell morphology	• Centrifugation and discarding the supernatant • Addition of ethyl alcohol	Protein coagulation
2.	Thin/serous fluids	Low cellularity	• Centrifugation • Addition of egg albumin powder	Coagulation
3.	Bloody aspirates	Plenty of RBCs can obstruct the diagnosis	Add either • 10% glacial acetic acid (few drops) • 0.1N HCl • Carnoy's fluid	Lysis of RBCs

○ **Alcohol fixation:** rapid fixation of smears in alcohol is important for Papanicolaou (pap) or H&E stain. As soon as the smears are made and labeled, they are fixed immediately in alcohol in a Coplin jar to prevent the drying artefacts, which may interfere with the diagnosis. Therefore to prevent the drying artefacts, air drying of the slide is avoided, and smears are fixed immediately in the alcohol. Pap stain is preferred for cytological smears as the cellular details are clearer with this stain.

Staining

Pap stain, named after Dr George N Papanicolaou, is the stain of choice used in cytology. It is a polychromatic stain, which shows variation in the staining color depending upon the cell's cellular maturity or metabolic activity.

Composition of Pap Stain

The components of Pap stain are OG-6 and EA-36 and Harris hematoxylin

○ OG-6 and EA-36 are synthetic cytoplasmic stains
○ OG-6 is a monochrome stain, while EA-36 is a polychrome stain.
○ Harris haematoxylin is a nuclear stain

Steps of staining (Table 6.5)

○ Fixation
○ Nuclear staining
○ Cytoplasmic staining
○ Dehydration

Table 6.5: Steps of Pap staining.

Step No.	Reagent	Duration in minutes
1.	90% Ethanol (fixation)	15
2.	80% Ethanol	2
3.	60% Ethanol	2
4.	Distilled water	5 dips
5.	Distilled water	5 dips
6.	Hematoxylin stain	2
7.	0.05% HCl solution	2
8.	Running tap water (Bluing)	10
9.	60 % Ethanol	2
10.	80% Ethanol	2
11.	80% Ethanol	2
12.	95% Ethanol	2
13.	OG-6 stain	2
14.	95% Ethanol	2
15.	95% Ethanol	2
16.	95% Ethanol	2
17.	EA-36 Stain	2
18.	95% Ethanol	2
19.	95% Ethanol	2
20.	95%Etanol	2
21.	95% Ethanol	2
22.	Absolute Ethanol	2

Contd...

Contd...

Step No.	Reagent	Duration in minutes
23.	Absolute Ethanol	2
24.	Absolute Ethanol	2
25.	Absolute Ethanol+ Xylene (1:1)	2
26.	Xylene	5
27.	Xylene	5
28.	Xylene	till clear
29.	Mounting in DPX	

○ Clearing
○ Mounting

CYTOLOGY OF FEMALE GENITAL TRACT (PAP SMEAR)

Smears in the female genital tract can be made from different organs like:
○ Cervical smear
○ Vaginal smear
○ Vaginal pool smear
○ Endometrial smear

A cervical smear or Pap smear is a screening test used for early detection of cervical cancer, even in the preinvasive state.

Advantages of Pap Smear

○ It is a painless and simple test
○ Can be done in OPD
○ Does not need anaesthesia
○ Can detect cancerous and precancerous lesions
○ Can identify non-specific and specific inflammations.

Normal Pap Smear

Also interpreted as "negative for intraepithelial lesion or malignancy" (NILM). Additional findings, such as reactive changes, infectious organisms, and inflammation can be there. Different types of cell seen in Pap smear are depicted in **Table 6.6**.

Microscopic findings in Pap smear: The microscopic findings in Pap smear are depict in **Table 6.7**.

Table 6.6: Types of cells seen in the Pap smear.

Type of cell	Shape	Nucleus	Cytoplasm	Common in
Superficial squamous cells (cells of superficial layer)	Large polygonal	Small, pyknotic	Transparent pink or green cytoplasm	Females of reproductive age group
Intermediate squamous cells (cells of middle layer)	Large polygonal	Larger nucleus, occasionally bi or multinucleated	Transparent pink or green cytoplasm	Females of reproductive age group
Parabasal and basal squamous cells also called as immature squamous metaplastic cells (cells of deep layer)	Round- to oval-shaped	50 µm with finely granular chromatin	Dense homogenous basophilic cytoplasm High nuclear to cytoplasmic ratio	Premenstrual, postpartum, women taking estrogen-restricting hormones, or postmenopausal
Squamous metaplastic cells	Round to polygonal	Round centrally located nuclei	Dense biphasic staining cytoplasm	Can be seen among women of reproductive age group

Contd...

Contd...

Type of cell	Shape	Nucleus	Cytoplasm	Common in
Endocervical cell	Tall, columnar-cells Present as Picket fence or honeycomb configuration	50 μm round basally placed nucleus with fine granular chromatin, occasional nucleoli	Granular or vacuolated cytoplasm	It is standard to have endocervical cells in the Pap smear
Endometrial cells	Small and cuboidal, averaging 10–20 μm	Hyperchromatic and may be round- to oval- to bean-shaped	Scant cytoplasm, dense or vacuolated	In cycling women, endometrial cells are expected to be seen on Pap tests from the first day bleeding starts through the twelfth day

Table 6.7: Microscopic findings in Pap smear.

Findings	Features	Causes
A. Non-neoplastic		
Inflammatory smear/NILM **(Fig. 6.3)**.	Neutrophils, lymphocytes, etc. Mild nuclear enlargement, fine and pale chromatin	Infection or inflammation.
Squamous metaplasia	Thick, "Dense" cytoplasm, sharply defined cell borders. Normal sized nucleus	Trauma, infection or inflammation
Hyperkeratosis	Anucleated squamous cells, may be present singly or in sheets	Trauma, infection or inflammation, use of diaphragm, cervical prolapse
Parakeratosis	Small superficial squamous cells having small, dense and pyknotic nucleus	Cervical atrophy, infections (most commonly HPV), preneoplastic lesions, neoplastic lesions as in squamous cell carcinoma
Tubal metaplasia	Endocervical cells are replaced by fallopian tube-like epithelium with cilia	Infection, trauma
Atrophy	Atrophic, small, keratinized degenerated squamous cells and many parabasal cells	Postmenopausal woman
Radiation effect	Enlarged, bizarre cells with variable sized nuclei (bi-or multinucleated), with smudged chromatin and prominent nucleoli	Radiation exposure
IUD associated changes	Cytoplasmic vacuolations, cracked nucleus with prominent nucleoli, *Actinomyces*-like organisms may be present	Females using IUDs
B. Epithelial cell abnormalities/neoplastic		
Atypical squamous cells of undetermined significance (ASCUS)	Increased N: C ratio, nuclei is 2.5–3 times the size of normal intermediate cell nucleus, mild hyperchromatic and irregular contours	Precursor lesion

Contd...

Contd...

Atypical squamous cells cannot exclude HSIL (ASC-H)	Atypical squamous cells present in crowded sheets	Precursor lesion
Low-grade squamous intra epithelial lesion (LSIL)/ mild dysplasia/cervical intraepithelial neoplasia (CIN) I	Nucleus is 3 times of normal intermediate cell nuclei, anisonucleosis, hyperchromasia, inconspicuous nucleoli and koilocytosis **(Fig. 6.4)**	Precancerous lesion
High-grade squamous intra epithelial lesion (HSIL)/ moderate-severe dysplasia/ cervical intraepithelial neoplasia (CIN) II/III	Cells in sheets, nucleus size is >3 times the normal, anisonucleosis, hyperchromasia **(Fig. 6.5)**	Precancerous lesion
Squamous cell carcinoma (SCC)	Cells in sheets with marked anisonucleosis, coarsely granular chromatin, irregular nuclear membrane tadpole cells	Cancerous lesion
Atypical Endocervical cells	Nuclear size is 3–5 times, hyperchromatic, anisocytosis, mitosis	Precancerous lesion
Atypical endometrial cells	Nuclear enlargement, hyperchromasia, occasional nucleoli, scant cytoplasm	Precancerous lesion
Endocervical adenocarcinoma in situ (AIS)	Neoplastic cells in clusters with nuclear stratification, enlargement, hyperchromasia, inconspicuous nucleoli, mitotic figures	Precancerous lesion
Endocervical adenocarcinoma	Marked pleomorphism with anisocytonucleosis, macronucleoli, hyperchromasia	Cancerous lesion
Endometrial adenocarcinoma	Marked pleomorphism with anisocytonucleosis, macronucleoli, hyperchromasia	Cancerous lesion

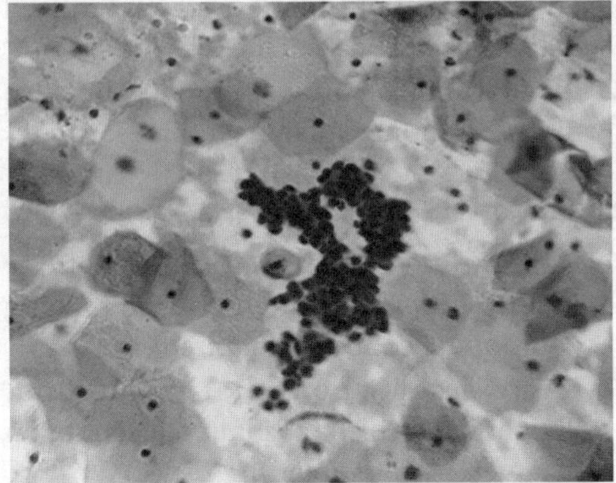

Fig. 6.3: Pap smear with squamous cells in the background and endocervical cells (in honeycomb pattern) in the center.

(For color version, see Plate 6)

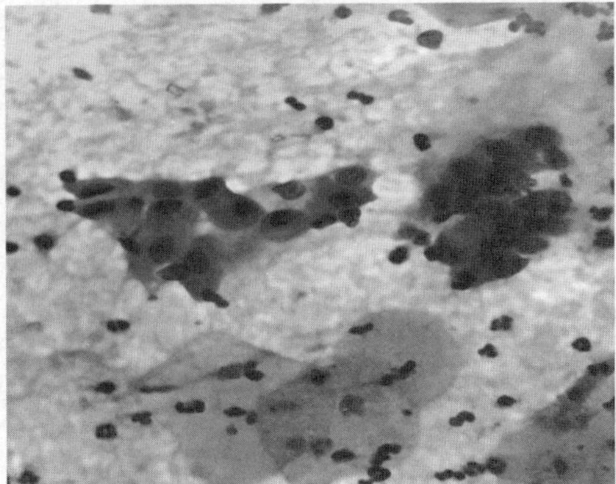

Fig. 6.4: Low-grade squamous intraepithelial lesion (LSIL).

(For color version, see Plate 6)

IMMUNOCYTOCHEMISTRY

Immunocytochemistry (ICC) is a technique used to identify antigenic (cellular or tissue) components with the help of primary or secondary labeled antibodies to detect the antigen-antibody interaction.

Types of ICC

Direct ICC

Involves the detection of antigens with the help of primary antibody.

Indirect ICC

In this, a secondary labeled antibody is used for the detection of the primary antibody.

Requirements

- Cells of interest/sample
- Microscopic slides
- Coverslips
- Primary antibody
- Fluorophore labeled secondary antibody
- Fluorescent microscope

ICC Steps

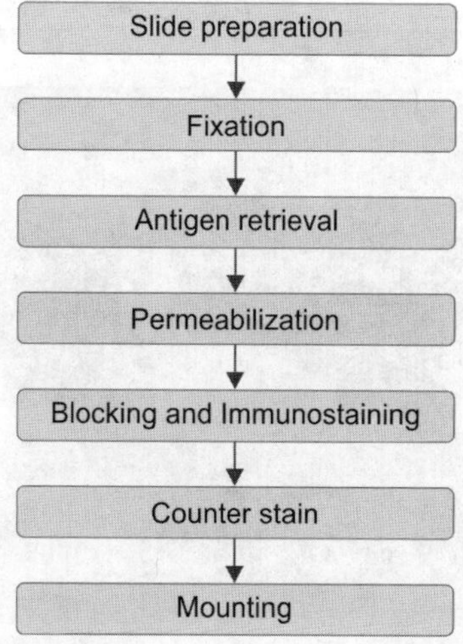

Applications of ICC

- To diagnose and classify benign and malignant tumors.

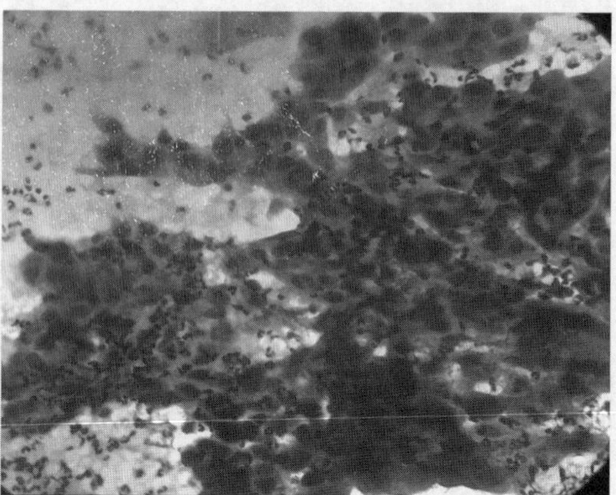

Fig. 6.5: High-grade squamous intraepithelial lesion (HSIL).

(For color version, see Plate 6)

- To determine the stage and grade of tumors.
- It is used as a prognostic marker in cancers.
- To identify the tumors of uncertain histogenesis.
- To predict the therapeutic response to therapy.
- For identification or confirmation of infective pathogens, such as like tubercular bacilli, HPV, HCV, etc.
- For identification of gene products involved in the pathogenesis of the disease.
- Identification of various neurodegenerative disorders or muscular dystrophies.

Limitations

- Due to the variations in the specificity of antibodies, thorough checking using appropriate control is required.
- Being a semi-quantitative method, determination of the absolute concentration of target is impossible.
- Being a multi-step procedure, a sample is processed at different stages resulting in the variation or loss of the natural state.

EXAMINATION OF URINE

Urine examination is an important non-invasive diagnostic tool that helps detect pathology in the genitourinary tract. It is a cost-effective and rapid technique for screening and semi-quantitative and qualitative urine analysis.

Normal Characteristics of Urine

Table 6.8 depicts the characteristics of normal urine.

Time for Sample Collection

Table 6.9 depicts the time for sample collection.

Table 6.8: Characteristics of normal urine.

Features	Normal value/range
Physical characteristics	
Volume	600–2000 mL/24 hours
Color	Pale yellow
Appearance	Clear
Odor	Aromatic (freshly voided)
Specific gravity	*1.003 to 1.030*
pH	4.6–8.0
Chemical characteristics	
Protein	<150 mg
Glucose	<0.5 g
Urobilinogen	0.5–4.0 mg
Creatinine	14–26 mg/kg in males and 11–20 mg/kg in females
Uric acid	250–750 mg
Sodium	40–220 mEq
Potassium	25–125 mEq
Microscopic characteristics	
Red blood cells	0–2/HPF
White blood cells	0–2/HPF
Epithelial cells	0–2/HPF
Hyaline cast	Occasional

Table 6.9: Time for sample collection.

Time of urine collection	Preferred for
Random collection	Routine urine examination
First morning sample	Routine urine examination
Post prandial sample	Glucose, urobilinogen estimation
24-hour sample	For quantitative estimation of protein and harmones
Catheter or plastic bag sample	Bacteriological examination from bed ridden patients, infants

The appropriate time of urine collection depends on the analysis being done. Urine collection can be done:

- Randomly (any time of the day);
- The first-morning sample
- Can be collected 2 hours after the meal, i.e., postprandial,
- 24-hour urine sample or
- Collected from the catheter or plastic bag.

Precautions to be taken During Specimen Handling and Collection

- The specimen should be collected in a wide-mouth container.
- The container should be labelled with the patient's Id.
- Midstream sample is ideal for examination.

- The specimen should be transported immediately to the laboratory.
- Examination and processing should be done within one to two hours of the collection of the sample.
- In case of delay, the sample should be refrigerated for a maximum of 8 hours at 4–6°C, or a chemical preservative can be used.

Chemical Preservatives

Some chemical preservatives that can be added to 24-hour urine samples are listed below:

- Toluene
- Hydrochloric acid
- Thymol
- Formic acid

MULTIPLE CHOICE QUESTIONS

1. **Pap smear is used for the screening of:**
   a. Colon cancer
   b. Cervical cancer
   c. Breast cancer
   d. Gastric cancer

2. **Cytology is the study of:**
   a. Cells
   b. Tissues
   c. Organs
   d. Systems

3. **The most common stain used for cytological smears:**
   a. H&E stain   b. Giemsa stain
   c. Pap stain   d. PAS stain

4. **The following characterises cytological features of malignancy, *except*:**
   a. Anisonucleosis
   b. Hyperchromasia
   c. Irregular nuclear margins
   d. Uniformly sized nucleus

5. **The ideal fixative used for cytological samples is:**
   a. 50% Ethanol
   b. 70% Ethanol
   c. 85% Ethanol
   d. 95% Ethanol

6. **What common fixative is used for transporting cytological smears to distant laboratories?**
   a. Coating fixative
   b. Aerosol fixative
   c. As such, without any fixative
   d. Both a and b

7. **The aerosol fixative is sprayed at a recommended distance of:**
   a. 4–6 inches
   b. 4–6 cm
   c. 10–12 inches
   d. 10–12 cm

8. **What is the most appropriate diagnostic procedure for palpable lesions/masses?**
   a. FNAC
   b. Excisional biopsy
   c. Pap smear
   d. None of the above

9. **The commonly used fixative for cytological smear is:**
   a. Xylene
   b. Ethanol
   c. Acetone
   d. Methanol

10. **Which of the following statement is incorrect about FNAC?**
    a. Is a minimally invasive procedure
    b. Produce speedy results
    c. Cannot differentiate between benign and malignant lesions
    d. Accurate when done by experienced hands

11. **All of the following statement/s are true about Carnoy's fixative, *except*:**
    a. It causes lysis of RBCs
    b. It is a basic fixative
    c. Preserves nuclear details and glycogen
    d. Performs a fast fixation

Answers:

1. b	2. a	3. c	4. d
5. d	6. d	7. c	8. a
9. b	10. c	11. b	

12. **Which fixative is commonly used for preserving nuclear details in cytology preparations?**
    a. Methanol
    b. Acetone
    c. Ethanol
    d. Buffered saline solution

13. **The clinical uses of FNAC is/are:**
    a. Diagnosis of neoplastic and non-neoplastic diseases
    b. Diagnosis of inflammatory disorders
    c. For microbiological and biochemical analysis
    d. All of the above

14. **Antigen retrieval is an important step in which of the following techniques?**
    a. Pap staining
    b. Diff quick staining
    c. Both a and b
    d. Immunocytochemistry

15. **All the statements about FNAC are correct, *except*:**
    a. It is an OPD procedure
    b. Clinical/radiological information is not necessary
    c. Can be done without the need for anaesthesia
    d. Is an essential component of pre-treatment/preoperative investigation

16. **What is the most common location where the non-aspiration technique is preferred?**
    a. Thyroid
    b. Breast
    c. Soft tissues
    d. None of the above

17. **Which of the following statement about non-aspiration technique is incorrect?**
    a. Is a preferred method for thyroid
    b. A syringe is attached to the needle
    c. Admixture of a sample with blood is generally less
    d. Smears are fixed in ethanol

18. **Which statement about the Pap stain is incorrect?**
    a. It is a polychromatic stain
    b. OG-6 and EA-36 and Harris hematoxylin are its components
    c. It is a monochromatic stain
    d. Is a preferred stain for cytological samples

19. **Immediate fixation of cytological smears is done in:**
    a. Ethanol
    b. Water
    c. Air dry
    d. None of the above

20. **Which of the following statement/s is false about FNAC?**
    a. It is a cost-effective method
    b. The extent and margins of the tumour can be evaluated
    c. Early screening of tumour is possible
    d. Is an OPD procedure

21. **Factor/s that can cause cellular damage depend upon the:**
    a. The duration between sample collection and smear preparation
    b. Enzymatic activity
    c. Protein content in the sample
    d. All of the above

Answers: 12. c   13. d   14. d   15. b
              16. a   17. b   18. c   19. a
              20. b   21. d

22. **Which one of the following is an example of a fluid with high mucus content?**
    a. Bronchial aspirates
    b. Cerebrospinal fluid
    c. Gastric fluid
    d. Pericardial fluid

23. **What is the ideal time technique for fluid fixation with high mucus content?**
    a. 6–8 hours
    b. 12–24 hours
    c. 24–48 hours
    d. 36–72 hours

24. **Specimens with high protein content is/are:**
    a. Pleural fluid
    b. Peritoneal fluid
    c. Pericardial fluid
    d. All of the above

25. **Rapid stain used for cytological smears is:**
    a. Diff-quick stain
    b. Pap stain
    c. PAS stain
    d. All of the above

26. **Specimen or fluid with low pH can be preserved for a maximum period of:**
    a. Few minutes
    b. 5–6 hours
    c. Both a and b
    d. None of the above

27. **The nuclear features of squamous cell carcinoma are:**
    a. Nuclear enlargement
    b. Hyperchromasia
    c. Anisonucleosis
    d. All of the above

28. **Which of the following is a characteristic of a malignant cell in cytology?**
    a. Hyperchromatic nuclei
    b. Well-defined cytoplasmic borders
    c. Uniform cell size and shape
    d. Low cellularity

29. **Which of the following is a characteristic finding in squamous cell carcinoma on a cervical Pap smear?**
    a. Irregularly-shaped cells with oran-geophilic cytoplasm
    b. Hyperchromatic nuclei
    c. Tadpole-shaped cells
    d. All of the above

30. **The Pap smear is primarily used for the detection of:**
    a. Bacterial infections
    b. Viral infections
    c. Fungal infections
    d. Precancerous and cancerous cells

31. **The method used for preparing a Pap smear is:**
    a. Liquid-based cytology
    b. Conventional smear
    c. Cellblock technique
    d. Both A & B

32. **The purpose of fixing the Pap smear slide is to:**
    a. Preserve cellular morphology
    b. Remove excess debris
    c. Enhance nuclear staining
    d. Improve cellularity

33. **The staining method commonly used in Pap smear preparation is:**
    a. Hematoxylin and eosin (H&E) stain
    b. Papanicolaou (Pap) stain
    c. Periodic acid-Schiff (PAS) stain
    d. Giemsa stain

Answers:	22. a	23. b	24. d	25. a
	26. a	27. d	28. a	29. d
	30. d	31. d	32. a	33. b

34. Which of the following is not included in the Pap staining protocol?
a. Counterstain with OG-6
b. Eosin Y to stain the nucleus
c. Ethanol fixation
d. Nuclear staining with hematoxylin

35. The use of a fixative, such as ethanol or spray fixative, is important in cytology smears to:
a. Enhance cellularity
b. Prevent cellular distortion
c. Remove excess debris
d. Improve nuclear staining

36. Which of the following is a common fixative for preserving cytology samples?
a. Formalin
b. Ethanol
c. Acetone
d. Methanol

37. The fixative used while mailing unstained cytological smears is/are:
a. Coating fixative
b. Carbowax
c. Spray fixative
d. All of the above

38. The accuracy of the cytological examination depends on:
a. Preparation of smears
b. Staining process
c. Both a & b
d. None of the above

39. Fine needle aspiration cytology (FNAC) is used for the diagnosis of:
a. Benign conditions
b. Infections
c. Malignancy
d. All of the above

40. The needle gauge commonly used for FNAC is:
a. 18 gauge
b. 21 gauge
c. 15 gauge
d. 20 gauge

41. The primary advantage of FNAC over open biopsy is:
a. Higher diagnostic accuracy
b. Lower risk of complications
c. Ability to assess tumour margins
d. Can assess the extent of tumor

42. The primary goal of using negative pressure during FNAC is to:
a. Increase sample yield
b. Minimise patient discomfort
c. Prevent sample contamination
d. Maintain needle stability

43. During the FNAC procedure, the "back and forth" or "to-and-fro" motion of the needle is performed to:
a. Maximise sample collection
b. Reduce the risk of bleeding
c. Create a vacuum effect
d. Prevent needle clogging

44. Non-aspiration cytology techniques are commonly used for sampling which of the following organs?
a. Thyroid
b. Breast
c. Lung
d. All of the above

45. The main advantage of non-aspiration cytology techniques over aspiration cytology is:
a. Higher diagnostic accuracy
b. Lower risk of complications
c. Ability to assess tumor margins
d. Low risk of hemorrhage

Answers:	34. b	35. b	36. b	37. d
	38. c	39. d	40. b	41. b
	42. a	43. a	44. a	45. d

46. **Effusion/fluid that is commonly sent to the laboratory for diagnostic purposes are:**
    a. Pleural fluid
    b. Peritoneal fluid
    c. Pericardial fluid
    d. All of the above

47. **Lumbar puncture (LP) is used for the collection of:**
    a. Cerebrospinal fluid (CSF)
    b. Pleural fluid
    c. Ascitic fluid
    d. Peritoneal fluid

48. **The presence of malignant cells in pleural fluid cytology is indicative of:**
    a. Malignancy
    b. Benign inflammatory condition
    c. Fungal infection
    d. Autoimmune disease

49. **The primary purpose of storing cytological samples at low temperatures is to:**
    a. Prevent microbial growth
    b. Maintain cellular morphology
    c. Enhance nuclear staining
    d. Reduce sample degradation

50. **Essential information/s that should accompany the specimen/sample include**
    a. Patient's name and date of collection
    b. Specimen type
    c. Clinical details
    d. All of the above

51. **The primary precaution to be taken when receiving/transporting cytological samples is/are:**
    a. Labeling of the container
    b. Timely transportation of the specimen
    c. Use of appropriate fixative
    d. All of the above

52. **The documentation required when receiving cytological samples includes:**
    a. Patient's name
    b. Type of specimen
    c. Requisition form details
    d. All of the above

53. **The initial step in processing cytological samples is:**
    a. Fixation
    b. Staining
    c. Washing
    d. Centrifugation

54. **The primary staining method used in cytology is:**
    a. Hematoxylin and eosin (H&E) staining
    b. Papanicolaou (Pap) staining
    c. Giemsa staining
    d. May Grünwald-Giemsa (MGG) staining

55. **The special stain commonly used to identify fungal organisms in cytology is:**
    a. H&E stain
    b. Gram stain
    c. Ziehl-Neelsen stain
    d. Gomori methenamine silver (GMS) stain

56. **The special stain used to detect amyloid deposits in cytology is:**
    a. Congo red stain
    b. Alizarin red stain
    c. Masson trichrome stain
    d. Wright-Giemsa stain

Answers:

46. d	47. a	48. a	49. a
50. d	51. d	52. d	53. a
54. b	55. d	56. a	

57. What should be done if a delay is expected in transporting fresh samples/fluid to the laboratory?
a. Refrigeration of sample
b. Addition of alcohol
c. Addition of xylene
d. None of the above

58. The primary precaution to be taken during FNAC is to:
a. Use sterile technique and maintain asepsis
b. Administer local anaesthesia to the patient
c. Both a & b
d. Perform the procedure under radio-logical guidance

59. Immunocytochemistry is a technique used to:
a. Detect specific antigens in cells
b. Identify cellular morphology
c. Evaluate nuclear staining patterns
d. Assess cellular viability

60. Which of the following is not the method of processing fluid/sample?
a. Centrifugation
b. Cytospin
c. Micropore filtration
d. Fixation

61. For hemorrhagic/bloody aspirates, the processing is done by adding:
a. Glacial acetic acid
b. 0.1N HCl
c. Carnoy's solution
d. Any of the above

62. Which of the following is used for the preparation of cell block?
a. Egg albumin
b. Blood plasma
c. Thrombin solution
d. All of the above

63. Which of the following method is used for the processing of CSF?
a. Cytocentrifuge
b. Cytospin
c. Slow sedimentation
d. All of the above

64. The most basic method used for the processing of urine specimens is:
a. Cytospin
b. Slow sedimentation
c. Membrane filters
d. Cytocentrifuge

65. The Saccomanno technique is used for:
a. Cervical cytology
b. Sputum cytology
c. Urine cytology
d. All of the above

66. Following is/are the method of collecting material from the respiratory tract:
a. Bronchial washings
b. Bronchial aspirates
c. Bronchoalveolar lavage
d. All of the above

67. Squash cytology is used for:
a. CNS tumors
b. Skin disorders
c. Cervical cancer
d. All of the above

68. Which of the following method is adjunct to the frozen section?
a. Imprint cytology
b. Excisional biopsy
c. FNAC
d. All of the above

Answers:	57. a	58. a	59. a	60. d
	61. d	62. d	63. d	64. d
	65. b	66. d	67. a	68. a

69. The limitation of imprint cytology over frozen sections is/are?
a. Cannot distinguish between in situ carcinoma from invasive
b. Depth of infiltration cannot be assessed
c. Both a & b
d. Only a

70. In the triple smear technique, the sample is collected from:
a. Ovary, vagina, cervix
b. Endocervix, oviduct, vagina
c. Vagina, cervix, endocervix
d. Endocervix, vagina, ectocervix

71. Method/s used for LBC (Liquid-based cytology)
a. Sure path
b. Thin prep
c. Both a & b
d. Only b

72. Which stain is also called a transparent stain?
a. H&E stain
b. PAS stain
c. Pap stain
d. Giemsa stain

73. Pap stain is also known as a transparent stain because:
a. It is transparent in appearance
b. Preserves the nuclear chromatin transparency
c. Cytoplasm appears transparent with this stain
d. Both b & c

74. 'G' in OG-6, one of the components of Pap stain, stands for:
a. Giemsa
b. Gelb
c. Galactin
d. Glycerin

75. The primary aim of the rapid fixation of cytological smears is?
a. To promote the enzymatic activity in the cells
b. To preserve the cytological details of cells
c. Both a & b
d. Only b

76. Which of the following statement/s is incorrect about ideal cytological fixative?
a. Do not excessively shrink or swell the cells
b. Activate the enzymes
c. Do not distort the cellular components
d. Preserves the nuclear details

77. The process of fixation of freshly prepared smears by submerging them in a liquid fixative is called as:
a. Dry fixation
b. Wet fixative
c. Microwave fixation
d. Heat fixation

78. Which of the following is/are coating fixative?
a. Carbowax
b. Polyethylene glycol
c. Both a & b
d. Only a

79. Which of the following method/s is used for processing of proteinaceous fluid?
a. Centrifugation and discarding the supernatant
b. Addition of ethyl alcohol
c. Both a & b
d. Only b

Answers:

69. c	**70.** c	**71.** c	**72.** c
73. b	**74.** b	**75.** b and d	**76.** b
77. b	**78.** c	**79.** c	

80. **To obtain an adequate sample during FNAC, it is important:**
    a. To maintain the negative pressure during aspiration
    b. Vigorously move the needle to and fro in the lesion
    c. Both a & b
    d. Only a

81. **Which of the following is used as a bluing solution during Pap staining?**
    a. Harris hematoxylin
    b. Alkaline running tap water
    c. Absolute alcohol
    d. Xylene

82. **Which of the following statement is true about Pap staining?**
    a. Immediate fixation of smears is important
    b. Xylene is used as a clearing agent
    c. Hematoxylin should be filtered before use
    d. All statements are true

83. **Fine needle aspiration cytology (FNAC) is primarily used for:**
    a. Obtaining tissue samples for histopathological examination
    b. Evaluating blood cell counts and morphology
    c. Diagnosis of benign and malignant lesions
    d. All of the above

84. **The purpose of counterstaining in cytological staining is to:**
    a. Provide contrast to the primary stain
    b. Enhance the visibility of nuclear details
    c. Differentiate different cell types
    d. Identify specific cellular structures

85. **The final step in the staining process of cytological smears is:**
    a. Dehydration
    b. Mounting
    c. Fixation
    d. Washing

86. **The components of the Pap stain include:**
    a. Hematoxylin, eosin, and orange G
    b. Hematoxylin, eosin, and safranin
    c. Hematoxylin, eosin, and methylene blue
    d. Hematoxylin, eosin, and Giemsa

87. **The differentiation step in the Pap stain involves:**
    a. Rinsing the slide in distilled water
    b. Immersing the slide in acid alcohol
    c. Counterstaining the slide with eosin Y
    d. Immersing the slides in xylene

88. **The process of overstaining the smears and removal of excess stains with the help of differentiating solution is called as:**
    a. Regressive method
    b. Progressive method
    c. Dehydration
    d. Counterstaining

89. **Which of the following is a cytoplasmic stain in Pap stain?**
    a. OG-6
    b. EA-36
    c. Both a & b
    d. Only b

90. **Cervical cancer cells can exhibit the following cellular features, *except*:**
    a. Nuclear enlargement and irregularity
    b. Increased nuclear-to-cytoplasmic ratio
    c. Hyperchromasia
    d. Presence of cilia on the cell surface

Answers:

80. c	81. b	82. d	83. c
84. a	85. b	86. a	87. b
88. a	89. c	90. d	

91. **The appropriate site preparation before performing FNAC includes:**
    a. Cleaning the skin with an antiseptic solution
    b. Applying a local anaesthetic at the puncture site
    c. Both a & b
    d. None of the above

92. **The number of passes or aspirations performed during FNAC depends on:**
    a. The size of the lesion
    b. The patient's pain tolerance
    c. The type of needle used
    d. The site of the lesion

93. **The primary purpose of ultrasound guidance in FNAC is to:**
    a. Locate the target lesion accurately
    b. Determine the size of the needle to be used
    c. Assess the vascularity of the lesion
    d. Determine the depth of the lesion

94. **The advantage of using ultrasound guidance in FNAC is:**
    a. Targeting the deep-seated lesion
    b. Reduced risk of complications
    c. Real-time visualisation during the procedure
    d. All of the above

95. **Possible complications of FNAC include:**
    a. Hemorrhage and hematoma formation
    b. Infection at the puncture site
    c. Nerve injury or damage to adjacent structures
    d. All of the above

96. **The main advantage of FNAC compared to other diagnostic procedures is:**
    a. Non-invasiveness and minimal risk of complications
    b. Ability to detect the extent of tumor
    c. Capability to assess tissue architecture
    d. Ability to detect subtle cellular changes

97. **Contraindications for FNAC include:**
    a. Coagulation disorders or bleeding tendencies
    b. Recent antibiotic use
    c. History of diabetes mellitus
    d. All of the above

98. **Patient preparation before FNAC includes:**
    a. Fasting for 12 hours
    b. Administering prophylactic antibiotics
    c. Obtaining informed consent
    d. All of the above

99. **The reagent used for clearing in the staining process is:**
    a. Xylene
    b. Alcohol
    c. Acetone
    d. Chloroform

100. **Direct immunocytochemistry is used to:**
    a. Identify specific cell types in a tissue sample
    b. Assessing the viability of cells in culture
    c. Analysing gene expression patterns
    d. Quantifying protein-protein interactions

Answers:	91. a	92. a	93. a	94. d
	95. d	96. a	97. a	98. c
	99. a	100. a		

101. The primary detection method used to visualize the target molecule in direct immunocytochemistry:
a. Fluorescence microscopy
b. Electron microscopy
c. Radioactive labelling
d. Light microscopy

102. Which of the following is a crucial step in the direct immunocytochemistry procedure?
a. Blocking non-specific binding sites
b. Cell fixation with paraformaldehyde
c. Protein denaturation with heat treatment
d. DNA staining with DAPI

103. The primary antibody used in direct immunocytochemistry is typically raised against:
a. The target molecule of interest
b. The secondary antibody
c. The substrate used for the detection
d. The fluorophore used for labelling

104. Which of the following is an advantage of direct immunocytochemistry?
a. Enhanced signal amplification
b. Ability to detect multiple targets simultaneously
c. Reduced background staining
d. High spatial resolution

105. Which of the following is an advantage of using indirect immunocytochemistry?
a. Increased sensitivity
b. Shorter incubation times
c. Direct visualisation of the target molecule
d. Elimination of background staining

106. What is the primary purpose of the secondary antibody in indirect immunocytochemistry?
a. To bind directly to the target molecule
b. To amplify the signal for detection
c. To label the substrate used for the detection
d. To block non-specific binding sites

107. Which antibodies are used in the indirect immunocytochemistry technique?
a. Polygonal antibody
b. Tertiary antibody
c. Secondary antibody
d. Monoclonal antibody

108. Indirect immunocytochemistry allows for signal amplification due to the potential binding of multiple secondary antibodies to a single primary antibody. This phenomenon is known as:
a. Cross-reactivity
b. Signal transduction
c. Signal amplification
d. Signal suppression

109. The detection of the target molecule in indirect immunocytochemistry is typically visualised using which of the following methods?
a. Fluorescence microscopy
b. Electron microscopy
c. Radioactive labelling
d. Light microscopy

110. **Which techniques are commonly used to detect cell surface antigens in immunocytochemistry?**
    a. Immunofluorescence staining
    b. Immunohistochemistry
    c. Immunoperoxidase staining
    d. Immunoelectron microscopy

111. **Which of the following techniques is commonly used for studying tissue sections?**
    a. Immunohistochemistry
    b. Immunocytochemistry
    c. Immunoperoxidase staining
    d. Immunofluorescence staining

112. **Which of the following is the first step in immunocytochemistry?**
    a. Cell fixation
    b. Blocking non-specific binding
    c. Primary antibody incubation
    d. Secondary antibody incubation

113. **What is the purpose of cell fixation in immunocytochemistry?**
    a. To preserve cellular morphology
    b. To enhance antigen accessibility
    c. To block non-specific binding sites
    d. To amplify the signal for detection

114. **After blocking, which antibody is typically incubated with the sample in immunocytochemistry:**
    a. Primary antibody
    b. Secondary antibody
    c. Tertiary antibody
    d. Conjugated antibody

115. **What is the final step in immunocytochemistry before visualization?**
    a. Washing excess antibodies
    b. Protein denaturation
    c. Signal amplification
    d. Cell permeabilization

116. **To minimize non-specific binding during immunocytochemistry, which of the following steps is crucial?**
    a. Blocking non-specific binding sites
    b. Increasing the antibody concentration
    c. Using a secondary antibody with a higher affinity
    d. Increasing the incubation time

117. **During the washing steps in immunocytochemistry, what precautions should be taken to avoid excessive background staining?**
    a. Ensure gentle and thorough washing.
    b. Increase the washing buffer concentration.
    c. Extend the duration of washing steps.
    d. Skip the washing steps altogether.

118. **Which of the following parameters is commonly evaluated to assess the adequacy of the cytological sample?**
    a. Cell morphology
    b. Sample color
    c. Sample pH
    d. All of the above

119. **In fine-needle aspiration (FNA) cytology, adequacy is primarily assessed based on:**
    a. Cellular yield
    b. Cellular composition
    c. Sample viscosity
    d. Sample odor

Answers:	110. a	111. a	112. a	113. a
	114. a	115. a	116. a	117. a
	118. a	119. a		

120. Which of the following is a commonly used criterion to assess the adequacy of a cervical Pap smear sample?
a. Presence of endocervical cells
b. Stain intensity
c. Slide thickness
d. Sample transparency

121. Which parameter is used to evaluate the adequacy of the liquid-based cytology (LBC) sample?
a. Presence of microbial contamination
b. Cellularity
c. Hemoglobin content
d. Sample viscosity

122. Adequacy assessment of bronchial brushings or washings involves evaluating the presence of:
a. Mucus
b. Air bubbles
c. Squamous cells
d. Ciliated columnar cells

Answers: 120. a   121. b   122. d

5

SECTION

Microbiology

Section Outline

GENERAL MICROBIOLOGY

Louis Pasteur is also known as the father of microbiology. He described fermentation, pasteurization, germ theory of diseases, anthrax vaccine and rabies vaccine.

Robert Koch discovered the anthrax disease and the bacteria responsible for tuberculosis and cholera.

Koch's postulates: (1) The microorganism should be constantly associated with the lesions of the disease; (2) It should be possible to isolate the organism in pure culture from the lesions of the disease; (3) Inoculation of a laboratory animal with the cultured microorganism must recapitulate the disease; (4) It should be possible to re-isolate the organism in pure culture from the lesions in the experimental animal.

Molecular Koch' postulate: A gene found in a pathogenic microorganism encodes a product that contributes to the disease (virulence factor) caused by the pathogen.

Paul Ehrlich discovered the method of staining the tubercle bacillus. With his side-chain theory, Paul Ehrlich explained the basic principle of immunity. He is called the father of chemotherapy for formulating the arsenic compound, Salvarsan, which was used in the treatment of syphilis during the first half of this century until penicillin was discovered by Alexander Fleming.

Joseph Lister is called the father of antiseptic surgery.

Antoni van Leeuwenhoek: Father of microscopy.

Microscope: The parts of a microscope is shown in **Figure 7.1**.

Types of Microscopes

○ **Bright field:** Forms a dark image against a brighter background, used for stained samples.
○ **Dark field:** Used to illuminate and identify living, unstained cells bacteria causing them to appear brightly lit against a dark background, e.g., for *Spirochaetes*.
○ **Phase contrast:** It is possible to visualize certain cell organelles and structures that are invisible with bright-field. It is useful for studying motility, endospores and inclusion bodies.
○ **Fluorescent microscope:** It uses fluorescent molecules, fluorophores for the labelling of defined cellular structures which absorb light at a specific wavelength (excitation) and emit it at a specific higher wavelength (emission), e.g., acridine orange for malaria parasite and Auramine for *M. tuberculosis*.

Staining Techniques

○ **Simple stain:** Involves directly staining the bacterial cell with a positively charged dye (basic dye),e.g., basic fuchsin.
○ **Negative stain:** Where the bacteria remain unstained against a dark background, e.g., India Ink.

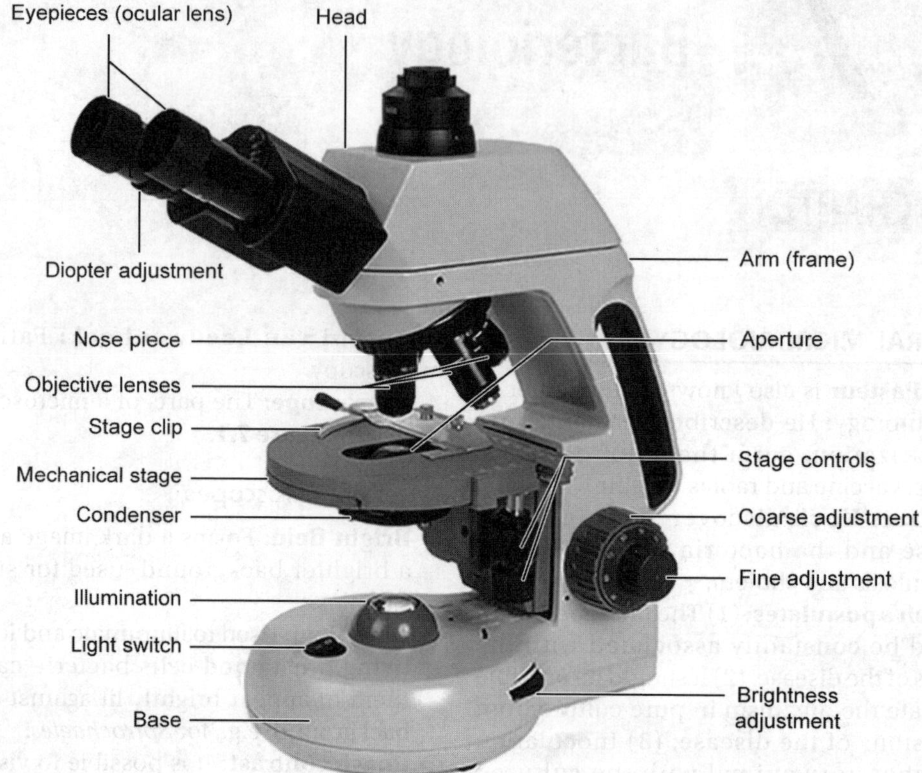

Fig. 7.1: Parts of microscope.

○ **Impregnation method:** Silver impregnation is the traditional method for detection of *T. pallidum* in formalin-fixed tissues. *Borrelia spp., Bartonella spp., Leptospira spp.,* and *Calymmatobacterium.* Weakly staining gram-negative bacteria, including *Legionella spp., Burkholderia spp., Francisella spp., and Helicobacter,* are also best demonstrated by silver impregnation.

○ **Differential stain:** It use more than one stain, which impart different appearance based on their structural properties. Some examples of differential stains are the Gram stain, acid-fast stain and the Kinyoun method of staining does not require heating.

○ **Endospore stain:** Schaeffer fulton method with malachite green 5% and 0.5% safranin, which results in the spore appear green and vegetative cells red. Acid-fast with 0.25% sulphuric acid.

○ **Flagellar stain:** The Leifson flagella stain method, all flagella stains use mordants, like tannic acid and potassium alum, to coat and thus thicken the flagellum in order to be observable by light microscopy.

○ **Capsular stain:** Wet-mount method using india ink where the capsule is visualized as a refractile zone surrounding a cell. Dry-mount method that precipitates copper sulfate and leaves the capsule as a pale blue zone. The polychrome methylene blue staining procedure for blood or tissue smears found from dead animals **(M'Fadyean's reaction)** rapid diagnostic test for anthrax bacilli bearing polypeptide capsule.

Acid-Fast Organisms

- Mycobacteria
- Nocardia
- Bacterial endospores
- Head of sperm
- *Cryptosporidium parvum*
- *Cryptoisospora belli*
- *Cyclospora cayetanensis*
- *Taenia saginata eggs*
- Hydatid hooklets

Demonstration of Bacterial Motility

- Hanging drop
- Semisolid agar
- Cragie tube method

Characteristic Motility of Bacteria

- **Darting motility:** *Vibrio cholerae* and *Campylobacter jejuni*
- **Tumbling motility:** *Listeria monocytogenes*
- **Corkscrew motility:** *Spirochetes*
- **Swarming:** *Proteus* and *Clostridium tetani*

Morphology of Bacteria

- **Cell wall:** Gram-negative bacteria are surrounded by a thin peptidoglycan cell wall, which itself is surrounded by an outer membrane containing lipopolysaccharide. A peptidoglycan monomer consists of two joined amino sugars, N-acetylglucosamine (NAG) and N-acetylmuramic acid (NAM). Gram-positive bacteria lack an outer membrane but are surrounded by layers of peptidoglycan many times thicker. Due to differences in the thickness of a peptidoglycan layer in the cell membrane between Gram positive and Gram negative bacteria, Gram positive bacteria (with a thicker peptidoglycan layer) retain crystal violet stain during the decolorization process, while gram negative bacteria lose the crystal violet stain. Teichoic acids acidic polymers found in the cell walls, capsules, and membranes of all gram-positive bacteria give them an overall negative charge due to the presence of phosphodiester bonds between teichoic acid monomers.
- **Capsule:** The bacterial capsule is usually a hydrated polysaccharide structure that covers the outer layer of the cell wall. The capsule of *Bacillus anthracis* is an exception its capsule is composed of polypeptide. Capsule resists phagocytosis from ingesting and destroying the bacterial cell.
- **Flagella:** They are the organelles for bacterial locomotion. It extends from the cytoplasm to the cell exterior and are composed of three major structural elements, the basal body, the hook and the filament.
- **Fimbriae or pili:** Fimbriae and pili are hair-like appendages present on the bacterial cell wall similar to flagella. They are shorter than flagella and more in number. They are involved in the bacterial conjugation, attachment to the surface and motility
- **Spores:** They are the most dormant form of bacteria since they exhibit minimal metabolism. Gram-positive bacteria produce intracellular spores called endospores as a survival mechanism. Spore forming bacteria include *Bacillus* (aerobic) and *Clostridium* (anaerobic) species.

Physiology of Bacteria

Bacterial Growth Curve (Fig. 7.2)

The bacterial growth curve represents the number of live cells in a bacterial population over a period of time. There are four distinct phases of the growth curve: lag, exponential

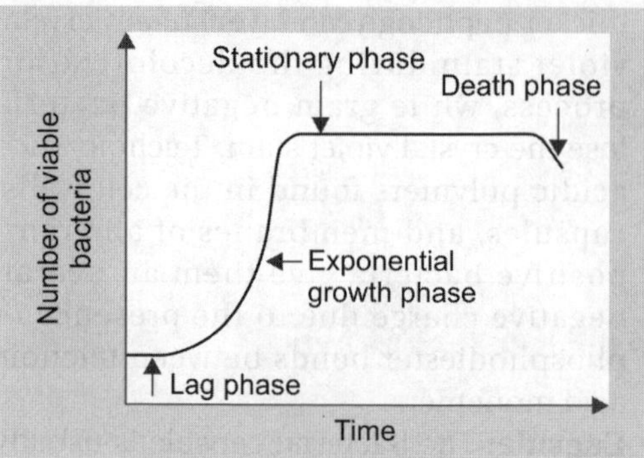

Fig. 7.2: Bacterial growth curve.

(log), stationary, and death. The initial phase is the lag phase where bacteria are metabolically active but not dividing.

Obligate Intracellular Organism

Obligate intracellular bacteria, which include *Chlamydia spp., Anaplasma spp., Ehrlichia spp., Rickettsia spp., Orientia spp,* and *Coxiella spp.*, replicate exclusively inside of eukaryotic host cells.

Endotoxin

Endotoxins or lipopolysaccharide (LPS)are the main component of the outer membrane of the cell wall of gram-negative bacteria.

Exotoxin

They are secreted proteins which act locally and at distance of the bacterial colonization site.

The pathogenic bacteria that produce exotoxins mainly include *Clostridium tetani, Clostridium botulinum, Clostridium perfringens, Corynebacterium diphtheriae, Group A streptococcus* and *Staphylococcus aureus.*

STERILIZATION AND DISINFECTION

Definition

○ **Sterilization:** A process that destroys or eliminates all forms of microbial life including viable spores with reduction of at least 10^6 log colony forming units.

○ **Disinfection:** Describes a process that eliminates many or all pathogenic microorganisms, except bacterial spores, on inanimate objects (10^3 log colony forming units).
○ **Cleaning:** Is the removal of visible soil (e.g., organic and inorganic material) from objects and surfaces.
○ **Asepsis:** It is a process where the chemical agent (antiseptic) applied to body surfaces will kill or inhibit the pathogenic microorganisms (and also commensals) present on skin.
○ **Decontamination:** It is reduction of pathogenic microbes to a level at which items are considered safe to handle and with reduction of atleast 1 log CFU of microorganism but not spores.

Factors Influencing Efficacy of Sterilant

○ Organism Load
○ **Nature of Organism:** Decreasing order of resistance of microorganisms: Prions > bacterial spores > coccidian cyst > mycobacteria > nonenveloped viruses > fungi > vegetative bacteria > enveloped viruses.
○ Concentration of the sterilant/disinfectant and temperature of the physical agent.
○ Nature of the sterilant/disinfectant
○ Duration of exposure
○ pH
○ Biofilm formation

The Spaulding Classification

This classification places reusable medical instruments or devices into three categories of ascending risk for infection **(Table 7.1)**.

Sterilization is carried out by physical or chemical methods (Table 7.2)
Physical:
Moist heat can be used:
○ At temperatures below 100°C.
○ At a temperature at 100°C.
○ At a temperature above 100°C (in saturated steam under increased pressure).

Table 7.1: Spaulding classification.

Spaulding classification	Medical device contacts	Disinfection level
Critical	Sterile tissue or the bloodstream, e.g., catheters	Sterilization
Semi-critical	Mucous membranes or nonintact skin, e.g., endoscopes	High level disinfection (HLD)
Noncritical	Intact skin only, e.g., thermometer	Intermediate level (ILD) or low level disinfection (LLD)

Table 7.2: Applications/limitations of different sterlization methods.

Process	Conditions	Applications/limitations
Heat sterilization		
Dry Heat		
Flaming	High temperature and short time processing	To sterilize loops and points of forceps in the flame of a bunsen burner until it is red
Hot air oven	160°C for 120 minutes	Powders and petroleum products
Infra-red rays	Infrared technology include short cycle time, low energy consumption, no cycle residuals, and no toxicologic or environmental effects.	For sterilization of selected heat-resistant instruments (not FDA approved) has longer wavelength and lower energy it cannot penetrate substances and can only be used in sterilizing surfaces
Radiation		
Nonionizing rays: Rays of wavelength longer than the visible light are nonionizing microbicidal wavelength of UV rays lie in the range of 200–280 nm, with 260 nm being most effective	UV rays are generated using a high-pressure mercury vapor lamp	UV light in biosafety cabinets can cause skin erythema and keratoconjunctivitis
Ionizing rays: Electron beams and gamma rays	Gamma rays have more penetrative power than electron beam but require longer time of exposure	To sterilize disposable petri dishes, plastic syringes, antibiotics, vitamins, hormones, glasswares and fabrics
Moist heat (below 100°C)		
Pasteurization	63°C for 30 minutes (the holder method) or 73°C for 20 seconds (the flash method)	Can destroy all nonspore forming pathogens in milk except *Coxiella burnetii* in holder method
Serum bath	Serum can be inactivated by heating in a water bath at 56 °C for 1 h on several successive days	Only vegetative bacteria are killed and spores survive. Proteins in the serum will coagulate at higher temperature
Vaccine bath	Vaccine preparation can be inactivated by heating in a water bath at 60 °C for 1 h	Only vegetative bacteria are killed and spores survive

Contd...

Contd...

Process	Conditions	Applications/limitations
Inspissation	The medium containing serum or egg are placed in the slopes of an inspissator and heated at 80–85°C for 30 minutes on three successive days. On the 1st day, the vegetative bacteria would die and those spores that germinate by next day are then killed the following day	LJ media/Loeffler's serum slope. If the spores fail to germinate then this technique cannot be considered sterilization
Moist heat (at 100°C)		
Boiling	Placing items like glassware in boiling water for 10–20 minutes	Certain bacterial toxins such as Staphylococcal enterotoxin are also heat resistant. Some bacterial spores are resistant to boiling and survive
Steam at 100°C (Arnold's and Koch's steamers) 100 °C	The articles are subjected to free steam at 100°C for 90 minutes	Media such as TCBS, DCA and selenite broth are sterilized by steaming. An autoclave (with discharge tap open) can also serve the same purpose
Tyndallization or fractional sterilization or intermittent sterilization	Free steaming for 20 minutes for three successive days. The vegetative bacteria are killed in the first exposure and the spores that germinate by next day are killed in subsequent days. The success of process depends on the germination of spores	Media containing sugar and gelatin
Moist heat (above 100°C)		
Steam sterilization (autoclave) types—gravity displacement and pre vacuum	121°C for 15 minutes at 15 psi or 134°C for 3 minutes (pre vacuum autoclave)	For sterilization of most culture media, glassware and other laboratory materials. Decontamination of microbiological waste may require at least 45 minutes at 121°C because the entrapped air remaining in a load of waste retards steam permeation and heating efficiency
Microwave	30-minute cycle with to 110°C. The microwave unit transmits energy as microwaves and this energy turns into heat inside the wet waste	Laboratory/hospital waste treatment
Chemical sterilization		
Glutaraldehyde 2%	For sterilization of medical instruments (exposure >10 hours is required)	Meticulous cleaning to remove organic matter. instruments should be rinsed with filtered water before use
Per acetic acid (0.2%)	0.2% for 12 minutes sterilize medical, (e.g., GI endoscopes) and surgical (e.g., flexible endoscopes) instruments	The instrument should be rinsed four times with filtered water before use
Gaseous sterilization		
Ethylene oxide (EtO) gas sterilization	Concentration of 450–1200 mg/L, at temperatures of 37–63°C and RH of 40–80% for 1–6 h	Heat-sensitive and moisture sensitive equipment and instruments

Contd...

Contd...

Process	Conditions	Applications/limitations
Hydrogen peroxide vapor (HPV) and hydrogen peroxide gas plasma (HPGP) sterilization	Concentration of 6 mg/L, temperature range of 37 time of 75 minutes	Heat-sensitive and moisture sensitive equipment and instruments
Ozone	The duration of the sterilization cycle is about 30–35°C; 4 h and 15 m	Processing reusable medical devices

○ **Principle of an autoclave:** There are four parameters of steam sterilization: steam, pressure, temperature, and time. Steam is admitted at the top or the sides of the autoclave chamber and, because the steam is lighter than air, forces air out the bottom of the chamber through the drain vent. By pushing the air out, the steam is able to make direct contact with the load and begin to sterilize it.

○ **Autoclave tape:** To indicate whether a specific temperature has been reached.

○ **Bowie-dick indicator:** A commercially available bowie-dick indicator **(Fig. 7.3)** is placed in the center of the autoclave in an empty cycle and run at 134°C for 3.5 minutes. Autoclave performance is acceptable if the sheet inside the test pack shows a uniform color change. Used in Central Sterile Supply Department (CSSD) department.

○ **Chemical indicators class 5 and 6 (Fig. 7.4):** They are devices used to monitor the presence or attainment of one or more of the parameters required for a satisfactory sterilization process. This change in color of the indicator is observed and interpreted as a pass or fail. Used in CSSD department.

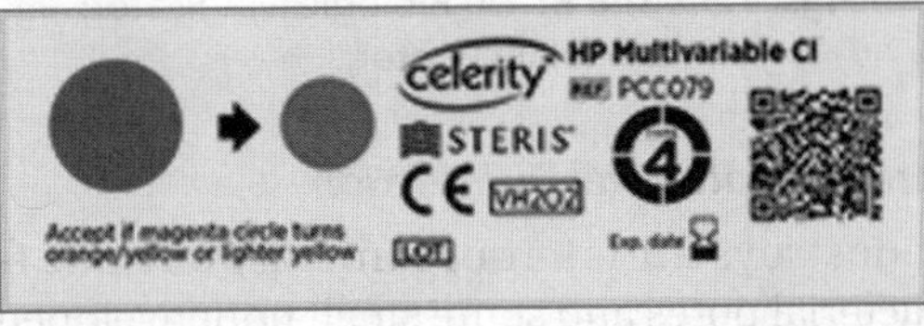

Fig. 7.4: Chemical indicators class 5 and 6.

Sterilization monitoring/Process control

See **Table 7.3**.

Disinfection in Healthcare

High-level Disinfection

It destroys all microorganisms but not bacterial spores, e.g., glutaraldehyde, hydrogen peroxide, etc.

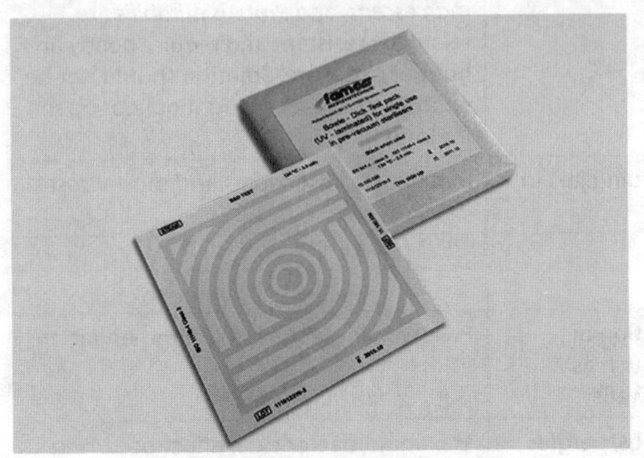

Fig. 7.3: Bowie-dick indicator.

Table 7.3: Different sterlization process and their biological indicator.

Process	Biological indicator (Figs. 7.5A and B)
Hot air oven	*B. atrophaeus*
Autoclave	*Geobacillus stearothermophilus spores*
ETO	*Bacillus atrophaeus*
Plasma sterilization	*Bacillus atrophaeus spores*
Ionizing radiation	*Bacillus pumilus*
Filtration	*Serratia marcescens Brevundimonas diminuta*

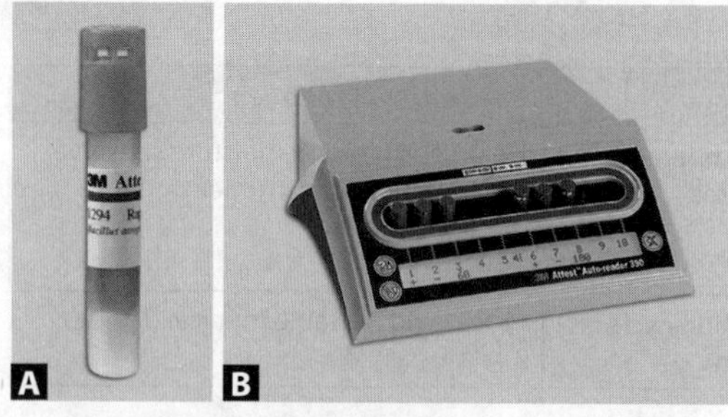

Figs. 7.5A and B: (A) Biological indicator; (B) Incubator.

Intermediate-level Disinfection

It destroys all microorganisms, but not is bacterial pores and some small nonenveloped viruses, e.g., alcohol, QACs. Intermediate-level disinfection is used for noncritical items.

Low-level Disinfection

It destroys most microorganisms and some viruses but has no action on *Mycobacterium tuberculosis* and spores, e.g., alcohol or QACs, etc., at lower exposures.

Commonly used Chemical Disinfectants in Health Care/Laboratory

See **Table 7.4**.

Testing of Disinfectants

Disinfectants are known to lose their activity on standing as well as in the presence of organic matter, their activity can be tested by the following methods:

- **Riedel Walker method (phenol coefficient):** For phenolic agents
- Chick Martin test

Table 7.4: Chemical disinfectants with their uses and limitations.		
Chemical	*Uses*	*Limitation*
Alcohols ethyl alcohol (ethanol, alcohol) and isopropyl alcohol, 60–90%	Environmental surface cleaning	No sporicidal activity, concentrations less than 50% have poor antimicrobial activity and skin irritant
Hypochlorite solutions: 0.1% (1,000 parts per million/ppm) for surface cleaning; (1.0 %) (10,000 ppm) for large (>10 mL) spills of blood and body fluids and *C. auris* and *C. difficile*	Environmental surface cleaning	Irritant of eyes, skin, and mucous membrane can cause asthma, corrosion of metal Fresh dilution should be prepared daily Solution should not be exposed to direct sunlight or kept open for long time
Hydrogen peroxide >0.5%	Environmental surface cleaning	Irritant for eyes organisms with high cellular catalase activity such as *Staphylococcus aureus*, *Serratia marcescens*, and *Proteus mirabilis* are relatively resistant and require nearly an hour of exposure. Solution should not be exposed to direct sunlight or kept open for long time
Phenols (5% phenol, 1–5% cresol, 5% lysol)	Can be used in discarding jars in TB laboratories	Inactive against spores and most viruses
Halogen-releasing agents—iodine and iodophors	Skin preparation	
Quaternary ammonium compounds (QACs)	Environmental sanitation of noncritical surfaces, such as floors, furniture, and walls	Follow manufacturer's recommendation
Chlorhexidine	Antimicrobial dressings, gargles or mouthwash	Maximum bactericidal effect occurring within 20 seconds

Contd...

Contd...

Chemical	Uses	Limitation
Heavy metals	1% silver nitrate solution; copper salts ; merthiolate	As treatment for ophthalmia neonatorum; copper salts are used as a fungicide Merthiolate at a concentration of 1:10,000 is used in preservation of serum
Cetrimide and benzalkonium chloride (cationic detergents)	They are widely used as disinfectants at dilution of 1–2% for domestic use and in hospitals	Pseudomonas can grow in cetrimide
Aniline dyes such as crystal violet	Bacteriostatic against gram positive bacteria	The dyes are used as selective agents in certain selective media. Malachite-green dye is added to LJ media to inhibit microorganisms other than mycobacteria and as a pH indicator

○ Capacity use dilution test (Kelsey-Sykes test)
○ In-use test

Filters (Table 7.5)

○ **Sporicidal agents:** Include gluteraldehyde, sodium hypochlorite, iodine iodophors, hydrogen peroxide and peracetic acid.
○ **Virucidal agents:** Ethyl alcohol 60%–80%, 3% hydrogen peroxide, povidone-iodine (PVP-I), sodium hypochlorite, glutaraldehyde and quaternary ammonium compounds (QACs)
○ **Mycobacteriocidal agents** 5% phenols, chlorine and alcohol.

○ **Bactericidal agents:** Alcohol, chlorine and chlorine compounds, formaldehyde, glutaraldehyde, hydrogen peroxide, iodophors, ortho-phthalaldehyde (OPA), peracetic acid.

Calculation of Sodium Hypochlorite Concentrations

[% chlorine in liquid sodium hypochlorite/% chlorine desired] – 1 = Total parts of water for each part sodium hypochlorite

Example: [4% in liquid sodium hypochlorite/1% chlorine desired]–1 = 3 parts of water for each part sodium

Table 7.5: Filters with their characteristics and uses and limitations.			
Type	Characteristic	Use	Limitation
Earthenware filters Pasteur-Chamberland filter/Berkefeld filter	Are made up of porcelain (sand and kaolin) or Kieselguhr	Used to remove microbes from heat labile liquids such as serum, antibiotic solutions, sugar solutions and urea solution	The disadvantages of depth filters are migration of filter material into the filtrate, absorption or retention of certain volume of liquid by the filters, pore sizes are not definite and viruses and mycoplasma could pass through
Asbestos filters	Magnesium silicate sterilized by autoclaving		Not reusable
Sintered glass filters	Pore diameter of 1–1.5 μm cleaned with warm concentrated H_2SO_4 and sterilized by autoclaving		

Contd...

Contd...

Type	Characteristic	Use	Limitation
Membrane filters	Cellulose diacetate; a pore diameter ranging from 0.015 μm to 12 μm		Little loading capacity and are fragile
HEPA (High Efficiency Particle Air) filters	99.97% efficient for removing particles >0.3 μm in diameter	Operating rooms and biosafety cabinets	

hypochlorite i.e., if 1 liter of 1% sodium hypochlorite is needed dilute 25 mL with 75 mL of water.

CULTURE MEDIA AND METHODS

○ **Liquid media:** It offers a uniform culture condition for the growth of bacteria producing general turbidity, e.g., nutrient broth and brain heart infusion broth.
○ **Semi-solid media:** They are prepared with lower agar concentrations of 0.2 to 0.5%. They have a soft and are used to cultivate microaerophilic bacteria or determine bacterial motility by cultivation in stab tubes, e.g., Hugh and Leifson's oxidation fermentation medium, Stuart's and Amies media, and Mannitol motility media.
○ **Solid media:** They are prepared by adding 1 to 2% agar. They make it possible to obtain isolated colonies of different bacterial species, which can be identified, e.g., MacConkey agar and nutrient agar.

Media are Classified into Six Types

1. Basal media
2. Enriched media
3. Selective
4. Indicator media/differential media
5. Transport media
6. Storage media
1. **Basal media:** Media do not require enrichment sources and are suitable for growing nonfastidious bacteria like *Staphylococcus* and Enterobacteriaceae. They are generally used to isolate microorganisms in labs or in sub-culturing processes, e.g., are nutrient broth, nutrient agar, and peptone water.
2. **Enriched media:** Addition of extra nutrients in the form of blood, serum, egg yolk, etc., to basal medium makes them enriched media for the growth of fastidious bacteria, e.g., are blood agar, chocolate agar, loeffler's serum, MacConkey agar and Lowenstein-jensen media.
3. **Selective:** A selective medium is a medium that allows the growth of one or more types of microorganisms while inhibiting the growth of other flora with the help of additives such as antibiotics. Cetrimide agar base is a culture medium used to selectively isolate and identify *Pseudomonas aeruginosa*.
4. **Indicator media/differential media:** These media thus allow to differentiate various kinds of microorganisms on the same agar plate, e.g., is blood agar.
   MacConkey agar is a selective and differential culture medium as it is designed to selectively isolate gram-negative and enteric bacteria and differentiate them based on lactose fermentation. MacConkey medium include crystal violet dye, bile salts, lactose, and neutral red (pH indicator). Crystal violet dye and bile salts halt the growth of gram-positive bacteria.
   TCBS agar (thiosulfate-citrate-bile-sucrose agar) is a selective differential medium for isolating and cultivating *Vibrio cholerae*.

Cystine-lactose-electrolyte-deficient agar (**CLED agar**) supports the growth of urinary pathogens but prevents undue swarming of *Proteus species* due to its lack of electrolytes.

5. **Transport media:** They are essentially buffer solutions containing carbohydrates, peptones and other nutrients (excluding growth factors) designed to preserve the viability of bacteria during transport without allowing them to multiply. Cary-Blair medium and Venkatraman Ramakrishnan (VR) medium for fecal and rectal samples, is ideal for transport *V. cholerae;*amies medium (*Neisseria gonorrheae)*, stuart medium (*Neisseria gonorrheae)*, pike's medium *(Streptococci)*

6. **Storage media:** Media used for storing the bacteria for a long period of time, e.g., egg saline medium and chalk cooked meat broth.

   Enrichment Broth: Liquid medium that only permits a specific species (pathogen) of a microbe to grow in it while inhibiting others (normal flora), e.g., selenite F. broth and tetrathionate broth for *Salmonella* and *Shigella,* alkaline peptone water (APW) for *V. cholerae.*

   Agar which is extracted from species of Gelidium and Gracilaria is a commonly used solidifying agent (1–2%) in microbiological media. Agar is an ideal solidifying agent for microbiological media because of its melting properties and because it has no nutritive value for the vast majority of bacteria. Solid agar melts at about 100°C; liquid agar solidifies at about 42°C. Smaller amounts (0.05–0.5%) are used in media for motility studies and for growth of anaerobes (0.1%) and microaerophiles.

Anaerobic Culture Media

1. Robertson's cooked meat broth (RCM)
2. Thioglycollate broth
3. Neomycin blood agar
4. PRAS (Prereduced anaerobically sterilized media)

RCM is suitable for growing anaerobic bacteria in air and also for the transport and preservation of their stock cultures.

Aerobic Culture Methods: Streak, Lawn, Stoke and Stab Method

Microaerophilic culture: Candle jars are used to grow bacteria requiring an increased (5–7%) CO_2 concentration (capnophilic bacteria), e.g., *Haemophilus influenzae, neisseria meningitidis and streptococcus pneumoniae.*

Anaerobic culture methods:

1. **McIntosh and Fildes anaerobic jar (Fig. 7.6)** works on the concept of replacement and evacuation, in which the air within the chamber is removed and replaced with a mixture made of gas (consisting of 5% CO_2, 10% H_2 and 85% N_2).

2. **GasPak system (Fig. 7.7)** generates an anaerobic environment by means of a gas generating pouch, the hydrogen thus produced reacts with oxygen present inside the jar producing water (which forms as condensation on the inside of the jar).
   $$2H_2 + O_2 + catalyst = 2H_2O$$

   Anaerobic indicator strips:

   ○ **Impregnated with methylene blue:** Remains colorless in anaerobic conditions, but turns blue on exposure to oxygen.

   ○ **Impregnated with resazurin, a redox indicator:** Colorless (white) in anaerobic conditions but turns to pink in the presence of oxygen.

   ○ **Biological indicator:** A plate inoculated with *Pseudomonas* is incubated along with other inoculated plates for anaerobic cultures.

3. **Anoxomat anaerobic culture system: Bacterial identification**

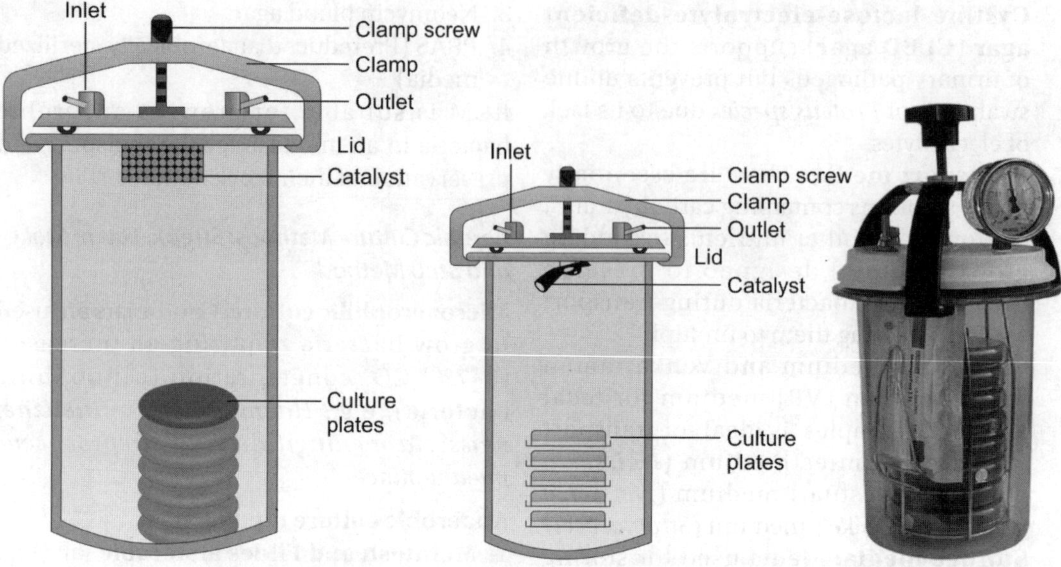

Fig. 7.6: McIntosh and Fildes anaerobic jar.

1. Conventional (identification by biochemical reactions).
2. Automated (VITEK 2, Phoenix, MicroScan WalkAway, MALDI-TOF)).
3. Molecular (PCR)

Biochemical Reactions

Gram Positive Cocci

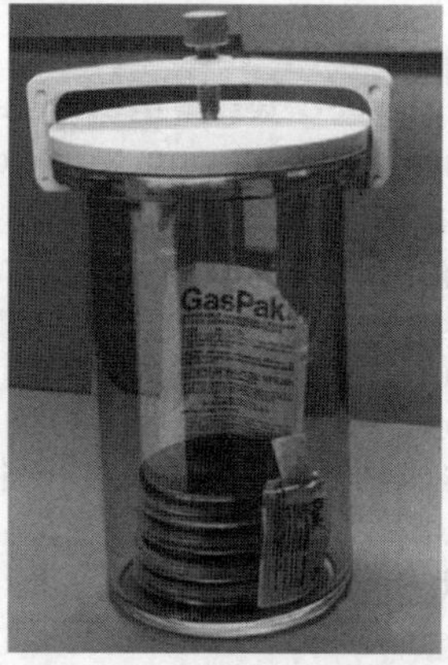

Fig. 7.7: GasPak system.

○ **Catalase (3% H_2O_2):** *Streptococcus species* (catalase-negative), *Staphylococcus species* (catalase-positive), and *Listeria species* (catalase-positive) can be differentiated. Positive organisms will evolve gas bubbles in the presence of H_2O_2.

○ **Coagulase (slide and tube):** Coagulase test is used to differentiate *Staphylococcus aureus* (positive) which produce the enzyme coagulase, from *S. epidermis* and *S. saprophyticus* (negative) which do not produce coagulase. Both tests utilize EDTA-treated rabbit plasma. Positive test will produce clumps of cells.

○ **CAMP test:** The Christie–atkins–munch-peterson(CAMP test) is a test to identify group B β-hemolytic *Streptococci* (*Streptococcus agalactiae*) based on their formation of a substance (CAMP factor) that enlarges the area of hemolysis formed by the β-hemolysin elaborated from *Staphylococcus aureus*.

○ **Bacitracin susceptibility test:** The bacitracin disc (0.04 units)is used to distinguish *Streptococcus pyogenes*, which forms a zone of inhibition around the bacitracin disc.

○ **Bile aesculin:** The bile-esculin test is widely used to differentiate *Enterococci* and group D. *Streptococci*, which are bile tolerant and can hydrolyze esculin to esculetin, from nongroup D. viridans group *Streptococci*, which grow poorly on bile.

○ **Bile solubility:** The test is used specifically to presumptively differentiate between *Streptococcus pneumoniae* (bile soluble) and other α-haemolytic *Streptococci* (not bile soluble) within 30 minutes of A 10% bile salt solution at 37°C.

Gram Negative Bacilli

○ **Oxidase test:** Tetra-methyl-p-phenylenediamine dihydrochloride, is the reagent which is an artificial electron donor for cytochrome c. When the reagent is oxidized by cytochrome c, it changes from colorless to a dark blue or purple compound, indophenol blue. *Pseudomonas aeruginosa, Pasteurella multocida, Vibrio spp., Aeromonas spp.* and *Neisseria spp.*

○ **Indole test:** The ability of an organism to degrade the amino acid tryptophan and produce indole. Addition of 5 drops of Kovács reagent to the top of the 24 hours of growth in peptone water. A positive indole test is indicated by the formation of a red color in the reagent layer on top of the agar deep within seconds of adding the reagent. *E. coli ,Vibrio, Aeromonas, Plesiomonas,* and *Pasteurella* and most strains of *P. vulgaris, M. morganii* and *Providenica* are indole positive.

○ **Methyl Red test:** If the tube turns red after adding the methyl red reagent, the test is positive for mixed acid fermentation(one or more organic acids formed during the fermentation of glucose). MR test positive

bacteria are *Escherichia coli*, while negative are *Klebsiella pneumoniae, Enterobacter species.*

○ **Vogues proskeur:** VP is a test used to detect acetoin in a bacterial broth culture. The test is performed by adding alpha-naphthol and potassium hydroxide to the Voges-proskauer broth, which is a glucose-phosphate broth that has been inoculated with bacteria. VP positive organisms include *Enterobacter* and *Klebsiella*.

○ **Urease test:** Identifies those organisms that are capable of hydrolyzing urea to produce ammonia and carbon dioxide. pH indicator phenol red, which changes the color to dark pink when positive (high pH). *Proteus, Helicobacter pylori, Klebsiella, Cryptococcus.* The rapid urease test (RUT) is a popular diagnostic test for diagnosis of *Helicobacter pylori.*

○ **Citrate test:** It screens the isolate for the ability to utilize citrate as its carbon and energy source. pH indicator bromothymol blue, which is green as neutral pH and changes to deep prussian blue at alkaline pH above 7.5. The green color indicates negative citrate test while the formation of blue color indicates positive citrate test. *Klebsiella, Enterobacter, Citrobacter, Providencia, Proteus, Serratia, Vibrio cholerae* and *Pseudomonas.*

○ **Phenylalanine deaminase test:** To test the ability of an organism to carry out oxidative deamination of phenylalanine by enzyme deaminase. This enzyme removes the amine group from the amino acid phenylalanine and produces phenylpyruvic acid (PPA) and ammonia. Phenylpyruvic acid reacts with ferric iron (10% ferric chloride is added to the medium) producing a visible green color. *Proteus sp., Morganella sp., Providenica sp* give positive PPA test.

○ **Triple Sugar Iron (TSI):** This tests ability of an organism to ferment glucose (0.1%), lactose (1%), and sucrose, (1%) and their ability to produce hydrogen sulfide due to sodium thiosulfate and ferrous ammonium sulphate present in the medium. The slant has an aerobic environment where, as the butt has an anaerobic environment under which fermentation patterns of organisms are determined. The acid base indicator phenol red is incorporated for detecting carbohydrate fermentation that is indicated by the change in color of the carbohydrate medium from orange red to yellow in the presence of acids. In case of oxidative decarboxylation of peptone, alkaline products are built and the pH rises and color of the medium from orange red to deep red. If the organism under identification ferments only glucose, the meagre amount of acid production in the slant of the tube during glucose fermentation oxidizes rapidly, causing the medium to remain orange red or revert to an alkaline pH. In contrast, the acid reaction (yellow) is maintained in the butt of the tube since it is under lower oxygen tension.

Interpretation

○ **An alkaline/acid (red slant/yellow butt) reaction:** It is indicative of glucose fermentation only *Shigella*.

○ **An acid/acid (yellow slant/yellow butt) reaction:** It indicates the fermentation of glucose, lactose and/or sucrose, *Escherichia* and *Klebsiella*.

○ **An alkaline/alkaline (red slant and red butt) reaction:** Absence of carbohydrate fermentation results and *Pseudomonas*.

○ **Blackening of the medium:** Occurs in the presence of H_2S Proteus, *Salmonella Typhimurium*.

○ **Gas production:** Bubbles or cracks in the agar indicate the production of gas (formation of CO_2 and H_2) *Escherichia* and *Klebsiella*.

○ **Oxidative fermentation test (Fig. 7.8):** The method described as the hugh and leifson test employs a semi-solid medium in tubes containing the carbohydrate under test (glucose) and a pH indicator bromthymol blue, the high acid concentration produced during fermentation will turn the indicator in OF media from green to yellow in the presence or absence of oxygen. Two tubes are inoculated and one is sealed immediately to produce anaerobic conditions. *Escherichia coli* (Fermentative); *Pseudomonas aeruginosa* (oxidative); *Alcaligenes fecalis* (negative OF test).

○ **String test:** It is used to differentiate *Vibrio cholerae* (positive) from *Vibrio* species and

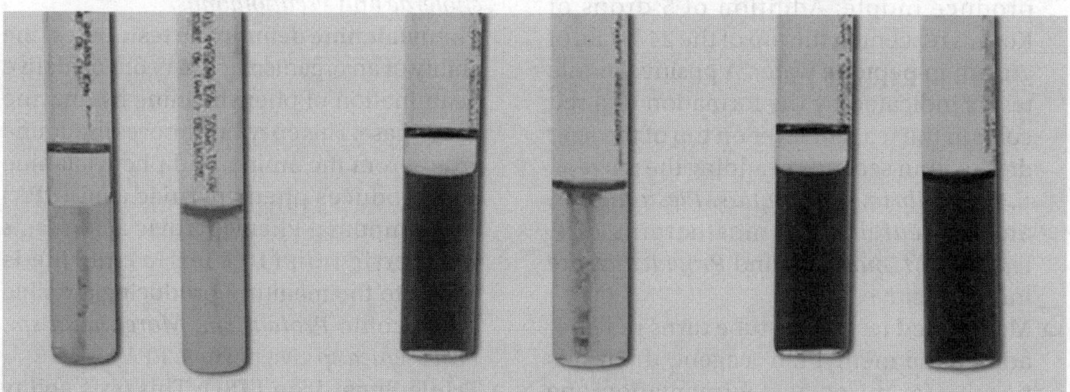

Fig. 7.8: Oxidative fermentation test.

(For color version, see Plate 7)

other bacteria like *aeromonas species* and *plesiomonas shigelloides*. The string test may be performed on a glass microscope slide by suspending 18–24 hours growth in a drop of 0.5% aqueous solution of sodium deoxycholate. If the cells lyse, the liberated cellular DNA makes the mixture viscous or "stringy."

IMMUNOLOGY

Immunity

Immunity refers to the body's ability to prevent the invasion of pathogens.

Classified as (Table 7.6):

○ **Innate:** This type of immunity is present in an organism by birth.

○ **Acquired/adaptive:** Acquired immunity or adaptive immunity is the immunity that our body acquires over time. Unlike the innate immunity, this is not present by birth.

T Lymphocyte

T lymphocytes (also called T cells) are produced in bone marrow and then move to the thymus through the bloodstream, where they mature. The "T" in their name comes from "thymus."

T cells have three main functions:

1. **T helper cells:** They use chemical messengers to activate other immune system cells in order to start the adaptive immune system.

2. **Cytotoxic T cells:** They detect cells infected by viruses or tumorous cells and destroy them.

3. **Memory T cells:** Some T helper cells become memory cells and activate the adapted immune system quickly if there is another infection.

B Lymphocytes

○ B lymphocytes (B cells) are made in the bone marrow and then mature there to become specialized immune system cells. They take their name from the "B" in "bone marrow." Like the T cells, there are many different types of B cells that match particular germs.

○ **The B cells are activated by the T helper cells:** This activates the B cells to multiply and to transform themselves into plasma cells which produce very large amounts of antibodies. Because only the B cells that match the attacking germs are activated, only the exact antibodies that are needed will be produced.

○ **Memory B cells:** Some of the activated B. cells transform into memory cells.

○ **Cytokines** are proteins and chemical messengers produced by different cells in the body.

Table 7.6: Difference between Innate and acquired immunity.	
Innate	**Acquired/adaptive**
From birth	Acquired during lifetime
It acts very quickly	Slower to respond
"Nonspecific"	Specific to the antigen
• Protection offered by the skin and mucous membranes • Immune system cells (natural killer cells)	T lymphocytes, B lymphocytes and antibodies
Memory absent	Memory responses are present
They use nonspecific receptors like "Toll-like receptors"	Host cell receptors are specific, T-cell and B cell receptors
Components are NK cells, phagocytes, acute phase reactant proteins, alternate and mannose binding pathways, cytokines—TNF	Components are T cell, B cell, classical complement pathway, cytokines (IL-2, IL-4, IL-5, IFN)

Table 7.7: Types of acquired immunity.

Active immunity	Passive immunity
Passive immunity is provided when a person is given antibodies to a disease rather than producing them through his or her own immune system	Active immunity results when exposure to a disease organism triggers the immune system to produce antibodies to that disease
Usually takes several weeks to develop	Immediate protection
Long-lasting	Lasts only for a few weeks or months
E.g., immunization of chickenpox, hepatitis, flu, and polio	**E.g.,** a baby receiving antibodies from her mother's breast milk and injection of antisera

Table 7.8: Difference between primary and secondary immune response.

Features	Primary immune response	Secondary immune response
Definition	Immune response that occurs following the first exposure to a foreign antigen	Immune response occurs following subsequent exposures
The threshold for activation (i.e., the dose of antigen needed to initiate response)	High	Low
Onset of response	Slow	Quick
Responding cells	Naïve B-cell and T cell	Memory B-cell and T cell
Lag phase (time between antigen exposure and antibody detection)	Long lag phase (4–7 days)	Short lag phase (1–3 days)
Antibody type	Low titer, IgM type and specific	High titer, IgG type and less specific

The various cells of the adaptive immune system communicate either directly or via cytokines.

Types of acquired/adaptive immunity: There are two types of adaptive immunity—active and passive **(Table 7.7)**.

Primary and secondary immune response **(Fig. 7.9)**.

The difference between primary and secondary immune response is depicted in **Table 7.8**.

Acute Phase Proteins (APP)

These are proteins (nonspecific markers) synthesized by liver in response to infection, inflammation, or trauma. Their levels in serum may be increased (positive APP) or reduced (e.g., albumin is a negative APP) within 90 minutes after the onset of a systemic inflammatory reaction, e.g., positive APP

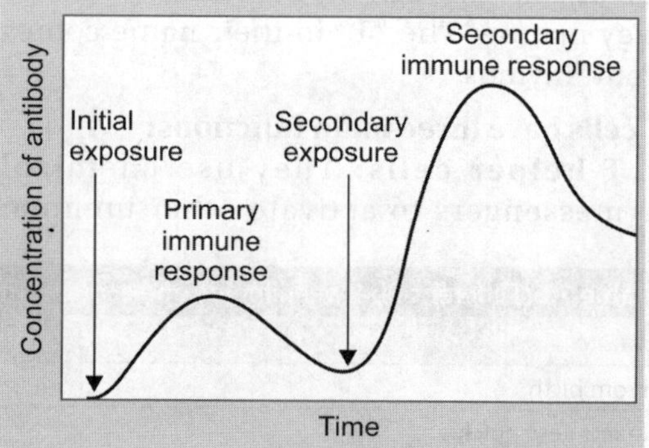

Fig. 7.9: Graph showing the time of primary and secondary immune response.

include: C-reactive protein (CRP), fibrinogen, ferritin, etc.

C-Reactive Protein Levels

○ **Less than 0.3 mg/dL:** Normal level

- **0.3 to 1.0 mg/dL:** Normal or minor elevation (can be seen in obesity, pregnancy, depression, diabetes, common cold, gingivitis, periodontitis, sedentary lifestyle and cigarette smoking)
- **Greater than 8 mg/L or 10 mg/L:** High (acuter bacterial infections, trauma, vasculitis)

Methods to Detect CRP

- Latex agglutination
- Immunoturbidimetry
- ELISA

Antigen: Any substance that causes the body to make an immune response against that substance.

Three types of antigens, classified based on where they are produced.

1. Self-antigens, or autoantigens, are produced in the body's own cells;
2. Endogenous antigens are produced in intracellular bacteria or viruses;
3. Exogenous antigens are produced outside the body and are foreign to the immune system.

Epitope is the part of an antigen that is recognized by the immune system.

Hapten: A hapten is essentially an incomplete antigen, that lacks antigenicity of its own but can elicit an immune response when attached to a large carrier such as a protein.

Antibody: Also known as an immunoglobulin (Ig), is a large, Y-shaped protein **(Fig. 7.10)** secreted by the immune system (B cells) to identify and neutralize pathogens encountered. It is composed of four polypeptide chains—two identical heavy chains and two identical light chains. The two antigen-binding sites (Fv) are identical, each formed by the N-terminal region of a light chain and the N-terminal region of a heavy chain. Both the tail (Fc) and hinge region are formed by the two heavy chains.

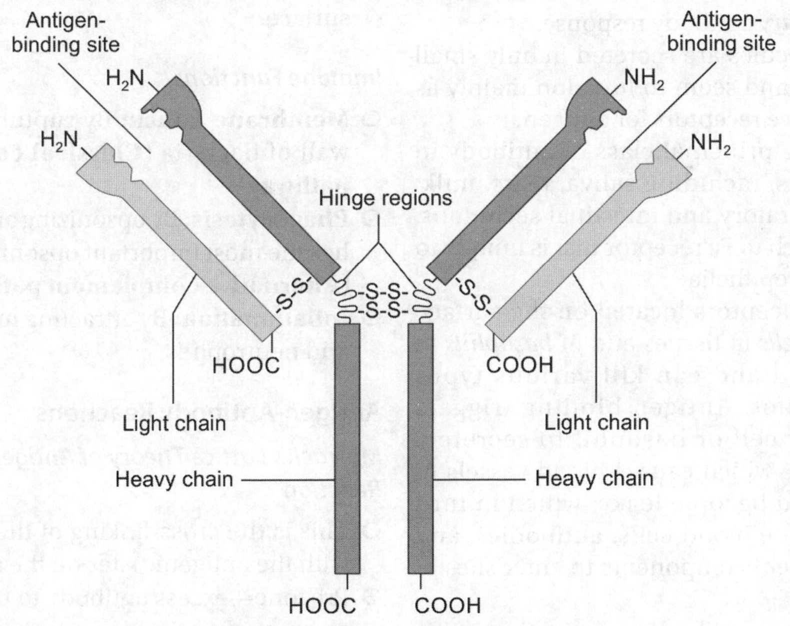

Fig. 7.10: Structure of an antibody.

There are five types of heavy chain constant regions in antibodies (immunoglobulin) and according to these types, they are classified into five *classes* of antibodies, IgA, IgD, IgE, IgG, and IgM, each with its own class of heavy chain—α, δ, ε, γ, and μ, respectively.

1. **IgG:** It is the major class of immunoglobulin in the blood is, which is a four-chain monomer produced in large quantities during *secondary* immune responses. Besides activating complement, the tail region (Fc) of an IgG molecule binds to specific receptors on (Fc receptors) macrophages and neutrophils which helps in phagocytosis. IgG molecules are the only antibodies that can pass from mother to via the placenta.

2. **IgM,** which has μ heavy chains, is always the first class of antibody made by a developing B cell.

   In secreted form, IgM is a pentamer composed of five four-chain units, giving it a total of 10 antigen-binding sites. It is secreted into the blood in the early stages of a *primary* antibody response.

3. **IgD** molecules are secreted in only small amounts and seem to function mainly as cell-surface receptors for antigen.

4. **IgA** is the principal class of antibody in secretions, including saliva, tears, milk, and respiratory and intestinal secretions. They attach to Fc receptor that is unique to secretory epithelia.

5. **IgE** Fc receptors located on the surface of *mast cells* in tissues and of *basophils* in the blood and can kill various types of parasites. Antigen binding triggers the mast cell or basophil to secrete a *histamine* which causes blood vessels to dilate and become leaky, which in turn helps white blood cells, antibodies, and complement components to enter sites of infection.

Monoclonal antibodies are monospecific antibodies that have the ability to bind to the same epitope. These antibodies are made in the laboratory by homogeneous hybrid cells (B cells) that are each clones of the same parent cell. treatment of many types of cancer, autoimmune conditions and in laboratory diagnostic tests.

Complement system A system of plasma proteins that can be activated directly by pathogens or indirectly antigen-antibody complex.

Complement system is composed of three different pathways.

1. **Classical pathway:** Activated by antigen-antibody complex; triggered by C1-complex

2. **Alternate pathway:** Activated by endotoxin (spontaneous C3 hydrolysis); does not rely on pathogen-binding antibodies like the other pathways hence part of innate immunity.

3. **Lectin pathway:** This pathway is activated by binding of mannose binding lectin to mannose residues on the pathogen surface.

Immune Functions

○ **Membrane attack:** By rupturing the cell wall of bacteria (**Classical complement pathway**).

○ **Phagocytosis:** By opsonizing antigens. C3b has the most important opsonizing activity (**Alternative complement pathway**).

○ **Inflammation:** By attracting macrophages and neutrophils

Antigen-Antibody Reactions

Marrack's Lattice Theory of Antigen-Antibody Reaction

○ This is the cross-linking of the antibodies with the antigenic sites on the antigens.

○ Prozone—excess antibody to the available amount of antigen (no agglutination is a result).

○ Zone of equivalence—optimal amounts of both antibody and antigen (results in agglutination).

○ Postzone—excess antigen to the available antibody (no agglutination is a result).

The types of antigen-antibody reactions are as follows:

○ **Precipitation reaction in liquid medium:** Soluble antigens combine with antibodies in presence of an electrolyte at suitable temperature and pH to form insoluble visible complex. This is called a precipitation reaction, e.g., slide flocculation test-VDRL and RPR for Syphilis.

○ **Precipitation reaction in gel (immunodiffusion):** The line of precipitation is visible as a band which can also be stained for preservation. There are two types of immunodiffusion tests in gels: Single immunodiffusion (antigen is then allowed to diffuse from wells cut into the agar gel). Double immunodiffusion (both the antibody and antigen are allowed to diffuse into the gel, called ouchterlony double diffusion Elek's Test). Other methods are radialimmunodiddusion, immunoelectrophoresis and counterimmunoelectrophoresis.

○ **Agglutination reaction: insoluble antigens:** Combine with antibodies in presence of an electrolyte at suitable temperature and pH to form visible clumps.

Example: Tube agglutination Widal Test; slide agglutination—serotyping, Coomb's test—Direct Coomb's test which detects antibodies that are adhered to the surface of the red blood cells as in autoimmune hemolytic anemias. The indirect Coombs detects antibodies that are circulating in the blood, done to diagnose reactions to a blood transfusion.

○ **Complement fixation:** Detect the presence of either specific antibody or

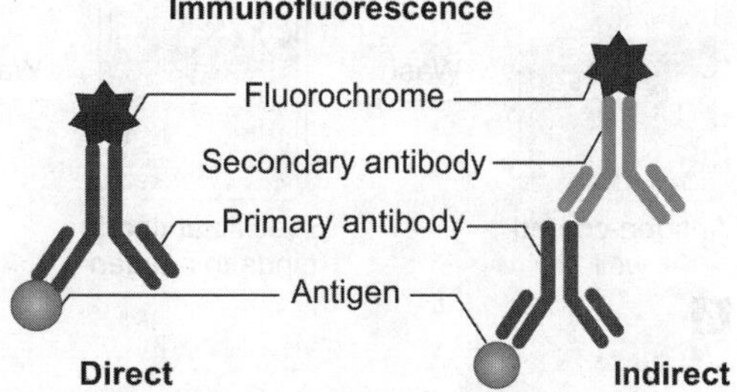

Fig. 7.11: Principle of immunofluorescence.

specific antigen in a patient's serum, based on complement fixation, e.g., the Wasserman reaction for syphilis

○ **Immunofluorescence:** Infected cells immobilized on a microscope slide act as the antigen, and bound antibodies of a sample are detected by a fluorophore-labelled secondary (antiimmunoglobulin) antibody **(Fig. 7.11)**, e.g., for detection of autoantibodies like Antinuclear Antibody (ANA).

ELISA—Enzyme-linked immunosorbent assay:

There are four major types of ELISA:

1. **Direct ELISA (antigen-coated plate; for screening antibody) (Fig, 7.12A)**
2. **Indirect ELISA (antigen-coated plate; for screening antigen/antibody)**
3. **Competitive ELISA (for screening antibody/antibody)**
4. **Sandwich ELISA (antibody-coated plate; for screening antigen) (Fig. 7.12B)**

Sandwich ELISAs are the most common type of ELISA. Two specific antibodies are used to sandwich the antigen, capture antibody which is coated on a microplate, and second antibody called as detector antibody. A disadvantage of the sandwich ELISA is the risk of cross reactivity and non-specific binding, which can be reduced by using primary monoclonal antibodies raised in different species. A competitive ELISA on the other hand is less sensitive and less prone

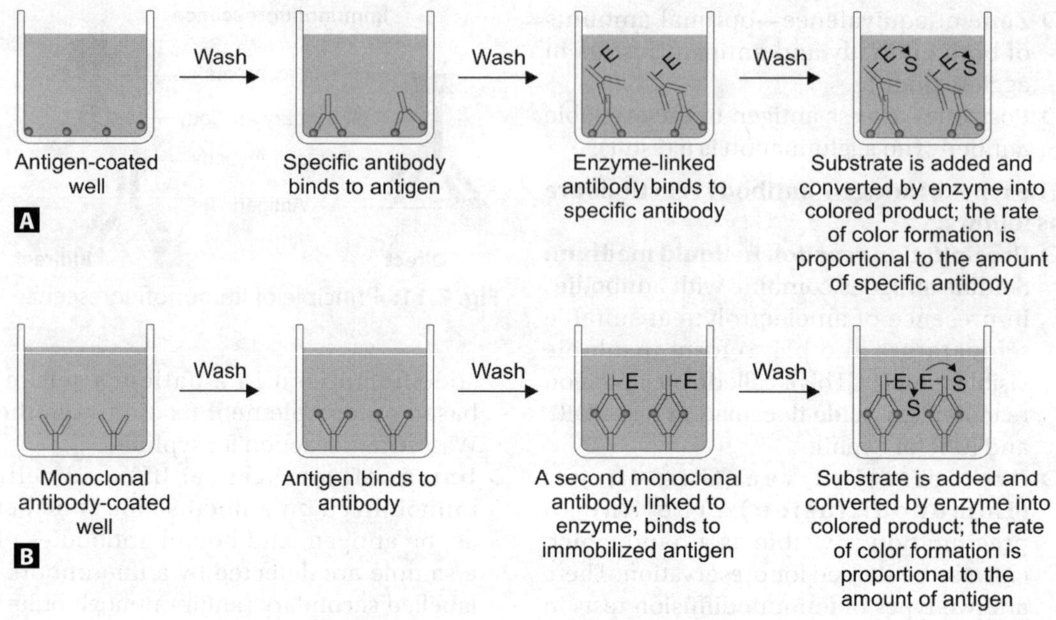

Figs. 7.12A and B: Indirect and sandwich ELISA.

to experimental errors. Also, It is quicker, more flexible and has good reproducibility.

The ELISA reader is a specialized **spectrophotometer**—an apparatus for measuring the intensity of light. The wavelength at which ELISA plate is read depends on the substrate. TMB (3,3',5,5'-tetramethylbenzidine) is the most common chromogen substrate used, that yields a blue color when oxidized by horseradish peroxidase (HRP) which is a label commonly conjugated to antibodies. The addition of an appropriate stop solution gives a clear yellow color that absorbs at 450 nm wavelength (highest sensitivity at this wavelength). A second wavelength to be used for subtraction (570–650 nm) from all values. This will correct for optical imperfections in the plates. Readings made directly at 450 nm without correction may be higher and less accurate. The greater the antigen/antibody concentration, the more light will be absorbed by the sample, resulting in a greater absorbance reading. The cutoff for ELISA is determined using kit literature. It is calculated by adding three standard deviations to the mean optical density (OD) value of ELISA runs on the samples of healthy volunteers. In general, a good standard curve should have the following characteristics:

1. R-squared value is greater than 0.95, and as close to 1 as possible.
2. The OD of the blank well should be lower than 0.25.
3. The maximum absorbance value should be higher than 0.8.

The endpoint titer is defined as the reciprocal of the highest analyte dilution that gives a reading above the cutoff.

Hypersensitivity—Classification and Different Skin Tests Used for Diagnosis

Types of hypersensitivity reaction: Hypersensitivity reactions are exaggerated or inappropriate immunologic responses occurring in response to an antigen or allergen. Type I, II and III hypersensitivity reactions are known as immediate hypersensitivity reactions because they occur within 24 hours of exposure to the antigen or allergen.

Gell and Coomb's Classification

- **Type I:** Reaction mediated by IgE antibodies. Fast response which occurs in minutes, rather than multiple hours or days. Free antigens cross link the IgE on mast cells and basophils which causes a release of vasoactive biomolecules, e.g., atopy, anaphylaxis and asthma.
- **Type II:** Cytotoxic reaction mediated by IgG or IgM antibodies, e.g., Autoimmune hemolytic anemia and thrombocytopenia.
- **Type III:** Reaction mediated by immune complexes, e.g., serum sickness.
- **Type IV:** Delayed reaction mediated by cellular response (T-cell), e.g., contact dermatitis.

Autoimmunity

Autoimmunity is when the immune responses of an organism runs against its own healthy cells, tissues and other normal body constituents. autoimmunity is initiated by a combination of genetic predisposition and environmental triggers. Autoimmune diseases, e.g., type 1 diabetes, Rheumatoid arthritis (RA), psoriasis/psoriatic arthritis, multiple sclerosis, systemic lupus erythematosus (SLE). Autoimmune tests may include antidsDNA, antiRNP, antiSm, anti-Sjogren's SSA and SSB, anti-scleroderma or antiScl-70, antiJo-1, and antiCCP

Vaccines

Vaccination is the most effective method of preventing infectious diseases. Smallpox was the first disease for which a vaccine was produced by **Edward Jenner**. He found out that people infected with cowpox were immune to smallpox.

Types of Vaccines

- Inactivated vaccines, e.g., polio, hepatitis A, and rabies vaccines.
- Live-attenuated vaccines, e.g., measles, mumps, rubella (MMR combined vaccine), BCG.
- Subunit, e.g., influenza and pneumococcal vaccines.
- Recombinant, e.g., hepatitis B, human papillomavirus [HPV], COVISHIELD.
- Polysaccharide, e.g., meningococcal polysaccharide vaccines Pneumococcal polysaccharide vaccine (PPSV23).
- Conjugate vaccines, e.g., *Haemophilus influenzae* conjugate vaccine (Hib) and pneumoccocal conjugate vaccine (Prevnar).
- Toxoid vaccines, e.g., diphtheria and tetanus toxoid.
- Viral vector vaccines, e.g., sputnik V (COVID-19).
- Messenger RNA (mRNA) vaccines, e.g., Pfizer-BioNTech and the moderna COVID-19 vaccines.

Immunization Schedule (Table 7.9)

Rabies Vaccine (Post-exposure Prophylaxis)

Standard Regimen

A regimen of five 1-mL doses of human diploid cell vaccine (HDCV) or purified chick-embryo cell vaccine (PCEC) vaccines should be administered intramuscularly to previously unvaccinated persons as soon as possible after exposure on days 0, 3, 7, 14, and 28 days.

Immunoprophylaxis

Homologous pooled human antibody, also known as immune globulin, is produced by combining the antibody fraction, specifically

Table 7.9: Immunization schedule.

Age	Vaccine	Comments
Birth	BCG OPV Hepatitis B-1 (BD)	BCG: Before discharge OPV: As soon as possible after birth Hep B should be administered within 24 hours of birth
6 weeks	DTwP/DTaP-1 IPV-1 Hib-1 Hep B-2 Rotavirus-1 PCV-1	DTwPor DTaP may be administered in primary immunization IPV: 6–14 weeks is the recommended schedule IfIPV, as part of a hexavalent combination vaccine, is unaffordable, the infant should be send to a government facility for primary immunization as per UIP schedule
10 weeks	DTwP/DTaP-2 IPV-2 Hib-2 hep B-3 Rotavirus-2 PCV-2	RV1: 2 dose schedule; all other rotavirus brands: 3 dose schedule
14 weeks	DTwP/DTaP-3 IPV-3 Hib-3 Hep B-4 Rotavirus-3 PCV-3	An additional 4th dose of hepatitis B vaccine is safe and is permitted as a component of a combination vaccine
6 months	Influenza (IIV)-1	Uniform dose of 0.5 mL for DCGI approved brands
7 months	Influenza (IIV)-2	To be repeated every year, in premonsoon period, till 5 year of age
6–9 months	Typhoid conjugate vaccine	As of available data, there is no recommendation for a booster dose
9 months	MMR-1	
12 months	Hepatitis A	Single dose for live attenuated vaccine
15 months	MMR-2, varicella-1, PCV booster	
16–18 months	DTwP/DTaP-B1, Hib-B1, IPV-B1	
18–19 months	Hep A-2, varicella-2	Only for inactivated HepA vaccine
4–6 years	DTwP/DTaP-B2, IPV-B2, MMR-3	
10–12 years	Tdap, HPV	Tdap is to be administered even if it has been administered earlier (as DTP-B2) HPV: 2 doses at 6 m interval between 9–14 year; doses: from 15 year or immunocompromised of any age (0–6 mo for HPV2, 0–6 month mo for HPV-4)

Age in completed weeks/months/years.

the class of antibody referred to as IgG, from the blood of thousands of adult donors. Because it comes from many different donors, it contains antibody to many different antigens. It is used primarily for prophylaxis for hepatitis A and measles, and treatment of certain congenital immunoglobulin deficiencies.

Source: Hyperimmune globulins can be of two types—homologous (human), heterologous (horse).

Uses: Treatment of botulism and diphtheria; postexposure prophylaxis for several diseases, including hepatitis B, rabies, tetanus, and varicella.

BACTERIOLOGY

Gram-positive cocci:

- **Gram-positive cocci in clusters (catalase-positive):** *Staphylococcus* (the staphylococci further subdivide into coagulase-positive (*S. aureus*) and coagulase-negative (*S. epidermidis* and *S. saprophyticus*) species.
- **Gram-positive cocci in chains (catalase negative):** *Streptococcus* (catalase-negative) Streptococcus bacteria subdivide into *Strep. pyogenes* (Group A), *Strep. agalactiae* (Group B), enterococci (Group D), *Strep viridans*, and *Strep pneumonia*.
- **Gram-positive bacilli (rods)** subdivide according to their ability to produce spores. *Bacillus* and *Clostridia* are spore-forming rods while *Listeria* and *Corynebacterium* are not. Spore-forming rods that produce spores can survive in environments for many years.
- **Branching filament rods:** *Nocardia* and *Actinomyces*.

Staphylococcus aureus is a gram-positive, catalase-positive, coagulase-positive cocci in clusters. *S. aureus* can cause inflammatory diseases, including skin infections, pneumonia, endocarditis, septic arthritis, osteomyelitis, and abscesses. *S. aureus* can also cause toxic shock syndrome (TSST-1), scalded skin syndrome (exfoliative toxin), and food poisoning (enterotoxin).

Staphylococcus epidermidis is a gram-positive, catalase-positive, coagulase-negative cocci in clusters and is novobiocin sensitive. *S. epidermidis* commonly infects prosthetic devices and IV catheters producing biofilms. *Staphylococcus saprophyticus* is novobiocin resistant and is a normal flora of the genital tract and perineum. *S. saprophyticus* accounts for the second most common cause of uncomplicated urinary tract infection (UTI).

Streptococci

Lancefield grouping is a serological method for classifying *Streptococci* into 20 groups (**A–U without I and J**) based on the presence of polysaccharide and teichoic acid antigens in the bacterial cell wall

Streptococcus pyogenes is a gram-positive group A cocci that can cause pyogenic infections (pharyngitis, cellulitis, impetigo, erysipelas), toxigenic infections (scarlet fever, necrotizing fasciitis), and immunologic infections (glomerulonephritis and rheumatic fever). ASO titer detects *S. pyogenes* infections.

Streptococcus agalactiae is a gram-positive group B cocci that colonize the vagina and is found mainly in babies. Pregnant women need screening for Group-B Strep (GBS) at 35–37 weeks of gestation.

Streptococcus pneumoniae is a gram-positive, encapsulated, lancet-shaped diplococci, most commonly causing otitis media, pneumonia, sinusitis, and meningitis.

Streptococcus viridans consist of **Strep. mutans** and **Strep mitis** found in the normal flora of the oropharynx commonly cause dental carries and subacute bacterial endocarditis (**Strep. sanguinis**).

Enterococci is a gram-positive group D cocci found mainly in the colonic flora and can cause biliary tract infections and UTIs. Vancomycin-resistant enterococci (VRE) are an important cause of nosocomial infections.

Gram-positive Rods

Clostridia is a gram-positive spore-forming rod consisting of *C. tetani*, *C. botulinum*, *C. perfringens*, and *C. difficile*. *C. difficile* is often secondary to antibiotic use (clindamycin/ampicillin), PPI use, and recent hospitalization.

Bacillus anthracis is a gram-positive spore-forming rod that produces anthrax toxin resulting in an ulcer with a black eschar.

Bacillus cereus is a gram-positive rod that can be acquired from spores surviving under-cooked or reheated rice. Symptoms include nausea, vomiting, and watery nonbloody diarrhea.

Corynebacterium diphtheria is a gram-positive club-shaped rod that can cause pseudomembranous pharyngitis, myocarditis, and arrhythmias. Toxoid vaccines prevent diphtheria.

Special Media (Table 7.10)

Listeria monocytogenes is a gram-positive rod acquired by the ingestion of cold deli meats and unpasteurized dairy products or by vaginal transmission during birth. *Listeria* can cause neonatal meningitis, meningitis in immunocompromised patients, gastroenteritis, and septicemia.

Gram Negative Bacteria

Enterobacteriaceae are nonsporulated, have variable motility, grow in the presence and absence of oxygen, ferment glucose, are oxidase negative, and can reduce nitrate to nitrite. Genus *Escherichia*, *Proteus*, *Enterobacter*, *Klebsiella*, *Citrobacter*, *Yersinia*, *Shigella*, and *Salmonella*,

Special media for G–bacteria are shown in **Table 7.11**.

The Kauffman and White scheme is a classification system that groups genus *Salmonella* into its serotypes on the basis of "O" antigen (polysaccharides associated with outer membrane) and "H" antigen (associated with bacterial flagella) and is determined by serotyping with antisera.

Nonmotile isolates may be "switched" to the motile phase using a Cragie tube—bacteria are inoculated down the center of a hollow tube in a semi-solid nutrient agar. Pathogenic strains of *Salmonella typhi* carry an additional antigen, "Vi", because of the enhanced **vi**rulence of strains that produce this antigen, which is associated with a bacterial capsule.

Table 7.10: Showing special media for G+ rods.

Medium	Ingredients	Growth characteristics
Loeffler's serum slope	Horse serum, beef extract, proteose peptones and dextrose	*Corynebacterium diphtheriae* show minute, cream-colored colonies with slightly raised centers; also abundant volutin in films from a moist loeffler serum slope
Tellurite blood agar	Meat extract, peptone sodium chloride, potassium tellurite, horse blood and agar	*C. diphtheriae* reduces potassium tellurite to tellurium and produce grey-black colored colonies

Table 7.11: Special media for G- bacteria.

Special media	Ingredients	Growth characteristics
MacConkey agar	Crystal violet dye, bile salts, lactose, and neutral red (pH indicator) pink colonies	Lactose fermenting pink colonies: *Escherichia coli, Enterobacter and Klebsiella* Lactose nonfermenting pale colonies: *Salmonella, Proteus* species, *Yersinia, Pseudomonas aeruginosa* and *Shigella*
Sorbitol-MacConkey agar	Crystal violet dye, bile salts, sorbitol and neutral red (pH indicator) pink colonies	Nonsorbitol fermenting colorless colonies, differentiation of enterohemorrhagic *E. coli*, serotype *E. coli* O157:H7
Deoxycholate citrate agar	Meat, peptone, lactose, sodium citrate, ferric ammonium citrate, sodium desoxycholate, neutral red indicator, and agar	*Salmonella* form colorless colonies with or without black centers. Shigella forms colorless colonies. *Shigella sonnei* becoming pale pink on further incubation due to late lactose fermentation

Contd...

Contd...

Special Media	Ingredients	Growth Characteristics
Xylose lysine deoxycholate (XLD) agar	Yeast extract, sodium chloride, xylose, lactose, sucrose, l-lysine hydrochloride, sodium thiosulfate, iron (III) ammonium citrate, phenol red, sodium deoxycholate, agar	Colonies of *Salmonella* will show a black center and a slightly red colored translucent zone due to the indicator color change. H_2S-negative Salmonella (e.g., *Salmonella paratyphi A.*) will grow pink with a dark pink center
TCBS Thiosulphate citrate bile-salt sucrose (TCBS) agar	Yeast extract, peptone, sodium thiosulfate, sodium citrate, ox bile, sucrose, sodium chloride, iron (III) citrate and bromothymol blue	Large yellow colonies of *Vibrio cholerae* Colonies with blue to green centers: *Vibrio parahaemolyticus*

A common set of working antisera is shown in **Table 7.12**.

Classification of *V. Cholerae*

Gardner and Venkatraman Classification

V. cholerae is classified into serogroups based on the composition of the O antigen of LPS. according to its major surface antigen into around 206 serogroups, of which O1 and O139 cause epidemic cholera. Strains belonging to the O1 serogroup are further divided into three serotypes, namely Ogawa, Hikojima, and Inaba. Serogrouping O1 has 2 biotypes-classical and ElTor. Currently all outbreaks are caused by ElTor biotype which is resistant to 50-IU polymyxin B disc.

Nonfermenters nonsporulated and aerobic, they are incapable of fermenting sugars, using them through the oxidative route. *Pseudomonas aeruginosa, Acinetobacter baumannii, Burkholderia cepacia, Burkholderia pseudomallei, Stenotrophomonas. Alcaligenes,* and *Moraxella.*

Sexually Transmitted Infections

The most common STIs are shown in Table 7.13.

Laboratory Diagnosis

Syphilis

A. Nontreponemal testing (screening tests for syphilis):
Venereal disease research laboratory (VDRL) and rapid plasma reagin (RPR) assays.
A negative test would be nonreactive, while a positive test would demonstrate a titer $\geq 1:8$. If the titer is $<1:8$, the test should be repeated, and a treponemal assay should be

Table 7.12: Common set of working antiseras.

O-antisera	H-antisera
polyvalent-O, groups A-G	polyvalent-H, specific and nonspecific
2-O, group A	polyvalent-H, nonspecific factors 1, 2, 5, 6, 7
4-O, group B	a-H (*S. paratyphi* A)
6, 7-O, group C1	b-H (*S. paratyphi* B)
8-O, group C2	c-H (*S. paratyphi* C)
9-O, group D	d-H (*S. typhi*)

Table 7.13: STIs and their causative agents.

Sexually transmitted infections	Etiological agent
Chancroid	*Haemophilus ducreyi*
Lymphogranuloma venereum	*Chlamydia trachomatis serovars L1, L2, and L3*
Pelvic inflammatory disease	*Chlamydia trachomatis serovars D-K*
Genital herpes	Herpes simplex virus 1(HSV-1) or herpes simplex virus 2 (HSV-2)
Gonorrhea	*Neisseria gonorrhoeae*
Granuloma inguinale	*Klebsiella granulomatis,*
Recurrent urethritis	*Mycoplasma genitalium*
Acquired immunodeficiency syndrome (AIDS)	HIV1
Anogenital warts	Human papillomavirus (HPV) types 6 and 11
Syphilis	*Treponema pallidum*
Trichomoniasis	*Trichomonas vaginalis*

performed as well. Nontreponemal tests are simple, inexpensive, and They will identify roughly 80% of patients with primary syphilis and close to 100% with secondary syphilis. They typically turn positive only after the appearance of the primary chancre. When quantified, they can be used for disease tracking as a fourfold change in activity is generally considered significant. However, they are not specific for syphilis and can often give false-positive results, so they are inadequate for a definitive diagnosis alone without confirmation from a treponemal test.

B. Treponemal testing: Fluorescent Treponemal Antibody Absorption (FTA-ABS) and the *Treponema Pallidum* Particle Agglutination (TP-PA) assays, while specific treponemal antibodies appear early, their level does not correlate well with disease activity or stage. They typically remain positive for life even after successful treatment, making them useless for disease tracking.

A positive result on at least one nontreponemal and one treponemal test is required to definitively confirm a syphilis diagnosis.

MYCOBACTERIA

Mycobacterium tuberculosis (*M. tuberculosis*), also known as **Koch's bacillus**. *M. tuberculosis* and seven very closely related mycobacterial species (*M. bovis, M. africanum, M. microti, M. caprae, M. pinnipedii, M. canetti* and *M. mungi*) together comprise *M. tuberculosis* complex. Majority of the tuberculosis (TB) cases are caused by *M. tuberculosis.*

Transmission

Aerosol transmission occurs when a person inhales **droplet nuclei** (1–5 microns in diameter) containing *M. tuberculosis*, and the droplet nuclei travel the upper respiratory tract, and bronchi to reach the alveoli of the lungs.

Pathogenesis

The physiology of *M. tuberculosis* is highly aerobic and requires high levels of oxygen. Therefore, it is primarily a pathogen of the mammalian respiratory system, affecting the lungs. TB patient may expel tubercle bacilli during coughing, sneezing, or talking and bacillary load is directly proportional to the infectiousness of the patient. The environmental risk factors are living or travelling in small, enclosed spaces without proper ventilation. Improper specimen handling procedures in laboratory that generate infectious droplet nuclei and pose hazard to the health care worker (HCW). The tubercle bacilli are ingested and destroyed by alveolar macrophages, however, a small number may multiply intracellularly and are released when the macrophages die. If alive, these bacilli may spread by way of lymphatic channels or through the bloodstream to more distant tissues and organs like regional lymph nodes, apex of the lung, kidneys, brain, and bone to cause extrapulmonary TB. Within 2–8 weeks, macrophages form a granuloma, that keeps the bacilli contained and under control, called as latent TB infection **(LTBI)**. Such patients cannot spread TB bacteria to others but are reservoirs of infection. LTBI can be detected by a tuberculin skin test **(TST)** or gamma-interferon assay **(IGRA)**. The National Tuberculosis Elimination Programme (NTEP), previously known as Revised National Tuberculosis Control Programme (RNTCP), aims to strategically reduce TB burden in India by 2025, considered treatment for LTBI to prevent TB disease with Rifamycin-based regimens, including 3 months of once-weekly isoniazid plus rifapentine, or 6 months of daily rifampin This is as per the recent guidelines for programmatic management of TB preventive treatment in India, 2021.

Reactivation of TB

If the immune system is weakened due to disease or malnutrition, the bacilli begin to multiply to cause TB disease. Other risk factors are persons for reactivation of TB is patients infected with HIV; children younger than 5 years of age; persons who were recently infected with *M. tuberculosis* (within the past

2 years); persons with a history of untreated or inadequately treated TB disease.

Laboratory Diagnosis

The methods used for the laboratory diagnosis of tuberculosis are:

Specimen Collection

Pulmonary TB: 2 specimens spot and early morning labelled as A and B, gastric aspirate in children.

Stool specimens from children are also recommended to be tested by Xpert MTB/RIF and Xpert MTB/RIF Ultra based on the fact that tuberculous bacteria are excreted in stool when bacteria are transported from the lungs to the oropharynx, are swallowed and then reach the gastrointestinal tract.

In extrapulmonary: specimen depending upon the site.

Digestion, decontamination and concentration of specimen: Petroff's (4% NaOH), NALC (N-acetyl-L-cysteine) + 2% NaOH.

Acid-fast staining by Ziehl Neelsen (ZN technique):

Principle

The presence of mycolic acid makes the bacilli acid-fast. *M. tb* is acid-alcohol (97% ethanol + 3% HCL) as well as acid (25% sulphuric acid) fast.

Procedure

1. Smear covered with primary stain and heated intermittently for 5 minutes.
2. Decolorize with 25% sulphuric acid for 3 minutes.
3. Counter stain with methylene blue for 1 minute.

M. tuberculosis appears as long, slender, beaded red colored bacilli. ZN stain is rapid, easy to perform and cheaper but with sensitivity of **10,000 bacilli/mL.**

Table 7.14: Grading of acid-fast bacilli.

Examination finding	No. of fields grading examined	Grading	Result
No AFB in 100 oil immersion fields	100	0	Neg
1–9 AFB per 100 oil immersion fields	100	Scanty (Record no. of bacilli seen)	Pos
10–99 AFB per 100 oil immersion fields	100	1+	Pos
1–10 AFB per oil immersion field	50	2+	Pos
More than 10 AFB per oil immersion field	20	3+	Pos

Grading of AFB Smears (Table 7.14)

Other Stains

Kinyoun's cold acid-fast staining
Auramine phenol technique (fluorescent stain).

Culture

Conventional (solid):

○ **Egg based:** The media include, Lowenstein Jensen, LJ with sodium pyruvate (LJ-P). Sodium pyruvate facilitates the growth of *M. bovis*. Others are: Dorset egg, Petragnani media. Colonies of *M. tuberculosis* appear buff, tough and rough. Whereas *M. bovis* appear smooth, white, and moist colonies. Culture is the gold standard for the diagnosis of tuberculosis.

○ **Agar based:** Middle brook 7H11 and 7H10 (preferred for isoniazid resistant strains).

Liquid

Kirchner's medium (selective) for culture of extrapulmonary specimens), middle brook 7H9, Dubos, Sula, Proskauer and Sauton media.

Automated

They monitor the growth continuously and detects faster growth (2–3 weeks).

Mycobacteria growth indicator tube (MGIT) uses oxygen sensitive fluorescent compound to detect mycobacterial growth and resistance to 1st line drugs.

BACT/ALERT microbial detection systems utilize a colorimetric sensor and reflected light to monitor the presence and production of carbon dioxide (CO_2) that is dissolved in the culture medium if microorganisms are present in the test sample.

Important points:

○ Samples for culture should never be collected in formalin.

○ If histopathological examination is required, two samples should be collected.

○ No preservative should be used for any extrapulmonary specimen for culture.

○ Extrapulmonary specimens should never be collected or transported in cetylpyridinium chloride (CPC). CPC otherwise, effectively sustains the viability of mycobacteria up to two weeks for sputum samples.

○ Isolation of mycobacteria from blood specimens by MGIT 960 has not been evaluated thoroughly.

○ If there are specific indications when a physician suspects disseminated TB in a HIV infected patient, blood can be collected provided, the culture systems for recovery of mycobacteria is available in that laboratory (BacT/Alert, MB Bact or Mycolytic F. medium on BACTEC 9050 systems).

○ Read all cultures used for isolating *M. tuberculosis* every week for up to 8 weeks.

○ Triple packing system should be utilized for transportation.

○ Swabs are always suboptimal specimens and not recommended because of risk of infection for specimen collector. Swabs except for laryngeal swabs or from discharging sinus should be avoided.

○ If two swabs are available, use one for smear and one for culture; if only one is available do only culture.

Antigen Detection

○ MPT 64 Ag by immune chromomatography test confirmation of *M. tuberculosis* culture isolates before proceeding for antitubercular sensitivity. The MPT64 test is a rapid test which can differentiate between NTM and TB disease, as the MPT64 protein is specific for *Mycobacterium tuberculosis* complex (MTBC) species.

○ Lipoarabinomannan (LAM) is the only WHO-endorsed TB biomarker that can be detected in urine. As replicating *Mtb* degrades, LAM which is a component of cell envelop, circulates in the blood and is filtered across the glomerular basement membrane of the kidneys into urine.

Molecular

Cartridge based nucleic acid amplification test (CB-NAAT) is an automated cartridge-based molecular (real-time PCR) technique which not only detects *Mycobacterium Tuberculosis* but also rifampicin resistance within two hours and has been endorsed by WHO as an initial diagnostic test, e.g., GeneXpert and TrueNat.

Truenat TB test is an indigenous chip-based real time polymerase chain reaction (PCR) test for the detection and diagnosis of *Mycobacterium tuberculosis complex* bacterial (MTB-complex) in sputum samples performed on portable, battery operated Truelab Real Time micro-PCR platform.

Xpert MTB/RIF is an automated in vitro diagnostic test using nested real-time PCR for the qualitative detection of MTB-complex and RIF resistance. The primers in this test amplify a portion of the rpoB gene containing the 81

base pair core region. The limit of detection of Ultra is lower (15.6 bacterial colony-forming units (CFU) per mL compared with 114 CFU per ml with Xpert)

Xpert Ultra has higher sensitivity and lower specificity than Xpert MTB/RIF for pulmonary tuberculosis, especially in smear-negative patients.

Xpert MTB/RIF should be preferred for testing CSF in patient with suspected tubercular meningitis in order to reach a quick diagnosis. Pleural biopsy is preferred over pleural fluid for bacterial confirmation.

Xpert MTB/XDR for detection of pulmonary tuberculosis and resistance to isoniazid, fluoroquinolones, ethionamide, and amikacin (second line injectable drugs).

Line Probe Assay

The line probe assay (LPA), which involves DNA extraction, multiplex PCR amplification, and reverse hybridization based on strip to diagnose TB and detect RIF as well as Isoniazid (INH) resistance due to mutations in rpoβ, and both inhA and katG genes. The detection limit of the LPA is 10,000 CFU/ml which is the same as that of smear microscopy. The turnaround time for the assay is 24–48 hour. First- and second-line line probe assays MTBDR*s* GenoType and MTBDR*plus* version 2 respectively detects resistance to 1st line and 2nd line drugs which helps in selection of appropriate tuberculosis (TB) treatment regimens.

All samples that test positive in TrueNat, are further going to be subjected to TrueNat — MTB Rif—Dx, to rule out rifampicin-resistance. Additionally, ruling out isoniazid or fluoroquinolone resistance by second line LPA (SL-LPA).

Tests for TB infection (TBI)

○ Tuberculin skin test (TST)
○ Interferon-gamma release assay (IGRA)

Both tests measure immune sensitization (type IV or delayed-type II hypersensitivity) to mycobacterial protein antigens that occurs following infection by *M. tuberculosis*. Testing for TBI by TST or IGRA is required for people living with HIV (PLHIV) or children aged < 5 years in contact with pulmonary TB patients. The **Mantoux tuberculin skin test** (TST) is one method of determining whether a person is infected with *Mycobacterium tuberculosis*. Reliable administration and reading of the TST requires standardization of procedures, training, supervision, and practice.

Procedure

The TST is performed by injecting 0.1 mL of tuberculin purified protein derivative (PPD) into the inner surface of the forearm. The injection should be made with a tuberculin syringe, with the needle bevel facing upward. The TST is an intradermal injection. When placed correctly, the injection should produce a pale elevation of the skin (a wheal) 6 to 10 mm in diameter.

Reading

The skin test reaction should be read between 48 and 72 hours after administration by a health care worker trained to read TST results. A patient who does not return within 72 hours will need to be rescheduled for another skin test. An **induration of 10 or more millimeters:** Positive.
An **induration of 6–9 millimeters:** Doubtful/equivocal.
An **induration of <5 millimeters:** Negative.

False Positive Reaction

- Previous TB vaccination with the bacille Calmette-Guérin (BCG) vaccine within 8–14 weeks).
- Infection with nontuberculosis mycobacteria (mycobacteria other than *M. tuberculosis*).

False Negative

- HIV
- Recent TB infection (within the past 8–10 weeks) or miliary TB.
- Very young age (younger than 6 months).
- Recent live-virus measles or smallpox vaccination.

IGRA

IGRAs measure the amount of interferon-gamma released in vitro by white blood cells when mixed with *M. tuberculosis* antigens or the number of T-lymphocytes producing interferon-gamma (within 8–30 hours to allow incubation depending on type of IGRA test used). The test has high specificity in BCG vaccinated, however, poor sensitivity in young age and requires history of HIV for interpretation.

Drug-Resistant TB (MDR and XDR)

Drug-resistant TB is caused by *M. tuberculosis* organisms that are resistant to the drugs normally used to treat the disease. Drug-resistant TB is transmitted in the same way as drug-susceptible TB, and is no more infectious than drug-susceptible TB. However, delay in the recognition of drug resistance or prolonged periods of infectiousness may facilitate increased transmission and further development of drug resistance.

MDR

Multi drug-resistant TB is resistance to at least the first-line drugs, i.e., isoniazid and rifampin.

Pre-XDR TB

Is defined as multi drug resistant/rifampicin-resistant (MDR/RR) TB with fluoroquinolone resistance.

XDR

XDR-TB is defined as Pre-XDR TB with additional resistance to bedaquiline and/or linezolid. Because XDR TB is resistant to first-line and second-line drugs, patients are left with treatment options that are more toxic, more expensive, and much less effective.

Drug-resistant TB disease can develop in two different ways, called **primary** and **secondary** resistance. Primary resistance occurs in persons who are initially infected with resistant organisms. Secondary resistance, or acquired resistance, develops during TB therapy, either because the patient was treated with an inadequate regimen, did **not** take the prescribed regimen appropriately, or because of other conditions such as drug malabsorption or drug-drug interactions that led to low serum levels.

There are two new drugs namely, **Bedaquiline (Bdq)** and **Delamanid** are being used to treat MDRand extensively drug-resistant tuberculosis XDR-TB.

Drug Susceptibility Testing

Drug susceptibility testing (DST) of Mycobacterium tuberculosi isolate is generally carried out *by proportion method which is the gold standard. Others are absolute concentration method and resistance ratio method.*

Molecular methods: Line probe assay and Xpert MTB/XDR assay.

Vaccine for TB

Bacille Calmette-Guerin(BCG) is an attenuated vaccine derived from *Mycobacterium bovis*, Danish strain 1331. The standard dose of BCG vaccine is 0.1mg reconstituted in 1 ml normal saline, administered intra dermally by 26 gauge tuberculin syringe within 1 hours The vaccine is given to newborn at birth. It is contraindicated and should not be given to HIV positive, or immunosuppressed child. Adverse local reactions, regional lymphadenitis, osteomyelitis and disseminated infection in immunocompromised children are known.

8

Virology

CHAPTER

VIROLOGY

General Properties of Viruses

- Viruses are the smallest infectious agents (ranging from about **20 to 300 nm** in diameter) and contain only one kind of nucleic acid (**RNA or DNA**) as their genome.
- The viral genome, often with associated basic proteins, is packaged inside a symmetric protein **capsid.** The nucleic acid-associated protein, called nucleoprotein, together with the genome, forms the **nucleocapsid**.
- A complete virus particle is called a **virion.**
- Viruses are **obligate intracellular** microorganisms.
- Cannot grow on artificial cell free media.
- Can pass through bacterial filters.
- In enveloped viruses, the nucleocapsid is surrounded by a **lipid bilayer** derived from the modified host cell membrane and studded with an outer layer of virus envelope glycoproteins.
- Viral polymerases. DNA viruses replicate their genomes using DNA-dependent DNA polymerases (also called DNA polymerases) and transcribe mRNA using DNA-dependent RNA polymerases (also called RNA polymerases).

DNA Viruses

DNA viruses contain usually double-stranded DNA (dsDNA) and rarely single-stranded DNA (ssDNA) example in bacteriophages.

- **Polyomaviruses:** BK virus and JC virus
- **Papilloma:** HPV 16, 18 are the most oncogenic viruses (cancer cervix in females).

HPV 6 and 11 are the most common strains associated with genital warts.

- **Parvovirus:** Parvovirus B19 erythema infectiosum, also known as fifth disease, is the most common clinical manifestation of B19 virus infection.
- **Adenovirus:** These viruses typically cause mild cold- or flu-like illness. Adenoviruses can cause illness in people of all ages any time of year.
- **Hepadnaviridae:** Hepatitis B virus (HBV)
- **Herpesviridae:** Herpes simplex virus type 1, herpes simplex virus type 2, varicella-zoster virus, cytomegalovirus, Epstein-Barr virus (HHV4), human herpesvirus 6, human herpesvirus 7, Human Herpesvirus-8 (HHV-8).

RNA Viruses

The nucleic acid is usually single-stranded RNA (ssRNA) but it may be double-stranded (dsRNA). RNA viruses can be subdivided into groups based on type of RNA that serves as the genome. **Positive or plus (+) strand RNA viruses** have genomes that are functional mRNAs. *Picornaviridae, Flaviviridae, Togaviridae, Hepeviridae, Coronaviridae* have positive sense genome. The genomes of negative sense RNA are NOT infectious and the first synthetic event in the replication cycle is mRNA synthesis. Example: *Orthomyxoviridae, Paramyxoviridae, Rhabdoviridae, Bornaviridae*, and *Filoviridae*.

Human diseases causing RNA viruses include:

○ **Orthomyxoviruses:** Influenza A, B, C and D
○ **Rhabdoviridae:** Rabies virus
○ **Flaviviridae:** Hepatitis C virus (HCV),
○ **Filoviridae:** Ebola disease,
○ **Coronaviridae:** SARS, MERS
○ **Picornaviridae:** Polio virus
○ **Paramyxoviridae:** Measles virus
○ **Arboviruses:** Dengue virus, Chikungunya virus, Zika virus
○ **Retroviridae:** Including adult human T-cell lymphotropic virus type 1 (HTLV-1) and human immunodeficiency virus (HIV).

Envelope

Most viruses are enveloped except nonenveloped DNA virus are—parvovirus, adenovirus and papovavirus. Non-enveloped RNA viruses are—picornavirus, reovirus, calcivirus, hepatitis A virus and hepatitis E virus. Enveloped viruses also tend to be more sensitive to extreme pH, heat, dryness, and simple disinfectants.

Shapes of the Viruses

○ **Rabies virus:** Bullet shape
○ **Ebola virus:** Filamentous
○ **Poxvirus:** Brick-shaped
○ **Adenovirus:** Space vehicle shaped
○ **Rotavirus:** Wheel shaped
○ **Tobacco mosaic virus:** Rod shaped
○ **Viroid:** RNA molecules without protein coat or capsid
○ **Prions:** Abnormal protein molecules without nucleic acids which are highly resistant to sterilization and cause neurodegenerative disease called prion disease, e.g., Creutzfeldt-Jakob disease.

Sample Collection

NP/OP Swab for Influenza Virus/SARS Coronavirus-2 Testing

Combined nasal and throat swab are collected by tilting patient's head back,

inserting the swab in the nostril parallel (1–2 cm) to the palate until the resistance is met at nasal turbinates using dacron swab in viral transport medium (VTM). If patient is intubated/tracheostomized—combine nasal swab in VTM along with tracheal aspirate in a sterile screw capped container. The swab is kept there for few seconds and then withdraw slowly in a firmly rotating motion (5 times clockwise and 5 times anti-clockwise).

Transport of NP/OP swab: The VTM sample is kept in a zip lock bag and putting in an outer zip lock bag. The outer zip lock bag with sample is kept in the thermocol box (with biohazard label) outer container with ice/frozen gel packs to achieve triple layer packing. The specimen requisition form is carried separately (not inside the sample container). Samples are kept on ice as soon as collected and transported to the laboratory with completed requisition form 44 ICMR, without delay as temperature affects the viability of the virus and hence, testing results are affected.

Cultivation of Viruses (Table 8.1)

Embryonated eggs may be inoculated by depositing virus into various sites **(Table 8.1)**.

Cell Culture

Cell monolayers are prepared using trypsin. After the cells have dispersed into a single-cell suspension, they are washed, counted, diluted in a growth medium (Eagle's media) and permitted to settle on the flat surface of

Table 8.1: Route of inoculation for cultivation of virus.

Route of inoculation	Virus
Yolk sac	Avian infectious bronchitis virus
Chorioallantoic membrane	Orthopoxviruses
Amniotic	Influenza virus
Allantoic	Influenza virus

a glass or plastic container. Eagle's media is an isotonic salt solution with added glucose, vitamins, and amino acids, buffered at pH 7.4, and containing antibiotics to inhibit the growth of bacteria and fungi with added serum.

Three main types of cultured cells:

1. **Primary monkey kidney epithelium:** Capable of only limited growth *in vitro*.
2. **Diploid strain of fetal fibroblasts:** A number of divisions in culture that is roughly related to the life span of the species of animal—about 50 for fetal human cells and about 10 for fetal cells from horses and cows.
3. **Continuous line of epithelial cells:** These are cells of a single type that are capable of indefinite propagation *in vitro. For example, continuous* cell lines derived from monkey (e.g., the Vero cell line), dog (MDCK).

Cell Culture Uses

○ Isolation of viruses from clinical specimens.
○ Production of vaccines and antigens for serological diagnosis.
○ Biochemical studies of viral replication.

Cytopathic Effects

Many viruses kill the cells in which they replicate, so that infected cell monolayers gradually develop visible evidence of cell damage, as newly formed virions spread to involve more and more cells in the culture. These changes are known as *cytopathic effects* (CPE).

1. **Enterovirus:** Rapid rounding of cells.
2. **Herpesvirus:** Focal areas of enlarged, rounded cells.
3. **Paramyxovirus:** Cells fused to form syncytia or giant cells.

Hemadsorption: Erythrocytes adsorb to those cells in the monolayer that are infected.

Viral inclusion bodies (Table 8.2): They are unique structures generated by viral proteins together with some cellular proteins as a platform for efficient viral replication.

Laboratory Animals

Infant mice are used for the isolation of arboviruses.

Assay of Viral Infectivity

1. **Plaque assays:** Measures exact numbers of infectious virus particles. The cell monolayers are usually stained with neutral red or crystal violet; the living (uninfected) cells take up the stain and the plaques appear as clear areas against a red or purple background.
2. **Negative staining** with potassium phosphotungstate makes it possible to

Table 8.2: Intracytoplasmic inclusion bodies in virus.

Intracytoplasmic inclusion bodies	Virus
Negri bodies	Rabies virus
Paschen bodies	Variola
Guarnieri bodies	Vaccinia
Bollinger bodies	Fowl pox
Molluscum bodies	Molluscum contagiosum
Intranuclear inclusion bodies	
Cowdry type A	Yellow fever, herpes simplex
Intracytoplasmic and intranuclear	
Measles	Warthin-Finkeldey
Cytomegalovirus	Owl's eye appearance

count the number of particles in viral suspensions by electron microscopy.

Important Viruses

Transmission

1. **Feco-oral route:** Hepatitis A, hepatitis E, rotavirus, polio virus, adenovirus 40,41, cytomegalovirus, calicivirus, astrovirus, Epstein-Barr virus.
2. **Blood transfusion:** Hepatitis B, hepatitis C, HIV, parvovirus.
3. **Transplacental route:** rubella, mumps, poliomyelitis, smallpox, rubeola, CMV, hepatitis B, hepatitis C, HIV, parvovirus, herpes virus, varicella-zoster virus.
4. **Respiratory route:** Measles, adenovirus, rhinovirus, influenza virus, SARS-CoV, MERS Co-V virus, RSV.
5. **Sexual route:** Hepatitis B, hepatitis C, HIV, HSV-2, HPV.

Hepatitis B Virus Laboratory Markers

HBsAg

○ If negative, chronic HBV infection is typically ruled out.
○ If positive, the patient is considered HBV-infected. Chronic infection is diagnosed when the HBsAg remains detectable for greater than six months.

Anti-HBs

If negative, the patient has no apparent immunity to HBV. If positive, the patient is considered immune to HBV (either because of resolved infection or vaccination).

Anti-HBc-IgM

This antibody is the only marker of infection in the 'window period' when the HBsAg and anti-HBs tests are both undetectable and its presence can assist in defining an acute infection.

HBeAg

The presence of this marker correlates with high infectivity and, in chronic carriers, with an enhanced risk of progression to cirrhosis.

Antibody to Hepatitis B e Antigen

The presence of this marker in chronic carriers generally denotes a less infectious state and a partial resolution of HBV infection.

HBV-DNA

The presence of HBV-DNA in serum or plasma denotes active HBV infection.

Markers of Hepatitis C Virus

○ **The qualitative HCV-RNA test** is typically positive within two weeks after infection can be used to diagnose acute infection if anti-HCV test is negative.
○ **The anti-HCV** is positive in the patient infected with HCV.

Arboviruses/Arthropod-borne Viruses

Are a group of RNA viruses that are transmitted by blood sucking arthropods (insect vectors) from one vertebrate host to the other.

Arboviral Infections Prevalent in India

Dengue, Japanese B encephalitis, West Nile fever, chikungunya fever, zika virus, hemorrhagic fevers, such as Crimean-Congo hemorrhagic fever, Kyasanur forest disease **(Table 8.3)**.

HIV Virus

There are two distinct serotypes of HIV virus: type 1 and type 2. HIV-2 is found largely in west Africa and vertical transmission of HIV-2 is unusual.

HIV Antigens

Core protein p 24, envelope (ENV) precursor protein gp 160 and the final ENV proteins (gp 120 and gp 41), (antibodies to gp 41 and

Table 8.3: Arbovirus and their vector, serology and molecular tests.

Arbovirus virus	Vector	Serology	Molecular
Dengue	Aedes aegypti	NS-1 antigen detection (day 1-day 18 of fever) by ICT/Mac ELISA, dengue specific IgM (day 5–90 days of fever)	RT PCR
Chikungunya fever	Aedes aegypti	IgM Mac ELISA	RT PCR
Japanese B encephalitis	Culex tritaeniorhynchus	IgM ELISA	RT PCR
Zika Virus	Aedes aegypti	IgM ELISA	RT PCR

p24 are the first detectable serologic markers following HIV infection) followed by polymerase (POL) gene products p31 (integrase), p51 (reverse transcriptase) and p66. Group-specific antigen (GAG) protein p24, and its precursor p55 (the glycoproteins and proteins are indicated by their mass in kilodaltons) are the earliest detected after infection (by Western blot) and tend to decrease or become undetectable with onset or progression of clinical symptoms.

Window Period

It is the time between first infection and when the test can reliably detect that infection. In antibody-based testing, the window period is dependent on the time taken for seroconversion (development of antibodies).

Testing Assays

1. **EIA (screening tests): 'Combination assays/4th generation ELISA',** which combine p24 Ag EIAs with traditional antibody EIAs, allows simultaneous detection of HIV antigen and antibodies using a single test thereby reducing window period, i.e., the interval between HIV infection and detectable HIV antigen/ antibodies.
2. **Rapid tests (screening tests):** These are visual tests in which a positive test appears as a dot on a tile or a comb.

3. **Western blotting (supplementary tests):** It consists of a multistep process similar to that of the EIA. HIV antigens are laid out—from the highest in molecular weight to the lowest—on a strip of nitrocellulose. When a specimen is incubated with the strip, any existing HIV antibodies bind to these HIV antigens. it is no longer essential as a confirmatory HIV test for adults or children.
4. **Virological testing (confirmatory tests):** These tests can be done on venous/ capillary whole blood dried on filter paper (DBS) or plasma.
   ○ **HIV DNA testing** by PCR for establishing HIV infection.
   ○ **HIV RNA testing** by **RT polymerase chain reaction** (RT-PCR), branched DNA (b-DNA), TMA or nucleic acid sequence-based amplification (NASBA) to quantify RNA and monitor HIV disease progression or response to ART.
   ○ **Ultrasensitive p24 antigen-based testing:** testing by ELISA after immune complex dissociation by (The formation of immune complexes with anti-p24 antibodies makes its quantification difficult beyond acute HIV-1 infection).

Window period of various tests are as follows:
○ **Nucleic acid test (NAT):** 10–33 days
○ **Antigen/antibody test:** 18–45 days
○ **Antibody test:** 23–90 days

HIV Strategies in Infant

Maternal HIV antibodies [immunoglobulin G (IgG)] are passively transferred across the placenta, HIV serological assays in infants are difficult to interpret. Infants born to HIV-infected women may therefore initially test seropositive, irrespective of their own infection status.

HIV DNA or HIV RNA on whole blood specimen on Dried Blood Spot (DBS), ultra-sensitive 24 Antigen assay (Up24 Ag) on plasma or DBS. Virological Test is the most reliable method for diagnosing HIV infection in infants and children less than 18 months of age.

Monitoring Treatment

- **CD4⁺ T-cell count:** Done by flow cytometry and is performed at diagnosis and every 3–6 months thereafter.
- **Viral load:** Detection of HIV RNA copies.
- **p24** Ag detection
- **Neopterin**

NACO Testing Strategies

- **Strategy I:** Only 1 test done for blood donors in blood banks.
- **Strategy IIa:** Seroprevalence or epidemiological purpose, 2 tests are done.
- **Strategy IIb:** For diagnosis of HIV/AIDS in symptomatic patients. 2 tests are done.

- **Strategy III:** For diagnosis of asymptomatic patients. Three tests are done.

SARS Co-V2

Real-time RT-PCR

- It is the gold standard for the diagnosis of COVID-19.
- **Gene targets for screening:** Spike protein (S), envelope protein (E), membrane protein (M), nucleocapsid (N).
- **Gene targets for confirmation:** RNA-dependent RNA polymerase (RdRP), open reading frames (ORF 1a/b), N2 nucleocapsid.
- A sample is considered positive below the Ct value of 37 cycles.
- **Automated real time systems:** CBNAAT/GeneXpert that uses E gene and N2 gene; Truenat uses E gene and RdRp gene.

Antigen Testing

It is a point of care test and highly specific, positive result is confirmatory; negative test should be retested with RT-PCR.

Antibody Detection

It is done for seroprevalence.

Genome Sequencing

To detect mutations in the virus.

Mycology

FUNGAL CELL WALL

Fungi possess chitinous cell walls, and plasma membranes containing ergosterol.

- **Yeast:** Yeasts are fungi that grow as solitary cells that reproduce by budding. Example: *Cryptococcus neoformans*.
- **Yeast like:** They exist as yeast cells along with pseudohyphae. Example: *Candida albicans*.
- **Molds:** Molds occur in long filaments known as hyphae, which grow by apical extension.
- **Dimorphic fungi:** Dimorphic fungi grow as yeasts or spherules in vivo, as well as in vitro at 37°C, but as molds at 25°C. Dimorphism is regulated by factors, such as temperature, CO_2 concentration, pH, and the levels of cysteine or other sulfhydryl-containing compounds.

Propagation in Fungi

- **Sexual spores:** Ascospores, basidiospores, oospores, and zygospores.
- **Asexual spores:** Sporangiospores (produced in sac-like cells called sporangia).

COMMON FUNGAL DISEASES

- **Pityriasis versicolor:** Condition characterized by lighter or darker patches on the skin.
- **Dermatophytosis:** Common infection of the epidermis (skin, hair, or nails) caused by dermatophyte molds.
  - *Trichophyton species:* Infect skin, hair and , nail. e.g., *T. rubrum*, *T.mentagrophytes*.
  - *Microsporum species.:* Infect skin, hair, e.g., M. audouinii, *M. canis*.
  - *Epidermophyton species:* Infect skin, and nail, e.g., *E. floccosum*.
- **Candidiasis:** Common superficial infections are oral cavity (thrush), vaginitis. *C. albicans, C. glabrata, C. krusei, C. parapsilosis, C. pseudotropicalis, C. stellatoidea,* and *C. tropicalis*. Direct microscopy of the lesion shows Gram positive yeast cell with pseudohyphae. On SDA, *Candida* shows white colored, smooth, and pasty appearance.
- **Mycetoma/Maduromycosis/Madura foot):** It is a chronic, progressive local infection caused by fungi (Eumycetoma) or bacteria (Actinomycetoma) and involving the feet, upper extremities, or back and characterized by the triad of **tumor formation**, **draining sinuses** and presence of **grains** in the exudates. Causative fungal agents are *M. mycetomatis* and *M. grisea;* bacterial agents are *Nocardia* species.
- **Chromoblastomycosis:** Chromoblasto-mycosis is a chronic fungal infection of the skin and the subcutaneous tissue caused by traumatic inoculation of a specific group of dematiaceous fungi (black fungi) (usually *Fonsecaea pedrosoi, Phialophora verrucosa, Cladosporium carrionii,* or *Fonsecaea compacta*) through the skin.

The sclerotic bodies (medlar bodies/muriform bodies/copper pennies) are extruded transepidermally, and they appear as black dots on the surface of the lesion (demonstrated microscopically as well); this is characteristic of chromoblastomycosis.

○ **Phaeohyphomycosis:** Subcutaneous phaeohyphomycosis is characterized by papulonodules, verrucous, hyperkeratotic or ulcerated plaques, cysts, abscesses, pyogranuloma, non-healing ulcers or sinuses. In India, commonly associated genera are *Exophiala, Phialophora, Cladosporium, Curvularia, Fonsecaea and Alternaria.*

○ **Rhinosporidiosis:** It is a granulomatous disease caused by ***Rhinosporidium seeberi*** affecting the mucous membrane of nasopharynx, oropharynx, conjunctiva, rectum and external genitalia. Characteristic histopathological features are several round or oval sporangia from which spores may be seen bursting through its chitinous wall.

Opportunistic fungal infections: Fungal diseases that affect people with weakened immune systems:
○ Aspergillosis
○ Candidiasis
○ Mucormycosis
○ Cryptococcal meningitis
○ *Pneumocystis jirovecii* pneumonia
○ Talaromycosis

LABORATORY DIAGNOSIS

Microscopy

1. **KOH Wet Mount Preparation**
   10% w/v KOH is used for the rapid detection of fungal elements in clinical specimens, as it clears the specimen making fungal elements more visible during direct microscopic examination. It is very useful for the presumptive diagnosis.

2. **Calcofluor white stain** is a fluorescent stain that is used for the rapid detection of yeasts, fungi, and parasitic organisms. It is a non-specific fluorochrome that binds to cellulose and chitin in cell walls.

3. **PAS (periodic-acid Schiff)** (Histopathological stain).

4. **GMS (Grocott's methenamine silver stain)** (Histopathological stain).

5. **India ink** preparation of cerebrospinal fluid (x400) shows a prominent clear zone around individual yeasts, consistent with the capsule of *Cryptococcus neoformans.*

Cultivation of Fungi

Culture Media

○ **Sabouraud Dextrose Agar (SDA)** is used for the isolation, cultivation, and maintenance of non-pathogenic and pathogenic species of fungi and yeasts. The constituents of the media are glucose, peptone, agar and pH is adjusted to 5.6 in order to enhance the growth of fungi. **Chloramphenicol** may be added as broad spectrum antimicrobials to inhibit the growth of a wide range of Gram-positive and Gram-negative bacteria. Cycloheximide may added to inhibit saprophytic fungi. **Emmons modification** of SDA (neutral pH) of the seems to enhance the growth of some pathogenic fungi, such as dermatophytes.

○ **Potato dextrose agar:** It promotes sporulation of dermatophytes.

○ **Cornmeal agar:** Identification of *C. albicans* by microscopic morphology or chlamydospore production.

○ **Czapek-Dox agar:** Identification of *Aspergillus* and *Penicillium* species.

○ **Dermatophyte test medium (DTM):** Primary and differential fungal cultures medium to isolate and identify dermatophytes.

○ **CHROMagar Candida medium:** Selective and differential chromogenic medium for the isolation and identification of various *Candida* species.

○ **Bird seed agar:** Selective and differential isolation of *Cryptococcus neoformans* from clinical specimens.

○ **Dixon's Agar:** Recommended for primary isolation and cultivation of *Malassezia furfur*.

Interpretation

1 SDA Slant each is incubated at 25°C and 37°C. Yeasts will grow as creamy to white colonies whereas molds will grow as filamentous colonies.

Thermally Dimorphic Fungi

Hyphal form is found in the environment on plants and the yeast form in the host. For example: *Sporothrix schenckii, Histoplasma capsulatum, Blastomyces dermatitidis, Coccidioides immitis* (distinct spherule-endospore phase in the host tissue), and *Paracoccidioides, Talaromyces marneffei, Malassezia furfur* (yeast phase in unaffected skin and mycelial phase in affected skin).

LPCB Mount

Lactophenol cotton blue wet mount preparation is commonly used for microscopic identification of fungi. Lactophenol serves as the mounting fluid and cotton blue as the dye. Lactic acid preserves the fungal structure and clears the tissue while phenol acts as a disinfectant.

○ **Germ tube test:** When the yeast is incubated in human or sheep serum at 37°C for 3 hours, they forms a germ tubes, which can be detected with a wet mount as filamentous outgrowth extending from yeast cells. It is positive for Candida albicans and Candida dubliniensis.

○ **Slide culture technique:** Riddel's method of slide culture allows fungi to be studied with as little disturbance as possible.

Fungal Serology

○ **Germ tube test:** When the yeast is incubated in human or sheep serum at 37°C for 3 hours, they forms a germ tubes, which can be detected with a wet mount as filamentous outgrowth extending from yeast cells. It is positive for *Candida albicans* and *Candida dubliniensis*.

○ **Galactomannan antigen test:** This test detects a polysaccharide that makes up part of the cell wall of *Aspergillus* species and other fungi. False positive tests have been reported in association with administration of certain antibiotics and cross reactivity exists with other fungal infections, such as those due to *Fusarium* species or *Histoplasma capsulatum*.

○ **Beta-d-glucan assay:** This test also detects a component in the cell wall of *Aspergillus* spp, as well as other fungi, such as *Candida*, and *Pneumocystis*.

○ **Cryptococcal antigen:** Lateral flow assay is a reliable, rapid, and inexpensive test that can be used on a s sample of blood or cerebrospinal fluid to detect cryptococcal antigen.

○ **Chlamydospores formation:** Corn Meal Agar is primarily used to elicit terminal chlamydospore production by *Candida albicans*.

Parasitology

PARASITOLOGY

- **Parasite:** An **organism** that lives in or on an organism of another species (its host) and derives nutrients directly from it without giving any benefit to the host.
- **Definite host:** Host where a parasite multiplies sexually and completes its life cycle.
- **Intermediate host:** Host where a parasite undergoes asexual cycle

Classification of Parasites

A. Protozoa are microscopic, one-celled organisms that can be free-living or parasitic in nature:
  - **Amoeba, e.g.,** *Entamoeba, free living amoeba (Naegleria, Acanthamoeba, Balamuthia)*
  - **Flagellates, e.g.,** Giardia, Leishmania, Trypanosoma
  - **Ciliates, e.g.,** *Balantidium*
  - **Sporozoa, e.g.,** *Plasmodium, Cryptosporidium*

B. Helminths are large, multicellular organisms that are generally visible to the naked eye in their adult stages. Helminths can also be either free-living or parasitic in nature. In their adult form, helminths cannot multiply in humans.
  - **Flatworms (platyhelminths):** These include the trematodes (flukes) and cestodes (tapeworms).
  - **Roundworms (nematodes):** Intestinal nematodes (*Trichuris, Strongyloides, Ascaris, Ancylostoma*) and somatic nematodes (*Filarial, Dracunculus, Trichinella*).

Transmission of Parasitic Diseases

- **Ingestion:** *Entamoeba, Giardia, Cryptosporidium, Taenia, Roundworms, Enterobius* (pinworm), *Trichuris* (whipworm).
- **Skin penetration:** *Hookworm, Strongyloides, Schistosoma.*
- **Vector borne:** *Leishmania, Plasmodium, Trypanosoma, Filaria.*
- **Sexual:** Trichomonas vaginalis.
- **Vertical:** *Toxoplasma gondii*
- **Blood transfusion:** *Toxoplasma gondii, Plasmodium.*
- **Autoinfection:** *Cryptosporidium, Strongyloides, Enterobius.*

Laboratory Diagnosis of Parasitic Diseases

Microscopic Examination of Stool

1. **Direct wet mount and iodine mount:** Saline for detection of trophozoites, cysts, eggs, larvae. Bile stained eggs appear golden brown. Liquid stool must be examined within 30 minutes of passage to visualize motile trophozoites, whereas soft specimens (which may contain both trophozoites and cysts) should be examined within one hour of passage. Lugol's iodine mount—nuclear details of cysts, eggs and larvae can be seen at the same time while iodine immobilizes the parasite.

Eggs of most of the intestinal parasites when pass through intestine are stained by bile. The exceptions are *Enterobius, hookworm,* and *Hymenolepis nana.*

2. **Permanent stained smears:** Iron-hematoxylin stain, Trichrome stain, Modified acid-fast stain for cysts of *Cryptosporidium, Cystoisospora* and *Cyclospora.*

   Preservation of stool specimens: Stool preserved in **formalin** can be tested for (wet mount, immunoassay, for fixed stained slide or can be concentrated prior to further testing. **Specimens preserved in PVA** are mostly used for permanent staining with trichrome.

Concentration Techniques of Stool

Morphology of the parasites are maintained and become easier to detect in concentrated specimen

- **Formalin-ethyl acetate sedimentation:** Easier to perform and less prone to errors. The parasitic organisms, have higher specific gravity than the solution, thus concentrating in the sediment.
- **Floatation (zinc sulfate or Sheather's sugar):** Use solutions which have higher specific gravity than the organisms so that the organisms rise to the top and float whereas the debris sinks to the bottom. This technique gives a cleaner material, however, some eggs may not float.

Blood Specimens

Specimen Collection

- **Timing of collection:** For malaria multiple blood smears taken at 8–12 hour intervals for 2–3 days should be obtained and examined without delay. If a filarial infection is suspected, the optimal collection time for demonstrating microfilariae is *Brugia* or *Wuchereria*—at night, after 8 PM (Species common in India), *Loa loa*—midday (10 AM to 2 PM) (species seen in West and Central Africa).

- **Type of sample:** Capillary blood obtained by fingerstick (pulp of the 3rd or 4th finger (alternate sites include ear lobe, or in infants large toe or heel) or EDTA blood.

- **Smears:**
  Two thick: A thick smear of proper density is one which, if placed (wet) over newsprint, allows you to barely read the words.
  Two thin smears (the cells should be in a monolayer at the tail end).

- **Special procedures for detecting microfilariae:** Centrifuge after adding 2% formaldehyde (Knott's technique) and examine as wet mounts.

- **Staining blood smears:** Giemsa stain/Leishman's stain For malaria diagnosis, WHO recommends that at least 100 fields, each containing approximately 20 WBCs, be screened before calling a thick smear negative.

- ***Quantitative buffy coat:*** (QBC; Becton Dickinson) method, blood samples are collected in a special tube containing acridine orange, an anticoagulant, and a float, and then are centrifuged in a microhematocrit centrifuge. After centrifugation, the tubes are examined using a fluorescence microscope.

- **Detection of parasite antigens:** Rapid immunochromatographic methods (ICT).
  HRP-II detect *P. falciparum* (remain positive for up to 2 weeks following treatment and even after parasite clearance).
  Lactate dehydrogenase (pLDH) detect: Distinguish *P. falciparum* from the non-falciparum species, but cannot distinguish between *P. malariae, P. ovale,* and *P. vivax* (negative following treatment).
  Aldolase: (pan-malarial antigen).

Thick and thin film microscopy should follow any positive RDT.

ICT Filaria Antigen Detection

ELISA: *Toxoplasma, Entamoeba histolytica* (Amoebic liver abscess), *Cysticercosis, Hydatid disease,* Triple antigen detection in stool *(Giardia, E.histolytica, cryptosporidium).*
- **Species-specific PCR for diagnosis of malaria.**
- **Culture of parasites: Leishmania**

Helminths (Table 9.1)

- **Cutaneous larva migrans:** Group of hookworms infecting animals can penetrate the human skin causing *A. braziliense, A. caninum, Uncinaria stenocephala.*
- **Larvae in stool:** Rhabditiform larvae of *Strongyloides stercoralis* or *Hook worm.*
- **Opportunistic parasitic infections in HIV patients:** Common protozoa-*Cryptosporidium parvum* and *Isospora belli.* Other infections reported are Leismaniasis, *strongyloidiasis* and toxoplasmosis.

Table 9.1: Helminths, their types, habitats and disease.

Nematodes	Habitat	Disease
Taenia saginata (beef tapeworm),	Intestine	Taeniasis
T. solium (pork tapeworm)	Cysticerci may develop in skeletal and heart muscle, skin, subcutaneous tissues, the lungs, liver, and other tissues, including the oral mucosa	Cysticercosis, Taeniasis
Hymenolepis nana (the dwarf tapeworm	Intestine	Asymptomatic commonly, heavy infections can cause weakness, headaches, anorexia, abdominal pain
Diphyllobothrium latum (the broad fish tapeworm)	Intestine	Asymptomatic, abdominal discomfort, diarrhea, vomiting, and weight loss. Vitamin B12 deficiency leading to pernicious anemia may occur
Echinococcus granulosus, *E. multilocularis*	Hydatid cysts in liver; dissemination to other organs (e.g., lungs, brain, heart, bone) may occur	Hydatid disease, alveolar echinococcosis respectively
Trematodes		
Liver flukes		
Fasciola hepatica (the sheep liver fluke), *Opisthorchis species,* *Clonorchis (oriental liver fluke)*	Liver and bile duct	Asymptomatic commonly
Blood flukes		
Schistosoma haematobium, *S. japonicum,* and *S. mansoni*	*S. haematobium* eggs lodge in the venous plexus of urinary tract; *S. mansoni* and *S. japonicum* eggs most commonly lodge in the blood vessels of the liver or intestine	Dysuria and hematuria; diarrhea, constipation, and blood in the stool
Intestinal flukes		
Fasciolopsis buski	Largest intestine	Mostly asymptomatic
Lung flukes		
Paragonimus westermani (the oriental lung fluke)	Lung	Cough, discolored sputum, hemoptysis, and chest radiographic abnormalities

Contd...

Contd...

Nematodes	Habitat	Disease
Nematodes		
Tissue nematodes		
Wuchereria bancrofti, Brugia malayi, B. timori		Peripheral hypereosinophilia, wheezing, chest pain, splenomegaly, lymphedema of the limbs (elephantiasis), genitalia (hydrocele) due to dysfunction of lymphatic vessels
Intestinal nematodes		
A. lumbricoides		Children-stunted growth via malnutrition, adult-abdominal pain and intestinal obstruction
Hookworm (Ancylostoma duodenale, and Necator americanicus), *Ascaris,* and *Trichuris trichiura whipworm* (soil transmitted helminths)	Hookworms live in the small intestine, *Trichuris trichiura* reside in large intestine	Iron deficiency anemia and protein deficiency caused by blood loss and serum protein loss at the site of the intestinal attachment of the adult worms. "Ground itch" associated with penetration of hookworm filariform (L3) larvae
Strongyloides stercoralis	Small intestine	Rash at the site of skin penetration, chronic malabsorption, duodenal obstruction, raised IgE, peripheral eosinophilia
Enterobius vermicularis (threadworm)	Large intestine	Perianal pruritus especially at night

Applied Microbiology

BIOHAZARD LEVELS

They are classifications of safety precautions necessary to be applied in the clinical microbiology laboratory depending on specific pathogens handled when performing laboratory procedures.

Four Classifications of Biosafety Levels (BSLs) Exist

1. **Biosafety level 1 (BSL-1)** controls microorganisms unusually known to cause disease with "minimal hazards" to the laboratory and the community. *Biohazard Level 1* usually includes viruses and bacteria, such as *Escherichia coli* and chickenpox and many noninfectious bacteria.
2. **Biosafety level 2 (BSL-2)** controls microorganisms generating "moderate hazards" to the laboratory and the community, such as hepatitis A, B, and C, Lyme disease, *Salmonella*, measles, mumps, HIV, and dengue. SARS CoV-2 for RT-PCR can be handled in BSL-2.
3. **Biosafety level 3 (BSL-3)** includes the control of infectious agents, which can cause both "serious hazards" and can cause a potential threat to the community via the respiratory transmission of the organism. A typical example of an organism under this classification is the *Mycobacterium tuberculosis*, the bacterial agent responsible for tuberculosis. SARS CoV-2 for culture can be handled in BSL-2.
4. **Biosafety level 4 (BSL-4)** is the highest and "most complex" biohazard level, involving a relatively few clinical microbiology laboratories. There is a high transmission via aerosol, making the pathogens more dangerous for the laboratory workforce and the surrounding community. Marburg and Ebola viruses fall into this risk group.

Biomedical Waste Management

- **Biomedical waste:** Wastes that are generated during the laboratory diagnosis, treatment or immunization of human beings or animals, or in research activities pertaining thereto, or in the production of biologicals.
  - **The waste generated falls into two categories:**
    1. General (nonhazardous solid waste, 80%).
    2. **Biomedical waste:** Includes infectious waste (10%) and chemical/radioactive waste (5%).
  - New BMW guideline—published in 2016—amendment added in 2018 and 2019.
  - According to BMW Rule (2016), segregation should be done by using containers of four different colors, each is designated for segregation of a particular waste category **(Table 10.1)**.

CPCB BMWM Guidelines for COVID–19 2020

- Mandatory labeling as "COVID-19": Use a dedicated collection bin labeled as

Table 10.1: Color coding for segregation of biomedical wastes.

Category	Type of waste	Type of bag/Container	Treatment/Disposal
Red	Infected plastic recyclable waste	Red colored non-chlorinated bags	Autoclaving/Microwaving/Hydroclaving followed by shredding
Yellow	Animal, human anatomical soiled waste	Yellow colored	Incineration/plasma pyrolysis/deep burial
White	Infected sharp waste	Puncture proof, leak proof, temper-proof containers	Autoclaving, followed by shredding/Mutilation; encapsulation in concrete sharp pit
Blue	Broken, contaminated glass	Puncture proof, temper-proof containers	Recycling

"COVID-19" to store and keep separately in storage room prior to handing over to staff of CBWTF OR be lifted directly from ward into CBWTF collection van. Also, use of dedicated trolleys with label "COVID-19 waste".

○ Double layered bags (2 bags) used for collection of BMW so as to ensure adequate strength and no-leaks.

○ Inner and outer surface of containers/bins/trolleys used for COVID-19 BMW—disinfect with 1% sodium hypochlorite solution daily.

○ Pretreat viral transport media, plastic vials, vacutainers, eppendorf tubes, plastic cryovials, pipette tips as per BMWM Rules 2016 and collect in red bags.

○ Maintain separate record of waste generated from COVID-19 wards/laboratory.

Bacteriology of Water

Indicator Organisms of Fecal Pollution

○ *E. coli is* the indicator of fecal contamination of water.

○ **Coliforms other than *E. coli*:** It shows that water has been in contact with soil, plants, septic tanks or sewerage lines/drain.

○ **Enterococci:** remote fecal contamination.

Methods of Bacteriological Water Analysis

○ **Multiple tube method (Presumptive coliform count):** This detects the probable number of coliform bacilli in 100 mL water in MacConkey broth (double and single strength. Coliforms are detected by color change to yellow and gas production within 48 h at 37°C. The MPN for a given pattern of results (e.g., 1–2–2 positive tubes out of a total set of 1 × 5 × 5) will be derived by MPN table (statistically).

○ Eijkman test, or differential coliform test, or confirmed *Escherichia coli* count, is a test used for the identification of coliform bacteria from warm-blooded animals based on the bacteria's ability to produce gas when grown in glucose media at 44°C.

○ **Methods for counting colony forming units (CFUs):** Membrane filtration method, pour plate method.

Method of Microbiological Examination of Milk

Chemical Tests

○ **Methylene blue test:** The milk is decolorized after reduction of methylene blue and rate of reduction is related to the degree of bacterial contamination.

○ **Alkaline phosphatase test:** It is used to indicate whether milk has been adequately pasteurized (enzyme gets destroyed).

○ **Milk ring test:** The test consists of mixing colored Brucella whole-cell antigen with fresh bulk/tank milk. In the presence of anti-*Brucella* antibodies, antigen-antibody complexes form and migrate to the cream layer, forming a purple ring on the surface.

Bacteriological Examination of Air

Settle plate method or slit sampler is used for testing bacteriological quality of air in surgical operation theaters and hospital wards.

Antimicrobial Susceptibility Testing

Methods

The **disc diffusion method (Kirby-Bauer agar)** is well documented and is the standardized method for determining antimicrobial susceptibility. This method is not reliable for the following antibiotics, such as colistin for GNB, vancomycin for GPC, azithromycin for *S. typhi* as these drugs diffuse poorly into agar resulting in smaller inhibition zones.

Stoke's method: This disc diffusion method allows each isolate to be compared against sensitive control of the same species on the same petri plate (that are subjected to the same conditions for medium, incubation duration and temperature, atmosphere and disc contents).

Factors Influencing the Size of Inhibition Zones

The size of the filter paper disk, the amount of antibiotic placed onto the disk, the type and concentration of the agar, the thickness and pH of the medium, the microbial strain tested, and the incubation temperature.

Broth Dilution Method

Media used for antimicrobial sensitivity testing: Mueller Hinton Agar (MHA)

Procedure

Preparation of a standardized inoculum from a bacterial culture from well-isolated colonies. The usual **McFarland standard** for the turbidity of the inoculum is 0.5. Inoculate the MHA plate with the swabbing three times after each rotation of the plate. Only 12 antimicrobial disks may be applied on a 150-millimeter diameter plate. Interpretation of AST results—the observed zone of inhibition is greater than or equal to the size of the standard zone (published in latest CLSI guidelines) the microorganism is considered to be sensitive to the antibiotic. Results of broth dilution method are commonly reported as the **minimal inhibitory concentration (MIC)**, which is the lowest concentration of drug that inhibits the growth of the organism.

The **E-test** (bioMérieux) is a method that integrates **disk diffusion and agar dilution** to determine the MIC and provides accurate, reproducible quantitative results. E-test offers a simple method for testing of anaerobes and fastidious bacteria.

The results of the above tests are reported as **susceptible, intermediate resistant, or resistant.**

Automated methods:

Vitek 2 compact, BD Phoenix, MALDI-TOF

MULTIPLE CHOICE QUESTIONS

GENERAL MICROBIOLOGY

1. Who is the father of immunology?
a. Louis Pasteur
b. Robert Koch
c. Paul Ehrlich
d. Edward Jenner

2. Which of the following is not capsulated?
a. *Bacillus anthracis*
b. *Klebsiella pneumoniae*
c. *Neisseria gonorrheae*
d. *Haemophilus influenzae*

3. Bacterial transduction occurs by:
a. Plasmids
b. Sex pili
c. Bacteriophage
d. Uptake of genetic material by other bacteria

4. Which of the following is the reason to reject a specimen for culture?
a. The specimen is in formalin
b. The information on the requisition slip does not match specimen label
c. Unsterile container
d. All of the above

5. All are examples of differential staining, *except:*
a. Gram stain
b. Acid fast stain
c. Spore staining
d. Methylene blue

6. Correct steps in acid fast staining procedure are:
a. Carbol fuschin-sulfuric acid-methylene blue
b. Carbolfuchsin-acetone-methylene blue
c. Gentian violet-acetone-safranin
d. Carbolfuchsin-acetone-safranin

7. Catalase production is negative in:
a. Streptococci
b. Staphylococci
c. *Proteus*
d. *Salmonella*

8. Which test detects the production of acid by fermentation of glucose so that pH of the medium falls below 4.5?
a. Methyl red test
b. Voges-Proskauer test
c. Indole test
d. Citrate utilization test

9. Which test detects the production of acetoin?
a. Methyl red test
b. Voges-Proskauer test
c. Indole test
d. Citrate utilization test

10. Nocardia resists decolorization with:
a. 1% sulfuric acid
b. 5% sulfuric acid
c. 20% sulfuric acid
d. Acid-alcohol

Answers:	1. d	2. c	3. c	4. d
	5. d	6. a	7. a	8. a
	9. b	10. a		

11. **Sporulation occurs in which phase of bacterial growth curve?**
    a. Lag phase
    b. Log phase
    c. Stationary phase
    d. Decline phase

12. **Which of the following helps in bacterial adhesion?**
    a. Cytoplasmic membrane
    b. Mesosomes
    c. Fimbriae
    d. Lipopolysaccharides

13. **Chinese letter arrangement is characteristic of:**
    a. *Mycobacterium tuberculosis*
    b. *Bacillus anthracis*
    c. *Corynebacterium diphtheriae*
    d. *Clostridium tetani*

14. **Correct regarding condenser of the microscope is:**
    a. Above the stage
    b. Below the stage
    c. Near the eyepiece
    d. Above the objective lens

15. **Rapid urease test (RUT) is a rapid diagnostic test used for:**
    a. *Proteus vulgaris*
    b. *Klebsiella pneumoniae*
    c. *Helicobacter pylori*
    d. *Cryptococcus*

16. **Methods used to detect motility in the laboratory is/are:**
    a. Craigie tube method
    b. Hanging drop method
    c. Both A and B
    d. None of the above

17. **Method of counting of total viable count of bacteria is:**
    a. Lawn culture
    b. Pour plate culture
    c. Stab culture
    d. Streak culture

18. **Lawn cultures are used to:**
    a. Test the susceptibility of bacteria
    b. Perform bacteriophage typing
    c. Prepare antigen
    d. All of the above

19. **India ink is an example of which stain:**
    a. Differential stain
    b. Positive stain
    c. Negative stain
    d. Basic stain

20. **Routine diagnostic testing procedures for SARS-CoV-2 can be handled in:**
    a. Biosafety Level 1 (BSL-1) laboratory
    b. Biosafety Level 2 (BSL-2) laboratory
    c. Biosafety Level 3 (BSL-3) laboratory
    d. Biosafety Level 4 (BSL-4) laboratory

Answers:

11. c	12. c	13. c	14. b
15. c	16. c	17. b	18. d
19. c	20. b		

CULTURE MEDIA

1. **Which of the following is not an enrichment medium?**
   a. Selenite F broth
   b. Tetrathionate broth
   c. Alkaline peptone water (APW)
   d. Loeffler's serum

2. **Which of the following is not a constituent of MacConkey Agar?**
   a. Peptone
   b. Lactose
   c. Phenol red
   d. Sodium taurocholate

3. **CLED agar (cystine–lactose–electrolyte-deficient agar or medium) is:**
   a. A differential medium
   b. Prevent the swarming of *Proteus* species
   c. Isolating and enumerating bacteria from urine
   d. All of the above

4. **Transport media used for gonococci are:**
   a. Amies and Stuart media supplemented with charcoal
   b. Cary and Blair Medium
   c. Venkatraman Ramakrishnan (VR) Medium
   d. Alkaline peptone water

5. **Which of the following is not a selective media:**
   a. Mannitol salt agar
   b. MacConkey's agar
   c. TCBS agar
   d. Blood agar

6. **Which of the following bacteria can grow in acidic pH?**
   a. Lactobacilli
   b. *Vibrio Cholerae*
   c. *Salmonella*
   d. *Shigella*

7. **All are basal media, *except*:**
   a. Nutrient broth
   b. Nutrient agar
   c. Glucose phosphate broth
   d. Peptone water

8. **A medium that is both selective and differential is:**
   a. Tryptic Soy Agar
   b. MacConkey Agar
   c. CLED Agar
   d. Chocolate Agar

9. **When a substance is added to a solid medium which inhibits the growth of unwanted bacteria but permits the growth of wanted bacteria, it is known as:**
   a. Selective medium
   b. Enrichment medium
   c. Enriched medium
   d. Differential medium

10. **All are capnophilic bacteria, *except*:**
    a. *Haemophilus influenzae*
    b. *Neisseria gonorrhoeae*
    c. *H. pylori*
    d. *Streptococci*

11. **One of them is a thermophilic bacteria:**
    a. *Escherichia coli*
    b. *Lactobacillus*
    c. *P. aeruginosa*
    d. None of the above

Answers:	1. d	2. c	3. d	4. a
	5. d	6. a	7. c	8. b
	9. a	10. d	11. b	

12. **Which culture medium is preferred for processing of urine specimens:**
    a. TCBS
    b. CLED
    c. Chocolate agar
    d. XLD agar

13. **Löffler's medium for *Corynebacterium diphtheriae* is a type of:**
    a. Enriched media
    b. Enrichment medium
    c. Selective media
    d. None of the above

14. **An example of an anerobic transport media is:**
    a. Cary-Blair medium
    b. Pike's medium
    c. Crystal violet medium
    d. Robertson cooked meat medium

15. **Agar-agar is used in microbiological media for:**
    a. Nutritive value
    b. Carbon source
    c. Solidifying media
    d. All of these

16. **Robertson cooked meat medium is used to grow:**
    a. Anaerobes
    b. Viruses
    c. Yeasts
    d. Aerobes

17. **Which of the following require chocolate agar to grow?**
    a. *E. coli*
    b. *Neisseria meningitis*
    c. *Mycoplasma pneumoniae*
    d. *Salmonella typhi*

18. **Triple sugar iron agar contains all sugars, *except*:**
    a. Glucose
    b. Sucrose
    c. Maltose
    d. Lactose

19. **The medium that does NOT support the growth of anerobic bacteria:**
    a. Robertson cooked meat broth
    b. Thioglycollate broth
    c. Neomycin blood agar
    d. Nutrient broth

20. **The CLED medium is preferred over MacConkey agar for the culture of organisms in case of UTI because:**
    a. It inhibits swarming
    b. It promotes the growth of candida, Streptococcus and Staphylococcus
    d. It differentiates between lactose fermenting and nonlactose fermenting bacteria
    d. It promotes growth of pseudomonas

Answers: 12. b   13. b   14. d   15. c
16. a   17. b   18. c   19. d
20. b

STERILIZATION AND DISINFECTION

1. **Which is a form of cold sterilization:**
   a. Infrared rays
   b. Steam sterilization
   c. Gamma rays
   d. UV rays

2. **What method is used to sterilize disposable plastic syringes?**
   a. Electromagnetic radiation
   b. Autoclave
   c. Ethylene oxide
   d. Boiling

3. **The process of eliminating or reducing harmful microorganisms from inanimate objects and surfaces is called as:**
   a. Disinfection
   b. Sterilization
   c. Decontamination
   d. All of the above

4. **Pasteurization of milk is done at ___________:**
   A. 73°C for 20 minutes
   b. 63°C for 30 minutes
   c. 72°C for 30 seconds
   d. 63°C for 30 seconds

5. **Which of the following methods of sterilization involves exposure to 100°C for 20 minutes on 3 successive days?**
   a. Autoclaving
   b. Tyndallization
   d. Pasteurization
   d. Inspissation

6. **Which of the following works by disrupting the cell membrane?**
   a. Lysol
   b. Povidone-iodine
   c. Thiomersal
   d. Ethylene oxide

7. **What sterilant is used in plasma sterilization?**
   a. Electromagnetic radiation
   b. Ethylene oxide
   c. Hydrogen peroxide
   d. Gamma radiation

8. **Biological control used in an autoclave is the spores of:**
   a. *Bacillus stearothermophilus*
   b. *Clostridium perfringens*
   d. *Bacillus cereus*
   d. *Clostridium histolyticum*

9. **What type of filter does a class II biologic safety cabinet use to filter infectious agents?**
   a. Millipore filters
   b. HEPA filters
   c. Charcoal filter
   d. Silica filter

10. **Alcohol has excellent in vitro bactericidal activity against most vegetative gram-positive and gram-negative bacteria; however, they are:**
    a. Not fast acting
    b. Not sporicidal
    c. Not bactericidal
    d. None of the above

11. **Blood spillage in the laboratory may be disinfected by:**
    a. Phenol
    b. Lysol
    c. Hypochlorite
    d. Formaldehyde

Answers: 1. c   2. c   3. a   4. b
             5. b   6. a   7. c   8. a
             9. b   10. b   11. c

12. **Which of the following is most resistant to sterilization?**
    a. Tubercle bacilli
    b. Viruses
    c. Spores
    d. Prions

13. **The statement which is false about hypochlorite is:**
    a. Inactivated by organic matter
    b. Corrosive
    c. Broad spectrum disinfectant
    d. Reducing agent

14. **The following method is used for sterilizing an antibiotic solution:**
    a. Dry heat sterilization
    b. Syringe filter
    c. Autoclaving
    d. Desiccation

15. **HEPA refers to:**
    a. High-efficiency particulate air
    b. Highly effective partition air
    c. Highly effective particulate air
    d. High-efficiency part aircycle

16. **sputum can be disinfected by all,** *except:*
    a. Autoclaving
    b. Boiling
    c. Cresol
    d. Chlorhexidine

17. **Best method for sterilization of sera is:**
    a. Filtration b. Autoclaving
    c. Radiation d. Heating

18. **All of the following are tests to check the efficiency of disinfectant,** *except:*
    a. Chick-Martin test
    b. Rideal-Walker test
    c. Hugh-Leifson test
    d. Kelsey-Sykes test

19. **Sporicidal agent is:**
    a. Glutaraldehyde
    b. Chlorine
    c. Benzalkonium chloride
    d. Cetrimide

20. **Phenol coefficient indicates:**
    a. Efficacy of a disinfectant
    b. Dilution of a disinfectant
    c. Quantity of a disinfectant
    d. Purity of a disinfectant

Answers:

12. d	13. d	14. c	15. a
16. d	17. a	18. c	19. a
20. a			

TUBERCULOSIS

1. **Which of the following is the component of mycobacteria which makes it acid fast?**
   a. Muramic acid
   b. Mycolic acid
   c. Teichoic acid
   d. Talosaminuronic acid

2. **A patient presents early in the morning to the DOTS centre to provide sputum samples. Which of the following reagents are used in the digestion and decontamination of his samples before smear preparation?**
   a. NaOH and KOH
   b. NaCl and N-acetyl cysteine
   c. N-acetyl cysteine and NaOH
   d. KOH and NaCl

3. **A patient with suspected tuberculosis gives a sputum sample for microscopic examination. What is the number of acid-fast bacilli that should be present in 1 mL of sputum for them to be detected by this method?**
   a. 100
   b. 1000
   c. 10000
   d. 10

4. **Which of the following media cannot be used to culture Mycobacterium tuberculosis?**
   a. BACTEC 460
   b. Middlebrook 7H10
   c. Loeffler's medium
   d. McLeod's medium

5. **Which of the following tests can be simultaneously detect TB and Rifampicin resistance in <2 hours?**
   a. LAM detection by ELISA
   b. Xpert MTB/RIF
   c. BACTEC MGIT
   d. Line probe assay

6. **Which of the following is not a method of testing drug susceptibility in Mycobacterium tuberculosis?**
   a. Proportion method
   b. Molecular method
   c. Disc diffusion method
   d. Radiometric broth method

7. **TB test done only on whole blood sample is __________:**
   a. TruNat TB
   b. GeneXpert
   c. Interferon gamma release assay
   d. All of the above

8. **A urine LAM (Lipoarabinomannan) assay was performed in an HIV +ve patient with a CD4+ count of 40/μL. Infection with which of the following organisms can be diagnosed using this test?**
   a. *M. tuberculosis*
   b. *M. liprae*
   c. *Mycoplasma*
   d. *Listeria monocytogenes*

9. **Positive tuberculin skin test is indicated by an area of induration:**
   a. <5 mm in diameter
   b. 6–9 mm in diameter
   c. No induration
   d. ≥10 mm in diameter

Answers:

1. b	2. c	3. c	4. d
5. b	6. c	7. c	8. a
9. a			

10. **What is correct about BCG vaccine:**
a. The route of administration is sub-cutaneous
b. WHO recommends Danish 1331 strain for vaccine
c. Killed strain of *Mycobacterium bovis*
d. All of the above

11. **Latent tuberculosis infection (LTBI) is diagnosed by:**
a. The tuberculin skin test (TST)
b. The interferon gamma release assay (IGRA)
c. None of the above
d. Both A & B

12. **Nikshay is a web-enabled patient management system for:**
a. TB control under the National Tuberculosis Elimination Programme (NTEP)
b. Seroprevalence of hepatitis B and hepatitis C
c. The National Leprosy Control Programme (NLCP)
d. None of the above

13. **Sputum smear grading of 3⁺ on Ziehl-Neelsen staining means:**
a. 1–9 AFB in 100 fields
b. 10–99 AFB in 100 fields
c. 1–10 AFB per field
d. More than 10 AFB per field

14. **According to Revised National Tuberculosis Control Programme (RNTCP), how many sputum samples are required for the diagnosis of pulmonary tuberculosis (TB) in India?**
a. Two sputum samples
b. One spot sample
c. 3 consecutive morning samples
d. None of the above

15. **Two sputum samples of TB suspect given one at spot and other in the morning are labeled as:**
a. A, B
b. 1, 2
c. Alpha, beta
d. Y, Z

16. **Which of the following stains are used for detection of *M. tuberculosis*?**
a. Auramine rhodamine
b. Ziehl-Neelsen
c. Kinyoun stain
d. All of the above

17. **Which is used in digestion and decontamination of sputum in smear preparation:**
a. N-acetyl-L-cysteine
b. KOH
c. NaCl
d. KCl

18. **Collection of urine sample of a patient of Tb/kidney:**
a. 24-hour urine
b. 12-hour urine
c. In early morning
d. Any time

19. **Tuberculosis bacilli was discovered by:**
a. Robert Koch
b. Edward Jenner
c. Louis Pasteur
d. Jonas Salk

20. **Multidrug resistance to tuberculosis is:**
a. Resistant to amikacin + ofloxacin
b. Resistant INH + rifampicin
c. Resistant INH + rifampicin + amikacin
d. Resistant rifampicin + amikacin + ofloxacin

Answers:

10. b	11. d	12. a	13. d
14. a	15. a	16. d	17. a
18. c	19. a	20. b	

BACTERIOLOGY

1. ***Salmonella Typhi* is the causative agent of typhoid fever. The infective dose of *S. typhi* is:**
   a. One bacillus
   b. 10^8–10^{10} bacilli
   c. 10^2–10^5 bacilli
   d. 1–10 bacilli

2. **All are correct regarding Widal test, *except*:**
   a. Baseline titer differs depending on the endemicity of the disease
   b. High titer value is a single Widal test is not confirmative
   c. O antibody last longer and hence is not indicative of recent infection
   d. O antibody cannot differentiate between types

3. **Drug commonly used against enteric fever are all, *except*:**
   a. Amikacin
   b. Ciprofloxacin
   c. Ceftriaxone
   d. Azithromycin

4. **There has been an outbreak of food born Salmonella gastroenteritis in the community and the stool samples have been received in the laboratory. Which is the enrichment medium of choice:**
   a. Cary Blair medium
   b. VR medium
   c. Selenite 'F' medium
   d. Thioglycollate medium

5. **A 24-year–old cook in a hostel mess suffered from enteric fever 2 years back. The chronic carrier state in this patient can be diagnosed by:**
   a. Vi agglutination test
   b. Blood culture in brain-heart infusion broth
   c. Widal test
   d. Bone marrow culture

6. **In a patient with typhoid, diagnosis within 5 days of onset of fever is best done by:**
   a. Blood culture   b. Widal test
   c. Stool culture   d. Urine culture

7. **Which of the following is not used to diagnose leptospirosis?**
   a. Microscopic agglutination test
   b. Dark field microscopy
   c. Macroscopic agglutination test
   d. Weil-Felix reaction

8. **A farmer presenting with fever off and on for the past 4 years was diagnosed to be suffering from chronic brucellosis. One of the following serological tests would be helpful in the diagnosis at this state:**
   a. Serum agglutination test (SAT)
   b. Weil-Felix reaction
   c. Microscopic agglutination test (MAT)
   d. Modified agglutination test

9. **Castaneda method of blood culture is usually used for diagnosis of:**
   a. Lobar pneumonia
   b. Toxic shock syndrome
   c. Relapsing fever
   d. Brucellosis

Answers:

1. c	2. c	3. a	4. c
5. a	6. a	7. d	8. a
9. d			

10. **Cholera can be diagnosed in the laboratory by all methods, *except:***
    a. Rapid diagnostic tests
    b. Hanging drop
    c. ELISA
    d. Stool culture

11. **Darting motility seen on stool examination, which organism may be present?**
    a. *Salmonella*
    b. *Shigella*
    c. *V. cholerae*
    d. *C. jejuni*

12. **Spore with drum stick appearance is produced by:**
    a. *C. bifermentans*
    b. *C. perfringens*
    c. *C. tetani*
    d. *C. tertium*

13. **Traveler's diarrhea is caused by:**
    a. ETEC
    b. EHEC
    c. EPEC
    d. EIEC

14. **Which of the following is the most common etiological agent of UTI:**
    a. *Escherichia coli*
    b. *Klebsiella*
    c. *Proteus*
    d. *Enterobacter*

15. **Following bacteria are late lactose fermenters:**
    a. *Serratia*
    b. *Citrobacter*
    c. *Shigella sonnei*
    d. All of the above

16. **False statement regarding Pseudomonas aeruginosa is:**
    a. Opportunistic pathogen
    b. Does not grow well at 42°C
    c. Pyocyanin produced
    d. Motile by polar flagella

17. **All are aerobic bacteria, *except:***
    a. *Nocardia sp.*
    b. *Pseudomonas aeruginosa*
    c. *E. coli*
    d. *Fusobacterium*

18. **Alfa-hemolysis on blood agar is produced by:**
    a. *Streptococcus pyogenes*
    b. *Streptococcus pneumoniae*
    c. *Streptococcus agalactiae*
    d. *Staphylococcus aureus*

19. **The capsule of Streptococcus pneumoniae in CSF can be demonstrated by:**
    a. India Ink
    b. Latex agglutination test
    c. Precipitation with antisera
    d. All of these

20. **Which of the following is a non-fermenter?**
    a. *Acinetobacter*
    b. *Kingella*
    c. *Burkholderia*
    d. *Serratia*

21. **Following is a nonspore forming bacteria:**
    a. *Bacillus*
    b. *Clostridium*
    c. *Bifidobacterium*
    d. *Sporolactobacillus*

Answers:

10. c	11. c	12. c	13. a
14. a	15. d	16. b	17. d
18. b	19. b	20. c	21. c

22. **The culture medium that is not used for isolating *Haemophilus influenzae* is:**
    a. Chocolate agar
    b. MacConkey's agar with *Staphylococcus aureus* streak
    c. Fildes agar
    d. Levinthal's medium

23. ***Mycoplasmas* are resistant to all, *except:***
    a. Tetracycline
    b. Penicillins
    c. Cephalosporins
    d. Lysozyme

24. **Which of the following bacteria can grow on nutrient agar?**
    a. *Neisseria gonorrhoeae*
    b. *Streptococcus agalactiae*
    c. *E. coli*
    d. *Haemophilus influenzae*

25. **Which organism has a beta-hemolytic reaction?**
    a. *Staphylococcus aureus*
    b. *Streptococcus pyogenes*
    c. *Pseudomonas aeruginosa*
    d. All of the above

26. **One rapid method for diagnosing brucellosis in cattle is:**
    a. Milk ring test
    b. Whey agglutination test
    c. Rose Bengal Card test
    d. ELISA

27. **Which of the following bacteria resist decolorisation with 5% sulfuric acid in acid fast staining?**
    a. *Nocardia*
    b. *Legionella*
    c. *Mycobacteria leprae*
    d. *Mycobacteria tuberculosis*

28. **McIntosh and Fildes agar anaerobic jar is used for the isolation of:**
    a. *Clostridium tetani*
    b. *Pseudomonas aeruginosa*
    c. *Nocardia asteroids*
    d. None of these

29. **One of the following is nonmotile:**
    a. *Salmonella*
    b. *E. coli*
    c. *Klebsiella*
    d. *Proteus*

Answers: 22. c   23. a   24. c   25. d
26. c   27. c   28. a   29. c

STD AND HIV

1. **Nontreponemal tests include:**
   a. RPR
   b. FTA-ABS
   c. TPHA
   d. TPI

2. **During the window period of patient with HIV, best diagnostic test is:**
   a. ELISA
   b. Western blot
   c. Rapid test
   d. RT-PCR

3. **Highest risk of transmission of HIV:**
   a. Sexual
   b. Blood product
   c. Needle/syringe
   d. Mother to fetus

4. **Lugol's iodine is used to stain the inclusion body of:**
   a. *Chlamydia trachomatis*
   b. *Chlamydophila psittaci*
   c. *Chlamydophila pneumoniae*
   d. All of the above

5. **The most commonly used method for isolation of Chlamydia:**
   a. Culture on artificial media
   b. Culture on vero cell line
   c. Inoculation into guinea pig
   d. Culture on McCoy cell line

6. **Which of the following tests is suitable for demonstration of *Treponema pallidum* in exudates?**
   a. Dark-ground microscopy
   b. Direct fluorescent-antibody staining for *treponema pallidum*
   c. Both of the above
   d. None of the above

7. **Which of the following techniques cannot be used for staining of *Treponema pallidum*?**
   a. Giemsa staining
   b. Gram's staining
   c. Silver impregnation staining
   d. Immunofluorescence staining

8. **Which of the specimen is optimal for the diagnosis of gonorrhoea by culture in males?**
   a. Urine
   b. Urethral swab
   c. Rectal swab
   d. Pharyngeal swab

9. **Which test for syphilis is good for screening treatment monitoring?**
   a. VDRL
   b. RPR
   d. TPHA
   d. Both A & B

10. **Venereal Disease Research Laboratory Test is preferred over the Rapid Plasma Reagin Test in the following situation:**
    a. For diagnosis of neurosyphilis
    b. Large serum sample load
    c. Cost constraints
    d. All of the above

11. **The method of collecting blood for HIV diagnosis in infants at ICTC is known as:**
    a. Dried blood spot (DBS)
    b. Rapid card testing
    c. Spot testing
    d. None of the above

Answers:	1. a	2. d	3. b	4. a
	5. d	6. c	7. b	8. b
	9. d	10. d	11. a	

12. Dried blood spot test may be used for the diagnosis of:
a. HIV
b. Hepatitis B
c. Hepatitis C
d. All of the above

13. Clue cells (epithelial cells heavily covered with adherent bacteria) are clue to the diagnosis of:
a. Herpes simplex infection
b. Bacterial vaginosis
c. Chlamydia infection
d. None of the above

14. Which of the following is a common pathogen of genitourinary tract?
a. *E. histolytica*
b. *T. vaginalis*
c. *S. stercoralis*
d. *T. brucei*

15. Stain for Treponema:
a. Fontana's
b. Acid-fast
c. Methenamine-silver
d. PAS

16. *T. pallidum* can be grown in:
a. Mice
b. Rodent
c. Armadillo
d. Cannot be grown

17. Genital herpes is an STD caused by:
a. Herpes simplex virus type 1 (HSV-1)
b. Herpes simplex virus type 2 (HSV-2)
c. Both A & B
d. None of the above

18. Painful genital ulcers are caused by all, *except*:
a. Herpes simplex infections
b. Syphilis
c. Chancroid
d. None of the above

19. The HPV test is a screening test for:
a. Breast cancer
b. Cervical cancer
c. STD
d. None of the above

Answers:	12. d	13. b	14. b	15. a
	16. d	17. c	18. b	19. c

IMMUNOLOGY

1. **What type of immunity is being conferred to a neonate receiving the BCG vaccine?**
   a. Natural active immunity
   b. Natural passive immunity
   c. Artificial active immunity
   d. Artificial passive immunity

2. **A 40-year-old man receives a tetanus immunoglobulin after a road traffic crush injury as he did not give history of tetanus toxoid. Which type of immunity is it?**
   a. Acquired
   b. Passive
   c. Both of the above
   d. None of the above

3. **Which of the following statements is false about IgG?**
   a. Ig G is used to diagnose fetal infection
   b. A positive test for Ig G indicates prior infection
   c. Cannot activate classical pathway of the complement system
   d. Most abundant in serum

4. **Which of the following is the secretory immunoglobulin?**
   a. IgG
   b. IgA
   c. IgM
   d. IgE

5. **Coomb's test is also known as:**
   a. Complement fixation test
   b. Agglutination test
   c. Neutralization test
   d. Antiglobulin test

6. **Rose-Waaler test is an example of:**
   a. Latex agglutination test
   b. Passive agglutination
   c. Reverse passive agglutination
   d. Co-agglutination test

7. **Prozone phenomenon of antibody excess is frequently seen in:**
   a. HIV
   b. Syphilis
   c. Both of the above
   d. None of the above

8. **Postzone phenomenon may be commonly seen in:**
   a. Cryptococcal antigen test
   b. Pregnancy test
   c. Both of the above
   d. None of the above

9. **Lateral flow assay is used to detect:**
   a. Antigen using fluorescent labelled antigen
   b. Antigen or antibody using nitrocellulose membrane
   c. Antigen or antibody using chemiluminescence
   d. Antibody using fluorescent labelled antigen

10. **Elevated serum immunoglobulin E (IgE) can be caused by:**
    a. Allergies
    b. Parasitic infections
    c. Immune conditions including hyper IgE syndrome (HIES)
    d. All of the above

Answers:

1. c	2. c	3. a	4. b
5. d	6. b	7. c	8. c
9. b	10. d		

11. **The edge effect in ELISA may be reduced by:**
    a. Bringing liquids (and plates) to the room temperature before the start of the assay
    b. Sealing plates with adhesive tape or placed in a 100% relative humidity environment during incubation
    c. Incubations in the dark at 37°C
    d. All of the above

12. **The cause of high background signal/noise in ELISA may be because of:**
    a. Nonspecific Ag-Ab binding
    b. Contamination of samples
    c. Cross-reactivity
    d. All of the above

13. **All are true about point-of-care testing (POCT),** *except:*
    a. It is faster than laboratory testing
    b. It provides a wider variety of laboratory tests
    c. It is beneficial in emergency situations
    d. It can be performed by any healthcare practitioner

14. **HLA-B27 is present in >90% of the following patients?**
    a. Spondyloarthritis
    b. Rheumatoid arthritis
    c. Both A & B
    d. None of the above

15. **Anti-cyclic citrullinated peptide (anti-CCP) antibody levels are characteristically elevated in:**
    a. Spondyloarthritis
    b. Rheumatoid arthritis
    c. Both A & B
    d. None of the above

16. **Which autoantibody is found in over 95% of patients of systemic lupus erythematosus (SLE)?**
    a. Antinuclear antibody tests
    b. Anti-dsDNA antibody
    c. Anti-Sm antibody
    d. Antiphospholipid antibodies

17. **The 2-mercaptoethanol test is used for the detection of:**
    a. IgM
    b. IgG
    c. Both IgM and IgG
    d. IgA

18. **Antistreptolysin O (ASO) titer used to measure antibodies against streptolysin O is used for the diagnosis of:**
    a. Rheumatoid arthritis
    b. Typhoid fever
    c. Rheumatic fever
    d. Rickettsial fever

19. **The sandwich ELISA is a type of enzyme-linked immunosorbent assay that uses:**
    a. A capture antibody
    b. A detection antibody
    c. A primary detection antibody
    d. A capture antibody and a detection antibody

20. **All are true for sandwich ELISA,** *except:*
    a. Sandwich ELISA has high sensitivity
    b. Sandwich ELISA is commonly used to detect and quantify antigens
    c. Sandwich ELISA is commonly used to detect and quantify antibody
    d. Sandwich ELISA has high specificity

Answers:

11. d	12. d	13. b	14. a
15. b	16. a	17. b	18. c
19. d	20. c		

21. **Following is true about Chemilumi-nescence immunoassay, *except*:**
    a. Measures relative light unit
    b. High sensitivity
    c. High-throughput processing
    d. Lower cost
22. **The earliest immunoglobulin to be synthesized by fetus is:**
    a. IgM   b. IgG
    c. Ig E   d. IgA
23. **The source of histamine in the im-mune system is:**
    a. Mast cells
    b. Basophils
    c. Both of the above
    d. None of the above

24. **Vaccine preventable infections are all, *except*:**
    a. Polio
    b. Hepatitis B
    c. Hepatitis C
    d. Hepatitis A
25. **C-reactive protein is:**
    a. Protein synthesized by the liver
    b. Level rises in response to infection
    c. Levels >10 mg/dL are considered a marked increase
    d. All of the above

Answers: **21. d**   **22. a**   **23. a**   **24. c**
         25. d

MEDICAL PARASITOLOGY

1. **Oocysts of *Toxoplasma gondii* are excreted in the feces of:**
   a. Cat
   b. Sheep
   c. Cattle
   d. Humans

2. **Which is the infective form of the malaria parasite to man?**
   a. Merozoite
   b. Sporozoite
   c. Gametocyte
   d. Trophozoite

3. ***Plasmodium* histidine-rich protein 2 (HRP2) test can detect:**
   a. *Plasmodium falciparum*
   b. *Plasmodium vivax*
   c. Both *P. vivax* and *P. falciparum*
   d. All forms of malaria

4. ***Leishmania donovani* can be cultivated in:**
   a. Blood agar
   b. NNN medium
   c. Diamond's medium
   d. RPMI 1640 medium

5. **The optimal blood collection time for demonstrating microfilariae is:**
   a. A blood sample is taken 30–45 minutes after 50–100 mg of DEC
   b. A blood sample is taken between 10:00 P.M. and 2:00 A.M
   c. Both A and B
   d. None of the above

6. **Modified acid-fast staining technique is used to visualize the oocyst of:**
   a. *Cryptosporidium*
   b. *Cystoisospora*
   c. *Cyclospora*
   d. All of the above

7. **NIH swab is used for the diagnosis of:**
   a. Pinworm
   b. Hookworm
   c. Roundworm
   d. Whipworm

8. **Which parasites can be transmitted by blood transfusion?**
   a. *Plasmodium species*
   b. *Toxoplasma gondii*
   c. *Leishmania species*
   d. All of the above

9. **Which of the following is a nematode?**
   a. *Ascaris lumbricoides*
   b. *Schistosoma haematobium*
   c. *Fasciola hepatica*
   d. *Entamoeba histolytica*

10. **What parasites can penetrate the skin?**
    a. *Strongyloides stercoralis*
    b. *Ancylostoma duodenale*
    c. *Necator americanus*
    d. All of the above

11. **Why is it important to perform stool concentration technique?**
    a. To detect the parasite when they are not found in wet mount
    b. To the detect the parasites which are few in number
    c. To separate parasites from fecal debris
    d. All of the above

12. **What are the methods of stool preservation?**
    a. 10% aqueous formalin
    b. PVA (polyvinyl-alcohol)
    c. Both A and B
    d. None of the above

Answers:	1. a	2. b	3. a	4. b
	5. c	6. d	7. a	8. d
	9. a	10. d	11. d	12. c

13. **What are the methods of stool concentration?**
    a. Saturated salt flotation
    b. Zinc sulfate centrifugal floatation
    c. Formol-ether concentration
    d. All of the above

14. **The common intestinal protozoan parasites are:**
    a. *Giardia intestinalis*
    b. *Entamoeba histolytica*
    c. *Cryptosporidium species*
    d. All of the above

15. **Hydatid disease is a parasitic infestation of:**
    a. *Echinococcus granulosus*
    b. *Hymenolepis nana*
    c. *Taenia solium*
    d. *Taenia saginata*

16. **Peripheral blood smear showing multiple ring forms within single red blood cells is suggestive of:**
    a. *P. vivax*
    b. *P. falciparum*
    c. *P. ovale*
    d. *P. malariae*

17. **Which parasite can be seen in urine?**
    a. *Taenia*
    b. *Ascaris*
    d. *Trichomonas vaginalis*
    d. *Trichuris*

18. **TORCH panel refers to the testing of congenital infections of the following parasitic disease:**
    a. *Taenia*
    b. Trichomonas
    c. Trichuris
    d. Toxoplasma

19. **Neurocysticercosis is a preventable parasitic infection caused by larval cysts of:**
    a. *Echinococcus granulosus*
    b. *Hymenolepis nana*
    c. *Taenia solium*
    d. *Taenia saginata*

20. **Which is the preferred stain for PVA fixed stool samples?**
    a. Trichrome stain
    b. Ziehl-Neelsen stain
    d. Giemsa stain
    d. Hematoxylin and eosin (H&E)

Answers: 13. d   14. d   15. a   16. b

17. c   18. d   19. c   20. a

MYCOLOGY

1. **Which of the following is a yeast?**
   a. *Candida*
   b. *Cryptococcus*
   c. *Fusarium*
   d. *Talaromyces*

2. **Which of the following is a component of fungal cell wall?**
   a. Ergosterol
   b. Lipoteichoic acid
   c. Mycolic acid
   d. Chitin

3. **Which of the following is true about dermatophytes?**
   a. *Epidermophyton* infects skin and hair
   b. *Microsporum* infects skin and hair
   c. Epidermophyton infects nails and hair
   d. *Microsporum* infects nails and hair

4. **Sabouraud's dextrose agar does not contain the following:**
   a. Taurocholate
   b. Cycloheximide
   c. Acidic pH
   d. Dextrose

5. **Stain used for identifying *Cryptococcus* is:**
   a. Giemsa stain
   b. Ziehl-Nielsen stain
   c. Gram stain
   d. Mucicarmine

6. **True about *Cryptococcus neoformans* is:**
   a. Cryptococcal antigen (CrAg) testing can be done on serum
   b. Niger seed agar is used to demonstrate melanin production
   c. Capsulated yeast
   d. All of the above

7. **Which of the following organism cannot be grown on any culture media?**
   1. *Paracoccidiodes brasiliensis*
   2. *Rhinosporidium seeberi*
   3. *Histoplasma capsulatum*
   4. *Pneumocystis jirovecii*
   5. *Rhizopus oryzae*
   a. 1 & 4
   b. 1, 3 & 5
   c. 1, 2 & 5
   d. 2 & 4

8. **Positive germ tube test is seen in:**
   a. *Candida albicans*
   b. *Candida glabrata*
   c. *Candida parapsilosis*
   d. *Candida tropicalis*

9. **Serum galactomannan is negative in:**
   a. Invasive aspergillosis
   b. Fusariosis
   c. Mucormycosis
   d. None of the above

10. **ß 1-3 glucan assay is positive in all, *except*:**
    a. Candidiasis
    b. Aspergillosis
    c. Pneumocystis pneumonia
    d. Mucormycosis

11. **Which of the following fungi is capsulated?**
    a. *Candida*
    b. *Rhodotorula*
    c. *Pneumocystis*
    d. *Cryptococcus*

Answers:

1. b	2. d	3. b	4. a
5. d	6. d	7. d	8. a
9. c	10. d	11. d	

12. **Which of the following is not a thermally dimorphic fungus?**
a. *Candida albicans*
b. *Histoplasma capsulatum*
c. *Blastomyces dermatitidis*
d. *Talaromyces marneffei*

13. **Which medium is best to recover the etiological agent from the skin scrapping with probable dermatophytosis?**
a. Sabouraud dextrose agar (SDA)
b. SDA with chloramphenicol
c. SDA with chloramphenicol and cycloheximide
d. Both B & C

14. **Dimorphic fungi are characterized by:**
a. Exist in the form of mould at 37°C and yeast at 25°C
b. Exist in the form of mould at 25°C and yeast at 37°C
c. Both mould and yeast at 25°C
d. Both mould and yeast at 37°C

15. **The function of cycloheximide in Sabouraud's dextrose agar is to prevent growth of:**
a. Gram positive bacteria
b. Gram negative bacteria
c. Saprophytic moulds
d. Yeasts

16. **The function of chloramphenicol in Sabouraud's dextrose agar is to prevent growth of:**
a. Contaminating bacteria
b. Yeasts
c. Saprophytic mould
d. All of the above

17. **Media used to demonstrate chlamydospore production is:**
a. Corn Meal agar
b. CHROMagar
c. Sabouraud Agar
d. All of the above

18. **The technique used to study undisturbed morphology of the fungi is:**
a. Cellophane tape mount
b. Slide culture technique
c. Both of the above
d. None of the above

19. **Aseptate, large diameter hyphae with wide branching angles in KOH mount slide are seen in:**
a. Mucormycosis
b. Aspergillosis
c. Fusariosis
d. None of the above

20. **All are true about mucormycosis, *except:***
a. Infection is caused by "Black fungus"
b. Transmission occurs through inhalation
c. Uncontrolled diabetes are under high risk
d. Amphotericin B is the drug of choice

21. **The most common direct microscopy method to visualize fungal elements in clinical sample is:**
a. KOH preparation
b. LPCB staining
c. Iodine mount
d. Albert stain

Answers:

12. a	13. d	14. b	15. c
16. a	17. a	18. c	19. a
20. a	21. a		

22. Which stain can be used to visualize fungi from culture?
a. ZN stain
b. KOH
c. Lactophenol cotton blue
d. Methenamine stain

23. Which of the following is not a medium to cultivate fungi from clinical samples?
a. Czapek-Dox medium
b. MacConkey agar
c. Bird seed agar
d. Brain-heart infusion agar

24. Which of the following is not a fungal stain?
a. Leishman stain
b. Calcoflour white
c. Periodic acid Schiff
d. Gomori's methenamine stain

25. Which of the following fungus is capsulated?
a. *Candida*
b. *Rhodotorula*
c. *Pneumocystis*
d. *Cryptococcus*

Answers: 22. c   23. b   24. a   25. d

VIROLOGY AND SARS COV-2

1. **What is the gold standard for diagnosis of COVID-19?**
   a. Antibody detection
   b. Real-time PCR
   c. Antigen detection
   d. All of the above

2. **Which hepatitis B marker is not detected in serum?**
   a. IgM anti-HBc
   b. IgG anti-HBc
   c. HBeAg
   d. HBcAg

3. **What does hepatitis B surface antibody detected mean?**
   a. A person is infected and can spread the hepatitis B virus
   b. A person is protected against the hepatitis B virus
   c. Both of the above
   d. None of the above

4. **What does presence of high level of anti HBeAg marker in the serum indicate?**
   a. High levels of HBV replication
   b. Greater infectivity
   c. Increased risk of hepatic fibrosis
   d. All of the above

5. **What is the first viral marker detected after infection with HBV?**
   a. HBV DNA
   b. HBsAg
   c. HBeAg
   d. IgM anti-HBc

6. **Which of the following hepatitis viruses is a DNA virus?**
   a. Hepatitis A
   b. Hepatitis B
   c. Hepatitis C
   d. Hepatitis G

7. **HCV can also be transmitted by:**
   a. Injection-drug use
   b. Blood, blood products, and organs
   c. Sexual transmission
   d. All of the above

8. **The decreasing order of the risk of transmission of following viruses in health care facility is:**
   a. HBV >HCV >HIV
   b. HIV >HCV >HBV
   c. HCV >HIV >HBV
   d. None of the above

9. **Laboratory confirmation of dengue fever can be made within 7 days after fever onset by:**
   a. rRT-PCR
   b. Nonstructural protein 1 (NS1) antigen by immunoassay
   c. Both A & B
   d. IgM MAC-ELISA against dengue virus

10. **The staining technique used for the demonstration of Negri bodies is:**
    a. Giemsa stain
    b. Wright's stain
    c. Field's stain
    d. Seller's stain

11. **All are true regarding SARS-CoV-2 Rapid Antigen Testing:**
    a. A positive test shows that the patient is actively infected with SARS-CoV-2
    b. A positive test should not be confirmed with a molecular test
    c. Detect SARS-CoV-2 nucleocapsid protein (N) antigens
    d. All of the above

Answers:	1. b	2. d	3. b	4. b
	5. a	6. b	7. d	8. a
	9. c	10. d	11. d	

12. Which one is true about transport of COVID-19 specimen to the laboratory?
a. Sample collected in VTM (viral transport medium)
b. Safely packed in triple container packing
c. Transported under cold chain
d. All of the above

13. What is the most effective way to prevent rabies infection?
a. Washing the wound thoroughly with soap and water
b. Applying a disinfectant to the wound
c. Receiving the rabies vaccine
d. Using antibiotics

14. The following rabies vaccine schedule should be followed for post-exposure prophylaxis in previously unimmunized individuals:

a. Intramuscular	1 mL dose	5 doses	Day 0, 3, 7, 14 and 28
b. Intradermal	0.1 mL dose	4 doses	Day 0, 3, 7 and 28

c. Both A & B
d. None of the above

15. Which arbovirus is NOT prevalent in India?
a. Dengue
b. Japanese encephalitis
c. Yellow Fever
d chikungunya fever

16. What level of anti-HBs antibody is protective?
a. (<10 mIU/mL)
b. (>10 mIU/mL)
c. (<5 mIU/mL)
d. (>100 mIU/mL)

17. Which of the following serologic markers suggests HDV–HBV coinfection?
a. Presence of both IgM anti-HBc and IgM anti-HDV
b. Presence of IgM anti-HDV alone
c. Both of the above
d. None of the above

18. All of the following statements regarding rotavirus gastroenteritis are true, *except:*
a. Common cause of severe, watery diarrhea and vomiting in infants and young children
b. Preventable by oral vaccine
c. The rotavirus antigen test detects rotavirus in the feces
d. Common cause of severe, watery diarrhea and vomiting in adults

19. SARS CoV-2 is a type of:
a. Rhinovirus
b. Flavivirus
c. Coronavirus
d. Enterovirus

20. A blood donor is screened for following viral infections:
a. HIV
b. hepatitis B
c. hepatitis C
d. All of the above

21. Monospot test, a heterophile antibody test is a rapid test for diagnosis of:
a. Epstein–Barr virus
b. Herpes virus
c. Hepatitis virus
d. Rhino virus

Answers:

12. d	13. c	14. c	15. c
16. b	17. a	18. d	19. c
20. d	21. a		

22. **From which of the following rhinovirus cannot be isolated?**
    a. Sputum
    b. Throat
    c. Feces
    d. Nasopharyngeal swab

23. **Which of the following viruses are best known for latent infections?**
    a. Herpesvirus
    b. Poliovirus
    c. HIV
    d. Rhinovirus

Answers: 22. c   23. a

MOLECULAR BIOLOGY

1. **What is the role of proteinase K in Viral RNA extraction?**
    a. It digests DNA
    b. Breaks down proteins and inactivates nucleases
    c. It lysis virus lipid membrane
    d. It acts as a buffer

2. **The minimum average inflow velocity of a class-2 biosafety cabinet is:**
    a. 10 ft/min
    b. 50 ft/min
    c. 75 ft/min
    d. 100 ft/min

3. **What is the role of lysis buffer in viral RNA extraction?**
    a. To lyse virus lipid membrane
    b. To lyse virus spike protein
    c. To lyse nucleoprotein
    d. To preserve RNA

4. **What happens to RNA when lysis buffer is added to the sample?**
    a. Stays inside the virus
    b. Comes out of the virus
    c. Precipitates
    d. Degrades

5. **What is IC (Internal Control) in viral RNA extraction?**
    a. Proteinase K   b. Protein
    c. RNA   d. Nucleases

6. **The role of ethanol in viral RNA extraction is:**
    a. To break the viral lipid membrane
    b. To sterilize virus lysate
    c. To dissolve RNA
    d. To precipitate RNA

7. **Which one is the example of elution buffer?**
    a. Tris-EDTA buffer
    b. 70% ethanol
    c. Proteinase K
    d. Detergent

8. **Following is the source of contamination during RNA extraction:**
    a. Contaminated gloves
    b. Contaminated tips
    c. Aerosol
    d. All of the above

9. **Sample contamination can be avoided by cleaning gloves frequently with:**
    a. Double distilled water
    b. Sodium hypochlorite
    c. 70% ethanol
    d. Tissue paper

10. **Cycle threshold (Ct) values represent the following:**
    a. PCR cycle number at which your sample's reaction curve intersects the threshold line
    b. The number of cycles in a RT PCR assay which determines the amount of nucleic acid in the sample
    c. The number of cycles required for the fluorescent signal to exceed background levels
    d. All of the above

11. **What is the principle of polymerase chain reaction of HIV DNA test requested for a neonate?**
    a. It detects target plasmids
    b. It can amplify small amounts of RNA
    c. It can amplify small amounts of DNA
    d. Reverse transcription of RNA

Answers:

1. b	2. d	3. a	4. b
5. b	6. d	7. a	8. d
9. c	10. d	11. c	

12. **Which of the following is not a step in PCR test:**
    a. DNA extraction
    b. DNA denaturation
    c. Primer annealing
    d. Downstream processing

13. **What type of bonds are broken during the denaturation step of a PCR cycle?**
    a. Hydrogen bonds
    b. Peptide bonds
    c. Both of the above
    d. None of the above

14. **The statement true about Taq DNA polymerase is:**
    a. It isolated from *Thermus aquaticus*
    b. It is a heat-resistant enzyme
    c. It amplifies the DNA for the production of its multiple copies
    d. All of the above

15. **All of the following are required in PCR reaction, *except:***
    a. Deoxyribonucleotides
    b. DNA polymerase
    c. Mg++
    d. All of the above

Answers: 12. **d**   13. **a**   14. **d**   15. **d**

APPLIED MICROBIOLOGY

1. **Which of the following requires treatment before disposal?**
   a. Laboratory waste
   b. Soiled dressings
   c. Human anatomical waste
   d. Contaminated plastic

2. **Eijkman test is also called as:**
   a. Presumptive coliform count
   b. Differential coliform test
   c. Colony plate count
   d. Methylene blue reduction test

3. **The test for recent contamination of water source is suggested by:**
   a. *Shigella*
   b. *Enterococcus*
   c. *Clostridium*
   d. *Staphylococcus*

4. **Which of the following test is not used for bacterial contamination of milk?**
   a. Methylene blue reduction test
   b. Phosphatase test
   c. Resazurin test
   d. Pasteurization

5. **Which of the following is both a diffusion and a dilution method of testing of antibiotic sensitivity?**
   a. Kirby-Bauer method
   b. Stokes method
   c. Epsilometer method
   d. Tube dilution method

6. **In which of the following is the disc diffusion method for antibiotic susceptibility testing applied?**
   a. Agar dilution method
   b. Kirby-Bauer method
   c. Broth dilution method
   d. PCR-based assay

7. **Which of the following methods of antibiotic susceptibility testing cannot be used to calculate the minimum inhibitory concentration of an antimicrobial drug?**
   a. Kirby-Bauer
   b. Tube dilution method
   c. Agar dilution method
   d. Epsilometer method

8. **Which of the following PCR should be performed for quantification of the template?**
   a. Multiplex PCR
   b. Nested PCR
   c. Reverse transcriptase PCR
   d. Real time PCR

9. **Which of the following is not used as an immediate test in the screening of urinary tract infections?**
   a. Pour plate culture
   b. Griess nitrite test
   c. Leukocyte esterase test
   d. Wet mount examination

10. **Most efficacious hand hygiene preparation in killing bacteria is:**
    a. Plain soap
    b. Antimicrobial soap
    c. Alcohol-based hand rub
    d. All of the above

11. **Which method is used to detect the presence of carbapenemase producing organisms?**
    a. Modified Hodge test
    b. Carba NP test
    c. Molecular testing
    d. All of the above

Answers:

1. a	2. b	3. b	4. d
5. c	6. b	7. a	8. d
9. a	10. c	11. d	

12. **What factors influence the size of the zone of inhibition?**
    a. The thickness and pH of the medium
    b. The size of the inoculum
    c. pathogen susceptibility
    d. All of the above

13. **The correct order of blood draw tubes for collection of venous blood specimens is:**
    a. Blood culture tube, sodium citrate tube, serum tubes, heparin tube, EDTA tube, sodium fluoride
    b. Sodium citrate tube, serum tubes, heparin tube, EDTA tube, sodium fluoride, blood culture tube
    c. Heparin tube, EDTA tube, sodium fluoride, blood culture tube, sodium citrate tube, serum tubes,
    d. None of the above

14. **All are specimen rejection criteria in Microbiology received for culture, *except:***
    a. Specimen in formalin
    b. Specimen in unsterile container
    c. specimens collected prior to administration of antimicrobial agents
    d. Samples in leaking container

15. **Blood culture bottle contamination during inoculation can be avoided by:**
    a. Proper skin antisepsis
    b. Disinfecting tops of the blood culture bottles with 70% isopropyl alcohol
    c. Both of the above
    d. None of the above

16. **Sodium polyanethol sulfonate, added to aerobic blood culture bottles:**
    a. As an anticoagulant
    b. Inhibit the antimicrobial agents in blood
    c. Both of the above
    d. None of the above

17. **The following clinical sample should never be refrigerated:**
    a. Urine
    b. Culture specimens
    c. Swab specimens
    d. CSF

18. **What is a significant bacterial count in urine culture?**
    a. 100,000 CFU of bacteria per mL of urine
    b. 100,000 CFU of bacteria per L of urine
    c. 10,000 CFU of bacteria per mL of urine
    d. 1,000 CFU of bacteria per mL of urine

19. **Freeze drying is also called as:**
    a. Lyophilization
    b. Cryopreservation
    c. Both of the above
    d. None of the above

20. **How many CFU ml is 0.5 McFarland turbidity for antimicrobial testing?**
    a. $1.5 \times 10^6\,\text{CFU/mL}$
    b. $1.5 \times 10^8\,\text{CFU/mL}$
    c. $1.5 \times 10^{10}\,\text{CFU/mL}$
    d. $1.5 \times 10^4\,\text{CFU/mL}$

Answers:

12. d	13. a	14. c	15. c
16. c	17. d	18. a	19. a
20. b